Morrison-Valfre's

FOUNDATIONS of MENTAL HEALTH CARE in CANADA

Morrison-Valfre's
FOUNDATIONS of MENTAL HEALTH CARE in CANADA

CANADIAN AUTHORS

Boris Bard, RN, MSc, ACMHN
Manager, Neurology Service
University Health Network
Toronto, Ontario

Eric MacMullin, RN, MSN
Professor
Bridging to University Nursing Program
School of Community and Health Studies
Centennial College
Toronto, Ontario

Jacqueline Williamson, RN, MEd, PhD
Professor
Practical Nursing Program
School of Health and Community Services
Durham College
Oshawa, Ontario

US AUTHOR

Michelle Morrison-Valfre, RN, BSN, MSN, FNP
Health Care Educator/Consultant
Health and Educational Consultants
Forest Grove, Oregon

ELSEVIER

Notice

Practitioners and researchers must always rely on their own experience and knowledge in evaluating and
using any information, methods, compounds or experiments described herein. Because of rapid advances
in the medical sciences, in particular, independent verification of diagnoses and drug dosages should be
made. To the fullest extent of the law, no responsibility is assumed by Elsevier, authors, editors or con-
tributors for any injury and/or damage to persons or property as a matter of products liability, negligence
or otherwise, or from any use or operation of any methods, products, instructions, or ideas contained in
the material herein.

Library of Congress Control Number: 2020947856

VP, Education Content: Kevonne Holloway
Content Strategist (Acquisitions, Canada): Roberta A. Spinosa-Millman
Director, Content Development: Laurie Gower
Content Development Specialist: Martina van de Velde
Publishing Services Manager: Catherine Jackson
Senior Project Manager: Claire Kramer
Design Direction: Bridget Hoette

Last digit is the print number: 9 8 7 6 5 4 3 2

Printed in India

Working together
to grow libraries in
developing countries

www.elsevier.com • www.bookaid.org

To my wife, Kira Bard, who always loves and supports me.
To the memory of 6 million Jewish victims of the Holocaust and the memory of
the Righteous Among the Nations who helped some to survive, leading, among
other things, to the new edition of this book.

Boris Bard

To my family, Rita, Bob, Rose, Colin, Linda, and Shirley for a lifetime
of support and encouragement. Special thanks to Chris Gray just for
being there and more thanks than I have words to express to my mentor
and friend, Professor Jonathon Bradshaw.

Eric MacMullin

To my beloved husband, Adolph; my cherished friend Marian
McCollum; and to you, dear reader.
May you leave this book richer in the knowledge of human behaviour.

Michelle Morrison-Valfre

REVIEWERS

Sharon Clegg, BSc(PT)
Physiotherapist
Faculty of Physiotherapy Technology
Dawson College
Montreal, Quebec

John Collins, PhD, MA, Dip. Ed(NT), BA(Hons), DPSN, CMS(dist.), RN, RPN
President/CEO, John Collins Consulting Inc.
Instructor, BSN Program
Vancouver Community College
Vancouver, British Columbia

Cheryl Derry, RN, CAE
Instructor, Practical Nursing
School of Health and Human Services
Assiniboine Community College
Brandon, Manitoba

Thomas Gantert, RN, MBA, PhD
Professor of Nursing
Fanshawe College
London, Ontario

Treva Job, RN, PHCNP, RN(EC), MEd, PhD(c)
Professor
Faculty of Nursing
Georgian College
Barrie, Ontario

Eric MacMullin, RN, MSN
Professor
Bridging to University Nursing Program
School of Community and Health Studies
Centennial College
Toronto, Ontario

Kelly McNaught, RN, MN
Nursing Faculty
Nursing Education and Health Studies
Grande Prairie Regional College
Grande Prairie, Alberta

Holldrid Odreman, RN, MScN-Ed, PhD
Professor of Nursing
School of Nursing
Niagara College
Welland, Ontario

Kathlyn Palafox, BSN, BCPID
Practical Nursing Program Coordinator
Secondary Senior Educational Administrator
Canadian Health Care Academy
Surrey, British Columbia

Angela Rintoul, NP, MN-ANP
Coordinator
Bachelor of Science in Nursing Program
Algonquin College
Pembroke, Ontario

TO THE INSTRUCTOR

Morrison-Valfre's Foundations of Mental Health Care in Canada, first edition, is intended for students and practitioners of the health care professions. Basic and advanced learners will find the information in this text useful and easy to apply in a variety of practice settings. Students in fields such as nursing, social work, respiratory therapy, physiotherapy, recreational therapy, occupational therapy, rehabilitation, and medical assisting will find concise explanations of adaptive and maladaptive human behaviours, as well as the most current therapeutic interventions and treatments.

Practising health care providers—all who care for patients in a therapeutic manner—will find this book a practical and useful guide in any health care setting.

At its core, this text has three main goals:

1. To help soften the social distinction between mental "health" and mental "illness"
2. To assist all health care providers in comfortably working with patients who exhibit a wide range of maladaptive behaviours
3. To apply the concepts of holistic care when assisting patients in developing more adaptive attitudes and behaviours

Unit I, Mental Health Care: Past and Present, provides a framework for understanding mental health care. The evolution of care for persons with mental challenges from primitive to current times is described. Selected ethical, legal, social, and cultural issues relating to mental health care are explored. Community mental health care is explained, followed by chapters pertaining to theories of mental illness and complementary and alternative therapies. A chapter on psychotherapeutic medication therapy ends the unit.

Unit II, The Caregiver's Therapeutic Skills, focuses on the skills and conditions necessary for working with patients. Eight principles of mental health care are discussed and then applied to the therapeutic environment, the helping relationship, and effective communications. Material devoted to self-awareness encourages readers to develop introspection—a necessary component for working with people who have behavioural difficulties. Readers explore common basic human needs, personality development, stress, anxiety, crisis, and coping behaviours. The section concludes with a description of the basic mental health assessment skills needed by every health care provider.

The patients for whom we care are the subject of **Unit III, Mental Health Challenges Across the Lifespan,** which focuses on the growth of "normal" (adaptive) mental health behaviours during each developmental stage. The most common mental health challenges associated with children, adolescents, adults, and older persons are discussed using the *Diagnostic and Statistical Manual of Mental Disorders* (DSM-5) as a framework. A chapter on dementia and Alzheimer's disease discusses the care of patients who have cognitive impairments.

Unit IV, Patients With Psychological Problems, explores common behavioural responses and therapeutic interventions for illness, hospitalization, loss, grief, and depression. Maladaptive behaviours and mental health disorders are described in chapters on somatoform, anxiety, eating, sleeping, mood, sexual, and dissociative disorders.

The chapters in **Unit V, Patients With Psychosocial Problems**, relate to the important social concerns of anger (and its expressions), suicide, abuse and neglect, acquired immunodeficiency syndrome (AIDS), and substance use. Sexual and personality disorders are also discussed. Chapters on schizophrenia and chronic mental illness focus on a multidisciplinary approach to treatment. The text concludes with a chapter titled "Challenges for the Future," which prepares students for the coming changes in mental health care.

STANDARD FEATURES

- Several key features are repeated throughout the text: **Objectives** stated in specific terms and a list of **Key Terms** (most with pronunciations) and page numbers.
- The **nursing process** is applied to specific mental health challenges throughout the text, with emphasis on multidisciplinary care. This helps readers understand the interactions of several health care disciplines and determine where they fit in the overall scheme of managed care.
- A **continuum of responses** describes the range of behaviours associated with each topic.
- **Development throughout the life cycle** relates to the aspect of each personality being studied.
- **Clinical disorders** include behavioural signs and symptoms based on the DSM-5.
- **Therapeutic interventions** include multidisciplinary treatment, medical management, application of the nursing process, and pharmacological therapy.
- Each chapter concludes with **Key Points** that serve as a useful review of the chapter's concepts.

FEATURES OF THE FIRST CANADIAN EDITION

The First Canadian Edition builds on the work of the venerable US-based text. Information specific to Canada and Canadian research, programs, and practices has been included, giving readers a current and clinically relevant perspective on the state of mental health care in Canada.

Throughout the text, a focus on the Canadian health care system and the influence of the *Canada Health Act* have been maintained. Medications referenced are currently used and available in Canada.

Where applicable, DSM-IV diagnoses and references from the American Psychiatric Association have been updated to the current *DSM-5*.

Increased attention to Indigenous health and healing practices has also been included, along with expanded exploration of other vulnerable populations in Canada.

An appendix featuring the *Canadian Standards for Psychiatric-Mental Health Nursing,* from the Canadian Federation of Mental Health Nurses, has been added to the end of the book for student reference.

The authors have worked from the perspective that mental health and addiction disorders are primarily chronic and genetic, setting treatment goals to maximum recovery as opposed to curative.

LEARNING AIDS

Because the majority of mental health care takes place outside the institution, the book emphasizes the importance of using therapeutic mental health interventions during every patient interaction. The following features encourage the reader's understanding and are designed to foster effective learning and comprehension:

- The two-colour design stimulates learning and calls attention to the important terms and concepts within the text.
- Selected **Key Terms** with phonetic pronunciations and a specific page reference to where the term can be found are listed at the beginning of each chapter, and each Key Term appears in colour at the first or most detailed mention in the text. Complete definitions are located in the **Glossary.** Terms with phonetic pronunciations were selected because they are either (1) difficult medical, nursing, or scientific terms or (2) words that may be difficult for students to pronounce.
- Throughout the text, cultural aspects of various mental health principles are explored in **Cultural Considerations** boxes to encourage further thought and discussion.
- **Critical Thinking** boxes pose questions designed to stimulate critical thinking.
- **Case Studies** with thought-provoking questions encourage readers to consider the psychosocial aspects of providing therapeutic care in both community and hospital settings.
- **Medication Alert** boxes prepare readers for the complexity of therapy with psychotherapeutic medications, including identifying drug interactions and potentially life-threatening side effects.
- Descriptions of each mental health disorder are drawn from *DSM-5* **criteria.**
- Multidisciplinary **Sample Patient Care Plans** demonstrate the application of the therapeutic (nursing) process to the care of individuals with various mental health disorders.
- **Nursing diagnoses** are stated in multidisciplinary terms within a holistic framework.

- The **holistic approach** to care offers readers a view of the "whole person" context of health care delivery.
- **NEW Critical Thinking Questions** at the end of each chapter encourage students to reflect on specific topics and scenarios, develop problem-solving skills, and consider how they might address current health care issues in practice. **Suggested Answers** to these questions, to guide class discussion, are found on the Evolve website.
- **References** encourage further exploration of the topics presented in the chapter. For easy access, the references are found at the end of each chapter in the book.
- The **Glossary** of Key Terms, written in an easy-to-understand format, follows the text and is also available on the Evolve website.

ANCILLARIES
For Instructors

We recognize that educators today have limited time to prepare for classroom and clinical activities. Therefore we provide a rich collection of supplemental resources for instructors within the Evolve Resources with TEACH Instructor Resource, including:

- **TEACH Lesson Plans,** based on textbook learning objectives and providing a roadmap to link and integrate all parts of the educational package. These straightforward lesson plans can be modified or combined to meet your unique teaching needs.
- **PowerPoint Presentations,** including approximately 800 slides with **i-clicker questions** and talking points for instructors.
- **ExamView Test Bank,** with more than 800 multiple-choice and alternate-format examination-style questions. Each question provides the correct answer, rationale, topic, client need category, step of the nursing process, objective, and cognitive level.
- **Open-Book Quizzes** for each chapter in the textbook, with separate answer guidelines.
- **Suggested Answers to the Textbook Critical Thinking Exercises** offer instructor guidance for classroom discussion about the Critical Thinking Questions found at the end of each chapter.
- **Answer Key** to the Study Guide.

For Students

In the Student Resources section of the Evolve website, there are more than 300 **Review Questions** with rationales for both correct and incorrect responses; an accompanying online **Study Guide**; Suggested Answers to the in-text Critical Thinking Questions; and an Audio Glossary.

READING AND REVIEW TOOLS

Objectives introduce the chapter topics.

Key Terms are listed with page number references, and selected difficult medical, nursing, or scientific terms are accompanied by simple phonetic pronunciations. Key terms are considered essential to understanding chapter content and are defined within the chapter. Key terms are boldfaced in the narrative and are briefly defined in the text, with complete definitions in the **Glossary**.

Each chapter ends with (1) **Key Points** that reiterate the chapter objectives and serve as a useful review of concepts, (2) **Additional Learning Resources**, and (3) **Critical Thinking Questions**.

Complete **References** at the end of each chapter cite evidence-informed information and provide resources for enhancing knowledge.

CHAPTER FEATURES

Case Studies contain critical thinking questions to help you develop problem-solving skills.

Critical Thinking Boxes contain thought-provoking scenarios and critical thinking questions.

Cultural Considerations address the mental health needs of culturally diverse patients.

Medication Alert boxes identify the risks and possible adverse reactions of psychotherapeutic medications.

Sample Patient Care Plans are multidisciplinary and address how members of the health care team work collaboratively to meet patient needs.

EVOLVE RESOURCES

Be sure to visit your textbook's Evolve website (http://evolve.elsevier.com/Canada/Morrison-Valfre/) for a Study Guide, an Audio Glossary, Review Questions, and more!

ACKNOWLEDGEMENTS

Canada is a country of immigrants. English is my fifth language. I am grateful to my daughter, Shelly Bard, for her help with this book.

Boris Bard

Much appreciation to Professor Lisa-Marie Forcier for her assistance with research and clinical scenarios and for her dedication to battling the stigma of mental illness.

Eric MacMullin

No text is written alone. The continued support of my husband, Adolph; of my friend Marian McCollum; and of other colleagues has provided the energy to complete this project when my own energy was low. The guidance, expertise, and encouragement from my editors Nancy O'Brien, Becky Leenhouts, and Mike Sheets are much appreciated. I also thank all the health care providers who so freely share their time and expertise with those who want to learn more about the dynamic and complex nature of human behaviour.

Michelle Morrison-Valfre

The product you are holding in your hands or viewing on your screen exists as a result of a great deal of work, research, and review. Although authors tend to get the most obvious credit (after all, it is our names that appear on the cover), a text of this nature would be entirely impossible if not for the work of many dedicated publishing professionals.

Although we have worked diligently to "Canadianize" the venerable Morrison-Valfre text, many other unsung heroes have toiled away to make this text as valuable to you, the reader, as humanly possible. Although it would be almost impossible to list them all, there are three individuals we would like to thank specifically.

Content Strategist/Acquisitions person extraordinaire Roberta Spinosa-Millman recognized the need for a specifically Canadian, fundamental text that addresses how we—as Canadians—approach, treat, and recognize mental health. Roberta pulled together three very different authors/mental health practitioners and set the foundation for us to work together to produce what we consider to be an excellent text and reference. Thank you, Roberta, for the dual opportunities of producing a text of this nature and of allowing us the honour to work together.

Somehow balancing Zen-like patience along with a subtle ability to kindly motivate and direct, Content Development Specialist Martina van de Velde worked extensively to ensure that our efforts were consistent and relevant. Many, many thanks to her for her collaboration, professionalism, and kindness. Again, for the times we did not get chapters completed on time, missed a deadline, or simply forgot, we offer apologies and, in equal measure, sincere admiration.

Finally, our "almost at the finish line" copy editor, Jerri Hurlbutt, who has a keen eye for detail, word, and idea flow and for use of reference and Internet-accessible information, took a sometimes rough draft and turned it into something of equal measures of accuracy and art. Jerri has also motivated and inspired us with her efficiency and work ethic. We simply cannot imagine this final product without Jerri's input and direction.

There are many, many others who were involved in getting this text from our brains into your hands, and to those far-too-anonymous people, we also give our sincere thanks. Sales staff, printers, clerical workers, technicians, and others have all played a vital role in making this text available.

Boris Bard
Eric MacMullin
Jacqueline Williamson

CONTENTS

Mental Health Care: Past and Present

1

The History of Mental Health Care

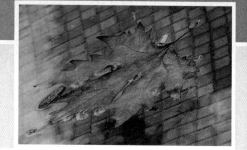

Mental/emotional health is interwoven with physical health. Behaviours relating to health exist over a broad spectrum, often referred to as the **health–illness continuum** (Fig. 1.1). People who enjoy robust health are placed at the higher-level wellness end of the continuum. Individuals with significant or multiple health challenges are typically placed at the continuum's opposite end. Most of us, however, function somewhere between these two extremes. As we meet with the stresses of life, our coping abilities are repeatedly challenged and we strive to adjust in appropriate ways. When stress is physical, the body calls forth its defence systems and wards off illness. When stress is emotional or developmental, we respond by using our established coping behaviours or sometimes creating new (and hopefully effective) coping behaviours.

Mental health is the ability to exist in "a state of well-being in which the individual realizes his or her own abilities, can cope with the normal stresses of life, can work productively

and fruitfully, and is able to make a contribution to his or her community" (World Health Organization [WHO], 2018). Mentally healthy people successfully carry out their activities of daily living, adapt to change, solve problems, set goals, prioritize challenges, and enjoy life. They are self-aware, directed, and responsible for their actions. People who are able to cope well are generally considered to be mentally healthy.

Mental health is influenced by three factors: inherited characteristics, childhood nurturing, and life circumstances. The risk for developing ineffective coping behaviours increases when problems or deficits exist in any one of these areas. **Mental illness** can impact an individual's ability to cope effectively, carry out daily activities, accurately interpret reality, execute sound judgement, and have accurate insights into the many challenges of daily life.

Society's understanding of the causes of mental health challenges has changed dramatically throughout our history

(Table 1.1). As we have advanced in our knowledge of anatomy and physiology, our beliefs around mental health disorders have gone from being based in superstition to grounded in biochemical and behavioural investigations.

EARLY YEARS

Illness, injury, and mental illness have concerned humanity throughout history. Physical illness and injury were easy to detect with nothing but the five senses. Mental illness was something different—something where the cause could not be seen, felt, or obviously understood—and therefore a condition to be feared.

Ancient Societies

Although historical records on ancient societies are vague, it can be assumed that some care was given to sick or injured people. Some early societies believed that everything in nature was alive with spirits. Illness was sometimes thought to be caused by the influence of evil spirits or demons.

Treatments for mental illness focused on removing the demons or evil spirits. Magical therapies made use of "frightening

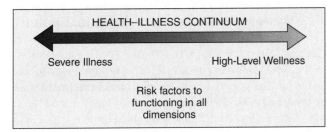

Fig. 1.1 The health–illness continuum, ranging from high-level wellness to severe illness, provides a method of identifying a patient's level of health.

masks and noises, incantations, vile odours, charms, spells, sacrifices, and fetishes" (Kelly, 1991). Physical treatments included blood-letting, massage, blistering, inducing vomiting, and the practice of **trephining**—cutting holes in the skull to encourage the evil spirits to leave. Generally, members of primitive societies with bizarre behaviours were allowed to remain within their communities as long as their behaviours were not disruptive. Severely ill or violent members of the group were often driven into the wilderness to fend for themselves, away from the safety and support the community offered.

Greece and Rome

Superstitions and magical beliefs dominated thinking until the Greeks introduced the idea that mental illness could be rationally explained through observation. The Greeks incorporated many ideas about illness from other cultures. By the sixth century BCE, medical schools were well established. The greatest physician in Greek medicine, Hippocrates, was born in 460 BCE. He was the first to base treatment on the belief that nature is a strong healing force. He felt that the role of the physician was to assist in, rather than direct, the healing process. Proper diet, exercise, and personal hygiene were his mainstays of treatment. Hippocrates viewed mental illness as a result of an imbalance of humors—the fundamental elements of air, fire, water, and earth. Each basic element had a related humor or part in the body. An overabundance or lack of one or more humors resulted in illness. This view (the **humoral theory of disease**) persisted for centuries.

Plato (427–347 BCE), a Greek philosopher, recognized life as a dynamic balance maintained by the soul. According to Plato a "rational soul" resided in the head and an "irrational soul" was found in the heart and abdomen. He believed that if the rational soul was unable to control the undirected parts of the irrational soul, mental illness resulted.

TABLE 1.1	**History at a Glance**	
History at a Glance	**View of Mental Illness**	**Events**
Greece and Rome	Imbalance of humors	Plagues, the (Christian) Church cared for mentally ill
Middle Ages	Demonic possession	Bedlam institution for mentally ill, 1247; witch hunts
Renaissance	Brain disorder, possession by devil	Treatment remains inhumane
Reformation	Demonic possession, some reasoning	Church stopped caring for the sick
Seventeenth and eighteenth centuries	Demonic possession	Quakers opened asylums Pinel advocated humane care Treatment remained harsh
Nineteenth century	Disease of the mind, may be curable	D. Dix, Dr. C.K. Clarke advocated humane care B. Rush wrote first text on mental illness Two-class system of private and public care
Twentieth century	Freud's psychoanalytical theories, behaviour can be changed	Effects of World Wars I and II advance study of mental illness Psychotherapeutic medications were introduced Mentally ill were deinstitutionalized
Twenty-first century	Biochemical imbalances	Lawmakers defining national health policies Physical causes of mental illness investigated

The principles and practices of Greek medicine became established in Rome around 100 BCE, but most physicians still thought that demons caused mental illness. The practice of frightening away evil spirits to cure mental illness was reintroduced, and its use continued well into the Middle Ages. Based on historical evidence, Romans seemed to have shown little interest in the body or mind. Most Roman physicians provided symptomatic relief and "wanted to make their patients comfortable by pleasant physical therapies" (Alexander & Selesnick, 1966), such as warm baths, massage, music, and peaceful surroundings.

By 300 CE, multiple epidemics killed hundreds of thousands of people and desolated the land (Alexander & Selesnick, 1966). Churches often became sanctuaries for the sick, and soon hospitals were built to accommodate the high numbers of sufferers. By 370 CE, Saint Basil's Hospital in England offered services for sick, orphaned, crippled, and mentally troubled people.

Middle Ages
Dark Ages

From about 500 CE to 1100 CE (in the Western world), priests cared for the sick as the (Christian) Church developed into a highly organized and powerful institution. Early Christians believed that disease was "God's retribution for personal or hereditary sin" (Ferngren, 2016). To cure mental illness, priests performed **demonic exorcisms**—religious ceremonies in which patients were physically punished to drive away the evil possessing spirit. Fortunately, Christian charity tempered these practices as members of the community cared for the mentally ill with concern and sympathy.

As time passed, medieval society declined. Repeated attacks from barbaric tribes led to chaos and moral decay. Epidemics, natural disasters, and overwhelming taxes significantly reduced the size and influence of the middle class. Cities, industries, and commerce disappeared or became much reduced. "The population declined, crime waves occurred, poverty was abysmal, and torture and imprisonment became prominent as civilization seemed to slip back into semi-barbarianism" (Donahue, 1996). Only monasteries remained as the last refuge of care and knowledge.

Throughout the Middle Ages, medicine and religion were interwoven. However, by 1130 laws were passed forbidding monks to practise medicine because it was considered too disruptive to their way of life (Amundsen, 1978). As a result, responsibility for the care of sick people once again fell to family members and the community at large.

In the late 1100s, a strong Arabic influence was felt in Europe. Knowledge of the Greek legacy had been retained and improved upon by the Arabs. They had extensive knowledge of drugs, mathematics, astronomy, and chemistry, as well as an awareness of the relationship between emotions and disease. The Arabic influence resulted in the establishment of learning centres, called *universities*. Many were devoted to the study of medicine, surgery, and care of the sick.

Problems of the mind, however, received only spiritual attention. Church doctrine still stated that if a person was insane, it had to be the result of some external force. The moon and lunar cycles were often associated with aberrant behaviour, thus the term **lunacy** was coined, meaning "a disorder caused by a lunar body" (Alexander & Selesnick, 1966). In time, large institutions were established, and mentally ill individuals were housed in "lunatic asylums." Despite some improvements in caring for such individuals, magical influences were still used to explain the torments of the mind.

Superstitions, Witches, and Hunters

The Church's doctrine of imposed celibacy failed to curtail many of the clergy's sexual behaviours, and so began an antierotic movement that focused on women as the cause of men's lust. Women were thought to be easily influenced by the devil and other external magical forces that stirred men's passions. As the historians Alexander and Selesnick (1966) note, "Psychotic women with little control over voicing their sexual fantasies and sacrilegious feelings were the clearest examples of demoniacal possession." This campaign, in turn, flamed the public's mounting fear of mentally troubled people.

Witch-hunting was officially launched in 1487 with the publication of the book the *Malleus Maleficarum,* or *The Witches' Hammer.* This was considered to be a guidebook on the prosecution of witches in a court of law (Kramer, 2019). Soon thereafter, Pope Innocent VIII and the University of Cologne voiced support for this "textbook of the Inquisition." As a result of this one publication, women as well as children and mentally ill persons were tortured and burned at the stake by the thousands. There were few safe havens for individuals with mental illness during these troubled times.

The first English institution for mentally ill people was initially a hospice founded in 1247 by the sheriff of London. By 1330, Bethlehem Royal Hospital had developed into a lunatic asylum that eventually became infamous for its brutal treatments. Violently ill patients were chained to walls in small cells and were often used to provide entertainment for the public. Hospital staff would charge fees and conduct tours through the institution. Less violent patients were forced to wear identifying metal armbands and beg on the streets. Individuals who had mental health challenges were harshly treated in those times, but Bethlehem Royal Hospital, commonly called *Bedlam* (Fig. 1.2), even with the documented abuses, was a moderately preferable option.

By the middle of the fourteenth century, the European continent had endured several devastating plagues and epidemics. One quarter of the earth's population, more than 60 million people, perished from infectious diseases during this period. The feudal system lost power and declined. Cities began to flourish and housed a growing middle class. As nursing historian Donahue (1996) notes, "Luxury and misery, learning and ignorance existed side by side." Society was beginning to demand social reforms around employment and payment for work done. Ironically, as the age of art, medicine, and science dawned, the hunting of "witches" became even more popular. It was a time of great contradictions.

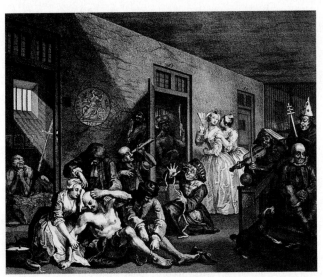

Fig. 1.2 Bethlehem Royal Hospital in London. (William Hogarth, "The Rake in Bedlam," c. 1735. From the series titled The Rake's Progress. Copyright The British Museum, London.)

The Renaissance

The Renaissance began in Italy around 1400 and spread throughout the European continent within a century. Upheavals in economics, politics, education, and commerce brought the world into focus. The power of the Church declined to some degree, as an intense interest in material gain and worldly affairs developed. At the same time, the medieval view of the naked body as sinful changed into more positive perceptions of the human form as a result of work by artists such as da Vinci, Raphael, and Michelangelo. Thousand-year-old anatomy books were replaced by volumes with art displaying realistic anatomical drawings. Observation, rather than ancient theories, revolutionized many of the ideas of the day.

Sixteenth-century physicians, relying on observation, began to record what they saw. Mental illness was at last being recognized with much less bias than before. By the mid-1500s, behaviours were accurately recorded for melancholia (depression), mania, and psychopathic behaviours. Precise observations led to classifications for different abnormal behaviours. Mental problems were now thought to be caused by some sort of brain disorder—except in the case of sexual fantasies, which were still considered to be God's punishment or to be possession by the devil. However, despite great advances in knowledge about the brain and mental illness, the actual treatment of mentally troubled people remained ineffective and inhumane.

The Reformation

Another movement that influenced the care of the sick—the Protestant Reformation—occurred from 1517 to 1648. Many people were displeased with the conduct of the clergy and widespread abuses occurring within the Catholic Church. Martin Luther (1483–1546), a monk who had questioned many of the teachings, philosophy, and restrictions of the church, and his followers broke away from the Catholic Church and became known as Protestants. As a result of this separation, many hospitals operated by the Catholic Church began to close. Once again, the poor, sick, and mentally ill were turned out into the streets.

Seventeenth Century

During the seventeenth and eighteenth centuries, developments in science, literature, philosophy, and the arts laid the foundations for the world we know today. Reason slowly began to replace magical thinking, but a strong belief in demons nonetheless persisted. The 1600s produced many great thinkers, and knowledge of the secrets of nature brought a sense of self-reliance. However, many people remained uncomfortable with these changes in the sciences and other areas and once again moved toward the security of witch-hunting as a means of protecting themselves from the unexplainable.

In the seventeenth century, conditions for the mentally ill were at their worst. While physicians and theorists were making observations and speculations about insanity, patients were bled, starved, and beaten into submission. Treatments for the mentally troubled remained in this unhappy state until the late eighteenth century.

Eighteenth Century

During the latter part of the eighteenth century, psychiatry developed as a separate branch of medicine. Inhumane treatment and vicious practices were openly questioned. In 1792, Philippe Pinel (1745–1826), the director of two Paris hospitals, liberated patients from their chains "and advocated acceptance of the mentally ill as human beings in need of medical assistance, nursing care, and social services" (Donahue, 1996). During this period, William Tuke, a member of a religious order called the Quakers, helped to established asylums of humane care in England. Initially a businessman, Mr. Tuke devoted much of his time to raising funds to open the York Retreat, a residential treatment centre where the mentally ill were to be cared for with kindness, dignity, and decency (Reisman, 1991).

In the American colonies the Philadelphia Almshouse was erected in 1731. It accepted sick, infirm, and insane patients as well as prisoners and orphans. In 1794, Bellevue Hospital in New York City was opened as a pesthouse (a shelter or hospital for people who were suffering from infectious diseases) for the victims of yellow fever. By 1816 the hospital had enlarged to contain an almshouse for poor people, wards for the sick and insane, staff quarters, and even a penitentiary. In 1835, in New Brunswick, on the site of a former cholera hospital, a provincial lunatic asylum was established, making it the first dedicated mental health facility in British North America (Austin, Kunyk, Peternelj-Taylor, et al., 2019).

In spite of some advances, the care and treatment of people with mental illness remained harsh and indifferent. The practice of allowing poor people and family members to care for the mentally ill continued well into the late 1800s and was only slowly abandoned. Actual care of mentally ill persons in the United States did not begin to improve until the arrival of Alice Fisher, a Florence Nightingale–trained nurse, in

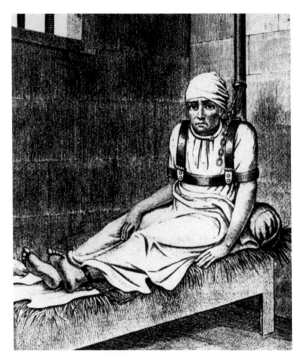

Fig. 1.3 A patient in chains in Bedlam, London's notorious Bethlehem Royal Hospital. (Courtesy U.S. National Library of Medicine, Bethesda, MD.)

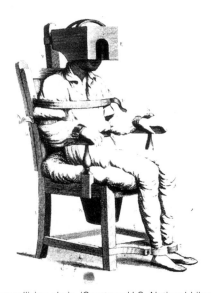

Fig. 1.4 Tranquilizing chair. (Courtesy U.S. National Library of Medicine, Bethesda, MD.)

1884. In Canada, the Hôtel Dieu, located in Quebec, provided some institutional care for "indigents, the crippled, and idiots"; however, standards of care remained low (Hurd, 1973; Sussman, 1998).

By the close of the eighteenth century, treatments for people with mental illness still included the medieval practices of bloodletting, purging, and confinement (Fig. 1.3). Newer therapies included demon-expelling tranquilizing chairs (Fig. 1.4) and whirling devices (Fig. 1.5). The study of psychiatry was in its infancy, and those who actually cared for insane people still relied heavily on the methods of their ancestors.

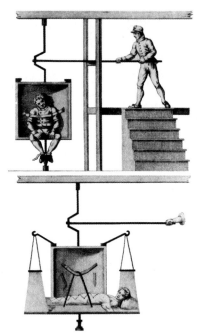

Fig. 1.5 Circulating swing and bed. (Redrawn from U.S. National Library of Medicine, Bethesda, MD.)

NINETEENTH CENTURY

Changes that occurred during the early 1800s had an enormous impact on the care of the mentally ill population. In the early to middle parts of that century, events like the attempted US invasion of Canada and ongoing rebellions against British rule in Upper and Lower Canada resulted in countermeasures to usher in political stability. Quebec, Ontario, Nova Scotia, and New Brunswick became the first four provinces to form a confederation. Many political processes became stable as a result of this confederation, including a more organized and structured medical care for their populations, which included the mentally ill.

One of the most important figures in nineteenth-century psychiatry was Dr. Benjamin Rush (1745–1813). His book, *Diseases of the Mind,* was the first psychiatric text written in the United States, advocating clean conditions (good air, lighting, and food) and kindness. As a result of Rush's efforts, mentally troubled people were no longer caged in the basements of general hospitals. However, only a few institutions for insane persons were available in the United States at this time, and even fewer were in Canada.

During the 1830s, attitudes toward mental illness slowly began to change. The "once insane, always insane" concept was replaced with the notion that cure might be possible in some circumstances. A few mental hospitals were built, but the actual living conditions for most patients remained deplorable.

It was not until 1841 that a 40-year-old schoolteacher exposed the inherent cruelty and inhumanity of the system. Dorothea Dix was contracted to teach Sunday school at a jail in Massachusetts. While there, she saw both criminals and mentally ill prisoners living in squalid conditions. For the next 20 years, Dix surveyed asylums, jails, and almshouses throughout Canada, the United States, and Scotland. It was not uncommon for her to find mentally ill people "confined in cages, closets, cellars, stalls, and pens . . . chained, naked, beaten with rods and lashed into obedience" (Dolan, 1968).

Dix presented her findings to anyone who would listen. The public responded so well to Dix's efforts that millions of dollars were raised, more than 30 mental hospitals throughout the United States were constructed, and care of the mentally ill greatly improved.

By the late 1800s, a two-class system of psychiatric care had emerged: private care for the wealthy and publicly provided care for the remainder of society. The newly constructed mental institutions were quickly filled, and soon chronic overcrowding began to strain the system. Cure rates fell dramatically. The public became disenchanted, and mental illness once again was viewed as incurable. Only small, private facilities that catered to the wealthy had some degree of success. In the absence of funding from the government, some facilities had evolved into large, remote institutions that became partially self-reliant, while still dependent on donations and benefactors.

By the close of the nineteenth century, many of the gains in the care of mentally ill persons had been lost. Overpopulated institutions could offer no more than minimal custodial care. Theories of the day gave no satisfactory explanations about the causes of mental health challenges, and current treatments remained ineffective. It was a time of despair for mentally troubled people and those who cared for them.

Dr. C.K. Clarke, a graduate of the University of Toronto, became highly influential in the delivery of mental health services in Ontario and, ultimately, Canada. As early as 1881, Dr. Clarke and his brother-in-law, Dr. William Metcalfe, advocated for the removal of restraints as a regular practice in mental health institutions. Sadly, Dr. Metcalfe was attacked by a paranoid patient and killed; however, Dr. Clarke continued to advocate for more humane treatment for the mentally ill (Pos, Walters, & Sommers, 1975). The Clarke Institute of Psychiatry, a world-renowned treatment facility, opened in Toronto in 1966 and was named in honour of Dr. Clarke. In 2002, the Clarke Institute became part of the Canadian Mental Health Association (CMHA).

TWENTIETH CENTURY

The 1900s were ushered in by reform movements, marked by the beginnings of political, economic, and social changes. For the first time in history, disease prevention was emphasized. For the mentally ill population, however, conditions remained intolerable, until 1908 when a single individual began a crusade that would improve the lives of millions of mentally ill individuals.

Clifford Beers was a young student at Yale University when he attempted suicide. Consequently, he spent 3 years as a patient in mental hospitals in Connecticut. Upon his release in 1908, Beers wrote a book that would set the wheels of the mental hygiene movement in motion. His book, *A Mind That Found Itself*, recounted the beatings, isolation, and confinement of a mentally ill person. As a direct result of Beers's work, the *Committee for Mental Hygiene* was formed in 1909. In addition to prevention, the group focused on removing the stigma attached to mental illness. Under Beers's energetic guidance, the movement grew nationwide and ultimately had a global impact. The social consciousness of a nation had finally been awakened.

Psychoanalysis

In the early 1900s, a neurophysiologist named Sigmund Freud published an article that introduced the term **psychoanalysis** to the world's vocabulary. Freud believed that forces both within and outside the personality were responsible for mental illness. He developed elaborate theories around the theme of repressed sexual energies. Freud was the first to succeed in "explaining human behavior in psychologic terms and in demonstrating that behavior can be changed under the proper circumstances" (Alexander & Selesnick, 1966). The first comprehensive theory of mental illness based on observation had emerged, and psychoanalysis began to gain a strong foothold in America (see Chapter 5).

Influences of War

During the first World War, in the United States and to a lesser degree in Canada, men were drafted into military service as rapidly as they could be processed. Some, however, were considered to be unfit mentally to engage in battle. As a result, the US government called on Beers's Committee for Mental Hygiene to develop a more efficient process for screening and treating mentally ill soldiers. The completed plan included methods for early identification of mental problems, removal of mentally troubled personnel from combat duty, and early treatment close to the fighting front. The committee also recommended that psychiatrists be assigned to station hospitals to treat combat veterans with acute behavioural problems and provide ongoing psychiatric care after soldiers returned to their homes.

Because of the war, a renewed interest in mental hygiene was sparked. During the 1930s, new therapies for treating insanity were developed. Insulin therapy for schizophrenia induced 50-hour comas through the administration of massive doses of insulin. Passing electricity through the patient's head (**electroconvulsive therapy [ECT]**) helped to improve severe depression, and **lobotomy** (a surgical procedure that severs the frontal lobes of the brain from the thalamus) almost eliminated violent behaviours. A new class of medications that lifted spirits of depressed people, the amphetamines, was introduced. All these therapies improved behaviours and made patients more receptive to Freud's psychotherapy.

During World War II, many draftees were still rejected for enlistment because of mental health problems. A large number of soldiers received early discharges based on psychiatric disorders, and many active-duty personnel received treatment for psychiatric issues.

The effects of the Korean War of the 1950s, the Vietnam War of the 1960s and 1970s, and other armed conflicts contributed significant knowledge to the understanding of stress-related problems. Post-traumatic stress disorders became recognized among soldiers fighting wars. Today, stress disorders are considered the basis of many emotional and mental health problems.

Introduction of Psychotherapeutic Medications

Psychotherapeutic medications are essentially chemicals that exert an effect on the mind. These drugs alter emotions, perceptions, and consciousness in several ways. They are used in combination with various therapies for treating mental illness. Psychotherapeutic medications are also called *psychopharmacological agents, psychotropic drugs,* and *psychoactive drugs.*

Even by the 1950s, despite the many significant gains in treatment options, effective therapies were still limited. Treatments consisted primarily of psychoanalysis, insulin therapy, ECT, and water/ice therapy. More violent patients were physically restrained in straitjackets or underwent lobotomies. Medication therapy consisted of sedatives (chloral hydrate and paraldehyde), barbiturates (phenobarbital), and amphetamines that quieted patients and rendered them less of a nuisance to the public and caregivers but did little to treat their illnesses.

In 1949, an Australian physician, John Cade, discovered that lithium carbonate was effective in controlling the severe mood swings seen in bipolar (manic-depressive) illness. With lithium therapy, many chronically ill patients were again able to lead normal lives and were released from mental institutions. Encouraged by the apparent success of lithium, researchers began to explore the possibility of controlling mental illness with the use of various new drugs.

Chlorpromazine (Thorazine) was introduced in 1956 and proved to control or reduce many of the bizarre behaviours observed in schizophrenia and other psychoses (Keltner & Folks, 2005). The 1950s concluded with the introduction of imipramine, the first antidepressant. Soon other drugs, such as antianxiety agents, became available for use in treatment.

As more patients were able to control their behaviours with drug therapy, the demand for hospitalization decreased. Many people with mental disorders could now live and function outside the institution. At this time, governments began the movement called **deinstitutionalization**, the release of large numbers of mentally ill persons into the community. The introduction of psychotherapeutic drugs opened the doors of institutions and set the stage for a new delivery approach, community-based mental health care.

The 1960s were filled with social changes. With the introduction of psychotherapeutic drugs came the concept of the "least restrictive alternative." If patients could, with medication, control their behaviours and cooperate with treatment plans, then the controlled environment of the institution was

no longer necessary. It was believed that people with mental disorders could live within their communities and work with their therapists on an outpatient basis.

Adult Community Mental Health Programs

As the population of people with mental illnesses shifted from the institution to the community, the demand for community mental health supports expanded. To meet this demand, adult community mental health programs were developed.

At these centres, the needs of people with mental health challenges might be met. Physicians (psychiatrists), nurses, and various therapists would develop therapeutic relationships with patients and monitor their progress within the community setting. Each centre was to provide comprehensive mental health services for all residents within a certain geographic region, called a **catchment area**.

It was believed that community mental health centres would provide the link in helping mentally ill people make the transition from the institution to the community, thus meeting the goal of humane care delivered in the least restrictive way. Unfortunately, most chronically mentally ill people were "dumped" into their communities before realistic strategies, programs, and facilities were in place.

Community mental health centres expanded throughout the 1980s, but funding remained inadequate and sporadic. Demands for services overwhelmed the system and many services began to close their doors, reduce supports, or limit the number of patients they would see, leaving a large population of vulnerable people on their own with little to no support.

TWENTY-FIRST CENTURY

In 2006, the National Alliance for Mental Illness (NAMI) conducted the "first comprehensive survey and grading of adult mental health care systems conducted in more than 15 years" in the United States (it was updated in 2009) (NAMI, 2009). The results revealed a fragmented system, poorly equipped to meet the needs of its target population. Recommendations focused on increased funding, availability of care, access to care, and greater involvement of consumers and their families.

Today, many of our population's most severely mentally ill people still wander the streets in abject poverty and homelessness as a result of an inability to access resources. Adult community mental health centres have closed their doors or drastically reduced their services. The original goals of comprehensive care, education, rehabilitation, prevention, training, and research were lost in the efforts to curtail costs.

Countries such as Canada, the United States, the United Kingdom, New Zealand, and Australia are faced with similar mental health care issues. It is in the best interests of all countries to accept the challenge of providing for our societies' mental and physical health care needs.

KEY POINTS

- Mental health is the ability to cope with and adapt to the stresses of everyday life.
- Mentally healthy people are self-aware, directed, and responsible for their actions.
- Mental illness is an inability to cope that results in impaired functioning.
- Mental health is influenced by inherited characteristics, childhood nurturing, and life circumstances.
- The causes and treatments of mental illness were based in superstition, magical beliefs, and demonic possession from primitive societies into the 1800s.
- Priests cared for the sick and exorcised demons, but mentally troubled people were treated with care by the Christian community during the Middle Ages.
- By the late Middle Ages, large asylums housed the insane, and the belief that witches were the carriers of the devil led to the burning of thousands of women, children, and mentally ill people.
- By the 1500s, psychotic behaviours were being accurately observed and recorded, but the Reformation movement returned many insane people to the streets as church sanctuaries closed.
- During the 1800s, Americans Dr. Benjamin Rush and Dorothea Dix and Canadian Dr. C.K. Clarke advocated for the humane care of mentally ill people.
- Standards for the care of the insane population improved during the mid-1800s until huge waves of people overwhelmed the mental health care system, causing the conditions to deteriorate.
- A book written by Clifford Beers about his experience as a mental patient set the mental hygiene movement of the early 1900s into motion.
- By the 1920s, Sigmund Freud's psychoanalytic theories became a popular method for treating emotional problems.
- The psychological effects of the First and Second World Wars highlighted the need for comprehensive mental health care and focused research on post-traumatic stress disorder (PTSD).
- With the introduction of psychotherapeutic drug treatment, many psychiatric institutions closed.
- Community mental health centres were built during the 1970s, but a change in political climate and funding left the project uncompleted and countless mentally ill people with reduced or no treatment options.
- Today, ongoing cost restraints challenge us to develop comprehensive, fiscally conscious care for society's mentally ill members.

ADDITIONAL LEARNING RESOURCES

Go to your Evolve website (http://evolve.elsevier.com/Canada/Morrison-Valfre/) for additional online resources, including the online Study Guide for additional learning activities to help you master this chapter content.

CRITICAL THINKING QUESTIONS

1. What current mental health stigmas may have begun hundreds of years ago? How many can you think of? How would you respond to the family of a newly diagnosed schizophrenic, who may believe these stigmas to be true?

2. How has technology improved mental health care?

3. What current social processes help to preserve the rights and dignity of mental health patients? Do you believe those processes are adequate? If not, what more could be done?

REFERENCES

Alexander, F. G., & Selesnick, S. T. (1966). *The history of psychiatry.* The New American Library.

Amundsen, D. (1978). Medieval canon law on medical and surgical practice by the clergy. *Bulletin of the History of Medicine, 52*(1), 22–44. https://www.jstor.org/stable/44450442?seq=1

Austin, W., Peternelj-Taylor, C., Kunyk, D., et al. (2019). *Psychiatric & mental health nursing for Canadian practice* (4th ed.). Wolters Kluwer.

Dolan, J. (1968). *History of nursing.* Saunders.

Donahue, M. P. (1996). *Nursing: The finest art* (2nd ed.). Mosby.

Ferngren, G. B. (2016). *Medicine & health care in early Christianity.* The Johns Hopkins University Press.

Hurd, H. M. (Ed.). (1973, Originally printed 1916–1917). *The institutional care of the insane in the United States and Canada:* (Vol. IV). Arno Press.

Kelly, L. Y. (1991). *Dimensions of professional nursing* (6th ed.). Pergamon Press.

Keltner, N. L., & Folks, D. G. (2005). *Psychotropic drugs* (4th ed.). Mosby.

Kramer, H. (2019). *The hammer of witches: Malleus Maleficarum: The most influential book of witchcraft.* e-artnow.

National Alliance on Mental Illness (NAMI). (2009). *Grading the states: A report on America's health care system for serious mental illness.* https://www.nami.org/Support-Education/Publications-Reports/Public-Policy-Reports/Grading-the-States-2009

Pos, R., Walters, J. A., & Sommers, F. G. (1975). Historical note: D. Campbell Meyers, 1863–1927: Pioneer of Canadian general hospital psychiatry. *Canadian Psychiatric Association Journal, 20*(5), 393–403. https://journals.sagepub.com/doi/pdf/10.1177/070674377502000510

Reisman, J. M. (1991). *Series in clinical and community psychology. A history of clinical psychology* (2nd ed.). Hemisphere Publishing.

Sussman, S. (1998). The first asylums in Canada: A response to neglectful community care and current trends. *Canadian Journal of Psychiatry, 43*(3), 260–264. https://doi.org/10.1177/070674379804300304.

World Health Organization (WHO). (2018). *Mental health: Strengthening our response.* Author. https://www.who.int/news-room/fact-sheets/detail/mental-health-strengthening-our-response

2

Current Mental Health Care Systems

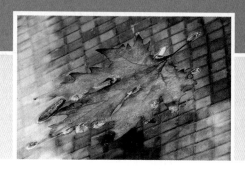

OBJECTIVES

Upon completion of this chapter, the student will be able to:

1. Describe the current mental health care systems in Canada, Norway, the United Kingdom, Australia, and the United States.
2. State one major difference between inpatient and outpatient psychiatric care.
3. Explain the community support systems model of care.
4. List settings for community mental health care delivery.
5. Describe components of the case management method of mental health care.
6. Discuss the roles and purpose of the multidisciplinary mental health care team.
7. Name high-risk populations served by community mental health centres.
8. List community-based mental health services for high-risk populations.

OUTLINE

KEY TERMS

advocacy (ĂD-və-kə-sē) (p. 15)
case management (KĀS MĂN-ăge-MĬNT) (p. 14)
community (kă-MŪN-ĭ-tē) **mental health centres** (p. 13)
community support (kă-MŪN-ĭ-tē să-PŎRT) **systems (CSS) model** (p. 12)
consultation (KŎN-sŬl-TĀ-shən) (p. 14)
crisis intervention (KRĪ-sĭs ĬN-tər-VəN-shən) (p. 15)
homelessness (HŌM-lĕs-nĕs) (p. 18)

inpatient psychiatric (ĬN-PĀ-shənt sī–k-Ē-ăt-rĭc) **care** (p. 12)
multidisciplinary (MŬL-tĭ-dĭ-sĭ-plə-nă-rē) **mental health care teams** (p. 16)
outpatient (ŎWT-PĀ-shənt) **mental health care** (p. 12)
psychosocial rehabilitation (sī-kō-SŌ-shəl RĒ-hă-bĭl-ə-TĀ-shən) (p. 14)
recidivism (rē-SĬD-ĭ-vĭz-əm) (p. 12)
resource linkage (RĒ-sŏrs LĔNK-əg) (p. 15)

Around the world, roughly 40% of countries have no mental health policy and 30% have no mental health care plan. The global median percentage of government health budget expenditures for mental health is just under 3%. In addition, many countries have poor coordination between mental health care and other health services (Dudley, Silove, & Gale, 2012).

MENTAL HEALTH CARE IN CANADA

By the late 1960s, Canada had adopted a **government-administered health insurance plan, which includes an array of mental health services.** Today a "single-payer arrangement" is used in the Canadian health care system, which is based on five principles: public administration, accessibility,

BOX 2.1 Principles of the Canada Health Act (1984)

- *Public Administration:* Provincial insurance programs must be publicly accountable for the funds they spend. Provincial governments determine the extent and amount of coverage of insured services. Moreover, management of provincial health insurance plans must be carried out by a not-for-profit authority, which can be part of government or an arm's-length agency.
- *Accessibility:* Canadians must have reasonable access to insured services without charge or paying user fees.
- *Comprehensiveness:* Provincial health insurance programs must include all *medically necessary* services. The Canada Health Act defines comprehensiveness broadly to include medically necessary services "for the purpose of maintaining health, preventing disease, or diagnosing or treating an injury, illness or disability."
- *Universality:* Provincial health insurance programs must insure Canadians for all medically necessary hospital and physician care. The condition also means that Canadians do not have to pay an insurance premium in order to be covered through provincial health insurance.
- *Portability:* Canadians are covered by a provincial insurance plan during short absences from that province.

Modified from Canadian Nurses Association (CNA). (2000). *Fact sheet: The Canada Health Act.* Author. https://www.cna-aiic.ca/~/media/cna/page-content/pdf-en/fs01_canada_health_act_june_2000_e.pdf

comprehensiveness, universality, and portability. Each guiding principle is explained in Box 2.1.

Each province or territory organizes, administers, and monitors the health care delivery system of its citizens. Benefits may vary, but all Canadian citizens are eligible for diagnostic, emergency, outpatient, medical, hospital, convalescent, and mental health services. The agency responsible for the health of Canadians is Health Canada. It provides technical and financial support for each provincial health care program, enforces federal food and drug laws, promotes health, and administers social welfare programs.

Across Canada, physician-provided mental health care is covered by provincial/territorial health care systems. This is not the case for other allied health professionals, such as psychologists, social workers, or mental health counsellors. Approximately 80% of psychologist consultations occur within the private for-profit system (Steele, Dewa, Lin et al., 2007; Government of Canada, 2006).

MENTAL HEALTH CARE IN INDUSTRIALIZED COUNTRIES

Norway

Like other European countries, Norway has adopted a national insurance system. The *National Insurance Act* of 1967 provides access to health care for everyone living in Norway. Employees contribute a percentage of their wages and pay out-of-pocket fees for health care until a "payment ceiling" (about $175) is reached. Thereafter, all services are covered except adult dental care.

Financing and delivery of health care services occur on three levels. Health policy is legislated, and health service delivery is monitored by national authorities. Hospitals and specialized medical services are managed by Norway's 19 counties, whereas primary health care services are organized on the municipal level. Mental health care is available to all citizens of Norway.

The United Kingdom

All British citizens are provided health care through a government-managed national health care system. The Secretary for Social Services is responsible for setting fees for private health care providers, budgets for hospitals, and salaries for hospital physicians. Parliament allocates funds for the health care system and regulates the rates at which general practitioners are paid. Tax revenues provide most of the financing for health care.

Mental health care is available for all British citizens as part of the standard benefit package. Physician services, emergency surgeries, hospital stays, and prescription drugs, along with preventive, home, and long-term care, are all provided by the government. Eye care is not included and dental care is limited, but all other basic health care needs are provided. Private insurance is also available.

Australia

Australians are provided an interesting mix of health care plans. The government provides a public health plan that covers all public hospitals and physician services. Also available is a national private plan, which supplements the basic public plan. In addition, numerous private insurance plans are available for eye care, rehabilitative services, and psychiatric treatment.

National health care is financed by a tax on all citizens above a certain income. Policy and budget decisions are made at the federal level. Individual states are responsible for the administration and delivery of health care services that are available through local government agencies, semi-voluntary agencies, and profit-oriented, nongovernmental organizations. The Mental Health Bill of 2013 addresses fairness, accountability, and inclusion of significant others when caring for the mentally ill in Australia's basic health plan.

The United States

Health care in the United States is based on the private insurance model. Currently, approximately 90% of US citizens are covered by private insurance or public programs (Medicare and/or Medicaid), leaving roughly 10% having no health care coverage. Rates vary by state, with Texas having the highest rate of uninsured and Massachusetts having almost 100% coverage. With the introduction of the *Affordable Care Act* (ACA; Obamacare) system of health care delivery, the rate of health care coverage increased; however, implementation of this model is at risk because of changes in government and individual states rejecting ACA coverage.

The distinction between public and private mental health care financing is beginning to blur. Federal funds (Medicare) and state funds (Medicaid) are being used to cover costs in both the private and public sectors. Currently, Medicare funds about 30 to 50% of all state mental health systems.

CARE SETTINGS

In Canada, admission rates to psychiatric inpatient facilities were at an all-time low by 1983 as mental health care was delivered primarily in community settings. However, by 1988, hospitalizations for mental illness were on the rise and emergency departments saw huge increases in patients with psychiatric issues. Today there are more people in need of care than there are treatment settings.

Inpatient Care

Individuals are admitted to **inpatient psychiatric care** based on need. The severity of the patient's illness, the level of dysfunction, the suitability of the setting for treating the problem, the level of patient cooperation, and the patient's ability to pay for services all enter into the decision regarding inpatient psychiatric care.

Inpatient care settings can include general mental health units that treat a wide variety of challenges, geriatric mental health units that specialize in the treatment of individuals over the age of 65, child and adolescent units focusing on those 18 and younger, and highly specialized psychiatric intensive care units for individuals who may experience periods of aggression and violence as part of their mental health challenges. Other even more specialized units provide expertise in areas such as eating disorders, developmental disorders, and even short-term inpatient resources for crisis intervention and stabilization. Patients may also be committed to psychiatric care by way of the criminal justice system. These settings are administered in a manner that is similar to a jail or correctional services facility. The legal aspects of involuntary commitment are discussed in Chapter 3.

Patients who receive inpatient care generally remain in a safe environment for 24 hours per day with all aspects of care focusing on providing therapeutic assistance. Discharge occurs when patient behaviour has improved and treatment goals have been attained. The majority of patients are discharged back into the community. Depending on individual housing options, some may be discharged to a group home or other structured setting or to another institution for longer-term psychiatric care.

The most important advantage of inpatient psychiatric care is that it provides patients with a safe and secure environment where they can focus and work on the challenges that brought them into the unit initially.

Outpatient Care

As the emphasis shifts to community mental health care, the demand for outpatient psychiatric service grows. An **outpatient mental health care** setting is a facility that provides services to people with mental health challenges within their home environments. With these services, psychiatric patients are able to remain within their communities, associating with normal aspects of everyday life, a considerably more therapeutic option than a mental health unit in a hospital.

Community-based mental health care occurs within a dynamic society. Supervision is limited, and the responsibility for controlling behaviour lies squarely with the individual. Patients are assessed in relation to their environment and therapies are designed to assist them in functioning appropriately within their communities. The number of outpatient

psychiatric care support services is sometimes outpaced by the mental health needs of a community or catchment area.

Mentally ill people make use of community services only sporadically. This "hit and miss" approach makes effective care difficult. Many wait until major problems occur before seeking treatment. When services are used, a "Band-Aid" approach that treats only the presenting concern is often utilized. As a result, many individuals who end up in the emergency departments of general hospitals or incarcerated in the corrections system are in need of inpatient psychiatric care.

According to the Office of the Correctional Investigator, Canadian offenders experience mental health challenges at a rate of two to three times more than the general population (Office of the Correctional Investigator, 2011). Approximately 11% of male offenders have a significant mental health diagnosis, with over 20% taking a prescribed medication for a mental health issue at the time they are arrested or apprehended. Slightly more than 6% were receiving some type of outpatient mental health treatment or support. Female offenders appear to be twice as likely as male offenders to have a mental health diagnosis at admission to a correctional facility, with over 30% having had a psychiatric admission to a hospital prior to admission to a correctional facility (Office of the Correctional Investigator, 2011).

Unable to cope in the community setting, people with chronic psychiatric issues often return to institutions or use community services on a revolving-door basis. This behaviour pattern is known as **recidivism** and means a relapse (return) of a symptom, disease, or behaviour, typically resulting in a visit (or revisit) to the local emergency department. Recidivism is a major problem in mental health care. It is associated with negative treatment outcomes, staff frustration, and inappropriate use of services. Lower rates of recidivism are seen in communities where coordination and cooperation among community agencies and mental hospitals exist.

Psychiatry and mental health care policies are often based on the medical treatment model: identify the symptom and then treat it. This point of view became inadequate once patients were released into the community. A broader, community-oriented, more flexible outlook was needed.

Community Support Systems Model

For mentally ill people to function well within their communities, a wide range of support services is necessary. The **community support systems (CSS) model** views patients holistically—as

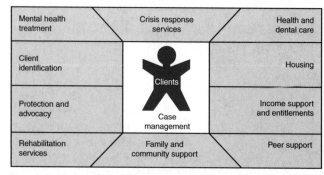

Fig. 2.1 Community support system. (Modified from Stuart, G. W. [2013]. *Principles and practice of psychiatric nursing* [10th ed.]. Mosby.)

BOX 2.2 Examples of Community Services

Serving Individuals
Rape crisis centres
Churches, synagogues, and mosques
Employment, job-training agencies
Recreational clubs
Adult education programs
Literacy programs
Mediation groups
Meals on Wheels
Colleges and universities
Mental health agencies

Serving Families
Women, Infants, and Children (WIC)
Children's groups (e.g., Boys and Girls Clubs)
Nutritional services
Church groups
Community "Welcome Wagon"

Recreation centres
Day care centres for young, disabled, or older people
Family planning agencies
Family recreation centres and groups
Shelters for victims of domestic violence

Serving the Community
Environmental groups
Education groups (e.g., Canadian Lung Association, Friends of
    Schizophrenics)
Utility companies
Community emergency shelters
Government agencies
Police and fire departments
Fair housing bureau or agency
Prisons
Performing arts centres
Public forests and parks

Data from Haber, J., McMahon, A. L., & Krainovich-Miller, B. (1997). *Comprehensive psychiatric nursing* (5th ed.). Mosby.

TABLE 2.1 Community Mental Health Care Delivery

Setting	Focus/Services	Staff Members	Comments
Emergency care (community hospital EDs, emergency psychiatric clinics)	Stabilization, assist with the crisis, refer to appropriate community resources	Nurses, social workers, therapists, psychologists, psychiatric technicians	Many chronically mentally ill persons use ED settings as an entry into the mental health care network
Residential programs (group homes)	Offer a protected, supervised environment within the community	Home care providers, therapists, nurses, technicians, physician	Provide food, shelter, clothing, supervision, counselling, vocational training, socialization
Partial hospitalization (day treatment centres)	Provides care and treatment for patients who are too ill to be independent; patients are gradually introduced into the community	Psychologists, therapists, nurses, counsellors, social workers, technicians	Multidisciplinary care and treatment have led to patient success and proven the effectiveness of these programs
Psychiatric home care	Delivers care to patients and families in their homes; helps patients and families transition from institution to home; crisis interventions; referral to resources	Psychiatric CNSs, home-care providers	Collaborates with patient, family, other mental health professionals to provide ongoing care
Community mental health centres	Services include crisis intervention, family counselling, education, care for the chronically mentally ill, medical care, vocational and skills training	Psychologists, therapists, nurses, counsellors, social workers, technicians	Lack of adequate financing has resulted in fragmented services

CNSs, clinical nurse specialists; *ED*, emergency department.

individuals with basic human needs, ambitions, and rights. The goal of the CSS model is to create a support system that fosters individual growth and movement toward independence through the use of coordinated social, medical, and psychiatric services. Effective community support systems are consumer oriented, culturally appropriate, flexible enough to meet individual needs, accountable, and coordinated. A typical program may include services such as health care, housing, food, income support, rehabilitation, advocacy, and crisis response (Fig. 2.1).

Community mental health centres are outpatient settings that reflect the CSS model by providing a comprehensive range of services. Many have forged strong links with community agencies, services, and government. Other centres have

developed slowly, but the CSS model of mental health care is proving to be one of the most comprehensive and workable concepts for aiding mentally ill persons (Johnson, 2017).

DELIVERY OF COMMUNITY MENTAL HEALTH SERVICES

Mental health services and support systems are available through a variety of community agencies, support groups, and civic organizations. Services focus on prevention, maintenance, and treatment of mental health conditions and rehabilitation of persons with mental health challenges. Some agencies or groups limit their focus to one area (e.g.,

Alcoholics Anonymous focuses on treatment of alcohol addiction). Individuals, families, and communities benefit from the activities of various groups. Box 2.2 lists examples of commonly available community services.

Community Care Settings

Community mental health services are based on the needs of specific populations. In addition, for best outcomes, mentally ill people must be treated in the least restrictive manner possible. Therefore, several services are available in various settings throughout the community. See Table 2.1 for examples.

With short institutional stays and the release of people with chronic mental illness into the community, the need for home psychiatric care providers to fill the gap between institution and community is rapidly growing.

Given the wide range of patient needs, multiple professions have evolved to offer services. *Social workers* provide support to individuals, families, and children in need. They also assist with everyday problems and challenges, connect their patients to community resources, and can diagnose and treat specific mental health, behavioural, and emotional issues. *Occupational therapists* have a strong focus on minimizing disability and social marginalization. Much of their work addresses a patient's level of ability and how that patient is able to function in their day-to-day activities as well as to meet the goals and aspirations they may have. Occupational therapists focus on "doing" as a means to encourage and support change. *Psychiatrists* are medical doctors with advanced education and training that allows them to diagnose and treat mental health conditions. Psychiatrists can also recommend and provide prescriptions for medications to treat or reduce the severity of many mental health disorders. *Peer support workers* are often individuals who themselves have been patients of the mental health and/or addictions treatment system at some time in their lives. They offer a unique perspective and use their own experience to support and guide others facing similar challenges. *Psychologists* work in a wide range of settings, from the community to prisons to mobile crisis teams, and can provide one-to-one counselling. Psychologists can assess behavioural and mental health challenges and provide treatment options to their patients. *Psychiatric clinical nurse specialists (CNSs)* ease the transition from hospital to home for patients and their families and assist patients in navigating the mental health care system. They also provide psychosocial crisis interventions and collaborate with patients, families, and other professionals to deliver the most appropriate and cost-accountable psychiatric care.

Case Management

Defined as a system of interventions, **case management** is designed to support mentally ill patients living in the community. The major components of case management are psychosocial rehabilitation, consultation, resource linkage (referral), advocacy, therapy, and crisis intervention. Patients are involved with the assessment, planning, and evaluation of their care. Goals are stated as patient outcomes. Success is measured in terms of patient satisfaction, improved coping behaviours, and appropriate use of services. The overall goal of case management is to have a successfully functioning patient able (with support) to avoid relapse and achieve

CASE STUDY

Joanne is a 59-year-old woman with severe depression, anorexia, and suicidal ideation. The psychiatric home care referral was an effort by her husband to prevent nursing home placement. Joanne presented with a 30-year history of scleroderma (a disfiguring skin condition), numerous surgeries and hospitalizations, and a 10-year psychiatric history with numerous suicide attempts. She has severe anxiety and agoraphobia (fear of crowds and open spaces). Her anorexia was severe, with her weight at 35 kg (77 lb). Medical and psychiatric problems were interwoven, and she needed comprehensive intervention.

Because Joanne could not leave home and needed medication management, a psychiatrist made home visits. Companion services were supplied while her husband was at work. Her husband was actively involved in the decision making regarding his wife's care, but he needed supportive interventions.

Over a 4-month period, Joanne progressed from a severely withdrawn, suicidal person to someone who was dealing with her panic attacks, agoraphobia, and scleroderma. Her weight had increased to 40 kg (90 lb). Although she would continue to cope with a chronic illness, her hopelessness was gone, and her ability to function in her daily life had markedly improved. She was able to continue living in her home and community with the help of community mental health services.
- What follow-up care would you plan for Joanne?
- What activities would help Joanne meet her social needs?
- What resources do you feel would be best for Joanne?
- What short-term and long-term goals might be appropriate for her and her husband?
- Do you think that institutional care might be the best option? Why or why not?

Modified from Mellon, S. K. (1994). Mental health clinical nurse specialist in home care for the 90s. *Issues in Mental Health Nursing, 15*(3), 229–237.

productive patterns of living. A look at each component of case management may help clarify the process.

Psychosocial Rehabilitation

Use of multidisciplinary services to help patients gain the skills needed to carry out the activities of daily living as actively and independently as possible best describes **psychosocial rehabilitation**. Patients are first assessed for physical, social, emotional, and intellectual levels of function. Then specific plans for teaching needed skills are developed. If patients are capable of work, vocational rehabilitation is offered.

The psychosocial rehabilitation model of care encourages decision making, thus empowering patients. This empowerment fosters a sense of self-esteem and mastery that results in improved coping abilities. As patients feel the success of making their own decisions, they are encouraged to take control of other areas of their lives. Education is also a strong component of psychosocial rehabilitation because mastering daily living skills motivates patients to practise more productive and independent ways of functioning.

Consultation

In mental health care, **consultation** is a process in which the assistance of a specialist is sought to help identify ways to work effectively with patient challenges. The case management system relies on the expertise of psychiatrists, nurses, psychologists, social workers, counsellors, and various therapists to find ways for patients to receive the services and support that help them to achieve their goals. For example, a nurse might work with a patient on reliably taking prescribed medication, while a social worker might locate supported housing, and a vocational counsellor could seek out an appropriate work setting. By covering all the bases, care providers hope to maintain patients in the least restrictive setting (the community) and assist them with their needs.

Resource Linkage

The process of matching patients' needs with the most appropriate community services best describes **resource linkage**. Health care providers have traditionally referred patients to other services, but resource linkage adds the component of periodic monitoring. The advantages of coordinating and linking services are several: patients can be more easily moved into different programs because background information moves with them; duplication of services is avoided; and as a patient's level of functioning improves, services can be tailored to support the new, more effective behaviours. With resource linkage, the focus for treatment of patients is on care instead of the more traditional emphasis on psychiatric symptoms and illness.

CRITICAL THINKING

You are a health care provider who has recently moved to this area. As a staff member in a community mental health clinic, you are responsible for helping refer patients to appropriate agencies.
- How would you go about locating agencies in the community that provide services for mentally ill individuals?

Advocacy

A critical concept of case management, **advocacy** is providing the patient with the information to make certain decisions. Advocacy for mentally ill people involves more than other areas of health care. Advocates work to protect patients' rights, help to clarify expectations, provide support, and act on behalf of patients' best interests. Every person involved in mental health care can act as an advocate by supporting community efforts and policies that encourage healthy living practices.

Therapy

Therapy is provided for each patient based on assessed needs, patient cooperation, and available services. Medications may be included as part of the overall plan of treatment. Therapies may include the use of counselling, support groups, vocational rehabilitation programs, and techniques to assist patients with problem-solving and adaptive behaviours.

Crisis Intervention

The crisis intervention component of case management is crucial to the success of the patient. People with chronic mental health challenges have great difficulty in coping with stress. What may be bothersome or inconvenient under normal circumstances could provoke a crisis for someone who has a significant mental health challenge. A crisis results whenever we feel that we have lost our ability to use our usual problem-solving and coping skills. Common sources of crisis include the loss of a loved one, change in employment circumstances, or being victimized. Experiencing a crisis is common to all people and is not limited only to individuals with previous or pre-existing mental health challenges.

Crisis intervention describes a short-term, active therapy that focuses on solving the immediate problem and restoring the patient's previous level of functioning. Crisis services help stabilize the patient, prevent further deterioration, and support the patient's readjustment process. The use of crisis services also results in better distribution of resources. Emergency department visits decrease, rehospitalization is reduced or prevented, and law enforcement resources are better focused on those who break the law instead of apprehending individuals with mental health challenges. For patients with severe, treatment-resistant mental challenges, a new approach, known as *continuous intensive case management,* is being used.

A highly flexible model of care, known as *assertive community treatment (ACT),* provides "medical, psychosocial, and rehabilitation services by a community-based team that operates 7 days a week, 24 hours a day" (Salkever, Domino, Burns, et al., 1999). The team usually consists of social workers, nurses, vocational specialists, occupational therapists, psychiatrists, peer support workers, and addictions specialists. Patients are seen individually and in supportive therapy groups. This team of professionals collaborates with the patient by providing 24-hour supports and assistance, including administration of medication, access to community services, attending various appointments and follow-up services, and even assistance with activities of daily living. Many patients also live in supervised housing arrangements. Table 2.2 provides a summary of the continuous care team's treatment activities. In short, care teams direct the patient's treatment during all encounters with the mental health care system.

Intensive case management programs have demonstrated that patients with chronic and severe mental illness can be effectively stabilized within the community with appropriate support systems. As the pressures of increased demand for services and cost restrictions force the system into trying new approaches, mental health care professionals must not lose sight of the most important element in the equation—the patient.

THE MULTIDISCIPLINARY MENTAL HEALTH CARE TEAM

Professionals working within the mental health system have various educational backgrounds. In the past, each would work with patients from his or her particular point of view or specialty. This approach resulted in disjointed, fragmented care. In some cases care providers worked at cross-purposes, leaving patients unsure and confused. The need for coordinated assessment and treatment was filled by the multidisciplinary mental health care team concept.

TABLE 2.2   Continuous Care Team Treatment Strategies

Setting	Mental Health Care Team Interventions
Community	Meets with patients 2–4 times per week Accompanies patient to appointments and other community activities Helps with daily living/social skill needs Monitors medications Nurtures relationships with persons interested in patient's well-being Encourages patient to call team instead of using ED
Emergency department	Prearranges for ED staff to notify clinician on arrival of continuous care patient Conducts assessment of patient and planning of care jointly with ED physician Avoids unnecessary hospitalizations
Hospital	Care team psychiatrist and primary therapist remain in charge of the patient's case Helps with decisions regarding admission, treatment, and discharge Coordinates treatment with inpatient staff

ED, emergency department.
Modified from Arana, J. D., Hastings, B., & Herron, E. (1991). Continuous care teams in intensive outpatient treatment of chronic mentally ill patients. *Hospital & Community Psychiatry, 42*(5), 503–507. ©American Psychiatric Association. Reprinted by permission.

Care Team

The main purpose of the team approach to treating mental illness is to provide effective patient care. The mental health care team "provides a forum where psychiatrists, social workers, psychologists, nurses, and others can democratically share their professional expertise and develop comprehensive therapeutic plans for patients" (Haber, McMahon, & Krainovich-Miller, 1997). The team approach can also be cost effective by preventing duplication of services and fragmentation of care. Patients and their significant others contribute to the plan of care and remain actively involved throughout the course of treatment.

Multidisciplinary mental health care teams exist in both inpatient and outpatient settings. The number of team members may vary, but the core of the team is usually composed of a psychiatrist, a psychologist, a nurse, and a social worker. Other team members, known as *adjunct therapists,* join the team as needed.

Each team member holds a degree or certificate in a specialized area of mental health. This approach allows patients to be assessed and treated from various points of view. As data are compiled, a broad, holistic picture of the patient emerges and individualized therapeutic plans are developed. Table 2.3 identifies care team members, their educational preparation, and their function.

Patient and Family

No discussion of the mental health team is complete without including the patient. As the consumers of services and the focus of therapeutic interventions, patients contribute important information that may make the difference between the success or failure of therapeutic plans. Including patients and their families in the treatment process reflects a fundamental change in attitude toward those with mental illness and their families. Today, mental illness is considered to be manageable and even treatable.

PATIENT POPULATIONS

Community mental health care was originally designed to provide prevention, education, and treatment services for all members living within an area or catchment. Community mental health services for the general public include crisis interventions, working with businesses to decrease costs and improve the effectiveness of mental health programs, and providing aid for individuals and families to adjust to life difficulties.

However, in every community, certain groups of people are at a higher risk for developing mental health challenges, large or small. They include more obvious populations, such as homeless people, and more subtle high-risk groups, such as children, families, adolescents, older people, people who are positive for human immunodeficiency virus (HIV) or are experiencing other debilitating chronic illnesses, and veterans of armed conflicts. People living in rural areas present a challenge because of the distance between services.

While often ignored, homeless people can be seen in every town and city in Canada. Studies indicate that between 25 and 75% of these individuals have a diagnosable mental health disorder, which can also include addictions to various substances. Who are the homeless? According to the organization Homeless Hub, a study in Toronto found that one third identified as being an immigrant, 45% identified as belonging to a racialized group, 22% identified as Black, and 9% as Indigenous (Aleman, 2016; Hwang, Ueng, Chiu, et al., 2010). While shelters and temporary housing might be available, many homeless individuals are reluctant or afraid to use them. Assaults, sexual abuse, and theft are common occurrences, making shelters less than ideal. Sadly, many homeless people feel safer on the street, making it more difficult to provide consistent and therapeutic services.

Patients with HIV infection or acquired immunodeficiency syndrome (AIDS) are using community mental health services in ever-growing numbers. People with AIDS face overwhelming physical, emotional, and social challenges. Mental health issues associated with HIV disease include organic problems, such as impairments in memory, judgement, or concentration progressing to dementia. Psychosocial difficulties include anxiety, depression, adjustment disorders, increased substance abuse, panic disorders, and suicidal thoughts. In addition, many researchers believe that stress directly affects the immune system. Fear of AIDS may hasten the onset of complications. AIDS-related anxiety can increase everyday apprehension in the lives of many noninfected people.

Comprehensive community mental health services for people with HIV/AIDS are not yet available in all areas.

TABLE 2.3   Mental Health Team Members

Team Member	Educational Preparation	Responsibilities and Functions
Psychiatrist	MD with residency in psychiatry	Physician; leader of the team; responsible for administration and planning; diagnostic and medical functions are main tasks
Clinical psychologist	PhD in clinical psychology	Specializes in study of mental processes and treatment of mental disorders; performs diagnostic testing; treats patients
Psychiatric social worker	Master's degree in social work (MSW)	Evaluates families; studies environmental and social causes of illness; conducts family therapy; admits new patients
Psychiatric nurse	Master's degree; advanced-level preparation; baccalaureate degree; diploma nurse; associate degree nurse; licensed practical nurse	Responsible for patient's activities of daily living/environment management and individual, family, and group psychotherapy; coordinates care team activities; supervises technicians and psychiatric assistants; active in various community roles
Psychiatric assistant or technician	High school education; special on-job training in setting of employment	Supervised by professional nurse; assists in providing basic needs of patients; carries out nursing functions; maintains the therapeutic environment; supervises leisure time activity; assists with individual/group therapy
Occupational therapist	Advanced degree in occupational therapy (OT)	Assesses potential for rehabilitation; provides socialization therapy and vocational retraining
Expressive therapist	Advanced degree and specialized training in art therapy	Helps make use of spontaneous creative work of the patient; works with groups; encourages members to analyze artwork; adjunct to care team in diagnosis and treatment of children
Recreational therapist	Advanced degree and specialized training in recreational therapy	Provides leisure time activities for patients; teaches hospitalized patients useful pastimes; uses pet therapy, psychodrama, poetry, and music therapy
Dietitian	Advanced degree and special training in dietetics (RD)	Provides attractive, nourishing meals; helps treat food-related illnesses
Auxiliary personnel (housekeepers, volunteers, clerks, secretaries)	Various backgrounds and on-job training	Assists patients with activities of daily living and other practical jobs; can be invaluable in helping patients
Chaplain	Seminary pastoral counsellor or rabbinical education	Attends to spiritual needs of patients and families; pastoral, marital counselling

Modified from Haber, J., McMahon, A. L., & Krainovich-Miller, B. (1997). *Comprehensive psychiatric nursing* (5th ed.). Mosby.

Treatment facilities that offer comprehensive services focus on persons with AIDS, their families and friends, and the public. Clinicians accept referrals from other agencies, provide mental status and suicide risk assessments, offer crisis intervention services, and provide individual or group therapies for patients with HIV/AIDS. Family members and significant others are encouraged to join support groups. Some mental health care centres train family members in techniques for keeping patients oriented or on task. Respite care (time off for the caregiver) services are sometimes coordinated through the centre. Some mental health care centres work with interested community groups to provide prevention strategies and education about AIDS for all citizens of the community.

Patients living in rural areas present a special challenge for mental health care providers. Small villages, settlements, and farms dot the landscape of a geographically expansive country like Canada. Often, rural residents define and relate to health differently than people in cities, often because of the difficulties they encounter with accessing resources. Children and adolescents living in rural areas have significantly less access to services as compared to their urban counterparts. Mental health care providers (e.g., nurses, therapists) who work in rural areas cope with patients of all ages and with all types of problems. They are also expected to provide and coordinate comprehensive mental health care with few available resources.

Military personnel who have served in war-affected areas of the world present special challenges in treating their mental health issues. According to Veterans Affairs Canada (2019), 24% of military personnel who are receiving disability benefits are doing so because of service-related psychiatric diagnoses. Of those, 71% have post-traumatic stress disorder (PTSD). Many return with stress-related problems severe enough to interfere with daily living. Historically, more than 10% of military personnel dispatched to Korea, and later Vietnam, suffered with chronic PTSD. War veterans have higher rates of depression, substance abuse, and homelessness than among the general population. Many have difficulty adjusting to life after military service.

Indigenous populations have unique mental health challenges. Suicide rates can be more than twice as high as those of the general population (non-Indigenous communities), with limited treatment and support resources being available in reserve communities. There is a recent trend of Indigenous communities taking ownership of treatment of addictions and mental health challenges in their communities, using their traditional understanding of holism and connection to the environment. Many Indigenous communities prefer to use a wellness approach, as opposed to a specific focus on mental illness.

Other populations, such as families, older persons, children, and adolescents, are also vulnerable to mental health problems. Community mental health services are a vital link to the well-being of a population. Social and economic changes will continue to influence community mental health care, but as the system matures, the goal of individualized, holistic mental health care for all people should not be forgotten.

IMPACT OF MENTAL ILLNESS

Mental illness affects everyone directly or indirectly. Many people personally know someone with behavioural problems or persistent, bizarre behaviour that affects their quality of life. Indirectly, mental illness costs Canadians annually roughly $15 billion in health care costs and lost productivity as the costs of care and number of patients needing care continue to escalate (Centre for Addiction and Mental Health [CAMH], 2020). Today health care reform is part of an overall strategy to distribute scarce resources and control expenses. Also, as a result of ongoing armed conflicts, the number of veterans requiring support for stress-related disorders has increased considerably. Sadly, the supportive services offered to veterans by Canada and many of its allies have proven to be inadequate.

Incidence of Mental Illness in Canada

One in four people in the world will be affected by mental or neurological disorders at some point in their lives. Around 450 million people currently suffer from such conditions, placing mental disorders among the leading causes of ill health and disability worldwide (WHO, 2001).

In Canada, according to the Canadian Mental Health Association (CMHA), one in five people in Canada will experience a mental health challenge, 8% of the population will experience a major depression at some point in their lives, and by age 40 about half of the population will have experienced a mental illness of some type. Suicide accounts for 24% of deaths for young adults aged 15 to 24, and 16% of deaths among individuals 25 to 44 years of age (CAMH, 2020; CMHA, 2020; Smetanin, Stiff, Briante, et al., 2011).

Chronic severe mental disorders, such as schizophrenia and depression, have emerged as major challenges to treatment. Substance abuse has become an international problem. The incidence of Alzheimer's disease and other dementias is expected to increase threefold over the next 15 years. Social problems such as AIDS, homelessness, violence, and abuse occur with mental problems. Millions of divorces each year place families in crisis situations.

Economic Issues

The nationwide movement to treat people with mental illness in the least restrictive environment is part of a plan to reduce mental health care costs while still providing ongoing care. Unfortunately, funding has not kept pace with the need for services.

The cost of treating mental illness in Canada is significant. In 2008, Canada spent $51 billion on the provision of direct care (Lim, Jacobs, & Ohinmaa, 2008), with an additional $30 billion provided through short- and long-term disability claims (Dewa, Chau, & Dermer, 2010). Costs have only increased since then, with a final value being undetermined at this time. Clearly, economic issues have and will continue to play a major role in the availability and delivery of mental health care.

Mental illness also influences economics in less direct ways. Unemployed, homeless, and troubled families cost society in many more ways than dollars. Loss of productivity and unfulfilled potential are difficult to appraise financially.

Social Issues

Many social problems are related to mental illness. Changing lifestyles, work patterns, family structures, and level of health are a few of the many changes that influence a society. Mentally ill individuals, however, are likely to be struggling with more basic issues, such as poverty, homelessness, and substance abuse.

According to Statistics Canada, in 2017, 3.4 million Canadians (or 9.5%) of the population lived below the poverty line (Statistics Canada, 2019). A significant number of persons in poverty are incapable of making a living as a result of mental problems. They exist along the fringes of society, attempting to meet the most basic needs of food, shelter, and clothing, frequently failing in their attempts to secure their most basic needs. Within this environment of poverty, hopelessness and alienation grows, making it even less likely that individuals in need will attempt to access available resources.

Homelessness and poverty are inextricably linked. The US National Academy of Sciences defines **homelessness** as the lack of a regular and adequate nighttime dwelling. Approximately 300 000 Canadians are homeless on any given day, including single mothers and children (Thompson, 2012), and as many as 85% of the homeless population suffer from addictions or mental disturbances (Walker, 1998).

Homelessness is a national problem that continues to grow. The actual number of homeless people is difficult to count because with no regular housing they tend to melt into society and disappear into the world of soup kitchens and temporary shelters. In the past, most homeless people were single men, usually with substance abuse problems. However, today's statistics present a different picture. Women, children, and families now account for many of those who are homeless.

Several factors contribute to homelessness. Social and economic conditions, such as a lack of low-income housing, public assistance eligibility requirements, and the movement of chronically mentally ill people into communities that lack adequate support systems, have all had an adverse effect on housing security. Access to and the quality of community resources relating to available housing, steady employment, and welfare services also affect homeless people. Family dysfunction, poverty, and health status all relate to the homelessness problem.

Many families live from paycheque to paycheque, with just enough money to scrape by until the next cheque. Even a small event can trigger a crisis. An increase in rent, for example, may force a family out of their home. Most community mental health centres offer services for homeless people. Currently, short-term strategies for working with the homeless population include temporary shelters, assisted-housing programs, and volunteer efforts such as Habitat for Humanity.

The common use of mind-altering chemicals has resulted in many mentally ill individuals becoming addicted to "recreational drugs," such as crack, cocaine, LSD, and heroin. When used in combination with prescribed psychotherapeutic drugs, overdose, permanent mental impairment, and death may occur. Street drugs also cost money; it is not uncommon for people with mental problems to spend money on drugs before they buy food. People with mental disorders and addiction suffer from two separate disorders, with each compounding the severity of the other. Illicit drug use and mental illness become a vicious circle.

The current mental health care system in Canada is undergoing major changes as government budgets change, social issues emerge, and needs for treatment grow. Improved organization and technology may address some of the system's problems, but provider–patient contact is, and will remain, the core of mental health treatment.

KEY POINTS

- The health care systems of many developed countries are undergoing financial challenges.
- Canada's health care system is administrated by each province or territory under the guidance of the Department of National Health and includes coverage for most medical, hospital, convalescent, and mental health services.
- Norway has a national insurance system that provides access to health care for everyone and covers all services, including mental health care.
- All British citizens are provided health care through a government-managed national health care system.
- Australians are provided a mix of health care plans that include a public health plan, a supplemental national private plan, and private insurance plans.
- Funds for health care in the United States are provided through federal (Medicare) and state (Medicaid) programs, private insurance coverage, and direct patient payments.
- Mental health care is offered in inpatient and outpatient (community) care settings.
- The community support systems (CSS) model for mental health care is an organized network of people committed to assisting those with mental illness within the community setting.
- Community mental health care settings include psychiatric clinics, general hospitals, residential care programs, day treatment facilities, and psychiatric home care.

- Case management is a holistic system of interventions designed to support the integration of mentally ill patients into the community.
- Psychosocial rehabilitation is the use of multidisciplinary services to help patients learn the skills and supports needed to carry out the activities of daily living as actively and independently as possible.
- Psychosocial rehabilitation, consultation, resource linkage, advocacy, crisis intervention, and therapy are the basic components of the case management system.
- Intensive case management may involve continuous care or assertive community treatment (ACT) teams who assume responsibility for the patient in and out of the hospital.
- Community mental health services serve high-risk populations such as children, people in crisis situations, homeless individuals, veterans, patients with HIV/AIDS, patients living in rural areas, and older people.
- Mental health services are commonly delivered by the multidisciplinary care team—a group of physicians, nurses, psychologists, therapists, and their assistants who each contribute to the patient's plan of care and treatment.
- Social and economic issues must be considered when discussing treatment of and resources for mentally troubled persons.

ADDITIONAL LEARNING RESOURCES

Go to your Evolve website (http://evolve.elsevier.com/Canada/Morrison-Valfre/) for additional online resources, including the online Study Guide for additional learning activities to help you master this chapter content.

CRITICAL THINKING QUESTIONS

1. Why does the "comprehensiveness" principle of the *Canada Health Act* (see Box 2.1) include that only medically necessary services are covered? What potential abuses is this clause attempting to prevent?
2. Many people with mental health challenges receive care at a community level. Do you think this is the best option, or should more inpatient facilities be made available?
3. Many homeless people are reluctant to stay at a shelter because of the potential for experiencing assaults, sexual abuse, and theft of belongings. If you were in charge of your city's homeless shelters, what could you do to address these concerns? How could you accomplish this in a financially responsible manner?

REFERENCES

Aleman, A. (2016). *What are the statistics on homelessness and mental health in Toronto?* Canadian Observatory on Homelessness/Homeless Hub. https://www.homelesshub.ca/blog/what-are-statistics-homelessness-and-mental-health-toronto

Canadian Mental Health Association (CMHA). (2020). *Fast facts about mental illness.* Author. https://cmha.ca/fast-facts-about-mental-illness

Centre for Addiction and Mental Health (CAMH). (2020). *Mental illness and addiction: Facts and statistics.* Author. https://www.camh.ca/en/driving-change/the-crisis-is-real/mental-health-statistics

Dewa, C. S., Chau, N., & Dermer, S. (2010). Examining the comparative incidence and costs of physical and mental health-related disabilities in an employed population. *Journal of Occupational and Environmental Medicine, 52*(7), 758–762. https://doi.org/10.1097/JOM.0b013e3181e8cfb5

Dudley, M., Silove, M., & Gale, F. (2012). *Mental health and human rights.* Oxford University Press.

Government of Canada. (2006). The human face of mental health and mental illness in Canada. Ottawa: Minister of Public Works and Government Services Canada.

Haber, J., McMahon, A. L., & Krainovich-Miller, B. (1997). *Comprehensive psychiatric nursing* (5th ed.). Mosby.

Hwang, S. W., Ueng, J. J. M., Chiu, S., et al. (2010). Universal health insurance and health care access for homeless persons. *American Journal of Public Health, 100*(8), 1454–1461.

Johnson, S. (2017). *Assertive community treatment: evidence-based practice or managed recovery.* Taylor and Francis.

Lim, K. L., Jacobs, P., Ohinmaa, A., et al. (2008). A new population-based measure of the economic burden of mental illness in Canada. *Chronic Diseases in Canada, 28*(3), 92–98.

Office of the Correctional Investigator. (2011). *Mental health and corrections.* Government of Canada. https://www.oci-bec.gc.ca/cnt/comm/presentations/presentations20120318-eng.aspx

Salkever, D., Domino, M. E., Burns, B. J., et al. (1999). Assertive community treatment for people with severe mental illness: the effect on hospital use and costs. *Health Services Research, 34*(2), 577–601.

Smetanin, P., Stiff, D., Briante, C., et al. (2011). *The life and economic impact of major mental illnesses in Canada: 2011–2041.* Prepared for the Mental Health Commission of Canada. RiskAnalytica. https://www.mentalhealthcommission.ca/sites/default/files/MHCC_Report_Base_Case_FINAL_ENG_0_0.pdf

Statistics Canada. (2019). *Canadian income survey, 2017. The Daily.* February 26. https://www150.statcan.gc.ca/n1/daily-quotidien/190226/dq190226b-eng.htm

Steele, L.S., Dewa, C.S., Lin, E., & Lee, K.L.K. (2007). Education level, income level, and mental health services use in Canada: Associations and policy implications. Healthcare Policy, 3(1), 96–106. doi: 10.12927/hcpol.2007.19177. https://www.longwoods.com/content/19H77/healthcare-policy/education-level-income-level-and-mental-health-services-use-in-canada-associations-and-policy-impl

Thompson, W. C. (2012). *The world today series, 2012.* Stryker-Post/Rowman & Littlefield.

Veterans Affairs Canada. (2019). *Veterans Affairs Canada statistics—facts and figures: 8.0 mental health.* Government of Canada. https://www.veterans.gc.ca/eng/about-vac/news-media/facts-figures/8-0

Walker, C. (1998). Homeless people and mental health. *American Journal of Nursing, 98*(11), 26.

World Health Organization (WHO). (2001). *Mental disorders affect one in four people.* Author. https://www.who.int/whr/2001/media_centre/press_release/en/

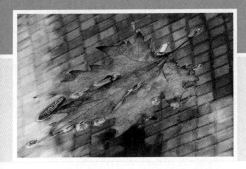

Ethical and Legal Issues

OBJECTIVES

Upon completion of this chapter, the student should be able to:
1. Compare the differences among values, rights, and ethics.
2. List six steps for making ethical decisions.
3. Identify the legal importance of practice acts.
4. Describe the process of involuntary psychiatric commitment.
5. Name four areas of potential legal liability for mental health care providers.
6. Know the difference between the legal terms *negligence* and *malpractice*.
7. Discuss three legal responsibilities that relate to nursing and health care providers.

OUTLINE

KEY TERMS

assault (p. 27)
attitudes (ĂT-ĭ-toodz) (p. 22)
autonomy (aw-TŎN-ə-mē) (p. 23)
battery (BĂ-tər-Ē) (p. 27)
belief (bĕ-LĒF) (p. 22)
beneficence (b-NĔ-fĬ-sən[t]s) (p. 23)
civil (SĬ-vĭl) law (p. 25)
codes of ethics (Ĕ-thĭks) (p. 24)
confidentiality (KŎN-fĭ-DĔN-shē-ĂL-ĭ-tē) (p. 24)
contract (KŎN-trăkt) law (p. 25)
controlled substances (KŎN-trŏld SŬB-stăn-səs) (p. 26)
criminal (KRĬM-ĭn-əl) law (p. 25)
defamation (dĕf-ə-Mā-shən) (p. 27)
duty (DŪ-tē) to warn (p. 28)
elopement (ĭ-LŌP-mənt) (p. 28)
ethical dilemmas (ĔTH-ĭ-kəl dĭ-LĔM-ăz) (p. 24)
ethics (ĔTH-ĭks) (p. 23)
felonies (FĔL-ə-nēs) (p. 25)
fidelity (p. 24)
fraud (frăwd) (p. 27)
informed consent (ĭn-FŎRMd cŭn-SĔNT) (p. 28)
invasion of privacy (ĭn-VĀ-shŭn PRĬ-vă-sē) (p. 27)

involuntary admission (ĭn-VŎL-ŭn-tăr-ē ăd-MĬ-shŭn) (p. 26)
justice (p. 23)
laws (p. 25)
liability (p. 26)
libel (LĬ-bəl) (p. 27)
malpractice (măl-PRĂC-tĭs) (p. 28)
misdemeanors (MĬS-dĭ-ME-nrs) (p. 25)
morals (MŎR-əls) (p. 22)
negligence (NĔG-lĭ-jĕns) (p. 28)
nonmaleficence (nŏn-mə-LĔF-ə-sən[t]s) (p. 23)
professional (prō-FĔ-shŭn-əl) (nurse) practice acts (p. 25)
public law (p. 25)
reasonable and prudent (PROO-dənt) care provider (p. 28)
restraint (p. 27)
right (RĬT) (p. 23)
slander (SLĂN-dər) (p. 27)
standards (STĂN-dərds) of practice (p. 25)
tort (tŏrt) law (p. 25)
value (VĂL-ŭ) (p. 22)
values clarification (VĂL-ŭs CLĂR-ĭ-fĭ-CĀ-shŭn) (p. 22)
veracity (p. 24)
voluntary admission (p. 26)

Health care professions are guided and defined by certain beliefs, rights, and principles that serve as the basis for ethical and legal concepts. The framework for delivering appropriate therapeutic interventions is rooted in these concepts.

Attitudes, beliefs, values, and morals influence who we are. To be effective with mental health patients, we must first appreciate these concepts within ourselves and then understand them as they apply to our patients and their support persons.

VALUES AND MORALS

Attitudes are ideas that help shape our points of view. The term can also describe one's outlook, such as, "He has a cheerful attitude." A **belief** is a conviction that is intellectually accepted as true, whether or not it is based in fact. A **value** is something that is held dear, a feeling about the worth of an item, idea, or behaviour. Values are formed in childhood. They shape our reactions, influence our behaviours, and reflect the society in which we live. Values are often used as a basis for making decisions. Values are individual, and they may change. **Morals** are based on one's attitudes, beliefs, and values. One's morals define right or wrong behaviour. Once established, morals become deeply ingrained and are not easily changed.

Acquiring Values

As children grow, they observe and take on the reactions of others in their environment. These adopted reactions become our earliest attitudes. Preschool children learn the difference between right and wrong behaviours. They adopt the family's beliefs and traditions. As attitudes and beliefs develop, values begin to form.

Children are exposed to a variety of values at school. They develop work habits and learn to solve problems, interact with others, and make decisions. Parental values are still modelled because the family remains the major source of values until adulthood.

During the teen years, adolescents begin to identify their own significant values. By early adulthood, an individual value system is established. Adults may feel secure with their values or discard them for new ones. Older persons may feel threatened by the changing social values, but they tend to hold onto their own value systems.

Culture, society, personality, and experiences all shape our values. How values are shared largely depends on the socio-cultural environment. Most societies use a combination of methods to transmit values (Potter, Perry, Stockert, et al., 2017). The methods of transmitting values are outlined in Table 3.1.

People who choose to work in the health care professions usually arrive with strong personal values. Human values that are important for care providers to embody include a concern for the welfare of others (altruism), respect for the uniqueness and worth of people (human dignity), equality, justice, truth, freedom, and acceptance. Caring is the foundation of health care, for if we do not care, we will be unable to effectively treat, teach, or work with patients.

Values Clarification

Every society has a value system. Habits, customs, and traditions are important to traditional societies. Modern societies rapidly

TABLE 3.1	How Values Are Transmitted
Mode of Transmission	**Definition**
Modelling	Copying an example: One person behaves in the ideal or preferred manner, and the other copies the behaviour.
Moralizing	Sets standards for right and wrong: Choice is not allowed.
Laissez-faire	Unrestricted choices: No direction is given. One is free to explore and learn from experiences. This mode of transmission may result in confusion or frustration.
Reward/ punishment	Rewards valued behaviours and punishes undesirable acts; authoritarian. Children learn that strength is right. This mode of transmission may send the message that violence is acceptable.
Responsible choice	A balance of freedom and restriction: One may choose among stated options. New behaviours and consequences are explored.

Modified from Potter, P. A., & Perry, A. G. (2001). *Fundamentals of nursing: Concepts, process, and practice* (5th ed.). Mosby.

TABLE 3.2	Values Clarification Process
Step	**Process**
Choosing	Consider all possible alternatives. Consider all possible consequences. Choose freely without pressure or coercion from others.
Prizing	Cherish or prize the choice. Share choice with others. Reaffirm importance of value.
Acting	Make value a part of behaviours (internalize value). Generalize value to all situations. Repeatedly act with a consistent behavioural pattern.

change, and people are often not aware of their values until they experience difficulties and their values are questioned.

Values clarification is a step-by-step process to help identify significant values. The process helps health care providers become aware of how their own values affect interactions with patients. Values clarification involves three steps: choosing, prizing, and acting (Table 3.2).

To illustrate, let us assume that you are working at the local clinic when a large, scruffy man who has not bathed in weeks presents himself for care. There is a wild look in his eyes, and he is arguing with himself as he approaches you. You realize that you are feeling afraid and want to run as far away as you can, but you also know you have an obligation to interact with this patient. How does the value of caring apply here?

First, by working in a helping profession, you have freely chosen to care about people; otherwise you would have selected another line of work. Second, you prize the value of caring because your patients see you as compassionate and concerned. Third, you act on your values by accepting the unkempt, scruffy man as a person worthy of care. You ask him what you can do to help. He begins to cry and tells you that since the death of his wife and children in a house fire, no one has cared if he lives or dies. By acting on your value (caring), you have touched this person and paved the way for him to improve his situation.

You have chosen to care. You cherish the value of caring enough to act, even when that value is threatened. Be clear about your values. Be aware of your patient's values, because they are the guidelines for one's lifestyle, conduct, and relationships.

RIGHTS

A **right** is described as a power, privilege, or existence to which one has a just claim. Rights have several roles in society—they can be used as expressions of power, to justify actions, and to settle disputes. Rights help define social interactions because they contain the principle of justice; they equally and fairly apply to all citizens. For example, we all have the right to be respected as human beings and treated with dignity. Rights also have obligations. You have the right to drive down the road, but inherent in this right is the obligation to obey traffic laws.

Patient Rights

The *Canada Health Act* is federal legislation pertaining to publicly funded health care. The Act's primary objective is "to protect, promote and restore the physical and mental well-being of residents of Canada and to facilitate reasonable access to health services without financial or other barriers." The purpose of the Act is to ensure that all eligible residents of Canada have reasonable access to insured health services on a prepaid basis, without direct charges at the point of service (Government of Canada, 1985).

People with mental illness tend to lose their rights in two ways. First, the problems with which they are coping require mental focus and energy, two attributes that are often reduced or eliminated during a period of moderate to severe mental illness. Often, as a result of the changes in mental processes, comprehension, and understanding, mental health patients are not able to recognize their rights, much less exercise them. Second, the mental health delivery system can impose limits on patients' abilities to exercise their rights.

Care Provider Rights

The rights of health care providers relate to respect, safety, and competent assistance. Care providers also have the right to being treated with respect as individuals. Care providers also have the right to full and equal participation as members of the health care team. All health care providers have the right to set standards for quality and develop policies that affect patient care.

Every health care provider has the right to function within a safe environment. This applies to both the physical environment (i.e., properly maintained equipment) and the affective or emotional environment. Care providers who strive to minimize the physical and emotional stresses of the working environment are exercising their right to function safely.

The right to competent assistance includes the right to receive assistance from people who are capable of performing at the stated level. For example, a registered practical nurse (RPN) working with other care providers is expected to be able to function adequately and safely within the full scope of practice for an RPN. All health care providers need to be aware of and exercise their rights. By doing this, we remind the system of the therapeutic values inherent in the care provider patient relationship.

ETHICS

Ethics are a set of rules or values that govern right behaviour. Ethics reflect values, morals, and principles of right and wrong. The purpose of ethical behaviour is to protect the rights of people. Health care ethics focus on the moral aspects of health care availability, delivery, and policy. They are also called *biomedical ethics, bioethics,* or *medical ethics.*

Ethical Principles

Ethical principles are the concepts that form the basis for professional codes of ethics (Edelman & Mandle, 2014). They are the behaviours that define what is good or right conduct. Ethical codes serve two purposes: (1) they act as guidelines for standards of practice, and (2) they let the public know what behaviour can be expected from their health care providers.

The concepts of autonomy, beneficence, nonmaleficence, and justice are the main ethical principles on which codes of ethics are established. Remember these principles. They will serve you well as you encounter the many ethical situations inherent in health care.

Autonomy refers to the right of people to act for themselves and make personal choices, including refusal of treatment. Care providers who practise the principle of autonomy encourage patients to participate in informed decision making. The procedure known as *informed consent* promotes autonomy by providing relevant information and choice for the patient.

Beneficence means to actively do good. Actions that promote patient health are beneficent. Choosing the action that is most therapeutic for the patient is an example of beneficence.

The principle of **nonmaleficence** can be stated in three words: *do no harm.* Perhaps it is the most important ethical principle of the caregiving professions. Although nurses must sometimes carry out procedures that result in pain, the inconvenience and discomfort are weighed against the benefits gained. Nobody likes the poke of the needle used to obtain routine blood work, but the information provided as a result has saved countless lives. In all cases, however, therapeutic interventions are delivered only after patient safety and comfort are considered. Nonmaleficence ensures that patients will not be harmed during care.

Justice implies that all patients are treated equally, fairly, and respectfully. Because health care resources are limited, the application of justice can be difficult. However, all patients deserve respect and a share of the available resources.

The concepts of *confidentiality, fidelity,* and *veracity* are other important ethical principles. The patient's rights to privacy, truth, and duty are protected by these ethical principles.

BOX 3.1   ICN Code of Ethics for Nurses

1. Nurses and People

The nurse's primary professional responsibility is to those requiring nursing care.

The nurse promotes an environment in which human rights, values, customs, and spiritual beliefs of the individual, family, and community are respected.

The nurse ensures that the patient receives accurate, sufficient, and timely information in a culturally appropriate manner on which to base consent for care and related treatment.

The nurse holds in confidence personal information and uses judgement in sharing this information.

The nurse shares with society the responsibility for initiating and supporting actions to meet health and social needs of the public, in particular those of vulnerable populations.

The nurse advocates for equity and social justice in resource allocation, access to health care, and other social and economic services.

The nurse demonstrates professional values such as respectfulness, responsiveness, compassion, trustworthiness, and integrity.

2. Nurses and Practice

The nurse carries personal responsibility and accountability for nursing practice, and for maintaining competence by continual learning.

The nurse maintains a standard of personal health such that the ability to provide care is not compromised.

The nurse uses judgement regarding individual competence when accepting and delegating responsibility.

The nurse at all times maintains standards of personal conduct that reflect well on the profession and enhance its image and public confidence.

The nurse, in providing care, ensures that the use of technology and scientific advances is compatible with the safety, dignity, and rights of people.

The nurse strives to foster and maintain a practice culture promoting ethical behaviour and open dialogue.

3. Nurses and the Profession

The nurse assumes a major role in determining and implementing acceptable standards of clinical nursing practice, management, research, and education.

The nurse is active in developing a core of research-based professional knowledge that supports evidence-based practice.

The nurse, acting through the professional organization, participates in creating a positive practice environment and maintaining safe, equitable social and economic working conditions in nursing.

The nurse contributes to an ethical organizational environment and challenges unethical practices and settings.

4. Nurses and Co-Workers

The nurse sustains a collaborative and respectful relationship with co-workers in nursing and other fields.

The nurse takes appropriate action to safeguard individuals, families, and communities when their health is endangered by a co-worker or any other person.

The nurse takes appropriate action to support and guide co-workers to advance ethical conduct.

Modified from the International Council of Nurses (ICN). (2012). *The ICN code of ethics for nurses.* Author. https://www.icn.ch/sites/default/files/inline-files/2012_ICN_Codeofethicsfornurses_%20eng.pdf

Confidentiality is the duty to respect private information. It is a legal and ethical duty of health care providers to keep all information about patients limited to only those directly involved with their care. Sharing private information not only is unethical but also may be grounds for legal action. All provinces and territories in Canada have laws pertaining to the requirement that health care workers maintain the utmost care to safeguard a patient's medical information. While transgressions are rare, care providers who violate these laws are subject to severe penalties, including financial, legal, and professional.

Fidelity is the obligation to keep your word. Telling the patient that you will return in 10 minutes is a promise. Keeping that appointment is essential, because the patient relies on you, and your credibility grows or diminishes based on how well you keep your promises.

The final principle, **veracity**, is the duty to tell the truth. Be careful here. Answer patient's questions honestly, but keep within your scope of practice.

Codes of Ethics

Codes of ethics for nurses have been developed by the International Council of Nurses, the Canadian Nurses Association, and regional nursing organizations (Box 3.1). Codes of ethics have been developed for other health care professions and may differ slightly, but all are based on the same ethical principles. Provide information to patients, be truthful, and support your patients, but consult your supervisor if there is any question of appropriateness. It is important to practise with ethical principles in mind.

Ethical Conflict

In today's world of advanced technologies and complex situations, no clear-cut answers exist for complicated questions that arise.

Ethical dilemmas (conflicts) exist when there is uncertainty or disagreement about the moral principles that endorse different courses of action.

In health care, ethical dilemmas arise when problems cannot easily be solved by decision making, logic, or use of scientific data. Answers to ethical dilemmas usually have broad effects. Because of this, many health care institutions have established bioethics committees to study, educate, and assist staff members in coping with ethical dilemmas.

Most of the time, no simple solutions exist for ethical dilemmas. Although each ethical dilemma is unique, the method for making ethical decisions can be applied to all situations. Guidelines for dealing with such dilemmas are given in Box 3.2. As Morrison (1993) notes, "Making ethical decisions in an orderly systematic manner increases one's ability to deal with the dynamic and sometimes complex issues relating to

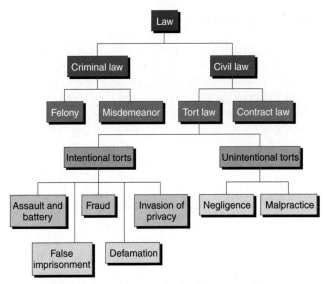

Fig. 3.1 Laws important for health care providers.

ethics. The quality of care depends on the skills and ethical integrity of the practitioner."

LAWS AND THE LEGAL SYSTEM

Every health care provider must be familiar with the basic concepts of the legal system.

Laws are the controls by which a society governs itself. They are derived from rules, regulations, and moral and ethical principles. Laws apply to every member of society.

General Concepts

Laws exist at every level of government and change as society changes, but they are all based on the principles of justice (fairness), change, standards, and individual rights and responsibilities. Laws have several functions in our society. They define relationships, describe appropriate and objectionable behaviour, and explain what kind of force is applied to maintain rules. Laws help provide solutions for many social and legal problems, and they serve to protect the rights of people while defining the limits of acceptable behaviour.

There are two types of law: public law and private law. **Public law** focuses on the relationship between the government and its citizens. The division of public law that is of importance to care providers is known as **criminal law**. Its main function is to protect members of society. Serious crimes, known as **felonies**, are punishable by imprisonment. Less serious crimes are called **misdemeanors**, with punishments ranging from fines to prison terms of less than 1 year.

Private law is also commonly called **civil law**. Its function is to deal with relationships between individuals. Two important types of civil law for care providers are contract law and tort law.

Contract law deals with agreements between individuals or institutions. These agreements or contracts may be written or implied. For example, on employment, health care providers enter into contracts with the employing institution.

"A *tort* is a legal wrong that is committed against the person or the property of another individual" (Morrison, 1993). **Tort law** relates to individuals' rights and includes the need to be compensated for a wrong. Tort law is especially important for care providers because many potential legal problems exist in every health care setting. Figure 3.1 lists the areas of law that are most significant for health care providers.

Legal Concepts in Health Care

The health care provider and health care system are governed by rules and standards. Nursing, for example, is regulated by provincial colleges of nursing that define the practice of nursing and regulate the profession through licensing procedures and disciplinary actions. Each provincial college of nursing identifies the limits and scope of practice through a series of regulations in provincial nurse practice acts. Nurses need to be familiar with their province's nurse practice act because it is the legal framework for practice in that province. Other health care providers are responsible for knowing their provincial governing regulations. Care providers are legally responsible for their actions. They are expected to know what is contained within their **professional (nurse) practice acts**.

Institutional policies also help to define health care practices. Policies are statements that define a course of action. *What* is to be done is stated in policies. *How* a task or skill is to be performed is defined in the institution's procedure manual. Job descriptions define the job, its functions, its qualifications, and to whom the care provider reports. Guidelines for sound health care delivery can be found in each province's practice act; professional standards; and the employing institution's policies, procedures, and job descriptions.

A *standard* is a measurement for comparison by which one evaluates an action. **Standards of practice** are developed by specific health care disciplines. Standards of nursing practice, for example, are a set of guidelines that provide measurable criteria for nurses, patients, and others to evaluate the quality and effectiveness of the nursing care provided. Psychiatric mental health standards for nursing practice can be found at the front of this book.

LAWS AND MENTAL HEALTH CARE

Historically, people with mental illnesses were afforded few legal rights. Only recently have mental health patients been able to exercise their claims to fair and adequate treatment in settings helpful to their care. Nurses and their colleagues need to be aware of patients' legal rights to freedom, privacy, and choice. Laws relating to mental health issues "attempt to balance the basic rights of the individual against society's interest in being protected from persons who, because of mental disorder, present a threat of harm" (Keltner & Steele, 2014).

Patient–Caregiver Relationship

An awareness of the obligations in the patient–care provider relationship ensures safe, legal practice. From a legal point of view, the care provider and patient enter into an *implied contract* on acceptance of service. The care provider provides services that are accepted by the patient. This idea of contractual obligations is one legal aspect of the care provider–patient relationship. Two other important aspects are liability and standards of care.

The concept of **liability** states that care providers are legally responsible for their professional obligations and behaviour. It includes the obligation to remain competent, maintain a current knowledge base, practise at a level appropriate to one's education, and practise unimpaired by drugs, disability, or illness.

Patients still retain their legal rights when they enter the mental health care system. Each province has acts that address a patient's rights to obtain information and treatment within a supportive, humane environment. These acts and legal expectations include patients of any category, mental health included. Individuals who are admitted to psychiatric facilities retain the right to vote, to buy and sell property, and to possess a driver's license.

People with mental illness may be unaware of their legal rights or unable to exercise them. Patients' judgements may be limited as a result of their illness and/or medications. It is important to recognize and safeguard patients' legal rights because behind every mental disorder lives a real person.

Adult Psychiatric Admissions

The decision to seek psychiatric care, whether made by the patient, family, or community, is difficult. When the patient originates the request for mental health services, it is considered a **voluntary admission**. Because they are often aware of their problems, most voluntarily admitted patients are active participants in their treatments and have a low potential for violence. Voluntarily admitted patients may legally discharge themselves at any time.

When an individual engages in behaviour that is harmful to themselves or others due to a suspected mental health concern, an **involuntary admission** process is undertaken. While each province has its own legal requirements around an involuntary psychiatric admission, the overall process is similar throughout the country. Because admitting an individual to a psychiatric facility involves a temporary suspension of their civil rights, very specific documentation and paperwork

must be completed. There are three usual mechanisms that can be utilized that will result in an involuntary individual receiving a mental health assessment (Ontario Psychiatric Patient Advocate Office, n.d.). The first mechanism involves a physician authorizing police to apprehend the identified person and transport them to a hospital, where they will be assessed by a physician. The second process involves family or significant other(s) giving testimony to a justice of the peace or a judge (typically at a court house). If the justice of the peace or a judge believes the concerns outlined to them, they may issue a document that allows the police or other authorized individuals to apprehend the person and bring them to a hospital. In both cases, once located, the person will be brought to a hospital, even if it is against their will. The third mechanism involves the police using their own judgement under the provincial mental health act. If a police officer encounters an individual who is behaving in a manner that suggests they are a risk to themselves or to others as a result of a potential or suspected mental health concern, that officer can apprehend the person under the *Mental Health Act*, even without a Form 1 or 2, and bring them to hospital.

The commitment process begins when a formal petition is filed. The patient is then assessed by one or two physicians, and a determination is made to either release or hospitalize the person (Stuart, 2013). If the person is hospitalized, the length of stay may be on an emergency, temporary, or indefinite basis. Patients who are indefinitely hospitalized must be gravely disabled and unable to provide for themselves. Indefinite commitments are most often an action of the courts that usually provide a guardian or conservator to protect the patient's rights. They are subject to yearly review, and patients retain the right to consult a lawyer and petition the court for discharge.

Areas of Potential Liability

Mental health care providers are placed in the unique position of balancing their patients' rights with the need to protect society. Many legal issues relate to the care of mentally ill individuals, and an awareness of the potential liabilities helps safeguard care providers' as well as patients' rights.

The most common crimes in health care settings are homicide, controlled substance violations, and theft. Legally, *homicide* is the killing of a human being, whereas *murder* is killing with intent. For example, a nurse who mistakenly gives a patient the wrong drug that causes death may have committed homicide. However, a nurse who knowingly administers a lethal drug may be guilty of murder.

The *Controlled Drugs and Substances Act* was passed in 1996 under the government of Prime Minister Jean Chrétien. The intention of the Act is to regulate the supply and distribution of certain powerful and potentially dangerous drugs. **Controlled substances** currently include narcotics, stimulants, depressants, hallucinogens, and some tranquilizers. As agents of the physician, nurses administer controlled drugs. They are responsible for adhering to their institution's policies and procedures regarding storage, distribution, and documentation of all controlled substances.

Robbery, theft, and larceny all describe the taking of another person's personal property. Patients who lose valuable items can hold the agency liable for theft. Ensuring that a valuables disposition list is completed for every patient is an important protection against theft.

Often, as part of clinical practice, health care providers enter into professionally intimate interactions with patients. Because professional boundaries can be violated, professional regulatory bodies have strict and specific guidelines regarding the type of relationship and interactions a health provider can have with a patient. The following excerpt from the British Columbia College of Nursing Professionals (BCNPP) practice standards is applicable to all health care providers:

> Within the nurse-patient relationship, the patient is often vulnerable because the nurse has more power than the patient. The nurse has influence, access to information, and specialized knowledge and skills. Nurses have the competencies to develop a therapeutic relationship and set appropriate boundaries with their patients. Nurses who put their personal needs ahead of their patients' needs misuse their power.
>
> The nurse who violates a boundary can harm both the nurse-patient relationship and the patient. A nurse may violate a boundary in terms of behaviour related to favouritism, physical contact, friendship, socializing, gifts, dating, intimacy, disclosure, chastising and coercion. (BCNPP, 2020)

Regulatory bodies like the BCCNP, the College of Psychologists of Ontario, or the Saskatchewan Association of Social Workers (SASW), for example, all publish guidelines and directives for members on maintaining appropriate, professional relationships. These same regulatory bodies have a mandate to protect the public and have the authority to investigate public complaints regarding their members. Their authority includes the ability to punish health care providers who knowingly transgress the guidelines of professional behaviour, and they can even revoke individual memberships, preventing that worker from being employed in the profession. Despite the thorough and well-published guidelines, however, transgressions do occur. All health-related colleges publish disciplinary decisions regarding members who have been investigated. Often this information is available through the regulatory body's website.

Fraud is the giving of false information with the knowledge that action will be taken based on the information. For example, a technician documents that a treatment was given when it was not. The physician then bases a decision on the patient's lack of response. The technician is guilty of fraud. Practising with the utmost honesty is the best protection against fraud.

Defamation is defined as a false communication that results in harm. It is subdivided into two categories: written defamation, or **libel**, and verbal defamation, referred to as **slander**. Psychiatric care providers should base their communications on objective data and clinical observations, not judgements or opinions.

Assault is any act that threatens a patient. No physical contact need occur, just a threatening action. Telling a patient that he or she will be physically forced to do something if uncooperative is an example of assault.

Battery is when touching occurs without the patient's permission. The best prevention against assault or battery is clear communication. Make sure patients understand what you intend to do before you begin.

Another important area of potential liability relates to **invasion of privacy**. "The right to privacy includes privacy related to the body, confidential information and the right to be left alone" (Morrison, 1993). An invasion of privacy occurs when a patient's space, body, or belongings are violated. Although care providers must be continually vigilant to protect a patient's privacy, those rights may occasionally be outweighed by the need to ensure safety. For example, a patient who behaves in a manner that suggests they could harm or kill themselves may have personal belongings searched or confiscated.

The patient's right to privacy also includes confidentiality, which is the sharing of information about the patient only with those persons who are directly involved in care. Discussing any patient with noninvolved people constitutes a breach of confidentiality.

CRITICIAL THINKING

You overhear two patient care attendants discussing Mrs. Samson while making the bed in Mr. Jones's room.
1. What are the ethical and legal principles being violated by the aides' behaviours?
2. How would you handle this situation?

Patient Restraint

A **restraint** is a limitation on a patient's or patient's movement. There are three general classifications of restraint used in Canadian health care settings: environmental, chemical, and physical restraints.

Environmental restraint involves a temporary management technique that involves environmental containment of a patient who is perceived to be in psychiatric crisis in a "room or in a space from which free exit is denied" (B.C. Ministry of Health, 2014; Mayers, Keet, Winkler, et al., 2010, p. 61). This type of restraint is considered to be a partial limitation or restriction on a patient's movements. Examples of this type of restraint include when a patient is placed in a locked room, maintained on a locked unit, or placed in a geriatric chair with a dinner tray secured.

A chemical restraint is the use of medication specifically intended to cause sedation, or a psychotropic medication used to change a patient's behaviour. The medication is specifically intended to address undesirable behaviour that may pose a risk to the patient or care providers. A chemical restraint is administered in response to concerns about safety and is separate from the patient's usual or typically prescribed medications.

A physical restraint is the most restrictive type of movement limitation. In circumstances where the patient's behaviour is escalating and an imminent risk to that patient or others in the area is obvious, a process involving the use of limb restraints is utilized. Typically, the patient's arms and legs are secured to a bed (or, very occasionally, to a chair) using leather or neoprene straps. Once the restraints are applied, the individual is prevented from leaving the bed or harming themselves or any others.

Any type of restraint must be considered a last resort, to be used only when all other approaches have failed. Environmental, chemical, and physical restraints should always be a temporary management technique and should never be used to punish a patient. Care providers risk malpractice and legal consequences on several levels as a result of the inappropriate use of patient restraints. As in all cases, facility-specific documentation about the restraints, patient behaviour, and events leading up to the restraint must be carefully documented.

The use of restraints in care facilities has changed considerably over the years. Unfortunately, many of these changes have come into place as a result of injuries and even the deaths of patients who have been restrained. Most facilities have implemented a "Least Restraint Policy" that requires care providers to utilize all available resources prior to restraint. Specific documentation is also required. Ensure that you are always compliant with the information provided by your regulatory body as well as your employer regarding patient restraint.

The concepts of both negligence and malpractice are rooted in the "reasonable and prudent person" theory. **Negligence** is defined as the omission (or commission) of an act that a reasonable and prudent person would (or would not) do. For example, a public swimming pool owner who did not repair a slide that then caused a child's injury could be guilty of negligence.

The concept of **malpractice** usually applies to professionals and is defined as a failure to exercise an accepted degree of professional skill that results in injury, loss, or damage. To be considered negligent, professional misconduct must meet four requirements:

1. The care provider owed a duty to the patient.
2. The care provider did not carry out the duty (breach).
3. The patient was injured as a result of the care provider's action or inaction (proximate cause).
4. Actual loss or damage resulted from the actions.

To illustrate, a suicidal patient is to be continuously observed (duty). The staff goes to lunch, leaving the patient alone (breach of duty). During this time, the patient commits suicide (proximate cause) and dies (damage). The staff is guilty of malpractice because no reasonable and prudent care provider would leave a patient unattended in a similar situation.

CARE PROVIDERS' RESPONSIBILITIES

The main responsibility of mental health care providers is to help patients cope with their problems. Dignified, humane treatment includes the protection of rights as human beings, citizens, and patients. Mental health patients have specific rights to treatment, refusal of treatment, informed consent, examination by the physician of their choice, confidentiality, and freedom from restraints.

Informed consent is an agreement between the patient and care providers that documents knowledge of and agreement to treatment. The patient must be aware, informed, and capable of consenting. Mental health patients are presumed competent and able to consent to treatment. Obtaining consent for treatment is the physician's responsibility, but nurses often assist in the process. Other legal issues that relate to psychiatric care include elopement and the duty to warn.

A special situation, known as **elopement**, sometimes arises during hospitalization when patients run away or elope from the institution. Care providers who fail to prevent patient elopement may be held liable if the patient is injured as a result of the elopement. Keeping patients under supervision, plus accurate documentation of patient behaviours and therapeutic actions, can prevent elopement from occurring.

All care providers have the **duty to warn**. In situations in which serious harm or death may occur, mental health care providers have a duty to protect potential victims from possible harm. For example, if your patient states that he intends to kill his barber, you have a duty to warn the barber. Contact the patient's physician and your supervisor, and be sure to document the situation.

In some provinces, nurses have a duty to report certain information. Examples of reportable data include suspected incidents of abuse, gunshot wounds, and certain communicable diseases. The rights of the patient are sometimes balanced by the right of the public to be protected.

Documentation in patient records is used in court to prove or disprove a claim. Data must be objective, with patient statements in quotation marks. Documentation should reflect the nursing process, standards of care, and patient responses. Accurate, objective documentation is one of the best defences against potential legal problems. Most health care facilities utilize some type of electronic documentation where dates and times often autopopulate. If you are required to document on paper, ensure that you are using ink, not pencil (black ink is generally preferred, as it photocopies better than blue ink) and that dates and times are indicated on the document.

The Reasonable and Prudent Care Provider Principle

The law judges professional actions by asking, "What would a **reasonable and prudent care provider** do under similar circumstances in a similar situation?" Then a comparison between behaviours is made. Engage in "reasonable and prudent" care by following standards of practice and the employing agency's policies, procedures, job descriptions, and contracts. Safe practice is based on your knowledge of the limits that define caregiving in your practice setting. Health care providers have the overall responsibility to practise in a competent, safe manner. This involves an active pursuit of new knowledge plus a willingness to conduct oneself according to ethical and legal standards. Areas of potential liability exist in many situations, and laws are not always clear when dealing with mental illness. To practise safely and effectively, be aware of your actions and develop an alertness to potential problems.

KEY POINTS

- Societies share common values, morals, and rights that serve as foundations for making decisions.
- Values clarification is a three-step process to identify one's significant values.
- Rights are defined as powers or privileges to which one has a just claim.
- Patients' rights are addressed by each province in its patient's bill of rights.
- Health care providers have the right to practise their professions in safety and with respect and competent assistance.
- Ethics is a shared set of codes, rules, or laws that govern right behaviour.
- Ethical principles for health care providers have been organized into codes of ethics based on primary and secondary ethical principles.
- The six-step ethical decision-making process helps health care providers in resolving ethical dilemmas.
- Laws are the controls by which a society governs itself. They function to define relationships, describe acceptable behaviours, maintain rules, and protect the public.
- Legal concepts that govern health care providers are found in provincial practice acts; standards of practice; and institutional policies, procedures, and job descriptions.
- The involuntary psychiatric commitment process consists of petitioning, examination, and a determination to either release or hospitalize.
- Areas of potential legal liability for mental health care providers include crimes, fraud, libel, slander, assault and battery, invasion of privacy, false imprisonment, negligence, and malpractice.
- Negligence is a failure to exercise an accepted degree of professional skill or learning that results in injury, loss, or damage.
- Health care practitioners have a legal responsibility to practise (1) in a safe, competent manner; (2) accurate and objective record keeping; and (3) within one's legal limitations. Nurses have the added responsibility to dispense controlled substances according to procedures.
- Any type of restraint must be considered a last resort, to be used only when all other approaches have failed.
- Care providers who work with mentally ill patients need to be aware of the potential liabilities inherent in patient care situations.

ADDITIONAL LEARNING RESOURCES

Go to your Evolve website (http://evolve.elsevier.com/Canada/ Morrison-Valfre/) for additional online resources, including the online Study Guide for additional learning activities to help you master this chapter content.

CRITICAL THINKING QUESTIONS

1. You return from your coffee break and are told by a colleague that your patient, Mrs. Mohammad, has been put in a geriatric chair. You inquire as to why this has happened, and your colleague explains that Mrs. Mohammad has been approaching the nursing station constantly, making ridiculous demands about her food and the cleanliness of her room. Do you feel this is an appropriate use of a restraint? Why or why not?

2. While returning to your unit, you hear two hospital workers discussing the admission of a local media celebrity to the facility in which you work. In the conversation, they mention the person's name and the individual's diagnosis and marital status. How would you respond to this?

3. You are working on an orthopedic unit. A staff member makes the following statement to you: "The unit clerk has made a few mistakes recently; I think she must be drinking on the job." The individual who is complaining to you has no proof that the clerk has been drinking, however, and is basing this opinion on the mistakes that have been made by the staff member. How would you respond to this accusation?

REFERENCES

B.C. Ministry of Health. (2014). *Provincial quality, health & safety standards and guidelines for secure rooms in designated mental health facilities under the B.C. Mental Health Ac*t. Author. https://www2.gov.bc.ca/assets/gov/health/managing-your-health/mental-health-substance-use/secure-rooms-standards-guidelines.pdf.

British Columbia College of Nursing Professionals (BCNPP). (2020). *Boundaries in the nurse-client relationship practice standard*. BCNPP. https://www.bccnp.ca/Standards/all_nurses/harmonized/Pages/boundaries.aspx

Edelman, C. L., & Mandle, C. L. (2014). *Health promotion throughout the lifespan* (8th ed.). Mosby.

Government of Canada. (1985). *The Canada health act (R.S.C., 1985, c. C-6)*. Library of Parliament, Research Branch. https://laws-lois.justice.gc.ca/eng/acts/c-6/fulltext.html

Keltner, N. L., & Steele, D. (2014). *Psychiatric nursing* (7th ed.). Mosby.

Mayers, P., Keet, N., Winkler, G., et al. (2010). Mental health service users' perceptions and experiences of sedation, seclusion and restraint. *International Journal of Social Psychiatry, 56*(1), 60–73. https://doi.org/10.1177/0020764008098293

Morrison, M. W. (1993). *Professional skills for leadership: Foundations of a successful career.* Mosby.

Ontario Psychiatric Patient Advocate Office. (n.d.). *Involuntary patients.* Queen's Printer for Ontario. https://www.sse.gov.on.ca/mohltc/ppao/en/Pages/InfoGuides/2016_Involuntary_Patients.aspx?openMenu=smenu_InfoGuides?

Potter, P. A., Perry, A. G., Stockert, P., et al. (2017). *Fundamentals of nursing* (9th ed.). Mosby.

Stuart, G. W. (2013). *Principles and practice of psychiatric nursing* (10th ed.). Mosby.

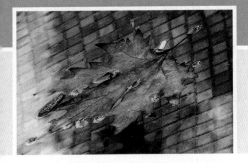

Sociocultural Issues

OBJECTIVES

Upon completion of this chapter, the student will be able to:

1. Compare the concepts of culture, ethnicity, and religion.
2. Explain the consequences of stereotyping mental health patients.
3. Describe seven characteristics of culture.
4. Identify three ways in which culture influences health and illness behaviours.
5. List the components of cultural assessment.
6. Explain the importance of recognizing patients' spiritual or religious practices.
7. Identify topics to be included in the assessment of a patient who is a refugee.
8. Integrate cultural factors into a holistic plan of therapeutic care.

OUTLINE

KEY TERMS

cultural assessment (p. 35)
cultural competence (KŎM-pa-tens) (p. 35)
culture (CŬL-chĕr) (p. 31)
disease (dĭ-ZĒZ) (p. 34)
environmental control (kŏn-TRŌL) (p. 36)
ethnicity (ĕth-NĬS-ĭ-tē) (p. 31)
extended (ĕk-STĔND-ĕd) family (p. 37)
gender (JĔN-dər) roles (p. 37)
illness (ĬL-nĕs) (p. 34)

norms (nŏrmz) (p. 32)
nuclear (NOO-klē-er) family (p. 37)
prejudice (PRĔ-jŭ-dĭs) (p. 32)
refugee (RĔF-ū-jē) (p. 38)
religion (rē-LĬ-jən) (p. 31)
role (p. 32)
spirituality (SPĬR-ĭ-choo-Ă-lĭ-tē) (p. 31)
stereotype (STĔR-ē-ō-tĭp) (p. 32)
territoriality (TĔR-ĭ-TŎR-ē-ĂL-ĭ-tē) (p. 37)

Culture has a profound influence on mental illness and its treatment. Mental illness is usually defined within a cultural context, based on what that culture considers to be normal. What may be appropriate behaviour in one culture might be considered insanity in another. This is an important point because an awareness of each patient's cultural background helps us understand the patient as a whole person and improves our therapeutic effectiveness.

THE NATURE OF CULTURE

An accurate understanding of any person is incomplete without consideration of the cultural, ethnic, moral, and religious concepts that define and guide that person's life.

Culture is the learned pattern of behaviour that shapes our thinking and serves as the basis for social, religious, and family structure. Culture is a shared system of values that provides a framework for who we are.

Ethnicity is a social term associated with the customs, cultural habits, and socialization patterns of a particular (ethnic) group. Ethnic groups can function as subsocieties within a larger society and play important roles in preserving cultures. The values, traditions, expectations, and customs of each ethnic group are passed from one generation to another. Ethnicity contributes to one's point of view; ethnic groups function as focal points for evaluating the value systems of other groups. A multicultural study in Great Britain revealed that ethnicity is "an important factor in influencing perceptions of schizophrenia" (Pote & Orrell, 2002).

Spirituality and religion play important roles in the concept of culture. The term **spirituality** refers to a belief in a power greater than any human being. **Religion** relates to a defined, organized, and practised system of worship. Religious groups may have values that range from allowing for individual variation to requiring a commitment to place the religion before family, work, and friends. Some mental health patients have religious components to their illnesses. Religious beliefs also impact the *perception* of mental illness, and sometimes become incorporated into the mental illness experience. "Delusions of religiosity" occur when delusional thought content emerges that is based on a person's experiences with religion. This creates a particular challenge for caregivers, as they may be required to "balance pathological behaviour with appropriate cultural expression of religion" (Taylor, 1994).

Characteristics of Culture

Culture is an abstract concept, composed of the values, beliefs, roles, and norms of a group. Large multicultural societies have many cultural variations and subgroups. Health care providers have varied cultural backgrounds themselves. Knowing how one's own culture relates to the patients' cultural backgrounds is important in establishing effective care.

Cultural values strongly influence a person's thinking and actions. A culture's belief system develops over generations, formed by the feelings and convictions that are believed to be true. Belief systems can be found in a culture's political, social, and religious practices. Conflicts in cultural value systems can lead to mental illness. People may also express one value and then act out another. Observing behaviours, rather than merely listening, allows caregivers to gain a more accurate picture of the patient's values. Because people of different cultures respond in various ways to time, activity, relationships, the supernatural, and nature, learning about the patient's cultural values is an important area of health care.

Beliefs about mental health have a strong effect on the outcome of treatment. When people believe in the treatment and in their care providers, successful outcomes are much more frequent. Thus it is important to know and respect the patient's beliefs. Some things that you might find strange may be of great cultural importance and significance to the patient.

Values and beliefs help define norms, which are a culture's behavioural standards. **Norms** are the established rules of conduct that define which behaviours are encouraged, accepted, tolerated, and forbidden within a particular culture. Simply put, norms are the generally accepted rules for behaviour.

A **role** is an expected pattern of behaviours associated with a certain position, status, or gender. Cultures commonly describe roles based on age, gender, marital status, and occupation. Individuals within the culture are expected to fulfill their roles and adapt their behaviours to meet the expectations defined by the role. Some cultures have clearly defined role expectations, whereas other cultures define their roles with vague and ambiguous terms.

"A **stereotype** is an oversimplified mental picture of a cultural group" (Haber et al., 1997). Some beliefs are passed on through generations and tend to colour the perceptions and influence the behaviours of people who hold them. Stereotyping may take negative, positive, or traditional forms. The extreme form of negative stereotyping is called **prejudice**.

Stereotyping occurs when one incorrectly assumes that all members of an identified group behave and respond in the same manner.

Stereotypes develop unconsciously in many people, especially those who have had little exposure to culturally diverse groups. Health care providers need to know and understand their own racial, ethnic, religious, and social stereotypes. Patients, especially those with mental health challenges, are very sensitive to discrimination. If they sense such treatment, they will resist receiving care. By removing stereotypes, each person can be treated as an individual with the respect and dignity that is their right. Caregivers who assess the behaviours of culturally different patients without personal biases are better able to distinguish adaptive behaviours from dysfunctional ones.

CASE STUDY

Hauni is a 22-year-old woman who recently arrived from Sumatra. She has been ill for 3 days and arrives at the clinic with a friend. Although Hauni speaks English, the nurse who is obtaining her history must frequently repeat her questions. With patience, Hauni responds to the questions, but she immediately freezes when Dr. Dankin, a male physician, enters the examination room. Although she feels very ill, she refuses to be examined. Sensing the patient's uneasiness, the nurse confers with Dr. Dankin, who recommends that the case be turned over to Dr. Linda Smith. Hauni responds immediately to Dr. Smith, even to the point where she becomes talkative.
- What difference did the recognition of the patient's cultural background make in her care?
- What do you think would have happened if the patient's culture were not considered?

Cultures vary greatly in values, beliefs, and behaviours, but they all share several characteristics. Table 4.1 presents a brief description of the main characteristics of culture.

Culture is a social phenomenon. It is learned through life experiences and transmitted or passed from one generation to another through language, symbols, and practices. Culture is shared. Values, beliefs, and standards of behaviour are known to all members and allow children to learn right from wrong and adjust their behaviours according to the cultural norms. Culture is integrated into an interwoven framework of political, social, religious, and health practices. Because a culture reflects its members, it is dynamic, changing, and adaptive. Cultural habits are satisfying. They fill a need within the society and result in gratification. Last, an individual's behaviour may or may not represent the culture. Individual behaviours may differ from the major behavioural patterns and still be tolerated to a certain extent. When a person's actions go beyond a culturally acceptable point, they may be considered eccentric, maladaptive, or deviant. Each of these characteristics helps to explain the framework of a culture. To deliver holistic, effective mental health care, all care providers must assess the effect and meaning that each cultural characteristic holds for the patient.

TABLE 4.1 Characteristics of Culture

Characteristics	Description	Example
Culture is learned.	A learned set of shared values, beliefs, and behaviours—not genetically inherited.	Cuban family members learn that humour is a way of making fun of people, situations, or things called *chateo*. It includes exaggeration, jokes, and satirical expressions or gestures.
Culture is transmitted.	Passed from one generation to another.	In Asian cultures the concept of family extends both backward and forward. An individual is seen as a product of all generations from the beginning of time. The concept is reinforced by rituals such as ancestor worship and family record books. Personal actions reflect on all generations.
Culture is shared.	A shared set of assumptions, values, beliefs, attitudes, and behaviours of a group. Members predict one another's actions and react accordingly.	In the Arab culture a woman will not make eye contact with a man other than her husband. All decisions are made by her husband. Because a woman may not be touched by another man, health care may be provided only by another woman.
Culture is integrated.	Includes religion, politics, economics, art, kinship, diet, health, and patterns of communication. All are interrelated.	In Ireland and North America, the primary cultural force and national unifier of Irish culture has been the Catholic Church. The parish, rather than the neighbourhood, has traditionally defined the family's social context.
Culture contains ideal and real components.	Behaviour may diverge from ideal behaviour and still be acceptable.	North American mainstream culture condemns the drinking of alcohol on a daily basis. However, those who do so but "hold their liquor well" are regarded with only minimal disapproval.
Culture is dynamic and continuously evolving.	Cultural change is an ongoing process. All aspects do not change at the same time. Habits and newer behaviours are easier to alter than deep-rooted values and beliefs.	Italian Canadian values regarding the family roles of men and women are often more traditional than those of other men and women in the workplace.
Individual behaviour is not necessarily representative of the culture.	Although culture defines the dominant values, beliefs, and behaviours, it does not determine all the behaviours in any group. Variation from the major pattern of behaviour is called *eccentric behaviour*. The meaning of this behaviour to the culture will determine whether it is regarded as normal, eccentric, or deviant.	Male and female roles are strictly defined in traditional Greek culture. Women are secondary; the man is the head of the family. Men work and provide for their families; it is a dishonour if the wife works outside the home. Within this cultural context, a Greek woman who is a proponent of the feminist movement might be viewed as eccentric or deviant.

Modified from Haber, J., McMahon, A. L., & Krainovich-Miller, B. (1997). *Comprehensive psychiatric nursing* (5th ed.). Mosby.

INFLUENCES OF CULTURE

People base many health decisions on both scientific and cultural values. As a result, many individuals seek health care from traditional healers as well as from medical practitioners.

Health and Illness Beliefs

The practice of Western medicine is based on scientific treatment methods and tends to disregard that which cannot be explained by research. Providers of health care are specifically licensed and trained in one area of expertise. Health care is offered in institutions and is often delivered in an impersonal, assembly-line manner.

Traditional medicine, by contrast, "embodies the beliefs, values and treatment approaches of a particular cultural group" (Edelman & Kudzma, 2017). Its foundation is based on empirical knowledge—observation and experience, without an understanding of cause or effect. Traditional practitioners explain disease culturally as an imbalance of energies. Caregivers may receive training through an experienced practitioner, religious groups, or self-study. Care is provided in the home or community in a personal, individualized manner. Providers of health care within the Western system of medicine need to know about patients' traditional medical practices, because many people seek out professional care only after seeking traditional healing (Table 4.2).

Traditional health beliefs involve explanations of the causes of health and disease. For example, Navajo and some traditional African cultures view health as a state of harmony with nature. The mind and body are one and function in harmony with the earth and the supernatural. Disease is caused by a state of disharmony.

Indigenous populations in Canada have traditional health and healing beliefs embedded in their culture; however, this is often combined with the use of Western healing modalities. There is a wide and varied belief structure, unique to each tribe and band.

The most noteworthy preface to any discussion of Indigenous health is that a universal Indigenous paradigm (i.e., belief system) does not exist. Nevertheless, despite diversity in geography, language, and social structure, Indigenous peoples do share certain values, which are philosophically distinct to Indigenous cultures (Rootman, 2012, p. 160).

TABLE 4.2   Comparison Between Traditional and Western Health Care Systems

Criteria	Western	Traditional
Philosophy of care	Curative	Curative
Approach to care	Fragmented specialization Often impersonal	Personalized
Setting for services	Institutions	Homes, community, other social places
Treatments	Technology Approved pharmacological agents	Herbs, charms, amulets, massage, meditation
Providers	Licensed professionals	Healers, shamans, spiritualists, priests, other lay unlicensed therapists
Support for care	Other ancillary personnel and agencies	Family, relatives, friends
Payment for services	Universal health care coverage Private insurance Personal funds	Negotiable
Philosophy of health	Influenced by the provider's definition and dealt with in terms of illness and treatment	Reflected as a quest for harmony with nature
Definition of disease	Result of cause–effect phenomena; cure is achieved by scientifically proven methods	Imbalance between person and physical, social, and spiritual worlds

Modified from Edelman, C. L., & Kudzma, E. C. (2017). *Health promotion throughout the life span* (9th ed.). Mosby.

Given their traumatic past involving colonization, removal from ancestral lands, and the residential school system, many Indigenous people have difficulty trusting established institutions, including those involving health care. While this remains a challenge today, efforts have been made to bridge the distance between mistrust of mainstream health care and the Indigenous population's use of it. The Truth and Reconciliation Commission (TRC) conducted interviews all across Canada in an attempt to understand the depth and extent of the challenges that exist. The Commission published 94 "Calls to Action," identifying priority concerns. For example, concern #1 is "the call upon the federal, provincial, territorial, and Aboriginal governments to commit to reducing the number of Aboriginal children in care" (TRC, 2015, p. 1). Another poignant example is #18: "We call upon the federal, provincial, territorial and Aboriginal governments to acknowledge that the current state of Aboriginal health in Canada is a direct result of previous Canadian government policies, including residential schools, and to recognize and implement the health-care rights of Aboriginal people as identified in international law, constitutional law, and under the Treaties" (TRC, 2015, p. 2)

Chinese cultures consider health to be a balance of positive and negative energy forces (yin and yang). An imbalance of yin or yang results in disease. People of Latin American descent may feel that good health is a gift from God, sprinkled with good luck. Illness is an imbalance of the hot and cold body properties and is considered God's punishment (D'Avanzo & Geissler, 2007). Low-income families may define health as the ability to work. Illness is seen as unpreventable.

Throughout the years, millions of people have sought health care from alternative (traditional) sources. Understanding and respecting the patient's cultural health beliefs and practices promote effective treatment for those who seek science-based health care.

Illness Behaviours

Disease is a condition in which a physical dysfunction exists and is essentially based in pathophysiology, whereas **illness** includes social, emotional, and intellectual dysfunctions. While culture has no effect on disease, illness and its attendant behaviours are strongly influenced by culture.

When the signs and symptoms of illness appear, an individual may choose one of four courses of action: (1) do something to relieve the symptoms, (2) do nothing, (3) vacillate without taking any real action, or (4) deny the existence of the problem.

The impact of culture on health and illness behaviour has been well summarized by Saunders (1954, p. 143): "an individual thus has cultural guides that enable him to know when he or others may be regarded as sick, something about the cause and nature of the sickness, what may be done to alleviate or remedy the condition, and the behaviour expected of him and of others in the situation."

Illness behaviours are also affected by beliefs (e.g., Christian Scientists do not seek medical help for illness) and culture. For example, if headaches were considered a sign of weakness, to seek treatment would be to act counter to the cultural heritage. To be effective, health care providers must assess each patient's attitudes and behaviours relating to illness.

On Mental Illness

Patients and their care providers may have very different belief systems about mental disorders. Members of a culture may define normal and abnormal behaviours differently from those outside the culture. To illustrate, in several cultures the practice of altered states of consciousness or trances is considered acceptable. Health care providers need to understand their patients' cultural definitions of mental health and illness.

Cultural descriptions of mental dysfunction are classified as *naturalistic* illness or *personality* illness. According to Haber et al. (1997), "naturalistic illnesses are caused by impersonal factors without regard for the individual." Forces that exist outside the individual cause mental illness. Personalistic illnesses are seen as aggression or punishment directed toward a specific person. Examples include voodoo, witchcraft, and the evil eye.

Beliefs in witchcraft are widespread in Haitian, Puerto Rican, African, and West Indian cultures. Spells, hexes, and incantations are used to cause a person injury, illness, or even death. The practice of voodoo calls the spirits of the dead back to the world of the living to bless or curse specific people. The chosen individual "takes on" or internalizes the behaviours associated with the hex. Mental illness in these cultures is considered to be the result of witchcraft, magic, or evil spells.

Stress and Coping

All cultures classify their members by gender and age. Age and gender roles contain certain norms, status, and expectations. Some cultures, for example, value older people and respect their acquired wisdom. Other cultures consider their elders as nonproductive burdens. Clearly, the role of elders in the latter example is associated with more stress. Adolescence in many cultures can be a stressful time. Societies that clearly define adolescence and its roles tend to be less stressful than cultures that lack a clear definition.

Women are often placed in stressful roles as a result of their culture. Traditional Greek culture, for example, sees the man as the breadwinner for the family. A Greek wife who works brings embarrassment to the entire family group. A great deal of stress would result for a working woman in this culture.

Stress is associated with various culturally defined roles. Ways of coping with stress are also culturally determined. Crying, screaming, and other displays of emotion are viewed as healthy outlets in one culture, whereas others expect quiet, unemotional responses to stress. Caregivers who are aware of patients' cultural stresses and their associated behaviours are better able to assist them in developing more effective coping skills.

CULTURAL ASSESSMENT

Cultural competence involves the process of continually learning about the cultures with which we work and developing cross-cultural therapeutic health care skills. A generally agreed-upon and frequently cited definition is as follows: "Cultural competence is a set of congruent behaviours, attitudes, and policies that come together in a system, agency or among professionals and enable that system, agency or those professions to work effectively in cross-cultural situations" (Cross, Bazron, Dennis, et al., 1989). A culturally competent mental health practitioner is one whose behaviours and attitudes promote effective resolution of a mental health issue for someone who is different, culturally, from themselves (Jackson, 2002).

So, what does it mean to be a culturally competent care provider? Being culturally competent simply means that you recognize that others may have a differing perspective on health, wellness, injury, and recovery, based on the influence of culture. Consider the following recommendations from *A Cultural Competence Guide for Primary Health Care Professionals in Nova Scotia:*

1. Examine your values, behaviours, beliefs, and assumptions.
2. Recognize racism and the institutions or behaviours that breed racism.
3. Engage in activities that help you to reframe your thinking, allowing you to hear and understand other world views and perspectives.
4. Familiarize yourself with core cultural elements of the communities you serve, including physical and biological variations; concepts of time, space and physical contact; styles and patterns of communication; physical and social expectations; social structures; and gender roles.
5. Engage patients to share how their reality is similar to, or different from, what you have learned about their core cultural elements. Unique experiences and histories will result in differences in behaviours, values, and needs.
6. Learn how different cultures define, name, and understand disease and treatment. Engage your patients to share with you how they define, name, and understand their ailments.
7. Develop a relationship of trust with patients and co-workers by interacting with openness, understanding, and a willingness to hear different perceptions.
8. Create a welcoming environment that reflects the diverse communities you serve (Davis-Murdoch, 2005, p. 6).

Transcultural health care delivery is the use of culturally sensitive therapeutic interventions. The care provider does not impose personal cultural values on others. The provider is an active listener and analyst who develops effective care plans based on the insights, knowledge, and beliefs of the patient's culture. All care providers must guard against the tendency to transfer their own cultural expectations onto patients or make generalizations based on their own cultural attitudes. Each patient is uniquely moulded by their culture.

Cultural assessments are tools that allow us to learn how patients perceive and cope within their world. Several tools have been developed, but all include six areas of assessment: communication, environmental control, space and territory, time, social orientation, and biological factors (Fig. 4.1) (Giger & Haddad, 2020). Box 4.1 summarizes a cultural assessment.

Communication

People of all cultures communicate. The process of communication, however, involves more than just the use of language. Communication is a complex, interwoven tapestry of voice, gesture, and touch. Both verbal and nonverbal components of communication have cultural meaning. To assess a patient's cultural communications, refer to Box 4.2.

Patients communicate their emotional states based on their cultural backgrounds. In some cultures, verbal expressions of emotion are approved, whereas other cultures value communicating indirectly and may resent the frankness of mental health care providers. Patients require sensitivity if we are to effectively understand each other. We all communicate; some of us are just louder than others.

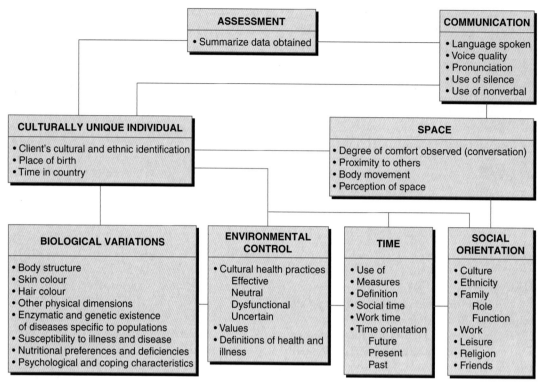

Fig. 4.1 Cultural assessment.

BOX 4.1 A Cultural Assessment

Use a narrative summary for the following categories:
- Cultural *identity* of the patient
- Cultural *explanations* of the problem or illness
- Cultural factors related to *stressors*
- Cultural factors relating to *psychosocial environment*
- Cultural factors relating to *level of functioning*
- Cultural elements of the *relationship* between patient and care provider
- *Overall cultural assessment* for diagnosis, planning, and care

---

Cultural traditions, practices, and kinship systems are also means of communication. A society's religious practices communicate its basic beliefs. Attitudes toward children, family, health care, and dying are all communicated through cultural behaviours. It is wise to learn the important customs of a culture if you are caring for its members.

CULTURAL CONSIDERATIONS

Your patient is a Xhosa from Southeastern Africa. His people believe that displeasing the ancestors results in illness.

Explain how this information will affect the patient's therapeutic care plan.

Environmental Control

Environmental control focuses on the individual's ability to perceive and control the environment. Does the patient feel that the power to effect change lies within, or is everything the result of fate, chance, or luck? What are the patient's values relating to

---

BOX 4.2 Cultural Communication Assessment

Verbal Communications
Language
Dialect
Pronunciation
Voice quality
Rate of speech
Style of speech
Volume of speech
Use of small talk, laughter
Music
Written language
Formal usage
Regional usage
Communicates emotions verbally
More verbally oriented

Nonverbal Communications
Touch
Use of touch
How touch is perceived and received
Space
Interpersonal distance
Use of silence, eye contact, facial gestures (e.g., smiles, frowns)
Communicates emotions nonverbally
More behaviourally oriented

---

the nature of humanity, the supernatural, health, and illness? How are the causes and treatments for mental illnesses viewed?

Environmental control includes an assessment of patients' cultural health practices. What is their definition of "good health," and what is done to maintain health? When alternative

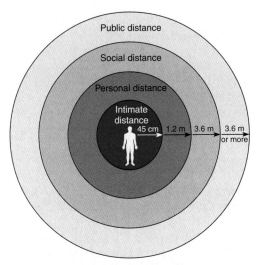

Fig. 4.2 Space and distance zones.

(traditional) practices are assessed, both patients and their care providers increase the potential for success.

Space, Territory, and Time

The concepts of space and territory are included in a cultural assessment. *Space* is the area that surrounds the patient—an invisible "bubble" that travels with a person. The physical distance that a person maintains between oneself and others is influenced by one's culture. People consciously maintain a "comfortable" distance from each other. Mental health patients often have additional perceptions about space. For example, some patients feel the need to be physically closer to people for feelings of safety and security. Space comfort areas are divided into four distances: public, social, personal, and intimate (Fig. 4.2). Observe and respect your patient's degree of comfort at each distance and their use of surrounding space.

Some patients have a need to establish a territory. **Territoriality** is the need to gain control over an area of space and claim it for oneself. For many, a territory helps to provide a sense of identity, security, autonomy, and control over the environment. People will protect their territory (even if it is the size of a hospital bed), and health care providers can be casually careless about invading these precious spaces. Caregivers, especially nurses, need to know and respect the patient's territorial space to provide culturally appropriate care.

The concept of time is rooted in a culture's basic orientation. Cultures oriented to the past (e.g., Chinese, Amish) strive to maintain the customs and traditions of previous generations. Present-oriented cultures focus on current daily events but may not follow a schedule. Many Indigenous cultures are present-oriented, but not necessarily to time. Cultures with future time orientations use today as a tool for meeting future goals. Schedules are established, and people are oriented to the time of day. An example of a future-oriented culture is the middle class of Canada and the United States. Western society's concept of time is linear. For individuals from some non-Western cultures, the linear concept of time is difficult to understand.

Patients with mental challenges frequently have misperceptions about time. They may have an inability to tell the difference between day and night, and difficulty following schedules is common. Problems with time may be based in the patient's cultural orientation or psychiatric illness. Until the caregiver can discover the difference, the delivery of effective care is difficult.

Social Organization

To assess a patient's social orientation, one must consider how the family unit and its importance in the society are culturally defined. The family unit imparts the culture's important traditions, beliefs, values, and customs. Social orientation also includes the meaning of work, gender roles, friends, and religion to the patient.

Although the functions of the family (e.g., caring for the young, providing identity, security) remain similar among most cultures, the size and composition differ. Middle-class North Americans tend to live within a **nuclear family** unit consisting of parents and one or more children. In many cultures, aunts, uncles, grandparents, cousins, and/or godparents are also included in the family. This family unit is called an **extended family**, and its importance to the patient is usually significant. To illustrate, the Inuit people view any separation from the family as traumatic. Many groups—such as traditional Chinese, Mexicans, and Puerto Ricans—believe the family to be the supreme social organization. Family causes take priority in these cultures. When care providers fail to consider the whole family, culturally sensitive care goals cannot be achieved.

Sexual orientation can also have an impact on both mental health and access to care. According to the US National Alliance on Mental Illness, lesbian, gay, bisexual, transgender, queer or questioning, and two-spirit (LGBTQ2) adults are twice as likely to experience a mental health condition, and they have a higher risk for suicide. LGBTQ2 adolescents are five times more likely to attempt suicide, and almost half of all transgender adults have considered suicide within a 12-month period. The risk of enduring a double stigma (sexual orientation and mental health challenges) decreases the likelihood that members of this community will seek out help or treatment.

Gender roles are expected behavioural patterns based on gender. The traditional roles for men and women in one society may collide with the expectations of another. Women who have learned to fill a serving, passive gender role may have great difficulty assuming the assertive and outspoken role of the modern Western woman. Be sensitive to this area of assessment. Few women will identify themselves as having a culturally based gender role conflict. Mental health challenges more frequently seen in women include eating disorders, phobias, and depression. Men, by contrast, tend to demonstrate more violent and aggressive behaviours. Cultural norms that identify gender roles often encourage the expression of conflict in different ways (Mood Disorders Society of Canada, 2009).

Assessment of social orientation also includes the patient's religious beliefs and practices. Religion serves many functions in a culture. Religious beliefs and practices bind people together in a common belief system. Religion helps to explain the

TABLE 4.3	The World's Largest Religions
Religious Body	**Number of Adherents**
Christianity	2.1 billion
Islam	1.5 billion
Secular/Nonreligious/Agnostic/ Atheist	1.1 billion
Hinduism	900 million
Traditional Chinese	394 million
Buddhism	376 million
Primal/Indigenous	300 million
African Traditional and Diasporic	100 million
Sikhism	23 million
Juche	19 million
Spiritism	15 million
Judaism	14 million
Baha'i	7 million
Jainism	4.2 million
Shinto	4 million
Cao Dai	4 million
Zoroastrianism	2.6 million
Tenrikyo	2 million
Neo-Paganism	1 million

Data from *Major religions of the world, ranked by number of adherents (2014).* https://www.adherents.com/Religions_By_Adherents.html

unexplainable, such as unexpected deaths or natural catastrophes, and it helps to provide meaning and guidance for living.

Religious beliefs and practices vary widely. Attitudes toward health, illness, death, burials, procreation, food, and stress all have religious components. Although it is impossible to discover the inner workings of every religion, it is necessary to be aware of the religious practices of those patients with whom you frequently interact. Table 4.3 lists the world's major religions by estimated numbers of adherents.

Biological Factors

The final area of cultural assessment focuses on the biological or physical differences that exist among different cultural groups. When assessing a cultural group for biological factors, consider the following: physical, enzymatic, and genetic variations; susceptibility to disease; and psychologic characteristics.

Physical variations include differences in body structure, eyes, ears, noses, teeth, muscle mass, and skin colour. People of some ethnicities are taller than others. The shape of the eyelids and nose varies from one ethnic group to another. Teeth may also vary in size and shape: Indigenous Australians have the largest teeth in the world, as well as four extra molars (Giger & Haddad, 2020). In contrast, White North Americans tend to have small teeth. Certain muscles of the wrist and foot are absent in some racial groups. Differences in skin colour range from pale white to black. Mongolian spots, for example, are bluish discolorations of the skin that may be found in Black, Asian, Mexican, and Indigenous newborns. In this

case, knowing the patient's cultural background may prevent possible misdiagnosis, because Mongolian spots can be mistaken for bruises resulting from child abuse.

Physical appearance, metabolic activities, enzyme functions, and susceptibility to disease are all influenced by hereditary and physical factors. To illustrate, sickle cell anemia is commonly found in Black people of African descent but rarely in White North Americans or Europeans. Lactose (milk) intolerance is common in Black, Indigenous, and Asian groups, yet is rare among White northern Europeans.

> ## ⚠ MEDICATION ALERT
>
> Culture and ethnicity play a role in the actions of medications. According to Flaskerud (2000), "there are dramatic ethnic differences in the metabolism of psychotropic medications and the effects of drugs on target organs." Monitor patients closely for adverse reactions to their medications.

Certain psychological characteristics may be associated with different cultural groups related to income. Low socioeconomic status can affect mental health when housing, education, and health care are substandard.

Feelings of insecurity can result when a patient's views of health are not considered in health care procedures. The Hmong people of Laos, for example, believe that "losing blood saps strength and may result in the soul leaving the body, causing death" (Rairdan & Higgs, 1992). Therefore, great anxiety is produced in a Hmong patient when blood is drawn.

In sum, cultural factors affect mental health. Nurses and their colleagues must become aware of group differences if they are to consistently deliver culturally appropriate mental health care.

CULTURE AND MENTAL HEALTH CARE

No society is immune to mental disorders, but research is needed to study mental illness from a worldwide perspective. The definition and treatments of mental illness vary among cultures. As stated earlier, in the attempt to understand and treat patients from diverse backgrounds, the concept of cultural competence has evolved. As the name implies, cultural competence involves delivering appropriate patient care based on knowledge of the patient's culture.

It is important here to understand the unique status of refugees. By definition, a **refugee** is a person who, because of war or persecution, flees from their home or country and seeks a safe refuge elsewhere. Many refugees have seen or experienced imprisonment, torture, and harrowing escapes. Some have lost family members, and all must learn to cope within a new and strange reality.

When assessing a person who is a refugee, be alert to the possibility of stress-related issues. In addition to the routine cultural assessment, tactfully obtain the following information: immigration history, a history of the flight and arrival in the new country, time in the new country, and who or what was lost. Because of a usually traumatic history, higher incidences of depression, anxiety, and stress disorders occur in refugee groups. Be sensitive to the special circumstances of refugees.

When attempting to assess immigrants for mental illness, practitioners must take into consideration the medical/psychological service climate of the country of origin. Historically, many individuals have faced an inability to access appropriate medical and mental health services in their country of origin and may never have been diagnosed previously or treated despite severe symptomology (Chang-Muy & Congress, 2016).

Patients from other cultures may evaluate their health care differently than the provider. Haitians, for example, may feel that improvement in health was not the result of good care but the mystical healing power of tree leaves kept close to the body. There exist many such customs and beliefs. If sensitive health care providers are able to view patients as unique, dynamically functioning individuals, then culturally effective health care is one step closer to becoming a reality.

CRITICAL THINKING

You are on vacation in Bali when you suddenly become ill with a high fever, vomiting, and diarrhea. After a long search, you finally locate a hospital. You enter the building and find that everything seems strange and uncomfortable to you. You cannot even speak the language, but you know you must be treated.
- How do you feel about this situation?
- What would you do to cope?

KEY POINTS

- Culture is a learned pattern of behaviours, values, beliefs, and customs shared by a group of people.
- Ethnicity is a social term associated with the customs, cultural habits, and socialization patterns of a particular (ethnic) group.
- Religion relates to a defined, organized, and practised system of worship.
- Stereotyping is basing one's behaviour on an oversimplified mental picture of a cultural group. Patients who sense such biases during treatment will resist receiving care.
- Culture is learned, transmitted, shared, integrated, dynamic, and satisfying.
- Culture influences people's health beliefs and practices, including patients' definitions of health and illness, attitudes about mental illness, stress and coping behaviours, and illness behaviours. When providing care, each area needs to be assessed.
- Cultural assessments focus on six areas: communication, environmental control, space and territory, time, social orientation, and biological factors.
- Religious beliefs and practices function to bind people together in a common belief system, help explain the unexplainable, and provide meaning and guidance for living.
- Religious beliefs and practices vary widely. Attitudes toward health, illness, death, burials, procreation, food, and stress all have religious components and implications for health care providers.
- Working with refugees requires extra sensitivity because of their frequently traumatic experiences and losses. In addition to the routine cultural assessment, obtain information about immigration history, a history of the flight and arrival in the new country, time in the new country, and who or what was lost.
- Because no universal descriptions of mental health and illness exist, the definition and treatment of mental illness vary among cultures.
- The aim of culturally competent health care is to deliver the diverse therapeutic actions necessary for appropriate, effective patient care.
- When caregivers are able to consistently view each patient as a unique, dynamic individual functioning within a sociocultural context, then culturally appropriate health care will become a reality.

ADDITIONAL LEARNING RESOURCES

Go to your Evolve website (http://evolve.elsevier.com/Canada/Morrison-Valfre/) for additional online resources, including the online Study Guide for additional learning activities to help you master this chapter content.

CRITICAL THINKING QUESTIONS

1. While working on an oncology unit, your patient of Métis descent informs you that she wishes to utilize smudging, a ceremony involving burning sacred herbs, in addition to chemotherapy. You are aware that the hospital has a strict anti-smoking policy. How would you respond to your patient?
2. At the clinic where you are employed, a co-worker identifies a new patient as being a member of a particular ethnic group. The co-worker advises others in the staff room that members of this group are known to steal things and can't be trusted. How would you respond to your co-worker?
3. In the emergency department, you attempt to assess your newly assigned patient. You observe that the new patient appears to be uncomfortable answering questions. You note that your patient speaks English proficiently, but with a thick accent from a region that you cannot identify. What methods could you utilize to establish trust with the patient?

REFERENCES

Chang-Muy, F., & Congress, E. P. (2016). *Social work with immigrants and refugees: Legal issues, clinical skills, and advocacy.* Springer.

Cross, T., Bazron, B., Dennis, K., et al. (1989). *Towards a culturally competent system of care* (Vol. I). Georgetown University Child Development Center/CASSP Technical Assistance Center [Seminal Reference].

D'Avanzo, C. E., & Geissler, E. M. (2007). *Mosby's pocket guide to cultural health assessment* (4th ed.). Mosby.

Davis-Murdoch, S. (2005). *A cultural competence guide for primary health care professionals in Nova Scotia.* Nova Scotia Department of Health, Primary Health Care Section. https://www.mycna.ca/~/media/nurseone/page-content/pdf-en/cultural_competence_guide_for_primary_health_care_professionals.pdf [Seminal Reference].

Edelman, C. L., & Kudzma, E. C. (2017). *Health promotion throughout the lifespan* (9th ed.). Mosby.

Flaskerud, J. H. (2000). Ethnicity, cultures, and neuropsychiatry. *Issues in Mental Health Nursing, 21*(1), 5 [Seminal Reference].

Giger, J. N., & Haddad, L. G. (2020). *Transcultural nursing: Assessment and intervention* (8th ed.). Mosby.

Haber, J., McMahon, A. L., & Krainovich-Miller, B. (1997). *Comprehensive psychiatric nursing* (5th ed.). Mosby.

Jackson, V. H. (2002). Cultural competency. *Behavioral Health Management, 22*(2), 21 [Seminal Reference].

Mood Disorders Society of Canada. (2009). *Quick facts: Mental illness and addiction in Canada* (3rd ed.). Author. https://mdsc.ca/documents/Media%20Room/Quick%20Facts%203rd%20Edition%20Referenced%20Plain%20Text.pdf

Pote, H. L., & Orrell, M. W. (2002). Perceptions of schizophrenia in multi-cultural Britain. *Ethnicity and Health, 7*(1), 7 [Seminal Reference].

Rairdan, B., & Higgs, Z. R. (1992). When your patient is a Hmong refugee. *American Journal of Nursing, 92*(3), 52 [Seminal Reference].

Rootman, I. (2012). *Health promotion in Canada: Critical perspectives on practice.* Canadian Scholars Press.

Saunders, L. (1954). *Cultural differences and medical care.* Russell Sage Foundation [Seminal Reference].

Taylor, C. M. (1994). *Essentials of psychiatric nursing* (14th ed.). Mosby.

Truth and Reconciliation Commission of Canada (TRC). (2015). *Truth and Reconciliation Commission of Canada: Calls to action.* Author. http://nctr.ca/assets/reports/Calls_to_Action_English2.pdf

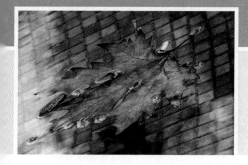

5

Theories and Therapies

OBJECTIVES

Upon completion of this chapter, the student will be able to:
1. Explain how theories can be applied to mental health care.
2. Discuss three psychoanalytic therapies that resulted from Freud's work.
3. Identify how developmental, humanistic, and behavioural theories differ in their viewpoints.
4. Discuss how Maslow's human needs theory can be used in the care of patients with emotional challenges.
5. Compare and contrast the main concepts of systems, cognitive, and sociocultural theories.
6. Describe the concept of homeostasis.
7. Explain how Selye's theories of stress and adaptation influence the delivery of health care.
8. Analyze how psychobiology is adding to our knowledge about mental health care.
9. Examine how nursing theories apply to mental health care.
10. Describe three kinds of psychotherapy used in the treatment of mental disorders.
11. Explain the difference between psychotherapies and somatic therapies for treating mental illness.

OUTLINE

KEY TERMS

affective (ă-FĔC-tĭv) (p. 45)
closed system (p. 49)
cognition (kŏg-NĬ-shŭn) (p. 50)
cognitive (kŏg-NĬ-tĭv) (p. 45)
countertransference (p. 44)
defence mechanisms (p. 43)
ego (Ē-gō) (p. 42)

equilibrium (Ē-kwĭ-LĬB-rē-ŭm) (p. 49)
homeostasis (HŌ-mē-ō-STĀ-sĭs) (p. 51)
id (ĬD) (p. 42)
inferiority (ĭn-FĒR-ē-ŌR-ĭ-tē) (p. 45)
libidinal (lĭ-BĬD-ĭ-nl) energy (p. 43)
life space (p. 49)
model (MŎD-əl) (p. 42)

A **theory** is defined as a statement that explains or describes a relationship among events, concepts, or ideas. Early theories evolved through observations and deductions. Modern theories are developed through observations and research. Many theorists use models to help explain their ideas more simply. A **model** is an example or pattern that helps explain a theory. For instance, a model of an airplane can be used to explain the theory of flight.

Models and theories about human behaviour help explain various aspects of human behaviour. They also describe the psychodynamics of basic needs, drives, conflicts, perceptions, values, attitudes, belief systems, and cultural influences that shape every individual. Helping professionals use theories as frameworks for describing relationships among people and various aspects of their environments.

HISTORICAL THEORIES

Symbolic and magical thinking was used to explain the workings of the world for many centuries. The belief that mentally ill people were possessed or controlled by evil spirits persisted until the late 1800s when radical new ideas were introduced (see Chapter 1).

Darwin's Theory

Charles Darwin (1809–1882) was a naturalist whose theory of evolution had a lasting impact on the emerging field of psychiatry. Basically, Darwin's theory stated that only the fittest organisms would adapt and survive. Through the process of natural selection, increasingly superior creatures evolved. In this way, nature culls the weak and preserves the strong.

Darwin's theory led to the persistent belief that people who were impaired or unsuccessful were, by nature, lower on the evolutionary scale. Poverty, disease, alcoholism, and mental illness were all claimed to be the product of inferior genetic makeup. High incidences of tuberculosis, rickets, infant mortality, and low adult life expectancies all indicated that nature was at work. This popular theory might have continued for many years had not the work of new theorists challenged the commonly held beliefs of the time.

Psychoanalytical Theories

By the middle 1800s, physicians everywhere were exploring new treatments for mental illness. Dr. Joseph Breuer (1842–1905) used hypnosis along with a new method of "talking out" symptoms. A brilliant young neurosurgeon, Sigmund Freud, heard of this and sought to work with the distinguished physician.

By 1902, Freud had become convinced of the talking cure's value and felt that unconscious thoughts and emotions had a strong effect on behaviour. Freud called this approach to therapy **psychoanalysis**, which means to explore the unconscious. Weekly discussions about psychoanalysis, attended by a number of Freud's colleagues (e.g., Alfred Adler, Otto Rank, Carl Jung), later provided the framework for several radical new theories.

Freud's theories focused on behaviours of which the patient was unaware. His study of the mind's unconscious processes evolved into theories about the development, structure, and dynamics of the personality. These ideas made psychoanalysis the most influential set of theories in the early twentieth century.

For the next 30 years, Freud developed and tested his theories. By the 1920s, the definition of psychoanalysis had broadened into three areas: Freud's theories of personality, a therapy for certain emotional disorders, and a method for investigating the workings of the mind. Today the term *psychotherapy* is used to describe a therapy relating to mental illness. Freud's theories that are important to health care providers relate to personality development, dynamics, and defences.

Freud believed that the mind was made up of three interacting structures, which he labelled id, ego, and superego. The **id** is a storage site for early childhood experiences and the instinctual drives for self-preservation, reproduction, and association with others. Freud stated that the id is governed by the "pleasure principle," by which a person seeks out immediate pleasure or avoids pain without regard to outcome. Because infants demand immediate attention, they are often described as "bundles of id."

The **ego** is the part of the mind in active awareness, the conscious mind. The ego develops when the child becomes aware of "self," usually around 2 years of age. The reality-based ego gradually gains control over the impulsive id and develops into the personality that copes with the external world.

The **superego** is the last to develop. Attitudes, values, role expectations, taboos, rules, ideals, and standards help form the superego. There are two parts to the superego: the conscience, which punishes through guilt and anxiety when behaviours move away from its standards, and the ego ideal, which rewards with feelings of satisfaction and well-being for "good" behaviours. The superego is not based in reality. It uses internal standards that were learned early in life. These standards, according to Freud, are primarily stored in the unconscious, where they remain unavailable to awareness but still influence the ego. The superego controls the id because of its strict and rigid moralistic rules. Freud stated that the ego must maintain the delicate balance of meeting id and superego needs within the limitations of the real world.

TABLE 5.1   Common Defence Mechanisms

Mechanism	Definition	Example
Compensation	Attempt to overcome feelings of inferiority or make up for deficiency	A girl who thinks she cannot sing studies to become an expert pianist.
Conversion	Channelling of unbearable anxieties into body signs and symptoms	A boy who injured an animal by kicking it develops a painful limp.
Denial	Refusal to acknowledge conflict and thus escapes reality of situation	A child covered with chocolate refuses to admit eating candy.
Displacement	Redirecting of energies to another person or object	A husband shouts at his wife, the wife then berates her child, who then scolds the dog.
Dissociation	Separation of emotions from situation; isolation of painful anxieties	A soldier casually describes the battle in which he lost his legs.
Fantasy	Distortion of unacceptable wishes, behaviours	A teenager doing poorly in school daydreams about owning a private jet.
Identification	Taking on of personal characteristics of admired person to conceal own feelings of inadequacy	Teenage adolescents dress and behave like the members of a popular singing group.
Intellectualization	Focusing of attention on technical or logical aspects of threatening situation	A wife describes the details of nurses' unsuccessful attempts to prevent the death of her husband.
Isolation	Separation of feelings from content to cope unemotionally with topics that would normally be overwhelming	A soldier humorously describes how he was seriously wounded in combat.
Projection	Putting of one's own unacceptable thoughts, wishes, emotions onto others	A woman is afraid to leave her house because she knows people will ridicule her.
Rationalization	Use of a "good" (but not real) reason to explain behaviour to make unacceptable motivation more acceptable	A student justifies failing an examination by saying that there was too much material to cover.
Reaction formation	Prevention of expression of threatening material by engaging in behaviours that are directly opposite to repressed material	A young man with homosexual feelings, which he finds to be threatening, engages in excessive heterosexual activities.
Regression	Coping with present conflict, stress by returning to earlier, more secure stage of life	A 4-year-old boy whose parents are going through a divorce starts to suck his thumb and wet his pants.
Restitution	Giving back to resolve guilt feelings	A man argues with his wife and then buys her roses.
Sublimation	Unconscious channelling of unacceptable behaviours into constructive, more socially approved areas	A hostile young man who enjoys fighting becomes a football player.
Substitution	Disguising of motivations by replacing inappropriate behaviour with one that is more acceptable	A man who is attracted to pornography campaigns to ban adult bookstores in his community.
Suppression	Removal of conflict by removing anxiety from consciousness	A woman with a family history of breast cancer "forgets" her appointment for a mammogram.
Symbolization	Use of an unrelated object to represent hidden idea	A girl who feels insignificant draws a picture of her family in which she is the smallest character.
Undoing	Inappropriate behaviour that is followed by acts to take away or reverse action and decrease guilt and anxiety	A man physically abuses his wife and then cleans her wounds and nurses her back to health.

The mentally healthy adult is said to be one who has achieved a dynamic balance among all the elements of the personality.

Freud's theory of personality development has the central theme of sexual instinct growth through four stages from newborn to adult. He believed that the most powerful motivation was the drive to reproduce and described this drive, which he called **libidinal energy**, as the need to seek sexual pleasure. Freud's stages became known as the psychosexual theory of personality development. Emotional disturbances, according to

Freud, arise from five sources: (1) instinctual-biological drives, (2) early childhood experiences, (3) deeply buried unconscious experiences and attitudes, (4) fixations (anxieties) arising from earlier psychosexual stages of development, and (5) defensive manoeuvres that help prevent the person from changing.

Freud believed that all individuals have conflict embedded within themselves and thus use tools to help to lessen negative feelings. He called these tools **defence mechanisms** and defined them as "psychological strategies by which persons reduce or avoid negative states such as conflict, frustration, anxiety, and stress" (Weiner & Craighead, 2010) (Table 5.1). Defence mechanisms are used to avoid negative emotional states. Individuals are not consciously aware of their use. No matter which mechanism is used, the goal is to reduce uncomfortable emotions. Commonly used defence mechanisms include denial, fantasy, projection, and repression. See Chapter 18 for a more complete discussion of defence mechanisms.

Psychoanalytical Therapies

Early therapies based on Freud's work were designed to assist patients in working through anxieties that resulted from unconscious, repressed conflicts. Freud used dream analysis to delve into patients' symptoms. He believed that during sleep, the individual's censor (superego) is less active; therefore, the unconscious (id) could express itself in dreams. Therapy centred on interpreting the dream's symbols to discover the unconscious wishes that were causing the conflicts.

The technique of free association soon followed. The patient was presented with a series of words or phrases and then asked to state the first words that came to mind. The therapist would then "interpret" each response and give the patient the "real" meaning behind each association.

Psychoanalysis was the main form of therapy for Freud and many of his followers. The process lasted for many sessions, sometimes for years. To achieve a cure in psychoanalysis, the patient must first recall past events and then develop insight into the meaning of each event. Many of Freud's theories are challenged today. However, his contributions have influenced the fields of psychiatry, psychology, the humanities, education, history, and the social sciences. Freud's revolutionary theories "brought about a new level of awareness and, for better or worse, a permanently altered image of humankind" (Weiner & Craighead, 2010).

Transference and Countertransference

One of the challenges of the therapeutic relationship is the issue of transference (see Chapter 11). Transference involves the unconscious association of a person significant in the patient's life onto the therapist. A simple example could involve a male patient projecting his feelings about his mother onto a female therapist. This can become evident when the patient reacts or responds in a manner that is not consistent with the interaction he is having with the therapist. For example, consider the following dialogue:

Therapist: John, unfortunately, I need to reschedule your next appointment. I have a personal obligation that is conflicting with it.

John: (becomes upset and yells) You never make me a priority! Everybody else is always more important to you than I am!!

In this exchange, John's reaction is excessive and likely reflects his feelings of disappointment in his mother and perhaps his own feelings of inadequacy. These feelings have been attached to this therapeutic relationship with his therapist.

The example above is considered to also be an example of *negative transference*. The assigning of negative feelings to the therapist suggests areas where further exploration within that therapeutic relationship should take place. Exploring

his patient's feelings about his mother, and his feelings about himself as a result, should become a therapeutic goal.

Conversely, *positive transference* involves the assignment of some previous positive experiences associated with an individual important to the patient onto the therapist. For example, a patient who has a particularly positive relationship with his sister identifies aspects of the therapist that remind him of his sister, and then attaches those feelings about his sister onto the therapist. Greene and Goodrich-Dunn (2014) describe three concerns that are specific to positive transference:

1. "The therapist is rendered less effective—if effective at all—because the patient's feelings are not based on the reality of the therapeutic relationship. Instead the feelings are based on another relationship.
2. Being at the centre of a positive transference can increase the likelihood that the therapist will engage in boundary violations, as well as damaging the therapist's objectivity regarding the patient.
3. Failing to redirect or acknowledge positive transference can increase the potential for a patient to begin to feel attracted to the therapist on a number of different levels, all of which can be damaging to the established goals of the therapeutic relationship."

Both positive and negative transference can involve aspects of sexual feelings. Often called an *erotic transference*, sexualized feelings from a patient's past can emerge and be assigned to the therapist. As with both negative and positive transference, sexual/erotic transference is counterproductive to the goals of a therapeutic relationship.

A skilled therapist can redirect positive, negative, and sexualized/erotic transference and can possibly even use these occurrences as sources for insight into the patient's behaviours and challenges.

While all of the above examples involve feelings that the patient has assigned to the therapist, what about the reverse? Countertransference refers to the automatic emotional reactions of the therapist toward a patient that occur within and because of the therapeutic encounter (Fortinash & Holoday-Worret, 2012; Rossberg, Karterud, Pedersen, et al., 2010; see Chapter 11). Countertransference is an emotional response to a specific patient, and is often irrational, inappropriate, highly charged, and generated by certain qualities of the patient. As with transference, countertransference can be negative, positive, and sexualized.

Analytical Psychotherapy

Carl Jung, the founder of analytical psychotherapy, differed from Freud in two basic respects: he believed (1) that the energy that Freud labelled "sexually based" was actually more of a general life energy and (2) that personality could change during adulthood and is actually influenced by future plans, goals, and dreams (Jung, 1968). Jung divided the mind into three levels: the conscious ego, the personal unconscious, and the deeper collective unconscious, which stores all the experiences of humans' ancestral past. The parts of the collective unconscious he called *archetypes*. He also coined the terms *extroversion* and *introversion* to describe outward-going and inward-focused personalities, respectively.

Jung's concept of the self focused on the importance of balance and wholeness. His ideas became known as the analytical theory. Jung used traditional psychoanalytic techniques but believed that the primary effort in life was to gain more awareness. He helped patients understand their problems and conflicts by uncovering the symbolic meanings of their disorders. The analytical view of psychotherapy did not survive as a separate discipline, but many of its concepts remain.

Other Theories

By the early 1900s, it was generally agreed that people were more than just physical bodies. The term **psyche**, borrowed from Plato, refers to the mental or spiritual part of an individual (compared with the term **soma**, which relates to the body). It was a time for several new, but related, theories about the nature of humans.

Individual Psychotherapy

Alfred Adler graduated from the Vienna School of Medicine in 1895 and attended Freud's weekly discussions on psychoanalysis. By 1918, he had developed a new way of thinking that became known as *individual psychology* (also called *Adlerian psychology*). Adler's personality theory states that the human infant, because of dependency and helplessness, starts out in this world in a position of **inferiority** (of being inadequate or less than others). The child must learn to master their world by assessing the environment and reaching certain conclusions. Each person wants to belong, to be considered as significant, and to be treated as an individual. Thus, as children grow, they find where they fit within the family. Adler believed that the perception of children's positions within the family helped to create the evaluations of self and other people that become incorporated into the adult lifestyle and that exert influence throughout life.

Adler theorized that the general goal of life is to gain mastery over the environment by coping with the tasks of work, belonging, social interactions, and interacting with members of the other gender. Later Adler added two additional life tasks, those of self and spirit. In the task of *self* people must define themselves and find meaning in their lives. Tasks of the *spirit* include considerations of religious, philosophical, and spiritual questions.

Adlerian or individual therapy views individuals as total organisms, functioning within the environment. Therefore, behaviour becomes meaningful only when viewed within the social setting. Because all behaviour is goal directed, people are capable of perceiving and assessing events to arrive at conclusions. However, each individual perceives the world from a unique point of view. To understand a person, the therapist "must be able to see with his eyes and listen with his ears" (Adler, 1964).

Adlerian proponents also believe that people have the ability to make choices and are responsible for their behaviour. They dislike the use of labels and do not consider people with mental dysfunctions as mentally ill. Patients are referred to as "discouraged." Therapy is designed to encourage them to assume responsibility for directing their lives in more positive ways.

The concept of a *value system* was introduced by Adler. The concepts of choice, individual responsibility, and finding

meaning in life evolved and later became the foundation for the humanistic school of psychology.

Other therapists during the early twentieth century also broke with the Freudian tradition. Karen Horney (1855–1952), an early follower of Freud, stressed the importance of social and environmental conditions on personality development. Her concept of basic anxiety stated that a child's isolation is not inherited but results from culture and social upbringing.

Erich Fromm (1900–1980) stressed human loneliness as the motivation for social interaction. His general theme of productive love is seen in many of his writings. Fromm also developed the concept of several personality or character types.

Interpersonal Psychology

Harry Stack Sullivan's (1892–1949) theory emphasizes the social nature of people and the critical role of anxiety in personality formation. He viewed the personality as a pattern of interpersonal relationships. Mental health problems were considered to be the result of distorted images of certain relationships. Sullivan called these distorted images **personifications** and believed that the images and behavioural patterns from one relationship spilled over into other relationships. Therapy is a matter of assisting the patient in discovering which personifications are unhealthy and substituting more effective behavioural patterns.

A central theme of Sullivan's theory is the concept of *anxiety*, which he defined as a vague feeling of uneasiness felt in response to stress. Sullivan also described six stages of psychological interpersonal development, beginning with infancy and ending with late adolescence. Many forms of therapy have benefited from his theories.

Often credited as the first published nursing theorist since Florence Nightingale, Hildegard Peplau (see Table 5.4) based much of her work on Harry Stack Sullivan's interpersonal relationship theory. Peplau was also the first documented nursing theorist to incorporate theories from fields outside of nursing. Peplau asserted that the therapeutic use of the self during nurse–patient relationships had a profound and significant impact on the outcome and the patient's overall well-being and recovery.

DEVELOPMENTAL THEORIES AND THERAPIES

Using Freud as a foundation, many theorists have offered their views of psychological development. Jean Piaget and Erik Erikson attempted to understand the relationships among the body, mind, and society throughout the life cycle. One of the most commonly used theories in health care is Erikson's eight stages of psychosocial development, which represents the first attempt to explain human behaviour throughout the entire life cycle.

Cognitive Development

Jean Piaget (1896–1980) devised a theory of intellectual (**cognitive**) development. He stated that personality is the result of interrelated cognitive and emotional (**affective**) functions. Growth is an increasing intellectual ability to organize and combine experiences. Piaget observed that certain behaviours occurred in

TABLE 5.2   Piaget's Stages of Intellectual (Cognitive) Development

Developmental Stage	Age	Developmental Task	Description
Sensorimotor	Birth–2 years	To recognize permanence of objects	Unable to do things or distinguish self from environment; reflexes evolve into repeated actions that become coordinated movements; learns that objects in environment are still present even when they are not seen, touched, tasted; begins goal-directed and imitative behaviour
Preoperational	2–7 years	To develop symbolic mental abilities	Thinking limited; centred on self; learns to use language as tool; establishes routines; thought is focused on only one part of situation; cannot understand more than one dimension of object; justifies own behaviour at all costs
Concrete operations	8–11 years	To develop logical, objective thinking	Understands numbers, length, mass, area, weight, time, and volume; can see interrelations; able to reflect and discover relationships in environment
Formal operations	12–15 years	To learn to think abstractly	Able to consider all possibilities of a situation; can think in terms of probability and proportions; uses problem-solving approach to conflicts

steps at certain age groups, so he divided these patterns into four main stages of intellectual growth (Table 5.2). Piaget believed that children struggle to find a balance between themselves and their environments. Although no specific therapies are based on Piaget's work, his theories have become essential in the understanding of intellectual growth and development.

Psychosocial Development

Erik Erikson (1902–1994) described the human life cycle in eight stages (Table 5.3), with each stage marked by a developmental or core task—a normal crisis that must be confronted and resolved. As each crisis is resolved, it leaves an impression

CASE STUDY

Susan is an attractive 42-year-old homemaker and mother of four teenage children. She has been married to Jeff, a long-haul truck driver and her high school sweetheart, for 22 years. The family is well respected in the community, and Susan frequently volunteers for charitable projects. The children are considered well behaved and polite. In all respects, Susan is a model wife, mother, and community member. Last week, however, Susan announced her unhappiness, left everything behind, and ran away with a 25-year-old travelling salesman.
• How would Erikson's theory of psychosocial development explain Susan's behaviour?

that contributes to one's total personality. The uniting of the personality occurs as each developmental psychosocial task is mastered. Erikson believed that success in one developmental stage prepares individuals to move into the next stage. Poorly resolved core tasks continue to haunt their owners until they are mastered. The case study above presents a person with an inadequately resolved developmental task. Erikson's theory is commonly used by care providers as a framework for assessing and planning individualized patient care.

Theories of personality development are an important tool for mental health practitioners. By understanding the patient's current level of development, we are better able to identify if that patient is functioning at, more or less, a normal level. In being able to identify when a patient is presenting in a manner that is inconsistent with what one might expect, more effective health care and individually tailored emotional and therapeutic supports can be provided.

BEHAVIOURAL THEORIES AND THERAPIES

The foundation for behaviourism lies in the assumption that all behaviour is learned. The behavioural school of thought states that behaviour is the result of past learning, current motivation, and biological differences. Learning is a behavioural change that results when individual actions repeatedly prove successful and are reinforced. Dysfunctional behaviours are the result of learned maladaptive behaviours. A mechanical approach to human behaviour is taken by focusing only on objective, observable, and measurable behaviours. The influence of the environment is stressed, but all behaviours are seen as responses to stimuli. Four important figures were instrumental in establishing the behavioural movement: Pavlov, Watson, Skinner, and Wolpe.

Ivan Pavlov (1849–1936) was the director of the physiology department at the Institute of Experimental Medicine in Saint Petersburg, Russia. There he pioneered research methods to evaluate the responses of dogs to various stimuli and discovered that a given behaviour was the response to a given stimulus. His famous experiment of conditioning dogs to salivate when they heard a bell demonstrated the mechanical aspects of behaviour. Pavlov then went on to discover that behaviours were more likely to be repeated when they were rewarded and they faded when ignored. His work on conditioning laid the foundation for the American behavioural movement.

The behavioural school of thought was established in the United States during the 1920s by John B. Watson (1878–1958).

TABLE 5.3 Erikson's Stages of Psychosocial Development

Core Task and Developmental Stage	Age	Associated Quality	Description
Oral-sensory (infancy)	Birth–1 year	Trust/mistrust Associated quality: hope	Dominated by biological drives and needs; learns to trust that needs will or will not be met; learns to trust or mistrust others and world in general
Anal-muscular (early childhood)	1–3 years	Autonomy/shame and doubt Associated quality: will (to do the expected)	Demands for self-control influence feelings of self-confidence vs. shame and doubt in own abilities; ego is developing; parallel play
Genital-locomotor (preschool years)	3–6 years	Initiative/guilt Associated quality: purpose	Actively explores environment; activities are directed with purpose; conscience develops; cooperative play; uses fantasy; imitates adults; beginning to evaluate own behaviour
Latency (school age)	6–12 years	Industry/inferiority Associated quality: competence (learning skills of adult)	Site of learning moves from home to school; masters skills and tasks valued by teachers and society; learns to behave according to rules; develops confidence and perseverance; practises self-restriction
Puberty (adolescence)	12–18 years	Identity/diffusion Associated quality: fidelity (commitment to value system)	Combines experiences to form sense of personal identity; forms sexual relationships; plans for future; feels confused and indecisive; if successful with prior crises, will develop strong sense of identity; peer groups important
Young adulthood	18–25 years	Intimacy/isolation Associated quality: love	If has strong sense of identity, is willing and able to unite own identity with another; develops devotion; commits to relationships, career. If weak sense of identity, has impersonal, short-term relationships; shows prejudice; becomes socially isolated
Middle adulthood	25–65 years	Generativity/stagnation Associated quality: caring	Strives to actualize identity that was formed in earlier stages; generates or produces children, ideas, products, services; is creative, productive, concerned for others; demonstrates caring through parenting, teaching, guiding others; adults who do not care become stagnant, self-indulgent, absorbed in themselves
Maturity	65 years–death	Integrity/despair Associated quality: wisdom (to accept one's life and value contributions that one has made)	Adjusts to changes; senses flow of time, past, present, and future; accepts worth and uniqueness of own life as it was and is; finds order and meaning in own life; despairs when life is viewed as waste; adults who focus on what "might have been" blame others, feel a sense of loss and contempt for others

He developed the basic viewpoint for behaviourism: psychology is an objective science—the science of behaviour. Watson published two books on behaviourism, and when he died in 1958, his views were a strong force in American psychology.

B.F. Skinner

Burhus Fredrick Skinner (1904–1990) was one of the most influential minds of the twentieth century. As a crusader for objective psychology, he stated that only observed behaviours in current situations were open to analysis. He pursued this idea by developing the theories of operant conditioning, positive and negative reinforcement, and shaping (Skinner, 1963).

Skinner's first research efforts were focused on developing a set of learning principles. He believed that all organisms moved toward pleasure and away from pain. His theory proposed that continual rewards strongly enforce desired behaviours, whereas negative reinforcements weaken and fade undesirable behaviours. The process of guiding patients to replace unacceptable responses with more desirable behaviours was called *shaping*, whereas the overall approach to changing observable behaviour became known as *operant conditioning*.

By 1953, Skinner published his book *Science and Human Behavior*. Throughout the 1960s, Skinner crusaded for improvements in the US educational system. He developed the concept of *programmed learning*, a process in which new knowledge is broken down into small bits of information and presented at the learner's pace. Today programmed learning techniques are commonly used in business and industrial training courses.

Other Behavioural Therapies

During the 1960s, Joseph Wolpe explained neuroses and anxiety as conditioned responses. Researchers Dollard and Miller developed their stimulus-response theory, which emphasized reward as the most important element in forming new behavioural responses. Today's behavioural therapists believe that emotional challenges stem from poor learning, conditioning, dysfunctional self-thinking, lack of skills, avoiding anxious situations, and misconceptions about reality. Therapeutic techniques focus on understanding the patient's current behaviour. The "past" is important only as it affects present actions.

Behavioural therapists teach patients to change dysfunctional thought and behavioural patterns by using behaviour modification therapies to replace undesirable behaviours with more appropriate actions. They also provide social skills and assertiveness training, which teaches patients to express themselves in constructive, nonaggressive ways. The behavioural school also promotes continual research as a tool for refining and improving treatment strategies.

HUMANISTIC THEORIES AND THERAPIES

By the mid-1950s, the two main schools of thought in the study of human behaviour were the psychoanalytic and the behavioural. Critics, however, believed that something was missing, and several began to look at human nature from a different point of view. This new outlook evolved into the field of humanistic psychology.

Humanistic theories are an important part of many of today's therapies because they emphasize the *total* individual. All realms of the human condition are considered important. Humanists also believe in the innate goodness of human nature and focus on the positive aspects of humanity. In short, people are holistic and multidimensional (many-sided) individuals—adapting to stress within a changing environment. These ideas serve as the foundation for the concept of holism and the model of comprehensive health care delivery.

Perls and Gestalt Therapy

The first contribution to the humanistic movement was made by Fredrick Perls (1893–1970), a German-born physician who worked with brain-injured soldiers after World War I. He studied psychoanalysis, but it was his years of work with his patients that sparked the idea of the *gestalt*, which means "whole." From this concept, Perls developed his psychotherapy, which he termed *gestalt therapy*. Perls accepted the notion of unresolved past conflicts, but he also stressed the present, freedom, responsibility, and attempts to become whole (or "actualized"). Perls's gestalt therapy paved the way for further exploration into human nature.

Maslow's Influence

Abraham Maslow (1908–1970) had a strong impact on the practice of nursing and health care. His ideas about holistic psychology were published extensively in theories of personality, motivation, self-actualization, and human nature. The core concept of Maslow's theories is that human nature is essentially good and contains the inherent potential for self-fulfillment (Maslow, 1971). He explored how people cope with and adapt to their situations. His investigations of people who function at highly successful levels led to a theory of motivation that has become widely adopted throughout the health care professions.

Maslow grouped human needs into a hierarchy or ranking (Fig. 5.1). Lower-order needs include physical and social requirements. Physical needs for air, water, food, elimination, and reproduction take first priority. The individual will perish if these needs are not filled. Second-priority needs relate to safety, security, and protection. Love and belonging needs come next. Everyone needs to feel accepted as part of a family or group. People who are lonely or isolated have unfulfilled belonging needs. Next are the needs for esteem, which include the needs for self-respect and the respect of others. Last is the need for self-actualization, or achieving one's full potential.

Maslow and the Blackfoot Nation Teepee Model

It is believed that Abraham Maslow formulated his hierarchy model based on aspects of Blackfoot First Nations culture (Grayshield & Del, 2020; Taylor, 2019). Some aspects of the hierarchical triangle appear to coincide with Blackfoot cultural ideas around paradigms of synergy and self-actualization. Narcisse Blood and Ryan Heavy Head from Red Crow Community College have concluded that "his Hierarchy of Needs model presents an inescapable resemblance to teepee designs, and his conceptualization of paradigms such as synergy and self-actualization seem to clearly derive from his epiphanies while among the Blackfoot Communities" (Kim-Prieto, 2014, p. 151).

Higher-order needs for optimal functioning include aesthetic and self-actualization needs. Aesthetic needs relate to the values of beauty, goodness, order, justice, and simplicity, whereas self-actualization needs encourage individuals to develop to their highest potential.

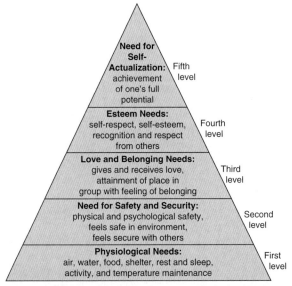

Fig. 5.1 Maslow's hierarchy of needs. (Data from Maslow, A. [1970]. *Motivation and personality* [2nd ed.]. Harper & Row.)

To understand the nature of self-actualized people, Maslow studied individuals who were highly successful. He found they had several similar characteristics (Box 5.1). Maslow also believed that when needs go unmet, illnesses can develop.

Today, Maslow's hierarchy of needs serves as a basis for planning and prioritizing patient care. To illustrate, maintaining a patient's airway (a physical need) takes priority over a need for socialization. Many patients in today's health care environments are experiencing unmet basic needs. Every nurse should be able to accurately assess and plan therapeutic interventions according to the patient's most critical unmet needs. Maslow was instrumental in the development of humanism, but he also gave us the tools for designing effective health care.

CRITICAL THINKING

The patient, a 22-year-old woman, has been admitted with anxiety, an inability to retain food or fluids, and shortness of breath. She has lived alone since her recent divorce.
- Using Maslow's hierarchy, list the patient's difficulties (unmet needs) in order of priority.

Rogers's Patient-Centred Therapy

Carl Rogers (1902–1987) developed a new approach to psychotherapy. During his work as a child guidance therapist, he became influenced by the theories of Otto Rank, a psychoanalyst who thought that people have a self-directing ability that emerges during therapy. Rank broke from the traditional techniques of therapy by stating that the patient should direct the therapeutic relationship using the therapist as a guide to self-understanding. Inspired by Rank's ideas, Rogers began work on a new system of psychotherapy.

Rogers also built on Maslow's work by stressing the goal of self-actualization. He believed that the goal of therapy is to assist patients in becoming increasingly more aware of their experiences and emotions. Rogers thought that the therapeutic relationship should foster an open and trusting climate in which patients can safely and freely express themselves. The therapist's task is to reflect patients' feelings and support work toward healthy functioning and self-actualization.

Rogers's efforts have benefited the disciplines of nursing, pastoral counselling, and education. He also worked with many leaders, policy makers, and groups experiencing conflict. However, his greatest legacy was his focus on the positive, achieving side of human nature, which gave people permission to accept themselves.

Current Humanistic Therapies

Many humanistic theories are with us today. The concept of holism has led to the development of a holistic health care model in which each patient is viewed as a unique person functioning within a changing environment. The concept of basic needs is used to plan and prioritize health care, to allocate scarce resources, and to assist patients in achieving their best.

Several therapies have evolved from the humanistic movement. Everett Shostrom developed a system of therapy based on the goal of self-actualization rather than cure. His actualizing therapy assists patients in learning to trust their inner or "core" selves despite life's negative influences.

Viktor Frankl's psychotherapy is based on a person's need to search for meaning and values in life. He called his system *logotherapy,* based on the Greek word for "meaning." His ideas of human worth and dignity grew out of his 3-year experience in a concentration camp (after having lost his entire family) during World War II.

Newer therapies continue to evolve, but each will be grounded in the basic premise of humanism: people are dynamic, multidimensional beings who strive for personal fulfillment.

SYSTEMS THEORIES

Systems theorists view humans as functioning within a set of related units (called *systems*). Royce and Powell (1983) developed the "open and closed systems" concept. They defined an **open system** as having boundaries that are permeable, passable, and accessible. Energy and information pass easily among open systems, and the organism grows and flourishes. A **closed system** has rigid, impermeable boundaries that shut out information and energy. If the system remains closed, the organism eventually will die.

Kurt Lewin (1890–1947) developed a field theory. He proposed that behaviour must be considered within the total situation. He rejected notions of past, future, or cause and effect and focused only on the immediate situation. He viewed people as systems who interact with other systems across boundaries. Lewin's concept of **equilibrium** states that each system attempts to maintain a balance, or steady state, within itself and among other systems.

Lewin also developed the concept of **life space**—the psychological field or space in which one moves. Life space includes oneself, other people, and objects. Behaviour is viewed as a function of life space. Lewin also proposed the concept of *psychological tension,* which results from the interaction of opposing systems. Although his work is complex, Lewin's theories influenced the development of several therapies.

In 1960, Maxwell Maltz published a popular book titled *Psycho-cybernetics,* which explained how "positive thinking" works by programming one's behaviour to achieve a desired self-image.

Systems theories differ from other approaches in that systems theorists believe that behaviour originates within the organism. All creatures are open systems with input, output, and regulating feedback mechanisms. People are open systems in a state of continual exchange, interacting within themselves, with other people, and with their environments.

COGNITIVE THEORIES AND THERAPIES

The word **cognition** is a general term that means "to know." It includes the mental activities of attention, language, imagery, memory, perception, and problem-solving. The development of modern cognitive psychology began in the 1890s with the work of Paul DuBois, a Swiss psychologist who believed that mental illness resulted from incorrect ideas. His rational psychotherapy changed the incorrect ideas through the use of reason and logic. Alfred Adler's individual therapy and Jean Piaget's work contributed to cognitive psychology by demonstrating the importance of intellectual factors in human development.

Albert Bandura's social learning theory established a relationship between cognition and behaviour. His work focused on the importance of learning through the use of symbols, imitation, and one's capacity for self-regulation through reflection and control. People learn by observing the outcomes of various situations (Bandura, 1986). These observations then develop into expectations and emotions. As a result, people compare themselves with others and make judgements based on their expectations and emotions. Thus our decisions act to determine our behaviours.

The main goal of all cognitive therapies is to replace dysfunctional beliefs and thoughts in order to cause a change in personal viewpoints. Patients develop successful self-control strategies by attacking dysfunctional behaviours and then learning specific coping skills. Current cognitive therapeutic techniques are grouped into three categories: cognitive restructuring, coping skills, and problem-solving skills.

Cognitive Restructuring Therapies

During the 1950s, Alfred Ellis developed a theory called *rational-emotive-behavioural therapy* (REBT) and treatment based on the irrational beliefs and unrealistic expectations people hold for themselves. He felt that it was not the event itself but the value placed on the event that determined behaviour. The goals of REBT were to help patients (1) gain insight into the irrational beliefs that cause their disturbed behaviours, (2) cease actively reinforcing the disturbed behaviours, (3) monitor the effects of their thoughts, and (4) adopt more appropriate outlooks by practising more effective thoughts.

By 1979, Aaron Beck had introduced *cognitive therapy* to help patients recognize their self-defeating tendencies and replace them with more adaptive thinking. Donald Meichenbaum's self-instructional training took a different approach to cognitive therapy. He believed that undesirable behaviours are the result of faulty instructions given in childhood. Therapy consists of using imagery, modelling, and anxiety control techniques to adopt new self-talk patterns. Today, cognitive remediation is used to help brain-injured children develop concentration, organization, and confidence (Graves, 2007).

Coping Skills Therapies

Several models have been introduced to teach patients how to develop more successful daily living skills. During the 1970s, Joseph Cautela described the process of *covert modelling*—the act of mentally rehearsing a difficult performance or event before actually doing the activity. This mental practice has been used by sport psychologists to improve the performance of their players. Coping skills training is similar to covert modelling except that anxiety is first induced and then the patient is trained to "relax the images away." Coping skills taught by cognitive therapists include training in anxiety management, assertiveness, progressive relaxation, and techniques to reduce physical responses to stress.

Problem-Solving Therapies

Some cognitive therapists see the cause of dysfunctional emotions as an inability to successfully solve problems. *Problem-solving therapy* teaches patients to solve their problems in more constructive and satisfying ways. Box 5.2 lists the steps in the problem-solving process. Note the similarities between this approach and the nursing (therapeutic) process.

Reality Therapy

William Glasser, MD, (1925–2013) founded the Institute for Reality Therapy to educate people about his therapeutic techniques. Glasser's theory, like Maslow's, states that people are born with certain basic needs. He thought that the most important needs are to be loved and belong, followed by needs to gain self-worth, respect, and recognition. Glasser believed that the specific issues of mental illness are rooted in failures within the social areas of functioning. He described people with mental illness as irresponsible and believed that values, ethics, and morals provide the basis for right behaviours. His "three Rs" of therapy encourage patients to do what is "realistic, responsible, and right" (Glasser, 1965).

BOX 5.2 Problem-Solving Process

1. State the problem.
2. Collect information about the problem.
3. Identify the causes or patterns of the problem.
4. Examine all possible options and outcomes.
5. Choose the best option and apply it to the problem.
6. Evaluate and revise actions based on outcomes.

Reality therapists help patients examine and evaluate the effectiveness of their behaviours and then develop more effective ways to satisfy their needs. Therapists and patients plan behavioural changes, and then contracts are made and both agree to abide by them. The use of contracts builds rapport, trust, and commitment. Reality therapy has become a valuable tool in treating chemical dependency problems. Glasser's methods have also been taught to thousands of educators who follow the principles of his book *Schools Without Failure*.

SOCIOCULTURAL THEORIES

Theories that focus on the social nature of people were introduced in the early twentieth century with the inquiries of George Mead. He believed that the social setting was extremely important in the development of one's self-concept. Mead stated that as children learn the rules and norms of their society, they take on approved behaviours. Breaking the rules results in social rejection and labelling if behaviours do not fall within acceptable social limits. Mead's concepts encouraged theorists to consider the social aspects of behaviour.

Mental Illness as Myth

In the 1950s, Thomas Szasz published a series of books and article attacking the concepts of mental illness by arguing that deviant (different) behaviours were culturally defined. Szasz stated that all societies have individuals whose behaviours are considered abnormal and ways of controlling their more undesirable members. Many societies do this by labelling people as "mentally ill" and removing them to institutions where they are taught to conform to more socially approved behaviours (Szasz, 1974). According to Szasz, *people are responsible for their behaviour*. Even those labelled mentally ill have the choice to take part in the labelling process by allowing it to occur. He also strongly stated that mental illness is not an illness but a socially defined condition.

Szasz believed that patients should be able to choose their therapist and treatment, define the problems they wanted to solve, and work with the therapist to change. Therapy was completed when the patient felt satisfied with the changes. His perspective has sparked a re-examination of the moral, legal, and political aspects of modern psychiatry.

The field of community psychology has evolved to focus on promoting changes in society at the community level. Community therapists work with local groups and organizations to improve social conditions, such as hunger, homelessness, teen pregnancies, and social conflict.

BIOBEHAVIOURAL THEORIES

Biobehavioural theories follow the medical model, which states that illness is the result of abnormalities in the structure, function, or chemistry of the body. A history, physical examination, laboratory tests, imaging techniques, and electroencephalograms (EEGs; brain wave recordings) are used to assist in diagnosis. The problem-solving approach is then applied to the data, and treatment plans are developed. Therapy is considered effective when the cause of the problem has been eliminated. Today, the fields of behavioural medicine and psychobiology are dedicated to uncovering new knowledge about the inner chemical and biological workings of the body.

Homeostasis

Walter Cannon, in the 1920s, was the first to consider the physical aspects of mental illness. His research on changes in the body's physiology during emotion led to the observation that the body always attempts to stabilize itself. Cannon believed that an emotion is a reaction that causes the body to use its resources. He described an emergency syndrome, which consists of a total body response that results in fright, fight, or flight behaviours when the individual is challenged or threatened. Cannon introduced the concept of **homeostasis**, which he defined as the tendency of the body to achieve and maintain a steady internal state. Disease, in his view, was the fight to maintain the body's homeostasis (balance) within an open system. The concept of homeostasis has also been applied to family systems, holistic health, and world ecology.

Stress Adaptation Theory

Hans Selye (1907–1982) was educated in France, Italy, Germany, and Canada. During his many years of study, he repeatedly observed students who were "just feeling sick." This led him to study Cannon's emergency syndrome and launched him toward years of research into the physical and biochemical changes associated with stress. The results of his studies led Selye to believe that many physical problems (e.g., hypertension, arthritis, coronary artery disease) are related to an inability to control stress (Selye, 1976).

Selye defined a **stressor** as a nonspecific response of the body to any demand placed on it. One's daily dose of stressors created what Selye called the "wear and tear" on the body. His studies revealed that people respond to stress in the same physical manner regardless of the stressor. Selye's *stress adaptation theory* (also called the *general adaptation syndrome*) describes the body's physical responses to stress and the process by which people adapt. The general adaptation syndrome consists of three stages: alarm, resistance, and exhaustion (Fig. 5.2).

When stress is first perceived, the brain triggers an alarm reaction that releases hormones that prepare the body to stand and defend itself or run away from the threat, the fight-or-flight response (Fig. 5.3). If the individual successfully adapts by coping with the stress, the body's heightened level of functioning returns to its usual state. However, if the stress cannot be resolved, the body continues to function at a high metabolic rate and progresses toward the next stage of adaptation.

The stage of *resistance* is the body's optimal attempt to cope with the stress. All coping skills and defence mechanisms are mobilized. Problem-solving becomes difficult. The individual becomes more susceptible to other, unrelated stresses. The person either adapts to the stress or progresses to the body's final attempt at homeostasis, the stage of *exhaustion*.

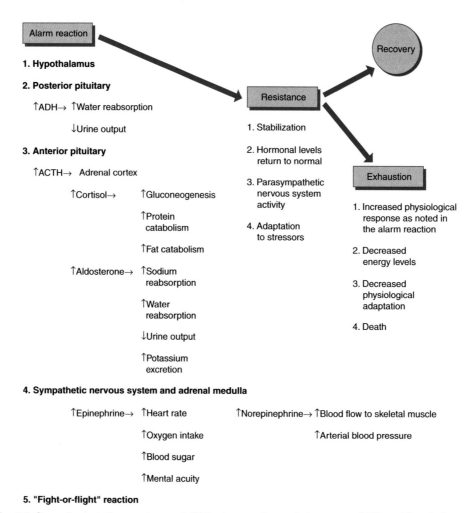

Fig. 5.2 General adaptation syndrome. *ACTH,* adrenocorticotropic hormone; *ADH,* antidiuretic hormone. (Modified from Potter, P. A., Perry, A. G., Stockert, P. et al. [2017]. *Fundamentals of nursing: Concepts, process, and practice* [9th ed.] Mosby.)

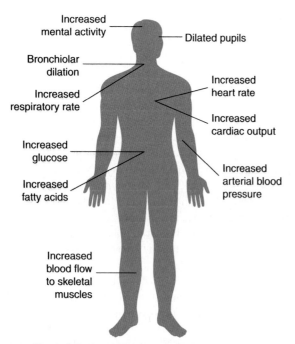

Fig. 5.3 Physical findings of the fight-or-flight response. (Modified from Potter, P. A., Perry, A. G., Stockert, P., et al. [2017]. *Fundamentals of nursing: Concepts, process, and practice* [9th ed.] Mosby.)

When stressors are overwhelming or last too long, the individual's resources become depleted and the organism begins to exhaust itself. Body processes break down as glands fail to produce the elevated levels of hormones required to meet the threat. Thinking becomes illogical and distorted. Problem-solving and communications are ineffective. Unless the stress is removed or adapted to, the individual continues to use all physical and emotional resources until death from exhaustion results. Chilling examples of Selye's general adaptation syndrome are seen in the accounts of prisoners of war and concentration camp survivors of World War II. Selye's work reminds us that effective health care can neither be given nor received if stress levels are ignored.

PSYCHOBIOLOGY

Psychobiology is the study of the biochemical foundations of thought, mood, emotion, and behaviour (Wilson, 1994). By applying the latest imaging technology and biochemistry, researchers are exploring human mental experiences and emotional states to learn about mood disorders, schizophrenia, language problems, and other conditions. Research is spawning new fields of study, theories, and therapies.

Psychobiological theories about the causes of mental illness relate to genetics, neurotransmitter activity, viruses, fetal development, and immune system dysfunction. The field of *neuropsychology* is devoted to the study and treatment of behaviours related to brain functioning. The interdisciplinary field of *cognitive psychophysiology* blends psychology and physiology to study mental processes by monitoring selective body systems, and the new science of *neurobehavioural toxicology* is exploring behavioural changes that result from exposure to toxins in the environment.

Psychoneuroimmunology

In the early 1960s, Jonas Salk developed a model of disease that encompassed the genetic, neurological, immune, and behavioural systems. Robert Ader (1981) later built on this model. His studies of the effects of stress on the immune system led him to coin the term **psychoneuroimmunology (PNI)**, the study of interactions among the body's central nervous system, its immune system, and aspects of the personality.

Ader's studies demonstrated that anxiety and depression can decrease immune system functions. Other researchers found that pain-relieving mechanisms in the brain could be activated by the body. Pain control by activating the opiate pathways in the brain has been seen in athletes, yogis, and women during labour. Some nurses are using this knowledge to help patients cope with severe pain by teaching them to turn on the body's pain-relieving mechanisms.

Research into **neurotransmitters** (the body's chemical messenger system) uncovered the existence of **neuropeptides**, neurotransmitters composed of amino acid strings. Further research showed that these amino acid strings actually connect the endocrine, immune, and nervous systems. It is believed this neurobiochemical system provides the pathway for emotional reactions. As research continues, there is mounting evidence that emotions, stress, and attitudes all have an impact on the body's immune response.

Studies are beginning to demonstrate that various interventions have a positive effect on the immune system. Research indicates that relaxation exercises increase the production of antibodies. Positive emotional states, humour, and laughter have been shown to increase an immune component in saliva (Dillon, Minchoff, & Baker, 1985). As the results of new research become known, our concepts of mental health and illness will change.

NURSING THEORIES

It is important for care providers to understand human behaviours from a helping point of view. Theories of nursing apply to the care of emotional as well as physical problems. The first nursing theory was developed by Florence Nightingale, who saw illness as the body's attempt to repair itself. Today's nursing theories view people as biopsychosocial beings who respond to stress in uniquely individual ways.

The focus of the therapeutic process in nursing is on assisting patients in using appropriate resources and abilities to effectively cope with their problems. Nurses may use many therapeutic techniques, but all therapy is designed to assist patients in achieving their highest possible level of wellness. Table 5.4 gives a brief explanation of the most common nursing theories.

As research increases our knowledge, our understanding of mental illness will broaden and new therapies will be introduced. Current mental health therapies are grouped into two basic categories: psychotherapy and somatic therapy.

PSYCHOTHERAPIES

Psychotherapy is the treating of mental and emotional disorders by psychological, rather than physical, means. Psychotherapies began with Freud's psychoanalysis and now include behaviour therapies, cognitive therapies, crisis intervention, hypnosis, and other therapies. Psychotherapeutic sessions take place on an individual basis or in a group setting.

Individual Therapies

Patients who work on a one-to-one basis with a therapist are involved in individual therapy. During psychoanalysis, patients analyze the meaning of certain behaviours and symbols and learn to cope by understanding the meaning or significance of their behaviours.

Patient-centred psychotherapy is based on the premise that "every person has within themselves the resources for constructive change" (Smoyak, 1993). Here the therapist expresses empathy to encourage growth and healthy change. Mobilizing the patient's inner resources through the therapeutic relationship is the goal of patient-centred therapy.

Cognitive therapy helps patients identify and correct their distorted thinking and dysfunctional beliefs. The therapist's role is focused on solving the problem within a limited time, as found in a solution-focused model. Studies have demonstrated that 6 to 12 sessions of therapy can be effective. The focus of therapy is on the issue that faces the patient at the moment. Solution-focused therapy has been effective for managing depression, stress, and marriage and family problems.

Behavioural therapy is tailored to each person's needs, behaviour, and environment. Behaviour-modification techniques are used by therapists and patients to define positive behaviours and reinforce behaviour changes. Behaviour modification has proven effective with developmentally disabled persons and those with severe forms of mental illness.

Group Therapies

Group psychotherapy was developed after World War II because of a shortage of psychiatrists. The central tasks of any therapeutic group are to (1) relieve emotional discomfort and human misery and (2) bring about psychological and behavioural changes.

Group therapy gatherings follow the medical model. Membership in the group is limited by the therapist. Group members are called "patients" who consider themselves "ill" and consequently exhibit "sick" behaviours. The goal of the therapist is to help patients resolve or better cope with their problems.

Self-help groups are limited to those who share a common problem, symptom, or life situation. Examples include Alcoholics Anonymous (alcohol use problems), The Mood

TABLE 5.4   Summary of Nursing Theories

Theorist	Goal of Nursing	Framework for Practice
Hildegard Peplau—1952	To develop interpersonal interaction between patient and nurse	Interpersonal model emphasizes relationship between patient and nurse
Ida Orlando—1954	To respond to patient's behaviour in terms of immediate needs	A nursing situation composed of patient behaviour, nurse reaction, and nurse action
Virginia Henderson—1955	To help patient gain independence as rapidly as possible	Henderson's 14 basic needs
Dorothy Johnson—1968	To reduce stress so that patient can recover as quickly as possible	Adaptation model based on seven behavioural subsystems
Martha Rogers—1970	To help patient achieve maximal level of wellness	"Unitary man" evolves along life process—humanistic nursing
Imogene King—1997	To use communication to re-establish positive adaptation to environment	Nursing process as dynamic interpersonal state between nurse and patient
Dorothea Orem—1971	To care for and help patient to attain self-care	Self-care deficit theory
Betty Neuman—1995	To assist individuals, families, and groups to attain and maintain maximal level of wellness by purposeful interventions	Systems model of nursing practice having stress reduction as its goal; nursing actions in one of three levels: primary, secondary, or tertiary
Myra Levine—1970	To use conservation activities aimed at optimal use of patient's resources	Adaptation model of human as integrated whole based on "four conservation principles of nursing"
Sister Callista Roy—1979	To identify types of demands placed on patient and patient's adaptation to them	Adaptation model based on four adaptive modes: physiological, psychological, sociological, and independence
Madeleine Leininger—1978	To care for individuals and groups in a culturally specific method meeting their health conditions	Cultural sensitivity with attention to the social structure through ethnonursing care
Jean Watson—1979	To promote health, restore patients to health, and prevent illness	Philosophy and science of caring: caring is an interpersonal process with interventions that result in meeting human needs

From Potter, P. A., & Perry, A. G. (2013). *Fundamentals of nursing* (8th ed.). Mosby.

Disorders Society of Canada, and support groups for families of persons with mental illness, such as the Schizophrenia Society of Ontario.

Last, consciousness-raising groups use the interactions among their members as a vehicle for achieving behavioural changes. The group is supportive of change, allowing individuals to analyze their interactions and then "try out" new behaviours with people from varied backgrounds.

Group therapy causes changes in behaviour through one or more change mechanisms (Table 5.5). The evidence compiled over 35 years demonstrates that many groups do provide benefits for their members. Emotional support for one another appears to be an effective therapeutic tool.

Online Therapy

A number of therapists have established online therapy practices. Online therapy is also known as *cyber-counselling, e-counselling, e-therapy,* and *tele-therapy.* Various therapies and services, ranging from answering a single question to ongoing counselling, are offered. Patients and therapists communicate via e-mail, instant messaging, Internet phone, real-time chats, and videoconferencing. Critics feel online therapy may be unethical and ineffective. People who believe in it see a way to reach individuals who are otherwise unable to seek counselling, particularly during times of pandemics. Web therapy has sparked fierce debates about its usefulness. At this time, there is a lack of research on the effectiveness of online therapy. Currently, the American Psychological Association is studying the issue, and has maintained recommendations on factors to consider when choosing online therapy (Novotney, 2017).

SOMATIC THERAPIES

The word *somatic* refers to the body. Historically, therapies for people with psychological distresses have been divided into those that work primarily with the mind (psychotherapies) and those that affect the body (**somatic therapies**). This division will soon fade as our knowledge of emotion and human physiology evolves.

Brain Stimulation Therapies

A group of somatic therapies "involve activating or touching the brain directly with electricity, magnets, or implants

TABLE 5.5 Group Change Mechanisms

Therapeutic Mechanism	Description
Expressiveness	Group members share emotional expression of positive and negative emotions.
Experience of intense emotion	Generating intense group emotion activates individual issues.
Altruism	The experience of helping others improves low self-esteem and poor self-concept.
Self-disclosure	The sharing of deeply personal material involves risk and develops trust.
Cognitive factors	Intellectual knowledge leads to a deeper understanding of self.
Communion	Groups foster a sense of oneness and belonging.
Discovering similarities	Relief is experienced when individuals discover that their problems are not unique.
Experimentation	Working with new behaviours within the low-risk group setting encourages change.
Feedback	Receiving information about how one is perceived by others is unique to groups.
Feelings of hope	Groups help individuals feel and believe that they can change with the group's help.

to treat depression and other disorders" (National Institute of Mental Health, 2016). Electroconvulsive therapy (ECT) was first used in 1938. After a general anaesthesia is administered, a seizure is induced by sending an electrical current through the brain. It is used to treat severe, long-lasting depression. See Chapter 21 for a more thorough discussion of ECT.

Vagus nerve stimulation (VNS) sends pulses to the vagus nerve using a device implanted under the skin. It was first used to treat seizures, but researchers discovered that treatments also affected mood regulation. Studies using VNS as a treatment for depression have had mixed results, so the therapy remains controversial.

Repetitive transcranial magnet stimulation (rTMS) involves use of magnets to stimulate the brain. Although it has been studied since the mid-1990s, clinical trials have had mixed results. It has been used to treat unresponsive major depression, psychosis, and other mental health challenges.

Magnetic seizure therapy (MST) uses magnetic pulses to induce a seizure. The patient is anaesthetized and given a muscle relaxant before treatment. Studies have shown that MST has fewer memory side effects than ECT. Studies are under way to evaluate the role of MST in treatment-resistant depression.

Deep brain stimulation (DBS) requires brain surgery to implant electrodes in the brain. A generator is implanted in the chest, and the brain is continually stimulated. DBS is being studied as a treatment for obsessive-compulsive disorders and depression. At present, DBS is available as an experimental treatment only.

Today the somatic treatment of mental illness is growing with the introduction of new therapies based on biochemical and physiological research. Drug treatment therapy was established years ago and plays a large role in treatment today. Biofeedback and **phototherapy** (treatment by exposure to light) are relatively recent developments. Acupuncture as a therapy for addictions involves the application of an ancient treatment method to modern problems.

Pharmacotherapy

The use of drugs to change behaviour dates back centuries, but it was not until the 1950s that medications for the control of mental illness were widely available. Currently, there are several groups of medicines that affect the mind. See Chapter 7 for a more detailed discussion of their use.

FUTURE DEVELOPMENTS

New therapies are currently being introduced. Feminist and women's therapy grew from the feminist movement of the 1970s; creative aggression therapy teaches patients to redirect their aggression and "fight fairly"; and movement therapy attempts to bring the body in tune with itself to restore balance. Therapies that complement traditional medicine, such as acupuncture, are being successfully used to treat mental health discomforts. Theories about the nature of human beings and their environments will continue to develop faster than our ability to make sense of it all. Evolving theories and their research activities now flow across many fields of study. Our understanding of human nature will continue to expand and encourage us to explore the most complex of all worlds, the one inside the self.

Many new developments utilizing technology offer fascinating resources to mental health consumers. Smartphone apps that remind users of up-and-coming appointments and medication times, self-administered mood assessments, along with text-based apps and face-to-face interactions through programs like Skype and Zoom keep consumers connected with supports in times of stability and in times of crisis.

KEY POINTS

- Theories and models help to explain human development and behaviour.
- Charles Darwin's theories led to the belief that mental illness was the result of inferior genetic makeup and a lower place on the evolutionary scale.
- Sigmund Freud's study of the unconscious processes of the mind evolved into theories about the structure, development, defences, and dynamics of personality.
- Analytical psychology was founded by Carl Jung, who recognized the spiritual and creative powers of people as well as their potential for growth.
- Alfred Adler's individual therapy focused on the ideas of choice, individual responsibility, and finding the meaning in life.
- Harry Stack Sullivan's interpersonal psychology described six stages of social development. He believed that the therapist's role was to sensitively assist patients in understanding how distorted images contribute to the anxiety and isolation in their lives.
- Jean Piaget's theory of cognitive development describes four stages of intellectual and emotional growth.
- Erik Erikson's stages of psychosocial development state that, as each developmental (core) task is mastered, individuals build and unite their personalities.
- The foundation for behavioural theories and their therapies is that all behaviour is learned and is seen as responses to stimuli.
- Ivan Pavlov developed the concept of conditioning.
- John B. Watson stated that psychology was the objective science of behaviour and began the movement known as behaviourism.
- B. F. Skinner's experiments found that positive reinforcement enforced behaviours, whereas negative reinforcement weakened behaviours.
- Behavioural therapies today assist patients in learning how to change their dysfunctional thoughts and behavioural patterns. Examples include behaviour modification techniques, assertiveness training, and training in social skills.
- Humanistic theories view the individual as a multidimensional person who adapts to stress within a dynamic environment while striving for self-fulfillment.
- The concept of gestalt led Fredrick Perls to develop a system of therapy that stressed the present, personal freedom, and attempts to become a whole person.
- Maslow's hierarchy of needs categorizes physical and psychological requirements for functioning and describes the characteristics of successful, highly self-actualized people.
- Carl Rogers built on Maslow's work by stressing the goals of self-actualization and awareness.
- Current humanistic theories have led to holistic health care, planning based on priorities of human needs, and therapies designed to assist patients in taking charge of their lives.
- Systems theories view humans as functioning within a set of interacting and related units called systems.
- Cognitive theories focus on the importance of intellectual factors in human development and function.
- Cognitive restructuring, coping skills techniques, and problem-solving skills help patients develop successful self-control strategies by reducing dysfunctional behaviours and then learning specific coping skills.
- Glasser's reality therapy teaches people how to fill their needs in effective, satisfying, and appropriate ways.
- Sociocultural theories focus on the impact of a society on people's behaviours and view mental illness as the result of social conditions.
- Thomas Szasz states that mental illness is a culturally defined myth with which people cooperate.
- Biobehavioural theories follow the medical model, which states that illness is the result of abnormalities in the structure, function, or chemistry of the body.
- The concept of homeostasis was developed during the 1920s by Walter Cannon, who found that the body has a tendency to achieve and maintain a steady internal state.
- The general adaptation syndrome, described by Hans Selye, consists of the stages of alarm, resistance, and exhaustion.
- Psychobiology is the study of the biochemical bases of thought, mood, emotion, and behaviour.
- Psychoneuroimmunology is the study of the interactions among an individual's central nervous system, immune system, and personality.
- Nursing theories view people as biopsychosocial beings who respond to stress in uniquely individual ways.
- Research has demonstrated that emotions affect immune functions.
- Current treatments for mental health challenges include various individual and group psychotherapies and somatic therapies, such as medications, brain stimulation therapies, biofeedback, phototherapy, and acupuncture.

ADDITIONAL LEARNING RESOURCES

Go to your Evolve website (http://evolve.elsevier.com/Canada/Morrison-Valfre/) for additional online resources, including the online Study Guide for additional learning activities to help you master this chapter content.

CRITICAL THINKING QUESTIONS

1. You are working on a mental health floor in the hospital, and one of your patients—a male who is close to your own age—brings you flowers from the gift shop and tells you that you remind him so much of his girlfriend from when he was in college. How would you classify this behaviour, and what would the most appropriate response be to this patient?

2. You volunteer to tutor a nursing student who has failed his first semester theory exam. The student tells you that he doesn't really get why theory is important, since nursing is a practice discipline. What could you tell the first-year student about theory and its relevance to nursing practice?

3. You are approached by a mental health patient who tells you that she is far too busy to schedule and attend regular follow-up sessions with a therapist. The patient asks you to recommend online therapy, which she feels would be more manageable once she is discharged. What might an appropriate response be to this patient?

REFERENCES

Ader, R. (1981). *Psychoneuroimmunology*. Academic Press.

Adler, A. (1964). *The individual psychology of Alfred Adler: a systematic presentation in selections from his writings* (2nd ed.). Harper & Row.

Bandura, A. (1986). *Social foundations of thought and action: A social cognitive theory*. Prentice-Hall.

Dillon, K. M., Minchoff, B., & Baker, K. H. (1985). Positive emotional states and enhancement of the immune system. *International Journal of Psychiatry in Medicine, 15*(1), 13.

Fortinash, K. M., & Holoday-Worret, P. A. (2012). *Psychiatric mental health nursing* (5th ed.). Mosby.

Glasser, W. (1965). *Reality therapy: A new approach to psychiatry*. Harper & Row.

Graves, B. (2007). Brain therapy study offers hope. *Oregonian, 157* (52, 468), B2.

Grayshield, L., & Del, C. R. (2020). *Indigenous ways of knowing in counseling: Theory, research, and practice*. Springer.

Greene, E., & Goodrich-Dunn, B. (2014). *The psychology of the body*. Wolters Kluwer Health/Lippincott Williams & Wilkins.

Jung, C. G. (1968). *Analytical psychology: Its theory and practice*. Random House.

Kim-Prieto, C. (Ed.). (2014). *Religion and spirituality across cultures*. Springer.

Maslow, A. H. (1971). *The farthest reaches of human nature*. Viking Press.

National Institute of Mental Health. (2016). *Brain stimulation therapies*. https://www.nimh.nih.gov/health/topics/brain-stimulation-therapies/brain-stimulation-therapies.shtml

Novotney, A. (2017). A growing wave of online therapy. *Monitor on Psychology, 48*(2), 48. https://www.apa.org/monitor/2017/02/online-therapy

Rossberg, J. I., Karterud, S., Pedersen, G., et al. (2010). Psychiatric symptoms and countertransference feelings: An empirical investigation. *Psychiatry Research, 178*(1), 191–195.

Selye, H. (1976). *Stress in health and disease*. Butterworth Press.

Skinner, B. F. (1963). Behaviorism at fifty. *Science, 140*, 951.

Smoyak, S. (1993). American psychiatric nursing: History and roles. *AAOHN Journal, 41*(7), 316.

Szasz, T. S. (1974). *The myth of mental illness: Foundations of a theory of personal conduct* (2nd ed.). Harper & Row.

Taylor, S. (2019). Original influences: How the ideals of America—and psychology itself—were shaped by Native Americans. *Psychology Today*. March 22. https://www.psychologytoday.com/us/blog/out-the-darkness/201903/original-influences

Weiner, I. B., & Craighead, W. E. (Eds.). (2010). *The Corsini encyclopedia of psychology* (Vol. 2, 4th ed.). Wiley.

Wilson, H. S. (1994). The 1990s as the decade of the brain. *Capsules and Comments in Psychiatric Nursing, 1*(1), 1.

6

Complementary and Alternative Therapies

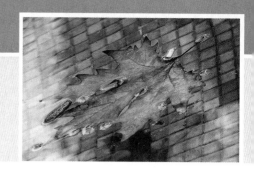

OBJECTIVES

Upon completion of this chapter, the student will be able to:

1. Explain the major differences between alternative and complementary therapies.
2. Analyze how the concept of holistic care relates to integrative medicine.
3. Discuss regulation of complementary and alternative medicines and therapies in Canada.
4. Examine what is meant by the term *whole medical systems.*
5. List three biologically based practices.
6. Discuss the basic premise of mind-body medicine.
7. Identify the theory underlying energy medicine therapies.
8. Describe four mental health challenges that may be helped by complementary and alternative medicine (CAM) therapies.
9. Examine seven alternative approaches to mental health care.
10. Specify two precautions relating to CAM therapies.

OUTLINE

KEY TERMS

acupuncture (ĂK-ū-PŬNK-chŭr) (p. 64)
allopathic (ăl-ō-PĂTH-ĭk) (p. 59)
alternative (ăl-TĔR-nă-tĭv) **medicine** (p. 59)
aromatherapy (ă-RŌ-mă THĔR-ă-pē) (p. 61)
Ayurveda (Ā-yŭr-vā-dă) (p. 61)
biofeedback (BĪ-ō-F ĔD-băk) (p. 64)

chelation (kē-LĀ-shŭn) (p. 62)
chiropractic (kī-rō-PRĂK-tĭk) (p. 62)
complementary (kŏm-plĕ-MĔN-tă-rē) **medicine** (p. 59)
dietary supplements (dĪ-ə-tĂ-rĒ SŬP-lə-mĕnts) (p. 61)
electromagnetic (ē-LĔC-trō-măg-NĔT-ĭc) **fields (EMF)** (p. 64)

expressive therapy (ĕk-SPRĔS-ĭv) (p. 63)
eye movement desensitization and reprocessing
    (EMDR) (p. 62)
homeopathy (hō-mē-ŎP-ă-thē) (p. 61)
hypnosis (hĭp-N Ō-sĭs) (p. 63)
integrative (ĬN-tĕ-grā-tĭv) medicine (p. 59)
massage (mŭ-SĂJ) (p. 62)
meditation (mĕd-ĭ-TĀ-shŭn) (p. 63)

naturopathy (nā-chŭr-ŎP-ă-thē) (p. 61)
prayer (p. 63)
Qi Gong (kē Gŏng) (p. 64)
Reiki (RĬ-kē) (p. 64)
spirituality (SPĬR-ĭ-tū-ĂL-ĭ-tē) (p. 63)
therapeutic (thĕr-ă-PŪ-tĭk) touch (p. 64)
traditional Chinese medicine (TCM) (p. 61)
whole medical systems (p. 60)

There are many systems of treatment for physical and mental problems in our world today. Some treatment systems are very old and play an important role in a culture. Other systems and practices are more recent developments. Some practices are rooted in objective (empirical) data, whereas others use energy fields as a basis for treatment. All, however, share the common goal of relieving pain and improving quality of life.

DEFINITION OF TERMS

Allopathic Medicine

Mainstream health care practices in the modern world are based on **allopathic** methods of treatment. Allopathic practitioners use medical and surgical methods to treat disease and injury by finding what is "wrong" and "fixing" it. Allopathic medicine is based on observation, scientific research, and objective explanations. Physicians (MDs), dentists, nurses, psychologists, and other therapists receive years of special training before they are allowed to practise.

Complementary Medicine

Complementary medicine includes practices and treatments that agree or "work with" allopathic therapies. They are used along with common medical treatments. Massage, for example, may ease pain and relax an injured body part. Complementary medicine practitioners usually undergo some type of formal training. Many medical practices are culturally based. Practitioners may or may not be formally educated.

Alternative Medicine

Alternative medicine refers to practices and treatments that are used instead of conventional (allopathic) medicine. The use of special herbs and following a certain diet to treat cancer and its symptoms are examples.

Integrative Medicine

Integrative medicine attempts to blend the most effective practices and treatments from both conventional and alternative treatment systems. Emphasis is on the interrelationship among body, mind, and spirit.

Holistic Care

Most current mental health care delivery systems are diagnosis and treatment oriented. Traditionally, most people received mental health care only after the onset of behavioural signs and symptoms. This approach resulted in acute conditions that were more difficult and expensive to treat. Emphasis was rarely placed on prevention or early diagnosis.

Since the 1980s, researchers have found that emotions cause chemical changes within the body that in turn affect the physical state. As health care models were developed to recognize the interrelatedness of mind, body, and environment, a movement (known as "holism") began to emerge.

The word *holism* is derived from the Greek word *holos*, meaning "whole." Holism today views a person as more than just the sum of their parts. The concept of holism helps to blend many aspects of mental health care. The primary goal of holistic mental health care providers is to "help clients develop strategies to achieve harmony within themselves and with others, nature, and the world" (Rawlins, Williams, & Beck, 1993). This statement reflects the holistic concept of care. We are no longer content simply to treat the illness; we are learning to treat the whole person (Fig. 6.1).

HEALTH CANADA'S LICENSED NATURAL HEALTH PRODUCTS DATABASE

The Licensed Natural Health Products Database is an online resource that provides information about natural health products that are licensed by Health Canada. As described on Health Canada's website, "Products with a license have been

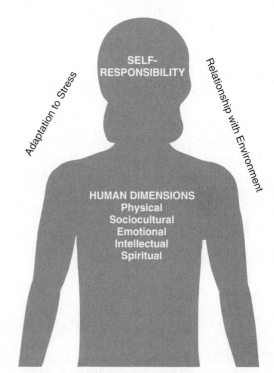

Fig. 6.1 Holistic health care concepts: relationship with human dimensions, self-responsibility, adaptation to stress, and environment.

assessed by Health Canada and found to be safe, effective and of high quality under their recommended conditions of use" (Government of Canada, 2019). The database allows for the entry of an eight-digit number which is found on the product, to locate licensing information. Products covered within this database include the following:

- Vitamin and mineral supplements
- Herbal and plant-based remedies
- Traditional medicines like traditional Chinese medicines or Ayurvedic (Indian) medicines
- Omega-3 and essential fatty acids
- Probiotics
- Homeopathic medicines
- Many everyday consumer products, like certain toothpastes, antiperspirants, shampoos, facial products, and mouthwashes (Government of Canada, 2019).

It is important for health care providers to be familiar with CAM therapies and their most appropriate uses. See Table 6.1 for an overview of medical treatments and CAM therapies.

BODY-BASED CAM THERAPIES

These therapies focus on working with the body's natural abilities to heal itself. They include a variety of therapies. Some, such as Chinese medicine, are very old, whereas others are of more recent origin. Here we briefly discuss the most commonly used CAM therapies.

Whole Medical Systems

Whole medical systems are built on complete systems of theory and practice. They include modern, Western medicine as well as osteopathy, homeopathy, naturopathy, and culturally

TABLE 6.1   Overview of CAM Therapies

Therapy	Example	Use in Mental Health Body-Based Therapies
Whole medical systems	Western medicine	Primary system of treatment
	Ayurveda	Diet, meditation, and other practices to bring body back into its innate harmony
	Homeopathy	Microdoses of natural substances
	Naturopathy	Supports the healing power of nature
	Traditional Chinese medicine	Balance of yin and yang forces
Biologically based practices	Aromatherapy	Uses scents to promote well-being
	Diet supplements	Vitamins and herbs to promote health
Body-based practices	Chiropractic	Spinal manipulation to restore balance
	Chelation	EDTA given to bind heavy metals
	Eye movement desensitization and reprocessing (EMDR)	Eye exercises therapy for post-traumatic stress disorder (PTSD)
	Massage	Muscle manipulation to relax body
	Phototherapy	Use of lights to treat seasonal affective disorder (SAD)
Energy-Based Therapies		
Mind-body medicine	Expressive therapy	Uses creative activities to reduce stress
	Hypnotherapy	Suggestions given when patient is in a relaxed, trancelike state
	Meditation	Attaining an altered state of consciousness through the focus of one's energies
	Prayer, spiritual healing	Appealing to a higher spiritual power
Energy medicine	Acupuncture	Focuses energies by inserting needles along energy pathways
	Biofeedback	Monitors physical responses during practice of relaxation techniques
	Qi Gong	Uses movement to balance energies
	Reiki	Balance of life force energies
	Therapeutic touch	Therapist reorients body energies
	Colour therapy	Rebalances energies with exposure to various colours
	Magnetic field therapy	Use of electromagnetic energy to treat illness
Technology-Based Practices		
Technology	Telemedicine	Video and computer to gain treatment information
	Text-based counselling, hotlines	Uses text messaging to help and support callers

based systems such as Ayurveda and Asian medicine. Several systems have developed outside of Western medicine, and some are much older. All systems, however, teach that wellness is a state of balance (physical, mental, spiritual) and illness is an imbalance. Herbal and natural remedies, along with good diet, exercise, and meditation/prayer, will correct the imbalance.

Ayurveda

Ayurveda is a healing system that was developed in India and literally means "the science of life." Ayurvedic medicine is described as "knowledge of how to live." Focus is on the innate harmony of the body, mind, and spirit. Therapies such as diet, meditation, herbs, yoga, exposure to sunlight, and controlled breathing are designed to restore balance, thus healing the individual.

Homeopathy

Homeopathy is "a therapeutic method that uses natural substances in microdoses to relieve symptoms" (Boiron, 2007). It is based on the "principle of similars." Its founder, German physician Samuel Hahnemann (1755–1843), developed treatments for his patients by choosing a very small portion of a substance that matched the patient's symptoms. Only one substance at a time is used, and the effects are closely monitored. Although the National Center for Complementary and Alternative Medicine (NCCAM) has found homeopathy to be unproven by scientific studies, there is anecdotal evidence for its effectiveness, as illustrated in the following Case Study.

CASE STUDY

Judy was a 33-year-old businesswoman with obsessive-compulsive disorder and complicated grief stemming from the unexpected loss of her 3-year-old daughter. She had been taking high doses of antidepressant medications but still felt that life was not worth living. She still blamed herself for the accident that took her beloved daughter and now was overprotective of her older child. Judy's overwhelming burden of guilt focused her thoughts of suicide.

Her obsessive-compulsive behaviours, with her since being sexually abused at age 7, increased dramatically. She began washing her hands 40 times a day and developed a constant fear of germs. The thought of contracting acquired immunodeficiency syndrome (AIDS) terrified her. She dreamed of being attacked and would not fall asleep until early morning. She started losing her hair and was compulsively eating candy.

Upon consulting a naturopath, Judy was started on homeopathic supplements. Within 6 weeks Judy's psychiatrist recommended she stop taking her antidepressant drugs. With continued therapy from both practitioners, Judy was able to control her compulsive behaviours and her obsessions with guilt and suicide.

Naturopathy

Originating in Europe, **naturopathy** views disease as an alteration in the process by which the body heals itself. The term *naturopathy* means "nature disease." Its focus is on the six principles described in Box 6.1. Practitioners use several therapies, including diet, herbs, nutritional supplements, hydrotherapy, massage, joint manipulation, and lifestyle counselling.

BOX 6.1 Principles of Naturopathy

1. The healing power of nature
2. Identification and treatment of the cause of disease
3. The concept of "do no harm"
4. The physician care provider as teacher
5. Treatment of the whole person
6. Prevention

Modified from Ullman, J., & Ullman, R. (2007). Healing with homeopathy. *Townsend Letter 2*, 7.

Traditional Chinese Medicine

Traditional Chinese medicine (TCM) can trace its beginnings to 200 BCE. It is based on the view that the body is a delicate balance of opposing forces: yin and yang. Yin is cold, slow, and passive, whereas yang is hot, fast, and active. Health is a balance between these two energies. Mental or physical problems arise when an imbalance of these vital energies (*qi*) results. This leads to blockage of energy and blood along the energy pathways (meridians).

Treatments are chosen on the basis of individual diagnosis and include acupuncture, the use of herbs, food therapy, massage, and body manipulation. The *Chinese Materia Medica* is an extremely old reference book of herbs and other medicinal substances.

Biologically Based Practices

The aim of biologically based practices is to improve the human condition through the use of substances extracted from nature. Treatments with these substances include aromatherapy, dietary supplements, and herbal therapies. Some are based on sound scientific evidence. Other therapies await the outcome of research before their usefulness can be examined.

Aromatherapy

Certain scents evoke certain responses in people. **Aromatherapy**, which involves treatment using scents, is the use of essential oils to promote health and well-being. Most essential oils are obtained from extracts or essences of flowers, herbs, trees, fruits, bark, grasses, and seeds. Each essential oil has distinct therapeutic, physical, and psychological properties. Certain aromas are said to prevent disease, whereas others produce a calming effect.

Aromatherapy has been practised for more than 6 000 years. Early Greeks, Romans, and Egyptians used fragrant oils for massage, bathing, healing the sick, and embalming the dead. It is thought that Hippocrates used aromatic fumigations in an attempt to cure Athens of a plague outbreak (Pinault, 1986).

Today aromatherapy is gaining greater acceptance because research is demonstrating that essential oils can exert specific effects on the individual. Lavender, for example, was found to promote relaxation and increase alpha brain waves, whereas jasmine increased alertness and beta brain waves. Further studies are being conducted.

Dietary Supplements

A **dietary supplement** is any product taken orally that contains one or more ingredients (such as vitamins or amino acids) that are intended to supplement one's diet but are not considered food.

Herbal Products

The use of certain plants (herbs) to treat disease and relieve suffering is an ancient, multicultural practice. Almost every culture uses some kind of plant substance to treat the sick. There are thousands of herbal treatments worldwide, but few are scientifically proven using clinical studies. Therefore, it becomes difficult to predict adverse effects or interactions with pharmaceutical medications or to judge the safety of using the herb. Researchers are currently studying the health claims of many commonly used herbal products.

Regulation of Health Products

In 2004, the Natural and Non-Prescription Health Products Directorate (NNHPD), a branch of Health Canada authorized under the existing *Food and Drugs Act*, was created. The purpose of this addition to the *Food and Drugs Act* is to strictly regulate all products that are categorized as natural health products, including non-prescription drugs. Oversight is achieved by requiring that all products have a product license before they can be sold in Canadian markets.

Body-Based Practices

CAM practices that involve moving some part of the body are termed *body-based*. These practices focus on moving the body into an improved state of function through treatment.

Chiropractic Treatment

The relationship between body structure (the spine) and function is the subject of study for **chiropractic** care. Practitioners use a therapy called *adjustments* to help improve the relationship and help the body heal. Many chiropractic treatments are not proven to be effective, however, and should be considered carefully by the patient prior to undertaking treatment.

Chelation

The chemical EDTA was synthesized in the 1930s by German scientists. Because of its ability to bind with heavy metals, "proponents claim that EDTA **chelation** therapy is effective against atherosclerosis and many other serious health conditions. However, there is no scientific evidence that this is so" (Green, 2013). Current international studies are being conducted to see whether chelation therapy is effective.

Eye Movement Desensitization

In 1987, Francine Shapiro, PhD, a practising psychologist in Palo Alto, California, introduced a new therapy to treat post-traumatic stress disorder (PTSD). **Eye movement desensitization and reprocessing (EMDR)** uses controlled eye movements to help reprocess traumatic memories. EMDR may be used to treat other disorders such as panic attacks, eating disorders, addictions, and anxiety. At first the scientific community dismissed this therapy, but published studies in more than 25 scientific journals have proved the value of EMDR. The therapy is gaining in popularity: "It has been endorsed by government mental health agencies in the United Kingdom and Israel, and is

in wide use throughout the United States and Europe" (Glaser, 2006). EMDR has been used to help victims of 9/11, Hurricane Katrina, and the 2004 South Asia tsunami.

Basically, the patient identifies a problem, such as flashbacks or nightmares of the event. The person also states what they would like to have happen instead. Then the therapist moves his or her hand or a baton in a certain pattern and the patient follows the movement with their eyes while recalling the disturbing event. Each "set" lasts 15 to 20 seconds and ends with the patient describing how their self-perceptions have changed. Some patients are helped with one treatment, but others require several. Most experience fewer negative emotions associated with the event after treatment.

According to Glaser (2006), "many therapists think EMDR helps the rational left side of the brain to 'knit' a disturbing memory from the emotional right side. Often, therapists describe this as *processing*." EMDR is proving to be a useful tool for treating those who suffer from the effects of overwhelming trauma.

Massage

Massage is the manipulation of muscles and connective tissue to relax the body and enhance well-being. It is one of the oldest healing arts, with written records in China that date back 3 000 years. Massage reduces stress, promotes relaxation, and improves circulation. It improves sleep, concentration, and energy. Many people with depression and anxiety are helped by the relaxing powers of massage. Each Canadian province and territory maintains the provision of massage therapy under its own specific regulatory acts and processes.

Phototherapy

A type of somatic therapy using bright lights for the treatment of depression, phototherapy, also known as light therapy, has been used with success in the treatment of seasonal affective disorder (SAD). During the winter months when the available daylight hours are fewer, many people become irritable, unable to concentrate, even depressed. Researchers found that exposure to full-spectrum light for at least 20 minutes per day resulted in an improvement of depressive symptoms (Rosenthal, 1993). Phototherapy appears to be a promising form of treatment for some disorders, but further studies and research are needed to determine its long-term effectiveness.

ENERGY-BASED CAM THERAPIES

Energy-based CAM therapies base their practices on two types of energy fields: the *veritable* and the *putative* (Table 6.2). Practitioners of energy medicine believe that illness results when the body's energies are out of balance. Therapies are intended to restore the amount and flow of body energy.

Mind-Body Medicine

Followers of mind-body medicine believe that the mind and spirit have the ability to affect the body and its functions. The concept of the mind influencing illness and bodily functions is an old one. Traditional Chinese and Ayurvedic medicine adherents practised the concept 2 000 years ago. Hippocrates, the father of allopathic medicine, believed that the mental,

TABLE 6.2	**Comparison of Energy Fields**
Veritable Energy	**Putative (Biofield) Energy**
• Uses mechanical vibration (sound) electromagnetic forces	• Based on concept that humans are infused with a form of energy
• Can be measured	• Cannot be measured
• Uses wavelengths and frequencies to treat patients	• Readjusts the energy flow to treat patients

moral, and spiritual aspects of the patient must be considered if treatment was to be successful. This mind-body approach was followed well into the sixteenth century, when Renaissance science tended toward separating the emotional and spiritual dimensions of humans from the body. As discoveries were made and technologies developed, the purpose became control over nature. Curing the illness became more important than healing the soul. The disease-based model and its search for pathological conditions became the dominant view.

However, in the 1920s, the work of Howard Cannon revealed the "fight or flight" response and demonstrated a direct relationship between stress and neuroendocrine responses in the body. During World War II, physician Henry Beecher showed the placebo effect when he injected wounded soldiers with saline instead of morphine and found that much of their pain was controlled. Later research found that as much as 35% of a therapeutic response to any medical procedure could be the result of the patient's belief about its effectiveness (Beecher, 1959).

Since the 1960s, research into the mind-body connection has been extensive. Much of the evidence demonstrates positive effects related to psychological functioning and improved quality of life. In addition, the risks of mind-body therapies are minimal.

Expressive therapies, such as music or dance, are thought to help people express thoughts and emotions that they are unable to state verbally. Hypnotherapy, meditation, prayer, and spiritual healing are believed to promote relaxation, decrease stress, and relieve emotional or physical pain.

Expressive Therapy

The use of creative activities to decrease stress is not new. Drawing, painting, and sculpting may help release inner conflicts and repressed emotions. Some mental health providers use **expressive therapy** to help diagnose and treat people with depression, schizophrenia, and trauma related to abuse. Dance and music therapy are helpful for those who are recovering from abuse to gain a sense of ease with their own bodies. Listening to music stimulates the body's neurotransmitter production (opiates and endorphins), which results in "feeling good." Music and sound therapy have been used successfully to treat stress, depression, grief, schizophrenia, and autism.

Hypnotherapy

The traditional definition of **hypnosis** is the induction of a relaxed, trancelike state in which the individual is receptive to appropriate suggestions. Brain scans of hypnotized persons document different patterns from those in people who are merely dozing. A typical hypnotherapy session lasts an hour. The therapist speaks softly and helps the patient become deeply relaxed and tuned out from outside distractions. Once the patient reaches "a state of hyperconcentration, the therapist makes suggestions" (Glower, 2005) that can alter the way one thinks and behaves. Smokers, for example, who use hypnosis are more likely to quit successfully. Hypnotherapy is being used to treat gastrointestinal problems, irritable bowel syndrome, pain, headaches, addictions, phobias, and anxiety. Self-induced hypnotic therapies are *relaxation* and *visualization*.

Hypnosis has everyday practical uses also. Bierman (a full-time emergency department physician) focuses on the concepts of human patterns and consciousness. He believes that hypnosis is just ideas and responses. His work with acutely traumatized patients demonstrates the power of the health care providers' words and actions (Bierman, 1995). The accompanying Case Study illustrates the use of Bierman's response-evoking hypnosis.

CASE STUDY

Larry, an alert 6-year-old, arrives at the clinic knowing that he will be on the receiving end of a "shot." He dreads the sight of the approaching nurse and begins to whimper. The nurse smiles and says, "I would like you, Larry, to hold still and look very closely at the circle over there. Tell me whether it is getting bigger or smaller, and really look! Just look hard, and tell me . . ." By this time, the injection has been given. "But I don't see it," says Larry. "That's right," says the nurse, "and you didn't feel it either!"

• What do you think made the outcome of this situation so positive?

Meditation

Meditation has been used in Eastern religions for more than 2 500 years. It has gained popularity in the West as a tool for combating stress. Many therapists who recommend meditation for their patients meditate daily themselves. There are many techniques for meditation, but all share four common elements: concentration, retraining the attention to one item while excluding all other thoughts, mindfulness, and an altered state of consciousness (Fig. 6.2). The physical effects of twice-daily meditation include "slower heart rate, decreased blood pressure, lower oxygen consumption, and increased alpha brain wave production" (Moore, 2010). Meditation techniques have been used successfully in the fields of education, business, medicine, and mental health care.

Prayer and Spiritual Healing

As a CAM therapy, prayer was utilized by only 15% of Canadians in 2016. **Prayer** is defined as an active process of appealing to a higher spiritual power, specifically for health reasons. **Spirituality** has a broader meaning that includes an individual's sense of meaning and purpose in life. Several studies are now being conducted to look at how prayer affects immune system functions and emotional well-being.

Mindfulness

Mindfulness is functioning, and being aware of oneself and one's immediate environment, in the moment. It is a process

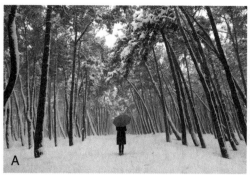 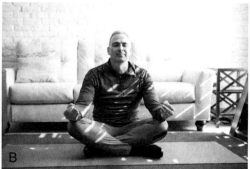

Fig. 6.2 Meditation can assume many forms. (A, iStockphoto/sguler; B, iStockphoto/Antonio_Diaz.)

TABLE 6.3	Life Force Energy*
Name	**Culture**
Qi	Traditional Chinese medicine
Ki	Japanese kampoo system
Doshas	Ayurvedic medicine

*Life force energy is also called *biofields, etheric energy, fohat, homeopathic resonance, mana, orgone force,* and *prana.*

of avoiding distractions and wandering thoughts, to fully immerse and experience what is happening to you—while it happens. "Mindfulness is a way of being that involves being fully present in the moment and observing one's own thoughts, feelings and actions without evaluating them or trying to change or avoid them" (Stein-Parbury, 2018, p. 320).

Energy Medicine

Practitioners of energy medicine believe in a vital, life force energy that flows through the human body. This life force is known by many names (Table 6.3). Although these energies have not been proven scientifically, therapists "claim they can work with this subtle energy, see it with their own eyes, and use it to effect changes in the physical body and influence health" (NCCAM, 2007). For the purposes of discussion, energy medicine is divided into two parts: biofield therapies and bioelectromagnetic field therapies.

Biofield Therapies

These are among some of the most used but unmeasured CAM therapies. Examples include acupuncture, biofeedback, Qi Gong, Reiki, therapeutic touch, and colour therapy.

Acupuncture. For more than 2 000 years, a treatment in Asian medicine has cured disease and alleviated suffering. **Acupuncture** is defined as the inserting of fine needles into the skin along specific sites on the body. These sites travel along energy channels called *meridians.* Stimulating these points is thought to restore the energy or *qi* balance within the body. More Western explanations of acupuncture relate to the release and movement of neurotransmitters, neuropeptides, and hormones. Acupuncture has been successfully used for the treatment of drug addictions and is proving to be a cost-effective and safe form of therapy.

Biofeedback. **Biofeedback** teaches patients to control their physical responses by providing visual or auditory information about autonomic body functions. Body functions such as respiration, pulse, or skin responses are monitored by machines while patients practise relaxation techniques and change the monitored data. For example, changes in respiratory or pulse rates that can be seen on a graph provide patients with objective feedback and encouragement. Biofeedback has proven useful in treating anxiety, hypertension, insomnia, headaches, and attention-deficit disorders.

Qi Gong. *Qi* is the Chinese name for vital energy. **Qi Gong** and Tai Chi are systems of movement, regulation of breathing, and meditation designed to enhance the flow of *qi* throughout the body.

Reiki. The word *Reiki* comes from the Japanese words *rei,* meaning "God's wisdom" or "Higher Power," and the word *ki,* which is "life force energy." **Reiki** is a life force energy that flows through one's body. When it is low, we are stressed or sick. When it is in abundance, we feel healthy and happy. Practitioners of Reiki use a "laying on of the hands" to promote relaxation and promote healing.

Therapeutic touch. **Therapeutic touch** is based on the practice of laying on of the hands. The healing energies of the therapist encourage the body's energies to return to a balanced state. Healers pass their hands over the body to identify the blockages or energy imbalances. The therapist then strengthens and reorients the body energies, thus restoring the biofield. Therapeutic touch is effective in stress-related conditions, such as migraine headaches and anxiety. Caution should be exercised, however, because mental health conditions such as paranoia, hallucinations, or delusions are associated with an impaired sense of touch.

Colour therapy. As stated earlier, high-intensity light has been used to successfully treat SAD. Colour therapy is still being studied, but practitioners believe that the energy fields that surround each of us (auras) are filled with constantly changing energies of colour. When one is sick, the aura is discoloured. Colour therapists scan the energy centres (chakras) for imbalances and expose the body to the appropriate healing colour to help heal the physical problem and rebalance energies.

Electromagnetic Field Therapies

Standard medicine has used electromagnetic field energy for years in magnetic resonance imaging (MRI), radiation therapy, cardiac pacemakers, and more. However, the use of that energy to treat illness with **electromagnetic fields (EMF)** is still under study.

TABLE 6.4 Complementary and Alternative Mental Health Therapies

Mental Health Issue	Complementary and Alternative Medicine Therapies
Stress, anxiety	Aromatherapy, diet, certain herbs, massage
Depression	Meditation, prayer, acupuncture, biofeedback, Reiki, therapeutic touch, music, dance, yoga, phototherapy, naturopathy
Post-traumatic stress disorder (PTSD)	Meditation, eye movement desensitization and reprocessing (EMDR), biofeedback, yoga
Sleep disorders	Aromatherapy, diet, certain herbs, massage, meditation, prayer, progressive relaxation

In magnetic therapy, magnets are placed over painful areas to relieve pain. Repetitive transcranial magnetic stimulation (TMS) has been successfully used to treat severe depression. Pulsating electromagnetic therapy enhances bone healing and is claimed to be effective with sleep disorders and headaches. Millimetre wave therapy has been used in Russia and other Eastern European countries to treat both physical and psychiatric illnesses. Exposure to low-power millimetre waves is thought to increase immunity and improve well-being. The main courses of action for these therapies are not well understood. Further investigations are being conducted.

TECHNOLOGY-BASED CAM APPLICATIONS

With the increasing use of electronic devices, mental health advice is just a text message away. Organizations like the Kids Help Phone and Crisis Services Canada offer 24-hour text-based crisis intervention. Electronic communications offer a wide range of information as well as a means of communicating with others using a medium that is known and comfortable for the user.

CAM APPROACHES TO MENTAL HEALTH CARE

An increasing number of people are seeking help for their emotional and mental health challenges through the use of nonmedical therapies and treatments. In fact, surveys have indicated that the number of "office visits to alternative medical practitioners already exceeds the number of visits to traditional medical physicians" (Sarnat, 2001). Table 6.4 lists some CAM therapies currently being used to treat several mental health conditions. Partnerships among CAM therapists and the traditional medical community are being formed in several areas of Canada and the United States. Many European nations have used some CAM therapies for years.

Many complementary and alternative therapies are proving to be effective and useful. Others are not. Some therapies have the potential to be dangerous, especially if used along with standard medical treatments. Ultimately, the consumer of health care services will make the choice. It is our responsibility to keep informed of the latest developments in CAM practices.

CAM Mental Health Therapies

Alternative approaches to mental illness emphasize the interactions of the body, mind, and spirit. Some therapies have long histories. Many remain unproven and controversial. The National Mental Health Information Center (www.mentalhealth.org) discusses several approaches to achieving mental wellness, discussed next.

Animal-Assisted Therapy

Animals are consistent and nonjudgemental. They are always accepting and help ease loneliness. Assistance dogs have helped people with physical disabilities for years. According to Vaughn (2007), "assistance dogs have been trained to aid those with certain conditions, such as severe social anxiety, young people with autism, and individuals prone to seizures." Many prisons now have programs that match inmates with shelter dogs. Working with animals has been found to promote socialization, increase empathy, encourage responsibility and commitment, and foster communication.

Culturally Based Healing

Acupuncture has been used to successfully treat individuals with stress, anxiety, and depression. It has been used in children with hyperactivity and attention-deficit disorders. Some therapists use it to assist the patient with detoxification from alcohol or drugs. Yoga and meditation can relieve stress and anxiety. Remember also that one's culture has a profound effect on the outcome of treatment.

Nutrition

The connection between mental health and nutrition has been theorized for thousands of years. Often individuals with mental health challenges consume lower-quality foods, possibly because the challenges of managing a mental health condition leave little energy or motivation to focus on nutritional needs. Poor-quality foods might have an impact on overall mental health. Research into the influences of and connection between nutrition and mental health has only recently begun. While many people feel that better quality nutrition makes them function better, more empirical, objective research is needed to identify and confirm why this is so.

Pastoral Counselling

Ministers, pastors, priests, and rabbis offer prayer and therapeutic listening. Many are not trained therapists, but most are wise in offering support and comfort. Pastoral counsellors work within a religious community where members work to help and support one another.

Self-Help Groups

People with related problems find great support and understanding with others with similar experiences. Those who "have

> ### BOX 6.2   Characteristics of Self-Help Groups
>
> Members have similar needs.
> The purpose is to help people cope with a life-changing event such as addiction, abuse, death, or diagnosis of a mental illness.
> Membership in the group is voluntary, confidential, and anonymous.
> Groups are informal, nonprofit, and free.
> Meetings are facilitated by a survivor or one familiar with the shared experience(s).
> Groups provide support, education, and ongoing encouragement.

products. Consult their database frequently at https://www.canada.ca/en/health-canada/services/drugs-health-products/natural-non-prescription/applications-submissions/product-licensing/licensed-natural-health-products-database.html for new information about CAM practices.

> ### CRITICAL THINKING
>
> You are monitoring the response of a patient who is taking an antipsychotic medication. He informs you that he has been taking an herbal preparation for his hallucinations and is now ready to stop taking his prescribed medications.
> • How would you respond to him?

been there" are invaluable resources for empowering others toward recovery. Box 6.2 describes the characteristics of self-help groups.

Stress Reduction and Relaxation

Learning to control the body's fight-or-flight response helps us to avoid the negative effects of stress. Techniques such as *guided imagery* and *creative visualization* teach the user to achieve a deep state of relaxation and then create a mental scenario of healing and wellness. Depression, alcohol and drug addictions, panic disorders, phobias, and stress have been treated with these techniques. Biofeedback offers objective evidence of relaxation. It has proven to be a useful tool in helping people with severe anxiety, phobias, and panic attacks.

WORDS OF CAUTION

Many CAM approaches to mental health care are based on years of observation, testing, and successful treatment; however, others are relatively new and unproven. Because we practise within an allopathic (traditional medical) framework, we use data derived from research and studies to draw conclusions. Health Canada licenses nontraditional drugs and

Adverse Effects

Some CAM therapies may have adverse or unwanted effects, especially if combined with traditional treatments. Prescription drugs can interact with certain herbs. Chelation therapy can deplete the body of potassium. Allergic reactions may result from inappropriate use of diet supplements or foods. Sometimes the individual is masking a serious need for medical help with an ineffective CAM therapy. It is important to fully explore a CAM therapy before engaging in any of its practices.

Implications for Care Providers

The use of CAM therapies to treat mental health challenges must be approached with caution. Always consult your supervisor and the patient's primary care provider before suggesting anything to the patient. Many times the whole picture is not apparent, and doing no harm is the care provider's first priority.

If a CAM therapy is used in your health care environment, learn as much as possible about it, including both the negative and positive aspects. Many changes and new discoveries are on the horizon as we attempt to learn more about one another and our complexities.

KEY POINTS

- Allopathic practitioners use medical and surgical methods to treat disease and injury by finding what is "wrong" and "fixing" it.
- Complementary medicine includes practices and treatments that agree or "work with" allopathic therapies. They are used along with common medical treatments.
- Alternative medicine refers to practices and treatments that are used instead of conventional (allopathic) medicine.
- Integrative medicine attempts to blend the most effective practices and treatments from both conventional and alternative treatment systems. Emphasis is on the interrelationship among body, mind, and spirit.
- The primary goal of holistic mental health care providers is to help patients develop strategies to achieve harmony within themselves and with others, nature, and the world.
- Whole medical systems are built on complete systems of theory and practice and include Western medicine,

osteopathy, homeopathy, naturopathy, and culturally based systems such as Ayurveda and Asian medicine.
- Biologically based practices use substances extracted from nature. Treatments include aromatherapy, dietary supplements, and herbal therapies.
- Body-based practices focus on moving the body into an improved state of function through treatment. They include chiropractic treatment, chelation, eye movement desensitization and reprocessing (EMDR), massage, and phototherapy.
- Energy-based therapies base their practices on two types of energy fields: the veritable and the putative.
- Followers of mind-body medicine believe that the mind and spirit have the ability to affect the body and its functions.
- Mind-body therapies include expressive therapies, such as music or dance, hypnotherapy, meditation, prayer, and spiritual healing.

- Practitioners of energy medicine believe in a vital, life force energy that flows through the human body.
- Energy medicine is divided into two areas: biofield therapies and bioelectromagnetic field therapies.
- Biofield therapies are among some of the most used but unmeasured CAM therapies.
- Examples of biofield therapies are acupuncture, biofeedback, Qi Gong, Tai Chi, Reiki, therapeutic touch, and colour therapy.
- Current bioelectromagnetic field theories operate on the theory that energy can treat illness.
- Magnetic therapy, repetitive transcranial magnetic stimulation (TMS), pulsating electromagnetic therapy, and millimetre wave therapy are bioelectromagnetic applications of this theory.
- Technology-based approaches to mental health care include telemedicine, telephone and text-based counselling, and hotlines.
- The use of CAM therapies to treat mental health challenges must be approached with caution because some CAM therapies may have adverse or unwanted effects.

ADDITIONAL LEARNING RESOURCES

Go to your Evolve website (http://evolve.elsevier.com/Canada/Morrison-Valfre/) for additional online resources, including the online Study Guide for additional learning activities to help you master this chapter content.

CRITICAL THINKING QUESTIONS

1. A mental health patient advises you that he plans to stop using his prescribed antidepressant, and instead will begin using an alternative product called St. John's wort. What would be an appropriate response to this patient?
2. A patient tells you that she is interested in the services of a registered massage therapist (RMT). She is nervous about the physical contact, however, and has a history of having experienced sexual abuse as a young child. What information about this profession could you provide?
3. A patient with a history of anxiety tells you that he would like to try an Indigenous sweat lodge experience, and has signed up for a weekend get-a-way to do so. The patient asks your opinion about this, and asks specifically if you think it will be worth the money.

REFERENCES

Beecher, H. (1959). *Measurement of subjective response*. Oxford University Press.

Bierman, S. F. (1995). Medical hypnosis. *Advances: The Journal of Mind-Body Health, 11*(1), 65.

Boiron, T. (2007). *Easy guide to homeopathy*. Boiron.

Glaser, G. (2006). Eye-catching therapy. *Oregonian, 155*(52,420) C1, August 23.

Glower, T. (2005). Your best alternative. *Health, 19*(6).

Government of Canada. (2019). *Licensed natural health products database (LNHPD)*. https://www.canada.ca/en/health-canada/services/drugs-health-products/natural-non-prescription/applications-submissions/product-licensing/licensed-natural-health-products-database.html

Green, S. (2013). *Chelation therapy: Unproven claims and unsound theories*. Quackwatch. https://www.quackwatch.org/01QuackeryRelatedTopics/chelation.html

Moore, S. (2010). Meditation. In I. B. Weiner, & W. E. Craighead (Eds.), *Corsini's encyclopedia of psychology* (4th ed.). Wiley.

National Center for Complementary and Alternative Medicine (NCCAM). (2007). *Biologically based practices: An overview*. https://www.nccam.nih.gov/health

Pinault, J. R. (1986). How Hippocrates cured the plague. *Journal of the History of Medicine and Allied Sciences, 41*(1), 52–75.

Rawlins, R. P., Williams, S. R., & Beck, C. K. (1993). *Mental health–psychiatric nursing: A holistic life-cycle approach* (3rd ed.). Mosby.

Rosenthal, N. (1993). *Winter blues: SAD—what it is and how to overcome it*. Guilford Press.

Sarnat, R. L. (2001). The future is now. *Total Health, 23*(2), 22.

Stein-Parbury, J. (2018). *Patient & person: Interpersonal skills in nursing* (6th ed.). Elsevier Australia.

Vaughn, D. (2007). Doggone helpful. *NurseWeek, 8*(13), 20.

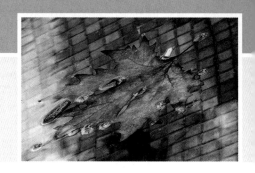

7

Psychotherapeutic Medication Therapy

OBJECTIVES

Upon completion of this text, the student will be able to:

1. Briefly explain how psychotherapeutic medications affect human beings.
2. Identify four classifications of psychotherapeutic medications.
3. Discuss three classes of antianxiety agents and the adverse effects associated with each.
4. Prepare a list of teaching points for patients who are beginning antidepressant therapy.
5. Explain the three major guidelines for care of patients taking lithium.
6. Identify one central nervous system and three peripheral nervous system adverse effects of antipsychotic (neuroleptic) medication therapy.
7. Describe five care guidelines for patients receiving psychotherapeutic medications.
8. Discuss three topics for teaching patients about their medications.
9. Explain how informed consent and nonadherence relate to psychotherapeutic medications.

OUTLINE

KEY TERMS

affective (ă-FĔC-tĭv) **disorder** (p. 72)
akathisia (ĂK-ə-THĒ-zhə) (p. 75)
akinesia (Ă-kĭ-NĒ-zh ə) (p. 75)
antipsychotics (ĂN-tī-sī-KŎT-ĭks) (p. 71)
autonomic nervous system (ANS) (ŏ-tō-NŎM-ĭk NŬR-vŭs SĬS-těm) (p. 69)
central nervous system (CNS) (SĔN-trŭl NŬR-vŭs SĬS-těm) (p. 69)
drug-induced parkinsonism (DRŬG-ĭn-doost PĂHR-kĬn-s ə n-ĭz-əm) (p. 75)
dyskinesia (DĬS-kĭ-NĒ-zhə) (p. 75)
dystonia (dĭs-TŌN-nē-ə) (p. 75)
extrapyramidal (ĔKS-tră-pĭ-RĂM-Ĭ-dĂl) **side effects** (EPSEs) (p. 75)
hypertensive crisis (hī-pĕr-TĔN-sĭv CRĬ-sĭs) (p. 72)
informed consent (p. 79)
lithium (LĬTH-ē-əm) (p. 73)

mania (MĀ-nē-ə) (p. 73)
monoamine oxidase inhibitors (MAOIs) (MŎN-ō-ă-MĒN ŎK-sĭ-dās ĭn-HĬB-ĭ-tors) (p. 72)
mood disorders (p. 72)
neuroleptic malignant syndrome (NMS) (NOOR-ō-LĔP-tĬk m -LĬG-nănt SĬN-drōm) (p. 75)
neuron (NOOR-ŏn) (p. 70)
neurotransmitter (NOOR-ō-TRĂNS-mĬ-tĔr) (p. 70)
nonadherence (p. 78)
parasympathetic (PAR-ă-SĬM-pă-THĒT-Ĭk) **nervous system** (p. 69)
peripheral (pĕ-RĬF-ĕr-ăl) **nervous system** (PNS) (p. 69)
psychotherapeutic (SĬ-kō-thĕr-ə-PYŪ-tĭk) **medications** (p. 69)
sympathetic nervous system (SĬM-pə -THĒT-ĭk) (p. 69)
tardive dyskinesia (TĂR-dĭv DĬS-kĭ-NĒ-zhă) (p. 75)

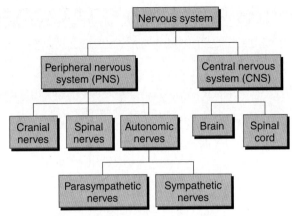

Fig. 7.1 Divisions of the nervous system.

Psychotherapeutic medications are powerful chemicals that produce profound effects on the mind, emotions, and body (Keltner & Folks, 2005). Their efficacy was first discovered as side effects of other medications, such as antihistamines for allergies. In 1949 lithium was found to be effective in treating the mania of bipolar illness. The 1950s brought the use of chlorpromazine (Thorazine) into the therapeutic regimen. The tranquilizer meprobamate (Miltown) became so popular in 1955 that drugstores were required to place signs in the window when they sold out (Keltner & Steele, 2019). By the early 1960s, tricyclic antidepressants, monoamine oxidase inhibitors (MAOIs), and haloperidol (Haldol) were on the market. The antianxiety medication called diazepam (Valium) became extremely popular, and soon it was the most often prescribed medication in the world. Newer psychotherapeutic drugs have been introduced, and even more will be available in the future. Health care providers who work with these drugs must remember that psychotherapeutic medications are powerful chemicals with many, sometimes severe, adverse effects.

HOW PSYCHOTHERAPEUTIC MEDICATION THERAPY WORKS

Psychiatric medications act on the body's central nervous system by altering the delicate chemical balances and imbalances within that system. Most psychotherapeutic medications interrupt the chemical messenger (neurotransmitter) pathways within the brain by suppressing major nerve pathways that connect the internal structures of the brain to the frontal lobes and limbic system.

The frontal lobes of the brain are the source of the higher human functions, such as love, creativity, insight, planning, judgement, and abstract reasoning. The limbic system is responsible for emotions, motivation, memory, and the fight-or-flight response. When these areas of the brain are affected by medications, profound changes in behaviour result. People usually experience more stable moods, but *many higher brain functions are impaired.* As with all medications, there is a trade-off between therapeutic effects and unwanted reactions. One of the primary responsibilities of health care providers (especially nurses) is to recognize therapeutic versus unwanted effects.

The human nervous system consists of an intricate network of structures that activates, coordinates, and controls all the functions of the body. All parts of the nervous system work together. It is important to remember that if a drug affects one part of the nervous system it will, without a doubt, have an impact on the other activities of the system. Figure 7.1 illustrates the divisions of the nervous system.

The **central nervous system (CNS)** is composed of the brain and spinal cord. Together they control all the motor and sensory functions of the body. Information travels from the brain down through the spinal cord, reaches the appropriate muscle group, and results in movement. Sensory information (e.g., touch, temperature, position) is relayed in the opposite direction: from the muscles and other body areas, *up* through the spinal cord, and into the brain. Throughout this process, the CNS combines all incoming (sensory) and outgoing (motor) data.

The **peripheral nervous system (PNS)** is composed of the 31 spinal cord nerves plus the 12 pairs of cranial nerves. The peripheral nervous system is further divided into a "motor" system and an "autonomic" (automatic) system. Each spinal nerve contains motor and sensory neurons (nerve cells). The motor portion of the spinal nerve activates heart, muscles, and glandular secretions, whereas sensations of touch, temperature, pain, and spatial perception are transmitted by the sensory portion. The cranial nerves carry a mixture of information; some nerves are mainly motor, others carry mainly sensory information, and a few perform both motor and sensory functions.

The **autonomic nervous system (ANS)** is responsible for regulating the vital functions of the body. The activities of the heart muscle, smooth muscles, and glandular secretions are all controlled "automatically" by this remarkable system. There are two divisions of the autonomic nervous system: the sympathetic and parasympathetic systems. They work together to monitor and govern "automatic" body responses.

The **sympathetic nervous system** prepares the body for immediate adaptation through the fight-or-flight mechanism. The heart rate and output increase, which moves blood into the muscles. Vessels to the stomach and other nonvital organs constrict and detour blood to the skeletal muscles. The pupils of the eyes dilate to improve visual acuity, and the bronchioles of the lungs expand to allow for greater exchange of airflow. Increases in blood sugar and fatty acid levels provide glucose for fuel, and all digestive and excretory processes are slowed. The result is greater cellular energy production and increased mental activity. Physically, the body is preparing to protect itself. People who are highly stressed demonstrate many sympathetic nervous system responses.

The **parasympathetic nervous system** is designed to conserve energy and provide the balance for the sympathetic system's excitability. The main functions of this system are to monitor and maintain control over the "regulatory" processes of the body, which it accomplishes by governing smooth muscle tone and glandular secretions. Parasympathetic stimulation slows the heart rate, decreases circulating blood volume, relaxes sphincters, and increases intestinal and glandular activity. Respiratory, circulatory, digestive, excretory, and

TABLE 7.1 Autonomic Nervous System Actions

Tissue	Parasympathetic (Cholinergic or Muscarinic) Response	Sympathetic (Adrenergic) Response
Eye	Constriction (miosis)	Dilation (mydriasis)
	Accommodation (focus on near objects)	
Glands	Increased salivation (copious, watery)	Increased sweating*
	Increased tears and secretions of respiratory and gastrointestinal tract	Increased salivation (thick, contains proteins)
Heart	Decreased rate	Increased rate
	Decreased strength of contraction	Increased strength of contraction
	Decreased conduction velocity through the atrioventricular node	Increased conduction velocity through the atrioventricular node
Bronchioles	Smooth muscle constriction (restricts airways)	Smooth muscle relaxation (opens airways)
Blood vessels	Constriction of vessels in heart (not a prominent effect in humans)	Dilation of vessels in heart and skeletal muscle
	Dilation of vessels in salivary gland and erectile tissues	Constriction of vessels in skin, viscera, salivary gland, erectile tissues, kidney
Gastrointestinal Tract		
Smooth muscle	Contraction	Relaxation
Sphincters	Relaxation	Contraction
Urinary Bladder		
Fundus	Contraction	Relaxation
Trigone and sphincter	Relaxation	Contraction
Uterus		Contraction
Liver		Glycogenolysis

*Acetylcholine is the neurotransmitter for this response.
Modified from Clark, J. F., Queener, S. F., & Karb, V. B. (2000). *The pharmacologic basis of nursing practice* (6th ed.). Mosby.

BOX 7.1 Neurotransmitters

Type	Examples
Amino acids	Glutamate, aspartate, glycine, D-serine, gamma-aminobutyric acid (GABA)
Biogenic amines	Monoamines, serotonin, norepinephrine, epinephrine, histamine, melatonin
Neuropeptides	Beta-endorphin, opioid peptides, somatostatin, calcitonin, vasopressin, oxytocin, glucagon
Others	Acetylcholine, dopamine, adenosine, nitric oxide

reproductive functions respond to parasympathetic messages. The parasympathetic nervous system uses the neurotransmitter acetylcholine to do its work, and it is often referred to as the *cholinergic nervous system.*

The sympathetic and parasympathetic divisions of the autonomic nervous system act in opposite ways. Fortunately, this excite-and-calm interaction provides a balance. Organs are rich in both adrenergic (sympathetic) and cholinergic (parasympathetic) receptor sites, and this allows the organism to maintain itself in a state of balance, or homeostasis. Table 7.1 lists the physical responses to parasympathetic

and sympathetic nervous system stimulation. It is wise to be familiar with these responses because many people who take psychotherapeutic medications demonstrate adverse effects related to autonomic nervous system functions.

The basic unit of the nervous system is the **neuron**, or nerve cell. Its function is to transmit electrical information to other neurons. Electrical information travelling through a neuron generates a chemical messenger called a **neurotransmitter**. Although nerve cells are found in great abundance throughout the body, they are not physically connected to one another. Each neuron is separated by a small space or gap called a *synapse.* Neurotransmitters travel across this gap, open a channel for the electrical information to pass, and then quickly become inactivated. Neurotransmitters are divided into groups: *biogenic amines* (monoamines), *amino acids,* and *neuropeptides* (Box 7.1). Many psychotherapeutic drugs alter the flow of message exchanges in or around the synapse. The study of the neurochemistry of behaviour has already altered the way in which mental–emotional conditions are considered.

CLASSIFICATIONS OF PSYCHOTHERAPEUTIC MEDICATIONS

The traditional four classes of psychotherapeutic medications are (1) antianxiety drugs; (2) antidepressants; (3) mood

TABLE 7.2 Antianxiety and Antidepressant Medications

Drug Class	Examples	Comments
Azapirones (for anxiety)	buspirone (BuSpar)	Takes 2–4 weeks to relieve symptoms of anxiety; not habit forming; does not impair memory, balance, or cause sedation; minimal adverse effects
Benzodiazepines (for anxiety)	triazolam (Halcion), lorazepam (Ativan), chlordiazepoxide (Librium), diazepam (Valium)	Oldest anxiolytic; fast acting; main adverse effect is drowsiness; potential for dependency; withdrawal symptoms if stopped abruptly
Beta-blockers (for anxiety)	propranolol (Inderal), atenolol (Tenormin)	Used to treat social phobias; reduces palpitations, sweating, tremors, blood pressure, and heart rate
Tricyclics (TCAs) (for depression, anxiety)	amitriptyline (Elavil), desipramine (Norpramin), doxepin (Sinequan Triadapin), imipramine (Tofranil), nortriptyline (Pamelor)	Takes 2–3 weeks to take effect; adverse effects: drowsiness, dry mouth, dizziness, weight gain, impaired sexual function; treats anxiety, depression, post-traumatic stress disorder (PTSD), obsessive-compulsive disorder
Monoamine oxidase inhibitors (MAOIs) (for depression)	phenelzine (Nardil), tranylcypromine (Parnate), selegiline (Carbex)	Not often prescribed because of serious adverse reactions and interactions with food and medications; strong dietary restrictions
Selective serotonin reuptake inhibitors (SSRIs) (for depression)	citalopram (Celexa), escitalopram (Cipralex), fluvoxamine (Luvox), fluoxetine (Prozac), paroxetine (Paxil), sertraline (Zoloft)	First choice for treating anxiety, depression, other problems; adverse effects: gastrointestinal distress, headache, dizziness, sexual dysfunction
Atypical antidepressants (for depression)	mirtazapine (Remeron), bupropion (Wellbutrin), maprotiline (Ludiomil), trazodone (Desyrel)	Agitation can occur with bupropion; common adverse effects: sleepiness, increased appetite, weight gain, dizziness
Selective serotonin/norepinephrine reuptake inhibitors (SNRIs) (for depression)	duloxetine (Cymbalta), venlafaxine (Effexor)	Adverse effects: nausea, dry mouth, dizziness, sedation, sweating, anorexia; monitor blood pressures

stabilizers, which are used to treat mood or emotional disorders; and (4) **antipsychotics**, which help curb hallucinations and loss of reality experienced by individuals with psychotic disorders.

Millions of people are currently being treated with psychotherapeutic medications. People receiving psychotherapeutic (also called *psychotropic*) medications must be routinely monitored for effectiveness, adverse effects, and life-threatening adverse reactions. Because of this need for close monitoring, *all* health care providers must be knowledgeable about the roles that these powerful chemicals play in treating mental illness.

Antianxiety Medications

Anxiety is common to us all, but when it interferes with one's ability to function it becomes an anxiety disorder. In today's world, anxiety disorders are a common mental health challenge. A thorough discussion of anxiety and its treatments can be found in Chapter 18. Here we consider the antianxiety medications that are a usual part of the therapeutic treatment plan.

Antianxiety drugs are medications that reduce the psychic tension of stress. They are also referred to as *anxiolytics* or *minor tranquilizers*. Medications in the antianxiety group are divided by their chemical formulas into categories. Table 7.2

lists the major medications used to treat anxiety and depression.

The benzodiazepines have "dominated clinical practice for more than three decades" (Keltner & Folks, 2005) in the treatment of anxiety disorders. They are effective, are generally well tolerated, and do not affect sleeping patterns (a common problem with many psychotherapeutic medications). Benzodiazepines are prescribed to provide sedation, induce sleep (called a *hypnotic*), prevent seizures, and prepare patients for general anaesthesia, but they are mainly used to decrease anxiety.

People with high levels of anxiety have low levels of a neurotransmitter called gamma-aminobutyric acid (GABA). Benzodiazepines act by increasing GABA activity, which results in decreased anxiety. They are fast acting, with the onset of action occurring within 1 hour. The medication exerts its action (duration) for about 4 to 6 hours. Thus, patients experience relief from symptoms within a fairly short span of time.

Benzodiazepines are metabolized by the liver and excreted by the kidneys. People with impaired liver or kidney function must be carefully monitored if this drug class is prescribed. Pregnant and nursing women are usually not treated with benzodiazepines because these medications enter the breast milk. Caution must also be used when administering

TABLE 7.3   Interactions With Monoamine Oxidase Inhibitors (MAOIs)

Type of Interaction	Signs/Symptoms
Anticholinergic reactions	Dry mouth, decreased tearing, blurred vision, constipation, urinary hesitancy or retention, excessive sweating
Hypertensive crisis	Throbbing, radiating headache, stiff neck, palpitations, tightness in chest, sweating, dilated pupils, very high blood pressure and pulse rate
CNS depression	Changes in level of consciousness; sedation, increasing lethargy, disorientation, confusion, agitation, hallucinations, lower seizure threshold

CNS, central nervous system.

antianxiety drugs to older or debilitated adults because of their slower metabolism.

The adverse effects of benzodiazepines are usually minimal, but they include fatigue, sedation, dizziness, and orthostatic hypotension (a drop in blood pressure on standing). Because long-term use of antianxiety medications can result in dependence, therapy for patients is usually limited to a few months.

The antianxiety drug called *buspirone* (BuSpar) differs from benzodiazepines in several ways. First, it belongs to a different chemical class, the azapirones, and does not cause the sleepiness or muscle relaxation associated with benzodiazepines. Second, therapeutic effects are not seen for 3 to 6 weeks after beginning treatment. Buspirone has less potential for abuse; however, patients are still cautioned to avoid alcohol. Third, the potential for overdose is lessened because the drug has a wide dosage range. Adverse effects are few: light-headedness, dizziness, headache, and nausea (Keltner & Steele, 2019).

The medication pregabalin (Lyrica) is classified as an anti-convulsant drug; however, it has also been found to exert a beneficial anxiolytic effect. It is currently being introduced to treat several kinds of anxiety disorders as well as seizures and neuropathic pain. Adverse effects are fewer than those of other antianxiety medications, so patients are more likely to adhere to their treatment.

Antianxiety drugs have several medication interactions, including CNS depression when they are combined with other CNS depressants, such as alcohol and street drugs (Skidmore-Roth, 2015). The combination can produce serious, even fatal, reactions. Concentrations of the cardiac drug digoxin may be increased during treatment with antianxiety medications, so patients taking this medication must be routinely assessed for signs or symptoms of digoxin toxicity. Antacids should not be taken because they interfere with absorption of the antianxiety drug into the bloodstream.

Nursing care for patients receiving antianxiety drugs includes frequent assessments for therapeutic actions and adverse effects. Many of these medications are prescribed on an "as needed" (prn) basis. Medications used on this basis require accurate patient assessments, good judgement, repeated evaluations of the medication's effects, and objective documentation.

Antidepressant Medications

Feelings of great joy and deep sadness are common human experiences. We are all familiar with these emotional extremes and think of them as the natural highs and lows of everyday life. But when one's mood begins to interfere with the ability to perform the routine activities of daily living, intervention is needed.

Mood disorders are ineffective emotional states, ranging from deep depression to excited elation. They are also called **affective disorders** because the word *affect* means "emotions." The major mood disorders are discussed in Chapter 21.

Antidepressant medications exert their action in the body by increasing certain neurotransmitter activities. Antidepressants are divided into categories based on their chemical formula: tricyclic antidepressants, **monoamine oxidase inhibitors** (MAOIs), selective serotonin reuptake inhibitors (SSRIs), atypical antidepressants, and selective serotonin/norepinephrine reuptake inhibitors (SNRIs) (see Table 7.2).

The physician's first choice for the treatment of depression is often an antidepressant. Antidepressants are also indicated for bipolar disorders, panic disorders, obsessive-compulsive disorders, enuresis (bed-wetting), bulimia, and neuropathic pain. Antidepressants have been used with success in post-traumatic stress disorder (PTSD), organic mood disorders, attention-deficit/hyperactivity disorder (ADHD), and conduct disorders in children.

Antidepressants interact with a variety of other substances. Because they block the destruction of specific major neurotransmitters, higher levels of these chemicals circulate throughout the body. Ingesting foods or medications that contain certain chemicals produces more neurotransmitters, which can result in overstimulation of the nervous system. Antidepressant medication interactions can produce serious cardiovascular and blood pressure reactions as well as CNS depression. Table 7.3 describes the more serious medication interactions encountered with the MAOI antidepressants.

Antidepressant medications require 1 to 4 weeks before relief is noticed. However, adverse effects may be experienced soon after beginning therapy. Some adverse effects are a nuisance, such as a dry mouth. Others, such as a **hypertensive crisis** (a sudden, severe elevation in blood pressure) can be life-threatening. Anticholinergic adverse effects include dryness of the mouth, nose, and eyes; urinary retention; and sedation. These discomforts can be so bothersome that some people refuse to take their medications regularly. Patients should be routinely monitored for physical and behavioural changes. Those experiencing postural hypotension should be protected from falls. Kidney and liver function should be assessed and monitored monthly. Any signs of toxicity (e.g.,

BOX 7.2 Dietary and Medication Interactions With Monoamine Oxidase Inhibitors (MAOIs)

Medications to Avoid

Prescription and over-the-counter medications: nasal and sinus decongestants; cold, allergy, and hay fever remedies; inhalants for asthma; weight-loss pills, pep pills, stimulants; narcotics, local anaesthetics

Any medication should be approved by the physician

Illicit drugs: cocaine, any amphetamine (uppers)

Foods to Avoid

Alcoholic drinks: beer, ale, red wines, sherry wines, liqueurs, cognac

Dairy products: aged cheese, sour cream

Fruits and vegetables: avocados, bananas, fava and broad beans, canned figs, any overripe fruit

Meats: pickled or smoked meat, bologna, chicken or beef liver, dried fish, meat tenderizer, salami, sausage

Other foods: large amounts of caffeinated coffee, tea, or cola; chocolate; licorice; soy sauce; yeast

BOX 7.3 Adverse Effects of Selective Serotonin Reuptake Inhibitor (SSRI) Antidepressants

Dry mouth, nausea, vomiting, constipation, diarrhea, anorexia, differences in taste; headache, changes in alertness, tremor, dizziness, weakness, fatigue, increased sweating; sexual dysfunction; visual disturbances; urinary disturbances

TABLE 7.4 Commonly Prescribed Antimanics

Generic Name	Trade Name
carbamazepine	Tegretol
clonazepam	Rivotril
gabapentin	Neurontin
lamotrigine	Lamictal
lithium	Carbolith
topiramate	Topamax
valproic acid	Depakene

Modified from Keltner, N. L., & Folks, D. G. (2005). *Psychotropic drugs* (4th ed.). Mosby.

headache, stiff neck, palpitations) should be reported to the physician immediately.

Patients should also be assessed for changes in attitudes and suicidal gestures. Frequently, depressed people attempt suicide when taking antidepressants because of increased energy levels that can lead to a renewed interest in suicide. Take precautions to protect patients if you believe that they may be suicidal. Changes in a patient's behaviour may indicate a therapeutic improvement, a medication adverse effect, a medication–food interaction, or an emerging psychosis. Good communication with patients helps in assessing subtle changes that may indicate problems.

No matter which medications they are taking, patients must be taught about their drug therapy. Instructions should include information about dosages, actions, and wanted and unwanted effects. Those who are taking MAOIs must understand their dietary and medication restrictions. Box 7.2 lists the foods and medications that must be avoided while taking MAOIs.

For many physicians SSRIs are the first choice in treatment because their adverse effects are more manageable (Box 7.3). Because of this, SSRIs are indicated for both short- and long-term therapy.

Mood-Stabilizer Medications

Mania is a state characterized by excitement, great elation, over-talkativeness, increased motor activity, fleeting grandiose ideas, and agitated behaviours. Some therapists refer to mania as *agitated depression* because it frequently occurs with severe depression. Antidepressant medication therapy helps patients cope with their depression, but it has little effect during the manic stage of behaviour.

Lithium is a naturally occurring salt. In 1949 lithium was found to be effective in the treatment of mania, but because of reports of fatal adverse effects, the medication was not available in the United States until 1970. Lithium is the mainstay treatment of the manic phase of bipolar depression. Newer products are currently available for patients who do not respond to or cannot tolerate lithium therapy because of distressing adverse effects such as nausea, diarrhea, tremors and weight gain, among others. Table 7.4 lists the major antimanic medications (mood-stabilizer medications that treat mania, not depression).

Lithium is currently used in Canada for the treatment of manic episodes. Because lithium stabilizes mood, it is indicated for the treatment of acute mania and as a prophylaxis (preventative) for patients with bipolar disorders. Lithium has also been investigated for the treatment of drug abuse, alcoholism, phobias, and eating disorders. Therapy is contraindicated (not prescribed) for pregnant women and people with kidney failure. Patients with physical health problems must be carefully monitored.

Lithium is well absorbed into the bloodstream and excreted faster than sodium by the kidneys. For this reason, patients who are taking lithium must be cautioned about balancing their salt intake, fluid intake, and activity. Lithium interacts with a variety of other medications. For a list of significant medication interactions associated with antimanic medications, consult a drug reference.

The difference between therapeutic and toxic levels of lithium is minimal. The medication is usually well tolerated by most patients, but how well the medication is excreted varies from patient to patient. The "narrow therapeutic index" of lithium requires close observation of patient responses. If the blood levels are too low, manic behaviour returns; if levels are too high, an uncomfortable and possibly life-threatening toxicity may result. Lithium levels higher than 1.5 mmol/L are considered toxic.

Clinical improvement commonly takes as long as 3 weeks. Patients in the acute manic stage usually require the addition of antipsychotic or sedative medications until the effects of

BOX 7.4 Guidelines for Patients Taking Lithium

To achieve a therapeutic effect and prevent lithium toxicity, patients taking lithium should be advised of the following:

1. Lithium must be taken on a regular basis at the same time daily. If the patient misses a dose, they need to wait until the next scheduled time to take the lithium.
2. When lithium treatment is started, mild adverse effects may develop, such as fine hand tremor, increased thirst and urination, nausea, anorexia, and diarrhea or constipation. Some foods, such as celery and butter fat, may have an unappealing taste. Most adverse effects will pass with time.
3. Serious adverse effects of lithium include vomiting, extreme hand tremor, sedation, muscle weakness, and dizziness. Notify the physician immediately if any of these effects occur.
4. Lithium and sodium compete for elimination from the body through the kidneys. An increase in salt intake increases lithium elimination, and a decrease in salt intake decreases lithium elimination. Thus, it is important that the patient maintain a balanced diet, liquid, and salt intake. The patient should consult the physician before making any dietary changes.
5. Various situations can require an adjustment in lithium doses—for example, the addition of a new medication to the patient's medication regimen, a new diet, or an illness with fever or excessive sweating.
6. Blood for determination of lithium levels should be drawn in the morning, approximately 8 to 14 hours after the last dose was taken.

TABLE 7.5 Commonly Prescribed Antipsychotics

Generic Name	Trade Name
Phenothiazines	
chlorpromazine	Thorazine
fluphenazine	Prolixin
mesoridazine	Serentil
perphenazine	Trilafon
prochlorperazine	Compazine
promazine	Sparine
thioridazine	Mellaril
trifluoperazine	Stelazine
Butyrophenone	
haloperidol	Haldol
Miscellaneous	
aripiprazole	Abilify
clozapine	Clozaril
loxapine	Loxitane
lurasidone	Latuda
olanzapine	Zyprexa
quetiapine	Seroquel
risperidone	Risperdal
thiothixene	Navane
ziprasidone	Geodon

lithium take hold. Patients are monitored monthly for thyroid and kidney functions because long-term use of lithium can cause altered thyroid function (hypothyroidism) and loss of the kidney's ability to concentrate urine. Great care must be taken to frequently assess and monitor each patient's responses to each medication because undesirable effects are present with every medication the patient receives.

The major guidelines for care of patients taking lithium relate to three areas: helping with the prelithium workup, educating the patient to maintain stable blood levels of the medication, and monitoring the patient for adverse effects and possible toxic reactions.

The prelithium workup consists of a complete physical, history, electrocardiogram (ECG), and numerous blood studies. Nurses are responsible for obtaining a complete functional assessment that describes the patient's habits and activities of daily living. They should also review the results of all diagnostic tests. Data from these assessments are used to plan appropriate care and forecast potential problems.

Stabilizing lithium levels involves teaching the patient and family about the following: expected adverse effects, the difference between common adverse effects and those requiring immediate notification of the physician, and coping with the lifestyle changes required by this medication. Box 7.4 lists the most important guidelines for patients who are receiving lithium.

Anticonvulsant medications are also used to help stabilize moods. Antipsychotic medications are sometimes prescribed, often in combination with other medications.

With every medication, ensure that the patient and family understand each bit of information. Ask them to repeat what they have learned, apply it to several "what if" situations, and describe the appropriate actions for each adverse effect. Reinforce the information with written instructions. The informed patient is a more willing participant in treatment.

Antipsychotic (Neuroleptic) Medications

Antipsychotics are also called *major tranquilizers* or *neuroleptics*. Most antipsychotic medications are available in tablet, liquid, and injectable forms. Every class of antipsychotics has profound effects on the most complex of all body systems—the brain and nervous system.

Most antipsychotic drugs are used to treat the symptoms of major mental disorders, such as schizophrenia, acute mania, and organic mental illnesses. They are also used with some resistant bipolar (manic-depressive), paranoid, and movement disorders. A few antipsychotics are used to treat nausea, vomiting, and intractable hiccups. Table 7.5 lists the most common antipsychotic medications.

The psychosis called *schizophrenia* is associated with two groups of symptoms: type 1, which are called *positive schizophrenic symptoms*, and type 2, which are called *negative schizophrenic symptoms* (Table 7.6). Antipsychotic medications appear

TABLE 7.6 Positive and Negative Symptoms of Schizophrenia

	Type I: Positive Symptoms	Type 2: Negative Symptoms
Signs and symptoms	Delusions, illusions, hallucinations	Anergia (lack of energy); anhedonia (inability to feel happiness or pleasure); apathy (does not care about anything); avolition (unable to choose or exert own will); flat affect (no emotional responses); will not speak unless spoken to
Anatomy and physiology	Hyperdopaminergic reactions (too much dopamine) Brain size and structure normal	Nondopaminergic reactions (too little dopamine) Brain has structural changes: decreased blood flow, increased size of ventricles, decrease in size of brain
Response to antipsychotic medications	Usually good	Usually poor

TABLE 7.7 Extrapyramidal Side Effects of Antipsychotics

Sign/Symptom	Definition
Akathisia	The inability to sit still
Akinesia	Absence of physical and mental movement
Drug-induced parkinsonism	Term used to describe a group of symptoms that mimic Parkinson's disease
Dyskinesia	The inability to execute voluntary movements
Dystonia	Impaired muscle tone (rigidity in the muscles that control gait, posture, and eye movements)
Tardive dyskinesia	Irreversible adverse effect of long-term treatment that produces involuntary, repeated movements of muscles in the face, trunk, arms, and legs

BOX 7.5 Medications Used to Treat Extrapyramidal Side Effects (EPSEs)

Anticholinergics	Beta-Blockers
benztropine (Cogentin) trihexyphenidyl (Artane)	propranolol (Inderal) atenolol (Tenormin)
Antihistamines diphenhydramine (Benadryl)	**Benzodiazepines** triazolam (Halcion), lorazepam (Ativan), chlordiazepoxide (Librium), diazepam (Valium)
Dopamine Agonists Pramipexole	

! MEDICATION ALERT

NEUROLEPTIC MALIGNANT SYNDROME

Neuroleptic malignant syndrome (NMS) is a potentially lethal adverse effect of antipsychotic drugs. The incidence of NMS was formerly much greater than it is today, but with today's careful scrutiny of patients by nurses and physicians, a significant reduction in its incidence and mortality has occurred.

NMS occurs most often when high-potency antipsychotic medications (e.g., haloperidol) are prescribed, but not always. NMS is not related to toxic drug levels and might occur after only a few doses. Typically, onset is within a week or so after initiation of an antipsychotic medication (Keltner & Steele, 2019).

to be much more effective in controlling the positive symptoms of acute schizophrenia. Studies have indicated that "antipsychotic medications, which seem so important in the early phase of psychosis, appeared to worsen prospects for recovery over the long-term" (Insel, 2013). Their use for patients with chronic brain disorders remains controversial because these medications block already depleted dopamine (a neurotransmitter) pathways.

Antipsychotic medications interact with many other chemicals. For example, antacids hinder the absorption of antipsychotic medications, so they must be administered 2 hours after the oral antipsychotic. Alcohol, antianxiety medications, antihistamines, antidepressants, barbiturates, meperidine (Demerol), and morphine produce severe CNS depression when mixed with antipsychotics. As a health care provider, you are responsible for the safety of your patients. Research every medication and over-the-counter drug for possible interactions with the prescribed antipsychotic, and monitor your patients' responses to each medication. If drug references do not contain enough information, consult the pharmacist or physician.

The adverse effects and adverse reactions of antipsychotic medications are numerous and troublesome for the patient. Both the central and peripheral nervous systems are affected by antipsychotics.

Extrapyramidal side effects (EPSEs), sometimes referred to as *extrapyramidal symptoms* (EPS), defined as abnormal movements produced by an imbalance of neurotransmitters in the brain, can be experienced by patients taking antipsychotic medications. The most common EPSEs are listed in Table 7.7.

EPSEs can progress to a permanent condition known as *tardive dyskinesia*. Decreasing the dosage or switching

TABLE 7.8   Commonly Prescribed Stimulants

Generic Name	Trade Name
amphetamine and dextroamphetamine	Adderall
atomoxetine	Strattera
bupropion	Wellbutrin
dextroamphetamine	Dexedrine
lisdexamfetamine	Vyvanse
methylphenidate	Ritalin, Concerta

to an atypical antipsychotic medication may help decrease symptoms. Medications that help treat EPSEs are listed in Box 7.5.

SIGNS AND SYMPTOMS

Symptoms begin most often during the first 2 weeks of treatment but may occur earlier or after many years. There are four characteristic symptoms that usually develop over a few days, and often occur in the following order:

- Altered mental status: Usually the earliest manifestation is a change in mental status, often an agitated delirium, that may progress to lethargy or unresponsiveness (reflecting encephalopathy).
- Motor abnormalities: Patients may have generalized, severe muscle rigidity (sometimes with simultaneous tremor, leading to cogwheel rigidity), or, less often, dystonias, chorea, or other abnormalities. Reflex responses tend to be decreased.
- Hyperthermia: Temperature is usually >38°C and often >40°C.
- Autonomic hyperactivity: Autonomic activity is increased, raising the potential for tachycardia, arrhythmias, tachypnea, and labile hypertension.

Peripheral nervous system adverse effects include dry mouth, blurred vision, photophobia (sensitivity to bright light), tachycardia, and hypotension. Care providers must protect patients from falls during the first few weeks of therapy because the chance for low blood pressure (hypotension) is greatest when patients stand up or change positions suddenly. These hypotensive episodes cause tachycardia (rapid heartbeat) as the body attempts to adapt to a lower blood pressure. Antipsychotic medications affect each person uniquely. They are powerful medications that must be administered with great care.

Stimulants are used to treat people with ADHD. Table 7.8 lists the most frequently prescribed stimulants.

PATIENT CARE GUIDELINES

Nurses and those who administer psychotherapeutic medications have five basic responsibilities relating to these medications: (1) to assess patients, (2) to coordinate care, (3) to administer medications, (4) to monitor and evaluate patient responses, and (5) to teach patients about their medications.

CASE STUDY

Gary, a 36-year-old man, is admitted to the mental health unit of the community hospital with a diagnosis of paranoid schizophrenia. He is considered a danger to others because of his aggressive and uncooperative behaviour. After receiving a major tranquilizer, he spent a relatively quiet night but cried out frequently. Today Mary is assigned to care for him.

After reviewing the change-of-shift report and Gary's record, Mary decides that he needs a thorough assessment, so she goes in search of her patient. She is surprised to find a rather burly, bearded man lying curled on his side and whimpering quietly to himself. While knocking on the door, she introduces herself and requests a few minutes of his time. "Hardly matters," he grumbles softly.

Mary approaches his bed carefully, remembering his tendency for physical aggression. As she seats herself near his bedside, she thinks that she caught an expression of pain. Acting on this nonverbal message, Mary gently questions, "Where are you hurting?"

Gary looks straight into her eyes and says through clenched teeth, "I think it's my back or legs or something. Ever since this pain started, I've been unable to control myself. All I want to do now is make everybody who is messin' with me hurt as much as I do."

This is the clue that sends Mary on the path of assessing Gary's pain. She discovers in his past medical history that Gary had fallen off a roof about 3 months ago. The injuries had not resolved, and attempts at treatment resulted in ever-increasing discomfort. Pain medications, even when combined with alcohol, had little effect on the pain. Mary's physical assessment reveals difficulties with walking, sitting, and changing positions. He is not able to lift his legs off the bed.

Mary knows that something is physically wrong. Her first priority of care is to help Gary find some relief from his pain. After sharing her findings with her supervisor, Mary consults the physician in charge of Gary's case, who orders several diagnostic tests. The results of the tests reveal a large herniated disk in his back. Gary is immediately transferred and prepared for surgery.

Weeks later, a large, burly man approaches Mary in the hallway. He reminds her of someone familiar, but she cannot quite place him. As he draws closer, she recognizes Gary, who has come to thank her for listening to him. "I told the others that I was hurtin', but they didn't listen, so I got upset. I guess I can be pretty rowdy when I'm hurtin'. But you listened to me and I had surgery and the pain is gone. I can be a nice guy again. If you hadn't listened to me, I'd really be crazy by now. Thanks."

Mary feels great but reminds herself to carefully and thoroughly (physically, emotionally, socioculturally, and spiritually) assess each patient as a unique individual. The answer to a complex problem may lie in a simple solution, but one must be alert enough to recognize the clues.

- What do you think might have happened if Mary had not assessed a physical problem in this mental health patient?

Each area of responsibility involves careful observation and an understanding of each medication's therapeutic and adverse actions. All care providers should be aware of their patients' medication regimens and report any unusual signs or symptoms to the nurse or physician.

Assessment

The first step of the nursing (therapeutic) process is the most important because an accurate and complete database enhances the quality and effectiveness of patient care. Many nurses are very skilled with the psychosocial and mental status assessments necessary for the care of patients with mental–emotional challenges. However, it is important to remember that physical difficulties are common companions of psychological issues. See the previous Case Study for a vivid example of this principle.

A history should be completed for every patient, whether the presenting problems are of physical or mental origin. A complete health history includes a profile of the patient's current living situation, family structure, and daily activities. Attention should also be paid to their past medical, family, and social histories. An investigation of the patient's chief complaint (problem) rounds out the basic database. Laboratory and other diagnostic studies may be ordered by the physician or nurse practitioner, and special medication assessments must be conducted for patients receiving psychotherapeutic medications (Stuart, 2013). Table 7.9 offers an example of a medication history assessment tool. Assessing patients is a continual process. Good physical and psychosocial assessments add an important dimension to the patient's overall plan of holistic care.

Coordination

Physicians and nurse practitioners prescribe treatments; psychologists recommend therapies; and social workers, psychologists, and other health care team members propose plans of care based on their area of expertise. Nurses coordinate and ensure that each component of the treatment plan is carried out while simultaneously conducting assessments. They juggle scheduling for tests, treatments, and therapies; monitor responses to medications; teach patients and their significant others about treatments, medications, and other aspects of therapy; and encourage patients to become actively engaged in their treatment. Nurses also act as advocates, consult with other members of the treatment team throughout the patient's stay, and provide care that encourages patients toward wellness.

Each health care team member coordinates patient care with others. Multidisciplinary care planning meetings are held frequently to discuss patient progress and challenges from each specialist's viewpoint. Treatment goals are discussed, and care plans are updated as patient behaviour changes.

Medication Administration

One traditional role of nurses is the administration of medications to patients. In some situations, medications can be given by family members and other nonregulated staff. Regardless of who administers the medication, it remains the responsibility of the nurse to monitor patients for medication effectiveness and adverse reactions. Other care providers should also be aware of the actions and adverse effects of their patients' medications to facilitate efficient communication with the nurse.

It is not uncommon for a patient to be taking two or more psychotherapeutic medications at the same time. In these instances, care provider must be especially vigilant for adverse effects and signs of medication interactions.

CRITICAL THINKING

You are monitoring the responses of three patients who are taking Haldol. The first patient is a 23-year-old woman, the second is a 50-year-old man, and the third is a 76-year-old man.
- Which patient is at greatest risk for developing adverse effects?
- What are your reasons for making this choice?

Monitoring patients' responses to their medications is an important, potentially life-saving intervention. Do not take this responsibility lightly, because your patients depend on your knowledge.

TABLE 7.9 Medication History Assessment Tool

Psychotherapeutic Medications	Other Prescriptions	Over-the-Counter Medications	Substance Use
Each medication ever taken	*Each medication in past 6 mo*	*Each medication in past 6 mo*	*Alcohol, caffeine, street drugs*
Medication name?	Medication name?	Medication name?	Substance(s)?
Reason for prescription?	Reason for prescription?	Reason for taking?	When used?
When started?	When started?	When started?	
Length of time taking medication?	Length of time taking medication?	Frequency of use?	Frequency of use?
Highest daily dose?	Highest daily dose?	Highest dose?	
Effectiveness?	Effectiveness?	Effectiveness?	Effects?
Adverse effects, adverse reactions?	Adverse effects, adverse reactions?	Adverse effects, adverse reactions?	Adverse effects, adverse reactions?
Any physical changes since starting medication?	Any physical changes since starting medication?		Any problems associated with use?
Was medication taken as prescribed (adherence)?	Was medication taken as prescribed (adherence)?		

Modified from Stuart, G. W., & Laraia, M. T. (2001). *Pocket guide to psychiatric nursing* (5th ed.). Mosby.

TABLE 7.10	**Teaching Guidelines: Psychotropic Medications**
Nursing Process	**Examples of Actions**
Assessment	Assess patient for the following: • Level of understanding • Ability to self-administer medications • Willingness to take medications on a daily basis • Level of cooperation • Ability to obtain and purchase medications • Support of family • Past medication history, including adverse effects of any medication taken
Planning	Nursing diagnoses: • Deficient knowledge: psychotherapeutic medications • Risk for nonadherence
Interventions	For each medication, teach patient to recognize the following: • Generic and brand names • Purpose and action • Therapeutic effects • Dosage, route, schedule of medication • Administration, what to do if a dose is missed • Specific precautions (driving, operation of power equipment) • Adverse effects and actions to take if they occur • Possible medication/food interactions • Signs of overdosage or underdosage • Medication storage, expiration dates Provide information in written form Develop written medication schedule Reinforce other data given by care team
Evaluation	Observe patient to evaluate effectiveness of teaching Reassess if any areas of instruction were not understood by patient or family

Monitoring and Evaluating

Physicians evaluate patient responses and adjust medical therapies, but care providers are in the best position to observe the physical and behavioural changes that accompany the administration of psychotherapeutic medications. All care providers should be familiar with the major adverse effects and adverse reactions for each class of psychotherapeutic medications used in their practice settings.

Interactions with other medications and substances can become life-threatening. For example, when alcohol is combined with antidepressant medications, severe CNS depression occurs. This in turn results in lethargy, progressing to respiratory depression, coma, and even death. Certain groups of people are at an increased risk for developing medication interactions, including older persons, debilitated people, people with immunosuppressed or compromised organ

systems (especially liver and kidneys), and patients who have physical illnesses.

Patient Teaching

Every individual has a right to be informed about their diagnosis and treatment plan. Each patient must be prepared to safely take each medication, monitor for adverse effects daily, and know what course of action to take when adverse effects do occur. See Table 7.10 for patient teaching guidelines.

Health care providers must be able to reach patients on their own level of understanding. To prevent miscommunication, the nurse must speak in terms that the patient can grasp and proceed at a pace that allows for understanding and the formulation of questions. Most psychotherapeutic medications slow the patient's ability to follow and understand a line of thought. Therefore, it is important to repeat essential points. Be sure the patient comprehends by having them repeat the most important information.

Provide information in writing. Having a written explanation gives the patient something tangible and real that can be reviewed and referred to when memory fails. Patients taking psychotherapeutic medications are likely to forget what has been taught. Preprinted medication information is helpful, but there is no substitute for individualized patient teaching. If possible, include the family or significant others. They can be very helpful in assisting the patient with following the medication routine.

Helping patients and their significant others to adapt to change is a health care provider's responsibility. Psychotherapeutic medications are designed to produce behavioural changes, and these changes affect the patient and the people within the patient's environment. A well-informed patient and family are able to cope more effectively with the life changes that result from psychiatric medication therapy.

SPECIAL CONSIDERATIONS

Because psychotropic medications affect the body's nervous system, they are potentially harmful chemicals. Professionals with prescriptive authority must weigh the benefits of therapy with the possible harm that may result from the adverse effects or adverse reactions of a medication.

Adverse Reactions

Health care providers, especially nurses, must constantly remain vigilant for the effects of psychotherapeutic medications. Patients who are taking psychotropic drugs (especially antipsychotics) are at risk for developing the serious problems of neuroleptic malignant syndrome (NMS) and tardive dyskinesia. Accurate identification of the signs and symptoms of each may prevent many complications. Detailed descriptions of these and other drug reactions are found in Chapter 31.

Nonadherence

An informed decision made by a patient not to follow a prescribed treatment program defines **nonadherence**. Many psychiatric patients choose to discontinue or reduce their medications because of the distressing adverse effects. Others have difficulty following treatment programs because of the nature of their illness. For example, paranoid or delusional people seldom cooperate with medication regimens or schedules. One study found that about 40% of patients stopped taking their prescribed medications within 1 year (Jarboe, 2002). Many outpatient patients do not take their medications as prescribed. Even patients within inpatient settings do not take their medications consistently. It is not uncommon for people to hide medications in their cheek or pretend to swallow and then discard or hoard them. The physician should be notified in these cases, and a liquid form of the medication should be requested.

The keys to improving patient adherence are education and an effective patient–care provider relationship. Work with your patients to find and eliminate the factors that lead to nonadherence. Simplify the medication routine, if possible. Teach about and monitor for adverse effects and adverse reactions.

Informed Consent

Another consideration relating to psychotherapeutic medications is the issue of informed consent. **Informed consent** is the process of presenting patients with information about the benefits, risks, and adverse effects of specific treatments, thus enabling them to make voluntary and knowledgeable decisions about their care. With the treatment of physical disorders, the process is straightforward: treatments are described, and the patient makes the decision to accept or reject the plan. However, with mental disorders, the picture is not so clear. In the past, psychiatric patients who were considered a danger to themselves or others were routinely medicated without their permission.

When patients stop taking their medications, care guidelines focus on ensuring safety and assessing for the return of symptoms. When caring for the patient within an inpatient setting, care providers should observe for any changes in behaviour, be prepared for the patient to become aggressive or act out, and protect the patient and others from harm. If the setting is the clinic, the care provider should instruct the patient's significant others about the return of psychiatric symptoms, the signs and symptoms of adverse effects and adverse reactions, and the available community resources. Although care providers cannot manipulate or force patients into taking medications, they can use their rapport and communication skills to assist patients in making decisions based on complete information and sound judgement. As Finkelman (2000) notes, "agency policies about informed consent must be followed to protect the patient, staff, and agency."

New medications are being developed, ones that act more specifically, have a shorter onset, and produce fewer adverse effects. Along with these developments, more treatments and therapies will be introduced. Complementary and alternative medicine will also play a growing role in mental health care. It is our responsibility to safely practise within these expansive and growing treatment options.

KEY POINTS

- Psychotherapeutic medications are powerful chemical substances that produce their effects on the nervous system by interrupting the chemical messenger (neurotransmitter) pathways within the brain.
- Four classes of psychotherapeutic medications are antianxiety drugs, antidepressants, antimanics, and antipsychotics.
- Medications for the treatment of anxiety include the benzodiazepines, the azapirones, and beta-blockers for social phobias. Their main adverse effects are sedation and gastrointestinal disturbances.
- Antidepressant medications treat depression and other mood disorders by increasing certain neurotransmitter activity within the brain and CNS.
- Mania and bipolar depressive illnesses are treated with lithium, a naturally occurring mood stabilizer.
- The major guidelines for care of patients taking lithium are helping with the prelithium workup, educating the patient to maintain stable blood levels of the drug, and monitoring the patient for adverse effects and possible toxic reactions.
- Antipsychotic medications are indicated for patients with schizophrenia, acute mania, organic mental illnesses, some resistant bipolar disorders, paranoid disorders, some disorders of movement, nausea and vomiting, and intractable hiccups.
- Extrapyramidal side effects (EPSEs) include CNS alterations that produce abnormal involuntary movement disorders. Peripheral nervous system side effects include dry mouth, blurred vision, photophobia (sensitivity to bright light), tachycardia, and hypotension.
- Patients who are receiving antipsychotics are at risk for developing the serious problems of NMS and tardive dyskinesia.
- Nurses who work with patients who are receiving psychotherapeutic medications have five basic responsibilities: to assess, to coordinate, to administer, to monitor and evaluate, and to teach.
- A special medication assessment (medication history) must be conducted for patients receiving psychotherapeutic medications.
- A primary responsibility of nurses is to monitor patients for medication effectiveness and adverse reactions.
- Patient education is a major role of nurses.
- Nonadherence is defined as an informed decision made by a patient not to follow a prescribed treatment program.
- Informed consent involves presenting patients with information about the benefits, risks, and adverse effects of specific treatments, thus enabling them to make decisions about their care.

ADDITIONAL LEARNING RESOURCES

Go to your Evolve website (http://evolve.elsevier.com/Canada/Morrison-Valfre/) for additional online resources, including the online Study Guide for additional learning activities to help you master this chapter content.

CRITICAL THINKING QUESTIONS

1. Your neighbour's son has a history of schizophrenia. He explains to you that he was prescribed a new atypical antipsychotic a few months ago and is feeling really good. He goes on to tell you that he plans to stop taking the atypical antipsychotic now, because it has cured his schizophrenia. How might you respond to this?

2. On the day of discharge, your mental health patient asks you for a taxi chit. Typically, the unit provides a bus ticket to provide otherwise healthy patients with transportation home. When you ask, your patient states that she thinks that "they" won't be able to follow her as easily in a taxi. On further discussion, your patient advises that she is been "cheeking" her medication, because she knows "they" have had them chemically altered. What is an appropriate response to this situation?

3. On routine rounds, you observe a patient who appears to be irritated and annoyed. She is sitting alone and has declined an invitation to play cards with another patient—an activity that she normally enjoys. On inquiry, the patient tells you that she is "very angry" that the nurses have been giving her a medication that isn't working. The patient explains further that she was started on a new medication, lithium, a few days ago, and expected to be feeling much better by now. She blames the nursing staff for giving her the wrong medication. How would you best address this patient's concerns?

REFERENCES

Finkelman, A. W. (2000). Psychopharmacology: An update for psychiatric home care. *Home Care Provider*, 5(5), 170 [Seminal Reference].

Insel, T. (2013). *Antipsychotics: Taking the long view.* National Institute of Mental Health. https://www.nimh.nih.gov/about/directors/thomas-insel/blog/2013/antipsychotics-taking-the-long-view.shtml

Jarboe, K. S. (2002). Treatment nonadherence: Causes and potential solutions. *Journal of the American Psychiatric Nurses Association*, 8(4), 18 [Seminal Reference].

Keltner, N. L., & Folks, D. G. (2005). *Psychotropic drugs* (4th ed.). Mosby.

Keltner, N. L., & Steele, D. (2019). *Psychiatric nursing* (8th ed.). Elsevier.

Skidmore-Roth, L. (2015). *Mosby's 2015 nursing drug reference* (28th ed.). Mosby.

Stuart, G. W. (2013). *Principles and practice of psychiatric nursing* (10th ed.). Mosby.

The Caregiver's Therapeutic Skills

8

Principles and Skills of Mental Health Care

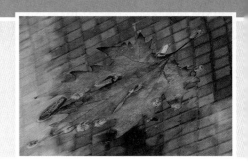

PRINCIPLES OF MENTAL HEALTH CARE

A **principle** is a code or standard that helps govern our conduct. Principles guide decisions and actions. Professional principles provide guidelines. Most health care professions are guided by standards of care, provincial regulatory bodies, and principles. This chapter examines the basic principles and skills for those who work with mentally or emotionally troubled patients.

The Mentally Healthy Adult

The concepts of mental health and mental illness are not easily defined. Health, by its very nature, is a changing state, influenced by genetics, behaviour, and the environment. Mental health is just as dynamic, changing as the stresses of life are encountered.

Most people manage to adapt to the changes in their lives and remain contributing members of their society. Problems exist, but mentally healthy adults are content with who and where they are in life. They are able to love and express love freely without the fear of losing their independence. Flexibility and a willingness to try something different lead to an eagerness for learning. Life is considered important, and special moments are cherished. Adversity is viewed as a challenge or opportunity for growth. To simplify, a **mentally healthy adult** is a person who can cope with and adjust to the recurrent stresses of daily living in an acceptable way. Although mentally healthy adults experience unhappiness, anxiety, or other psychic distresses, they manage to mobilize their resources, rise above the negativity, and continue on with their lives.

Citizens of industrialized cultures label a person as *mentally ill* only after the ability to function independently in society is impaired for a noticeable period of time (Giger & Haddad, 2020). In our culture, mental illness results when an individual's problems become so overwhelming that one is unable to carry out the activities of daily living or function independently. Other cultures have different definitions of mental illness.

CULTURAL CONSIDERATIONS

We typically use our own culture as a basis for understanding another person's culture. Sometimes, however, finding some commonality or basis for comparison is difficult. Consider this example:

Laos is a country in Southeast Asia. Its inhabitants, the Lao, believe that 32 spirits live within the body and govern its functions. Illnesses, including mental disturbances, are thought to be the result of an imbalance of the spirits, unhealthy air currents, or bad winds. Pinching or scratching parts of the body to produce red marks helps to let the bad winds out of the body and restore health. Strings are worn around the wrists, neck, ankles, or waist to prevent soul loss.

Keeping an open mind in all interactions with patients helps to build trust and understand vastly different cultural considerations.

Mental Health Care Practice

The helping professions are based on the care of the whole person. Practising the principles of mental health care is the

BOX 8.1 Principles of Mental Health Care

1. Do no harm.
2. Accept each patient as a whole person.
3. Develop mutual trust.
4. Explore behaviours and emotions.
5. Encourage responsibility.
6. Encourage effective adaptation.
7. Provide consistency.

responsibility of all health care providers. No matter which specialty or where the setting, every caregiver helps patients cope with their problems.

The world of health care is familiar and comfortable for those who practise within its realm. The sights, sounds, and smells of the health care environment become known and familiar. Daily routines are established, and the employees all understand what behaviours are expected of them. However, to a person who is ill (disabled, stressed), visiting a medical facility can be an uncomfortable experience. Anxiety results when illness or disability affects any individual. No matter how casual a patient may appear, a heightened stress level is present every time interactions with health care providers take place. Some people are so intimidated by the health care system that they wait until their problems become severe and difficult to treat. Sensitive care providers remember that patients are "out of their element" when seeking health care and need emotional support and effective care.

The skills developed when working with the mental and emotional needs of people will be used throughout your career, for yours is the profession of caring. The seven principles of mental health care listed in Box 8.1 will help guide you.

Do No Harm

The "do no harm" principle serves as a guide for all therapeutic actions. Care providers in every setting have the responsibility to protect patients, but for care providers working with mental health patients, this principle is especially important.

The main therapeutic tool of mental health care providers is the "self." Therapeutic use of the self can result in great improvements in patients' behaviours when the "do no harm" principle is applied. When it is overlooked or forgotten, the one who loses is the patient, the very person we are obligated to protect. No matter what the circumstances, avoid any action that may result in harm to your patient. This concept is derived from the ancient writings of Hippocrates, whose principle of "do no harm" proves to be as true and valid today as it was so long ago.

Accept Each Patient as a Whole Person

People living with mental health challenges suffer from a socially imposed stigma. The word **stigma** is defined as a sign or mark of shame, disapproval, or disgrace, of being shunned or rejected. Because people feel uneasy about discussing behaviours that are different, they generally shy away from mentally troubled individuals. One of the barriers in recovering from a mental illness is the social stigma that patients experience. Care providers should set examples by acting as advocates for patients and educating themselves about psychiatric illnesses.

The principle of **acceptance** (allowing others to be who they are without passing judgement) is important in health care because you will care for many different people. Those differences do not have to be understood, but they must be accepted. You may even disapprove of patients' attitudes and behaviours, but you must accept the person because it is the person who is the focus of your health care activities. This section discusses a point of view that encourages the principle of acceptance.

Holistic Framework

Holistic health care is based on the concept of "whole." Understanding patients in relation to their work, family, and social environments encourages care providers to consider their patients' many needs and tailor individualized interventions.

In a health-oriented model, patients are assessed for their strengths and abilities. Goals of care are mutually developed. Interventions are designed for the individual, and patients receive the services most important and relevant to them. Responsibility for success is shared among patients and care providers.

Health care providers who practise holistically realize that each person must be accepted for who and what he or she is, no more and no less. They accept the whole person and search for meaning in the patient's actions. Behaviours are attempts to fill needs. Your acceptance is communicated to the patients, and your actions will result in success. However, if you pass judgement, patients will sense your disapproval and therapeutic actions will not be successful.

Viewing patients holistically also involves an acceptance of their lifestyles, attitudes, social interactions, and living conditions. This can be difficult, especially when the environment or lifestyle is harmful. People with mental–emotional difficulties may display odd behaviours or verbalize unusual beliefs. They need to be accepted, just as patients with physical maladies are accepted. Our reactions to their behaviours can sometimes cloud their messages. Identify your reactions to patients. Work to develop an acceptance of each by considering the whole individual.

Progress may come slowly when working with patients who are experiencing mental health difficulties. A holistic point of view and a focus on the positive encourage both care providers and patients to strive for success. They allow psychiatric patients respect and help us accept all people regardless of how different they may be from ourselves.

Develop Mutual Trust

The word *trust* means assured hope and reliance on another. Erikson's theory (see Chapter 5) lists the development of trust as the first core task of the infant. Trust is an important concept for human beings, who are social and group oriented. Trust implies cooperation, support, and a willingness to work together. Trust occurs on many levels. For example, when you drive your vehicle, you are engaging in an act of trust: You trust that oncoming drivers will stay on their side of the small, painted yellow line that divides the road. Numerous other small acts of trust occur throughout the day, but we are usually too busy to notice. Yet to care providers, the concept of trust holds much importance.

Individuals who are unable to trust cannot rely on others for help. Many people with mental–emotional issues struggle with problems of trust. Care providers must routinely demonstrate that they can be trusted. To communicate the messages of trust, remember to do what you say you will do. If you tell a patient that you will return in 10 minutes, be back in 10 minutes (better yet, be there in 9 minutes). Patients soon learn which care providers follow their words with actions. Trust begins to grow when patients know they can depend on their care providers.

Trust is the foundation of therapeutic relationships. It forms the basis for the success or failure of all actions. People who become your patients, no matter what their diagnoses, need to trust that they will be cared for in a safe and supportive manner. The development of trust between patients and care providers involves three concepts: caring, empathy, and advocacy (Keltner & Steele, 2019).

For people living with mental illness, caring plays an especially important role in developing trust. They know, subconsciously, whether you actually care about them or regard them as just another patient. Before trust can be developed, patients must truly believe that their nurses and other providers care.

Empathy is the ability to recognize and share the emotions of another person without actually experiencing them. Empathy is a powerful therapeutic tool. If patients believe that you are willing to share their discomforts, they become more interested in learning to help themselves.

Advocacy is the process of providing a patient with the information, support, and feedback needed to make a decision (Keltner & Steele, 2019). Patient advocacy adds the obligation to act in the patient's best interest. People with mental–emotional difficulties are not always capable of making informed decisions. Here care providers can intervene to ensure that the patient's basic needs are being met. For example, if a patient decides not to eat, the care provider may act in the patient's best interest by making the food easily available. The patient cannot be forced to eat, but they can be encouraged to make more healthful choices. Patient advocacy also involves the concept of empowerment. Many mentally ill people are quite capable of taking part in their care and treatment. Some are not, but all deserve the opportunity to make the decisions they are capable of making. Nurses and other care providers act as advocates by assisting patients through the decision-making process. Providing information and education assists patients in making appropriate decisions about their care. When patients feel that their care providers understand and act in their best interests, trust is established. The therapeutic relationship is discussed more fully in Chapter 11.

Explore Behaviours and Emotions

Every behaviour serves a purpose and has meaning. Behaviours are attempts to fill personal needs and goals. Each of us lives within our own private world. Most people's private worlds (internal frames of reference) are agreeable with others. However, people with mental–emotional difficulties have private worlds that may be difficult for the average person to understand.

"**Behaviour** consists of perceptions, thoughts, feelings, and actions" (Stuart, 2013) (Fig. 8.1). A disruption in any one of these areas can result in behavioural problems. Distorted perceptions, impaired thought processes, and alterations of emotional expression lead to maladaptive actions. Behaviours also must be understood in terms of the context or setting in

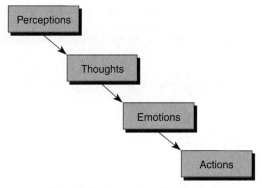

Fig. 8.1 Components of behaviour.

which they occur. A particular environment may be threatening because of uncomfortable past experiences in similar settings.

It is sometimes difficult to accurately interpret the messages a patient's behaviour is sending. Actions may be clouded with symbols or influenced by chemical substances. Alcohol and other drugs affect perceptions, emotional expression, and judgement, as well as behaviour.

An often-overlooked method of understanding the meaning of a patient's behaviour is to simply ask the individual. Many patients are willing to share themselves when (1) they have trust in you and (2) you are willing to take the time to listen. When people with mental health challenges can discuss their behaviours or share their emotions, they are not looking for approval or reproach. Acceptance and a gentle exploration of what the behaviours mean to them will help you develop and practise insight. Recognizing ineffective behaviours and replacing them with more appropriate actions are the first steps toward gaining some control over one's situation.

Explaining how you view the patient's behaviours allows for perception checks. Is the patient sending the same message that you are receiving? Does each of you see the same messages in the patient's symbols? If the patient says he feels like a duck, do you know what he is really trying to portray? Sharing your perceptions helps patients see how their behavioural messages are being received by other people. It also allows care providers the opportunity to gain insight into their worlds.

Some patients are unable to verbally share the meanings of their behaviours. They communicate with actions only. Care providers must develop acute observational skills with these individuals. Repeated behaviours are often attempts to undo or fix something. Other actions can be cries for help or forms of self-punishment for wrongful deeds. The meaning of a patient's behaviours may be shrouded in mystery, but time, trust, and persistent observations assist in discovering the real meanings that lie behind the messages.

Encourage Responsibility

Responsible people are capable of making and fulfilling obligations. They are accountable for their decisions or actions. **Responsibility** implies that a person is able to exercise capability and accountability. Individuals who are unable to make or keep obligations are not considered responsible. Health care providers work with patients who exhibit a wide variety of coping styles and behaviours. Encouraging responsibility is a primary mental health intervention because it helps build self-worth,

dignity, and confidence. It also assists patients in learning more successful coping behaviours. Responsibility is a cornerstone of modern societies and a goal of mental health care.

As children grow and develop the necessary skills for living within a society, so do their responsibilities. The assumption of responsibility starts when the child begins to explore and manipulate the environment. Responsibility is learned early. The primary instructor is the family, but the social group and culture exert strong influences. As children learn about "right behaviours," they develop the responsibility to engage in them. There is a saying that states, "If the family does not teach responsibility, then the school will. If the school does not teach responsibility, then the group will. If the group does not teach responsibility, then society will, and society sends irresponsible people to jail."

Many people living with mental–emotional problems have difficulty behaving in responsible ways. Some have never been taught responsibility because they grew up in a dysfunctional family or childhood experiences taught them otherwise or left this out. Others cannot remember or hold onto a logical picture long enough to be responsible. However, every person has the capacity for growth and thus some degree of responsibility. Nurses and other professionals who work with individuals who are mentally ill can plan and implement specific interventions designed to help patients achieve their highest possible level of responsibility.

The first step in developing self-responsibility relates to care of the self. The basic physical needs of life (Maslow's lower-order needs, refer to Fig. 5.1) must be met no matter what the circumstances. Every adult, and sadly many children, must procure food, clothing, and shelter for themselves. People living with mental–emotional problems commonly have difficulty meeting basic needs, so lessons of self-responsibility usually begin with something as basic as caring for one's daily personal hygiene needs.

Care providers should assess their patients' abilities to perform the skills associated with the activities of daily living. For example, sometimes the reason for poor hygiene is a lack of knowledge. A person may never have been taught to bathe frequently or brush their teeth after every meal. In such cases the care provider must teach, and the patient must learn, the basic skills of personal cleanliness. When the patient assumes responsibility for basic needs, it leads to improved feelings of self-worth. When one looks good, one feels better. Small successes become positive steps that help equip patients with the skills necessary for effective functioning.

The next step in assuming self-responsibility is to be accountable for one's emotions. "I'm sorry, I lost my temper" does not excuse the action. Mental health patients frequently have poor control over their emotions (called *poor impulse control*). They immediately react without considering the consequences of their behaviours. Becoming responsible for one's emotions involves the willingness to identify and then "own" the problems and emotions. It also requires a willingness and determination to try new and more effective ways of coping with emotional reactions.

When patients learn to replace an unacceptable behaviour with a more effective action, they achieve a degree of control over their lives. As individuals become responsible, they begin to succeed. Those small successes help remove them from the role of victim and to realize the value of becoming responsible.

BOX 8.2 Reality Therapy

Reality therapists do not accept the concept of mental illness. Calling people "irresponsible" rather than "mentally ill" and describing how they are irresponsible can help patients develop the responsibility to satisfy their needs.

Reality therapy differs from psychoanalysis in six ways:

1. Because reality therapy does not accept the notion of mental illness, patients are not accepted into therapy as mentally ill people who have no responsibility.
2. Reality therapy works in the present with an eye on the future. It does not accept the limitations of the past.
3. Reality therapists personally relate to patients, not as aloof professionals or transference objects.
4. Reality therapists do not look for unconscious conflicts. Patients cannot excuse their behaviours based on unconscious motivations.
5. The morality of behaviour is emphasized. Issues of right and wrong are defined and enforced.
6. The goal of reality therapy is to help patients help themselves fulfill their needs right now.

BOX 8.3 Cognitive-Behavioural Therapy and Dialectical Behaviour Therapy

Cognitive-behavioural therapy, or CBT, teaches people how their thoughts, feelings, and behaviours influence each other. For example, if you believe that people don't like you (thought), you might avoid social situations (behaviour) and feel lonely (feeling). CBT teaches people how to use these relationships to their advantage: A positive change in one factor (changing a thought or behaviour) can lead to positive changes in all factors. CBT is an approach that has been proven by research to work for many different mental health problems, including depression, anxiety disorders, eating disorders, and substance use problems.

Dialectical behaviour therapy (DBT) is based on CBT, but places a greater focus on emotional and social aspects of behaviour. DBT was developed to help people cope with extreme or unstable emotions and harmful behaviours. DBT is an evidence-informed approach that is used to help people regulate their emotions. It began as a treatment for borderline personality disorder, and current research shows it may also help with many different mental illnesses or concerns, particularly self-harm.

From Canadian Mental Health Association, B.C. Division. (2015). *What's the difference between CBT and DBT?* Author. https://www.heretohelp.bc.ca/q-and-a/whats-the-difference-between-cbt-and-dbt

People who seek treatment for mental or emotional problems must assume the responsibility for cooperating with and following their therapeutic plan of care. This involves a commitment to becoming actively involved, by sharing personal information, being open to new ideas, and being willing to try new ways of doing things.

Patients are also responsible for the effects of their actions on others. The enjoyment of social interactions is accompanied by the responsibility of behaving appropriately. People who have problems with emotional (impulse) control can become a threat to the safety of others when their behaviours are inappropriate. It is important for care providers to assist patients in controlling their behaviours because people who act in irresponsible ways are soon removed from social settings.

Responsibility is a fundamental concept in mental health care. It is a key to developing more effective behaviours and building self-worth. Some psychiatric therapies are designed around the concept of responsibility. For example, William Glasser's (1998) reality therapy (Box 8.2) and cognitive-behavioural therapy (Box 8.3) use responsibility as a therapeutic tool.

Encourage Effective Adaptation

Mental health patients may be labelled with one or more psychiatric diagnoses, but all have one thing in common: unsuccessful coping behaviours. The very nature of mental illness is characterized by actions that are not in keeping with society's definitions of appropriate behaviours. Mental health care providers provide patients with education about and opportunities to engage in more effective behaviours.

With some mental–emotional difficulties we can speak of cures. Situational depression, for example, is frequently cured. Many cases of confusion or delirium are cured when a physical problem is discovered and treated. However, some mental problems are chronic and force patients and their significant others to make permanent changes in how they live their lives. Despite this reality, many people living with

chronic illnesses (physical and mental) adapt and lead full, satisfying, and meaningful lives. Adaptation in this context is not the same as the "cure" of a medical illness. Here it means sufficient improvement to carry on everyday activities. In other words, if we can teach patients to replace maladaptive behaviours with more effective actions, they will improve in their abilities to live more successfully.

One Step at a Time

There is an old saying, "The longest journey begins with a single step." This was never more true than it is in mental health care. To people living with mental–emotional challenges, everything seems overwhelming. Even the simplest decisions can be monumental. People diagnosed with schizophrenia may not be able to differentiate one world from another long enough to follow a train of thought to a logical conclusion. Therefore, it is important for caregivers to give instructions simply and to repeat them often.

When planning therapeutic interventions, remember that it is important to master the first item before proceeding to more complex steps. This process involves breaking down a task or concept into small and simple units. For example, the goal is for the patient to arrive on time for appointments. This may involve wearing a watch, being able to tell time, remembering the appointment, and transporting themselves to the appointment. The first step in meeting the goal may be the purchase of a watch or learning to tell time.

There are two important points here. First, *do not assume; assess.* Using the preceding example, one assumes that every adult can tell time, but the results of this assessment might reveal that the patient could not tell time because of blurred

TABLE 8.1	**Types of Coping Behaviours**	
Mechanism	**Description**	**Example**
Psychomotor (physical)	Efforts to cope directly with problem	Confrontation, fighting, running away, negotiating
Cognitive (intellectual)	Efforts to neutralize threat by changing meaning of problem	Making comparisons, substituting rewards, ignoring, changing values, using problem-solving methods
Affective (emotional)	Actions taken to reduce emotional distress; no efforts are made to solve problem	Ego defence mechanisms such as denial and suppression; see Chapter 5 for other ego defence mechanisms

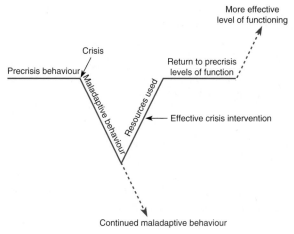

Fig. 8.2 Stages of crisis.

vision. Unless the care provider helps the patient deal with the visual problems, they will not be successful in meeting the goal of routinely keeping all appointments. Second, remember that *success is built on many small steps.* Breaking each learning experience into small units increases the chances of mastery. Make sure that the patient will succeed within the first few steps. The taste of success is especially sweet in the early stages, and it encourages people to continue trying. One small, successful step soon becomes two, and those small triumphs can become symbolic of the patient's potential for growth and change.

Crisis Intervention

When experiencing stress, people use their resources to decrease the discomfort. These efforts, called **coping mechanisms,** are defined as any thought or action aimed at reducing stress. We all use coping mechanisms as the tools that help us work through the ups and downs of daily living. Coping mechanisms are divided into three main types: *psychomotor* (physical), *cognitive* (intellectual), and *affective* (emotional). When coping mechanisms are successfully used, an individual is able to solve problems and reduce stress. These are adaptive or constructive coping mechanisms. However, when efforts to decrease stress are used without resolving the conflict, then the coping mechanism is labelled as *maladaptive* or *destructive.* Table 8.1 describes each type of coping mechanism.

A **crisis** is an upset in the homeostasis (steady state) of an individual. A crisis has several characteristics that separate it

from other stressful situations. First, the definition of crisis is an individual matter that depends on the perception of the event, the severity of the threat, and the available coping strategies and resources. Second, a crisis occurs when an individual's usual coping mechanisms are ineffective. The crisis demands new solutions with new coping strategies. Third, crisis is self-limiting. Because human organisms cannot endure high levels of continued stress, crises are usually resolved within a short time. Fourth, a crisis usually affects more than one person. Everyone within the person's support system is affected by the crisis.

As people experience a crisis, they travel through similar stages: perception, denial, crisis, disorganization, recovery, and reorganization (Fig. 8.2). Once an event is perceived as a crisis, an overwhelming feeling of denial is experienced. This emotion serves to protect the individual from sudden, intense stress. An increase in tension is felt as attempts are made to eliminate the problem. As efforts to cope are ineffective, the individual or family enters the stage of crisis in which everything seems to "fall apart."

During the disorganization phase, individuals become preoccupied with the crisis situation. Activities of daily living no longer continue. The individual becomes flooded with anxiety as attempts are made to reorganize or escape. They may blame others or pretend the situation does not exist, but nothing helps. Once all attempts to deny, solve, escape, or ignore the problem have failed, the individual slowly moves toward recovery. This is the stage at which most people seek help.

Recovery begins when attempts to cope with the problem result in success. One success provides encouragement and builds on another, and soon the stage of reorganization is entered. Normal activities are resumed. When a crisis is successfully resolved, the individual functions at a higher level than before. Growth has taken place, and the person becomes stronger and more capable.

Crises can also result in unsuccessful resolutions or pseudoresolutions. Unresolved crises result when maladaptive behaviours are used to hide the problem. An example is the husband who sends his wife to counselling for depression while he continues to abuse her when he drinks. Pseudoresolution occurs when nothing is learned from the crisis and the opportunity for growth was missed. However, new stressors may trigger buried conflicts of the unresolved crisis. The inability to solve future crises may be compounded by these old conflicts.

CRITICAL THINKING

List two crises you have personally experienced.
- What coping mechanisms did you use?
- How were they successful in helping you cope?
- What did you do to resolve each crisis?
- What was learned from each experience?

BOX 8.4   The Crisis Prevention Institute

The Crisis Prevention Institute (CPI) provides training for individuals in how to respond to potentially violent workplace situations. Most health care agencies require CPI training on an annual basis.

The mission of the Crisis Prevention Institute is to reduce the likelihood and severity of workplace violence incidents. This mission is advanced by training professionals in time-tested strategies, by equipping organizations with confident and productive employees, and by helping health care providers give the people they serve a safe and compassionate environment in which to live, learn, and thrive. Through staff training, premium resources, and unrivalled support, they set the global standard for behaviour management training, and help health care providers make life better for people all around the world.

From Crisis Prevention Institute. (2020). *About us.* https://www.crisisprevention.com/en-CA/About-Us

The main goal of **crisis intervention** is to help individuals and families manage their crisis situations by offering immediate emotional support (see Box 8.4 for one organization that provides training in this area). People are then assisted in developing effective coping mechanisms, which allows time to reorganize resources and support systems.

Victims of crisis are treated in settings such as emergency departments, clinics, jails, places of worship, homes, and even over the telephone. Crisis hotlines are 24-hour telephone lines that are staffed by volunteers trained in crisis intervention techniques. Emotional support and referral to various community resources are offered to any caller.

Guidelines relating to crisis intervention have been developed by the National Institute for Training in Crisis Intervention and other organizations. Because crisis situations are high-stress encounters for all parties, the following guidelines can assist in providing safe, effective crisis interventions:

1. **Care is needed immediately.** Actions must be taken to reduce anxiety levels. Sometimes this may require only reassurance. In other situations, interventions must be taken to ensure safety and prevent harm.
2. **Control.** People experiencing a crisis are often unable to exercise control. Safety for both patient and care provider must be considered. The care provider must quickly assume control but only until the patient is able to recover self-control. Again, the level of control is determined by each situation. Some people are relieved that someone else is in control, whereas others resort to physical aggression during a crisis. Control is important in a crisis because without it the patient cannot be helped to work with the problems that triggered the crisis.
3. **Assessment.** Although assessment usually is the first step in the care process, the issues of immediacy, safety, and control must be considered first in crisis. Thoroughly assess the situation. Ask direct questions, such as, "What happened?" Have the patient explain the situation and review the events of the past 2 weeks. A quick and accurate assessment helps to determine the best therapeutic interventions.
4. **The patient's disposition is determined.** A treatment plan is developed that assists the patient in working on the problems triggering the crisis. The focus of crisis intervention therapy is to help patients manage their problems more effectively.
5. **Referral.** Once emotionally stabilized and in control, patients are referred to professional, community, or support group resources. The most successful referrals match the patient's needs with the most appropriate service.

Know what resources are available within your community before interacting with the patient. Searching online or using reference material while a patient is experiencing a crisis does not provide the person in need with a sense of confidence in you as a care provider.

6. **Follow-up.** Care providers must see whether the referrals were actually contacted. A follow-up telephone call will often reveal new problems that prevent the patient from receiving needed care.

All people experience crises. When new coping mechanisms are needed but are unavailable because of immaturity, an individual experiences a developmental or maturational crisis. Severe stresses within one's environment may cause a situational crisis. Assisting people in crisis to mobilize their resources is an important step in encouraging effective adaptation.

Provide Consistency

The last principle for mental health care providers relates to the concept of **consistency,** which describes behaviours that imply being steady and regular, dependable. People living with mental illness often lack the security of someone who is there when needed. In some cases, the consistency and reliability of mental health care providers are their only stability. The link that serves as a bridge between the patient's world and the world of reality is frequently the reliability of the therapeutic relationship.

The concept of consistency is usually addressed in the patient's plan of care, but each therapeutic intervention must be routinely used by every member of the care team. Patients often test staff members by "playing one against the other" or attempting to manipulate the situation and gain control. However, when each care provider responds by giving the same message, patients learn that members of the care team can be relied on to do what they say they will do. Two general guidelines for providing consistency are to set limits and to focus on the positive changes that patients are making.

Setting limits involves patients, staff members, and institutional policies (Chenevert, 1994). As the plan of care is developed, each rule or limitation is established. Facility policies define some limitations. The remainder relate to therapeutic activities, social interactions, and personal behaviours. Whatever the limitations, the patient must be informed of and willing to cooperate with the plan of care.

Each member of the care team is responsible for understanding the purpose of each limitation and the methods for enforcing them. To illustrate, the facility's policy is for all patients to remain out of bed during the day. To accomplish this, the staff informs each patient every morning that the doors to the rooms will be locked by 9 a.m. Then the aide makes 9 a.m. rounds and locks the door to each room. The patients were first informed and then reminded of the rule. Then the enforcement or actual action demonstrated that the limitation would be enforced. Something as simple as providing a routine can teach patients about the values of reliability, consistency, and stability.

This brings us to a valuable point: Do not commit yourself unless you are able to fulfill the commitment. If your actions are not reliable, if you do not behaviourally demonstrate stability and consistency, then the therapeutic relationship will be established with great difficulty. Patients are people, and they need to know whether someone truly cares and is willing to make the connection that helps them to heal.

SKILLS FOR MENTAL HEALTH CARE

Care providers serve as therapeutic instruments, with each interaction designed to move patients toward the goals of care. They also act as role models for good mental and physical health. They are expected to help solve problems while graciously coping with the varied personalities of many individuals. Care providers work to instill confidence in their patients and encourage them to change and try new behaviours within the security of the therapeutic relationship.

To practise effectively, a care provider's approach to patients must continually be monitored and adjusted. Thought and consideration are given to each therapeutic action. Making a positive, therapeutic use of your personality requires "a consistent, thoughtful effort directed toward developing an awareness of self and others" (Taylor, 1994).

Self-Awareness

Simply defined, **self-awareness** is a consciousness of one's personality. It is the act of looking at oneself—of considering one's abilities, characteristics, aspirations, and concepts of self in relation to others. It is an awareness of one's personal and social behaviours and how they affect others (Morrison, 1993). In short, self-awareness is the ability to objectively look within.

The development of self-awareness requires time, patience, and a willingness to routinely consider one's behaviours, attitudes, and values. The rewards, however, are worth the efforts because both patients and care providers benefit when therapeutic goals are achieved. Personally, self-awareness allows

individuals to direct and mould the pattern of their lives, to be in charge of their own direction and development. Care providers who encourage the development of self-awareness in their patients must be ready to practise it themselves. To improve self-awareness requires caring, insight, acceptance, commitment, a positive outlook, and the willingness to nurture oneself. If you are willing to put effort into these areas, you will evolve into a person who is able to use your personality to achieve therapeutic change and personal fulfillment.

Caring

Everyone has the universal human need for love. Maslow's hierarchy of needs lists the need for love and belonging as the first nonphysical requirement after safety. Without love, infants fail to grow or thrive and adults become isolated, lonely, and depressed. Human beings are gregarious creatures. We are meant to live with others. Although physical appearances, behavioural patterns, and communication styles may differ, each person carries within the need to belong and be loved.

Caring is the energy on which the health care professions are built. It is defined as a concern for the well-being of another person, and it includes behaviours such as accepting, comforting, honesty, attentive listening, and sensitivity. Caring is the glue that binds individuals to one another. It is energy of the soul, freely given in hopes of helping another human being. Caring cannot be taught as a procedure or skill. It must be developed, encouraged, and moulded into the therapeutic personality of the care provider.

Caring serves as a thread that connects people and moves them toward recovery. For people with mental illness, caring plays an especially important role. They can perceive whether one actually cares about them or regards them as just other patients. Box 8.5 lists several therapeutic actions that demonstrate caring.

The caring qualities of empathy and advocacy are also particularly important when caring for mentally troubled individuals. Patients with mental illnesses frequently live in a lonely world of personal suffering, detached from society. Empathy, in these cases, becomes a powerful therapeutic tool that can help re-establish one's self-worth and dignity.

BOX 8.5 Therapeutic Actions: Caring

Address patient by Mr. or Ms. (last name) until otherwise instructed.
Respect the patient's unique personality.
Do not judge the patient's behaviours or attitudes.
Share often with the patient that every person has the potential for change.
Show interest in the whole person, not just the diagnosis.
Customize information to the patient's level of understanding.
Watch for nonverbal messages.
Promote self-esteem by recognizing and communicating that the patient is a worthwhile and valuable individual.
Assess your own interactions, nonverbal actions, and communications for expression of care.

BOX 8.6   Using Failure Positively

To use failure positively:
1. Realize that failure is a necessary part of growth.
2. Give yourself permission to fail.
3. Consider failure as a learning experience.
4. Discover new options and opportunities created by the failure.
5. Expect to succeed with the next attempt.

TABLE 8.2   Focus on Correcting Behaviour Versus Person

Focus on Behaviour	Focus on Person
"Sam, undressing in the dayroom is inappropriate."	"Sam, I've told you not to undress in the dayroom."
"Mariah, stop! No slapping is allowed here."	"Mariah, stop that! Why are you slapping him?"
"I find it difficult to be here when you . . ."	"You're disgusting when you do that."

Insight

We all are responsible for our own development, both professionally and personally. We gain insight and wisdom through experience. **Insight** is the ability to clearly see and understand the nature of things. Insight relies on common sense, good judgement, and prudence. Although not always comfortable, our insights provide us with new opportunities to take risks, explore our own potential, and fail as well as succeed. For care providers, insight includes sensitivity to people, the ability to make keen observations, and a willingness to seek new knowledge.

Self-awareness is developed through the practice of reflection—the process of looking into one's own mind. **Reflection** is an analysis of self—one's feelings, reactions, attitudes, opinions, values, and behaviours. Personal reflection is the process of learning who you are. This type of reflection may be accompanied by emotional discomfort, but for those individuals who can overcome their emotional defences, reflection serves as a valuable tool for developing self-awareness.

It is also a process for observing and analyzing one's behaviour in various situations. Reflection allows us to "step out" of the interaction and watch our own behaviours. This process is often assisted when care providers can view themselves interacting with various patients on video. This type of reflection allows care providers to identify both personal and professional learning needs. Practise professional reflection by keeping a small notebook. Throughout the day, jot down any questions or subjects that relate to the care of your patients—anything about which you feel you need to know more. After work, make it a point to research at least one question or topic every day. This practice will serve as a valuable aid for gaining new knowledge. Knowledge breeds competence, and from competence grows the confidence to provide the best possible care.

Risk Taking and Failure

The process of developing self-awareness includes the elements of risk and failure. If one is to grow, then one must take risks. Risk taking implies the possibility of **failure.** For most of us, the word *failure* has a negative meaning that implies defeat and a lack of success. However, failure can be filled with positive, growth-promoting experiences. Failure provides the opportunity for change. It encourages creativity, stimulates learning, and sharpens one's judgements. Failure is a price that must be paid for improvement. When used as a learning tool, the experience of failure can provide insight and the foundation for the next step toward success. The person who never fails cannot savour the rewards of success.

How do we grow from our failures? The first and most important step is to understand that *failure is a necessary part of change.* The second step is *to give yourself permission to fail.* The odds of a person living a lifetime without a failure are about zero. Failure, learning, and growth are all partners in the development of self-awareness. The third step is to *consider your failure as a learning experience.* Examine the elements of the failure, and discover what improvements could be made. More effective actions in the future can avoid the failures of the past. The fourth and last step is to *discover the opportunities that are created by failure.* Often a failure opens new doors or presents a problem in an entirely different light. Examining and learning from failure can create new options and opportunities. Box 8.6 lists several suggestions for using failure as a positive experience. Remember that one fails only when one refuses to grow from the experience.

Acceptance

Although people may engage in behaviours that are considered inappropriate, every individual has worth and some degree of dignity. Each patient must be given respect and the opportunity to participate in care if treatment is to be successful. Acceptance in this context means the receiving of the entire person and the world in which they function.

Accepting patients does not necessarily include approving of their behaviours. This is an important distinction; you must accept the person, but you do not have to accept the behaviour. Many care providers who work with mentally and emotionally troubled patients do not hesitate to tell a patient when their behaviour is inappropriate, but no mental health care provider should ever directly attack or correct the person. Table 8.2 presents examples of communications that focus on the difference between correcting the behaviour and correcting the person. The very reason patients with mental–emotional problems seek help is to correct their ineffective behaviours. As their care providers, we must accept the entire person as a complete package regardless of our own reactions. This acceptance then becomes the foundation on which other therapeutic actions are based.

Boundaries and Overinvolvement

Caregivers give of themselves in the care of others. To effectively care for others, we must care for ourselves and recharge our batteries if we are to maintain the necessary energy to therapeutically work with patients. One of the ways in which care providers maintain their energy levels is to define their helping boundaries.

We all have limits or boundaries that we will not cross. Personal boundaries provide order and security because they help to establish the limits of one's behaviour. A nurse, social worker, psychologist, or any care provider must take the lead in establishing the therapeutic boundaries in all professional interactions.

Professional boundaries define the needs of the care provider "as distinctly different from the needs of the patient: what is too helpful and what is not; and what fosters independence vs. unhealthy dependence" (Pilette, Berck, & Achber, 1995). Once patients stabilize, they are expected to begin functioning independently with guidance and encouragement from the health care team. Professional (helping) boundaries have been crossed when care providers become too helpful or controlling. The care provider may feel good, but the patient does not function better as a result of the interventions.

The need for professional boundaries must be continually balanced with one's need to be caring. To do this, care providers need to establish their own set of professional boundaries by defining the limits of both their personal and professional lives. The focus of the professional aspect is the patient, but the focus of the care provider's personal life is themselves. The boundaries of each remain distinct because one cannot focus on the patient and the self at the same time.

To maintain their professional boundaries, care providers frequently assess relationships with their patients. If they find themselves having difficulty setting limits or feel that they are the only one who "really understands" a certain patient (the beginnings of co-dependency), then cause for concern exists and help should be sought. Discussing the situation with appropriate persons can help provide perspective and increase one's therapeutic effectiveness. The therapeutic relationship is anchored in the effective management of professional (helping) boundaries. When the focus of interaction is the patient and progress is being made toward the therapeutic goals, the relationship is effective and satisfying for both the patient and the care provider.

Detecting boundary violations is often difficult because "a person's own needs stimulate and maintain the violation" (Pilette et al., 1995). However, early detection helps prevent larger problems in the future. Frequent self-assessments help in monitoring for problems. A delicate balance exists between knowing when to help and when not to help patients. Care providers who are aware of this balance keep the patient as the major focus of concern and maintain the professional boundaries that help individuals progress toward their therapeutic goals.

We have all had (or will have) special patients, those who have touched us deeply. Becoming overinvolved is not difficult to do. However, to thrive and grow, we must learn to walk the fine line between compassion and overinvolvement.

Care providers are people too, complete with their own attributes and problems. It is easier to form rapport with some patients than with others. Sometimes that rapport leads to an overinvolvement because the patient touches the care provider in some special way. This initial attraction can soon result in conflict because the care provider begins to have difficulty separating the professional relationship from the growing friendship with the patient. When the patient–care provider relationship begins to fulfill the care provider's needs, co-dependency results. The relationship loses its therapeutic effectiveness, and the care provider or patient withdraws, left with a mix of unresolved feelings and unmet goals.

To protect yourself from becoming co-dependent, remember this one rule of thumb: If you show a significantly greater level of concern for one patient than for others, then you are running the risk of becoming overinvolved. Recognize this risk early, and discuss it with your supervisor. Exploring your feelings in relation to the patient can help you regain the balance between professionalism and compassion. Often just the personal awareness of the potential of becoming overinvolved is enough to prevent it from occurring. Compassion, empathy, and acceptance are vital elements of health care, but they must be balanced by professionalism, judgement, and therapeutic actions that meet the patient's needs.

Commitment

A **commitment** is a personal bond to some course of action or cause. The health care professions are undergoing radical changes. If provision of high-quality care for every person is to remain a primary goal of our society, then a strong commitment from each health care provider will be needed to maintain the focus on our patients. Care providers must be committed to providing competent health care, no matter what the setting or circumstances.

The first and most important commitment is to *yourself*— the commitment to consciously take charge of your personal and professional growth. Self-commitment involves a promise to do the best you can in every situation and to be the best that you can be. Each person has a unique set of talents, an individual personality, and areas that need improvement. People who are committed to improving themselves are able to consider both the positive and negative aspects of their personalities without guilt or remorse. They realize their mistakes and attempt to profit from them by extracting the lessons hidden in each error. They then commit themselves to applying hard-earned lessons to new situations, which in turn enhances self-awareness and expands one's ability to cope with new experiences.

Health care providers have stronger commitments than most people. They are committed to caring about the welfare of humankind. They demonstrate this dedication by continually seeking out new knowledge, keeping up to date with the latest professional developments, and striving to improve their therapeutic effectiveness.

You are committed; otherwise, you would not be reading these words. Take the time to discover what you feel is most important in life. Then look behind the topic, and you will find yourself committed to a certain course of action. The exercise of describing one's commitments helps to expand

---
BOX 8.8   How To Develop a Positive Attitude

1. Recognize your negative thoughts, emotions, and attitudes. Reject them and remove them from your personality.
2. Replace each negative attitude by frequently repeating positive statements.
3. Repeat upbeat and enthusiastic words that help to build a feeling of success.
4. Visualize future successes.
5. Act the part.

---

self-awareness and reminds us of the interconnectedness of all human beings.

Positive Outlook

Distress of the human spirit can be far more damaging than a medical diagnosis. In contrast, a positive, health-oriented attitude alone can make a difference in functioning. Learn to approach problems with an attitude that employs the patient's strengths, assets, and resources. A focus on the positive aspects of a situation stands a greater chance of success. When it is assumed that the mental health patient will succeed, the patient usually lives up to expectations and does just that—succeeds. One small success fosters and breeds other triumphs. Keep your focus on the "can do." It can have surprising results.

One of the most effective and important tools for developing self-awareness is a positive or optimistic attitude. One's outlook affects every perception, thought, and emotion. People are attracted to individuals with positive attitudes. A person with a positive outlook radiates energy and well-being that cheers everyone in the vicinity. On the other hand, individuals with negative attitudes tend to discourage other people from interacting with them. Their attitude of doom and gloom can even foster the development of many physical and mental problems.

Positive attitudes and thoughts can act as buffers against stress and conflict. They can prevent caregiver burnout, the syndrome that results when care providers give too much without renewing their energies (Box 8.7). A positive outlook does not require one to be continually upbeat. The reality of each situation must be considered objectively, but there is no reason to harbour a negative attitude when a positive one is much more fulfilling. In addition, care providers who practise positive thinking act as role models for those patients who do not cope effectively within their worlds.

Achieving and maintaining a positive outlook is especially important for care providers who work with individuals who are mentally and emotionally troubled. A positive attitude is the secret weapon for coping with the adversity of life. It is the key to maintaining physical and emotional health, especially for those who share their energies therapeutically. Developing a positive attitude (Box 8.8) is a process that requires persistent and patient efforts because our current attitudes and habits that run counter to such an attitude are deeply ingrained.

However, the process can be assisted by following these five tips:

1. **Listen to your self-talk.** Pay attention to the words you use. Each word has an emotional attachment to it. The human brain is programmed by thoughts, which become feelings, which evolve into words and actions. Many people complain of being under too much stress or pressure. No one denies that modern life contains its share of stresses. However, it is how each stressor is defined that determines your point of view. If you do not define the event as stressful, then it is not. Practise listening to yourself. You may be surprised at what you discover.

2. **Change recurrent negative themes.** Any thought, emotion, word, or action that is self-defeating needs to be replaced with a positive, empowering one. Releasing and replacing one's negative attitudes lead to greater self-esteem, awareness, confidence, and happiness, not to mention the added benefits of a highly effective immune system. Practise changing your negative themes, because your outlook determines the success or failure of an action.

3. **Be your own cheerleader.** Give yourself a pep talk every morning and whenever you are coping with stresses. Present yourself with positive, inspiring thoughts. Your brain does not question your thoughts. Those stored thoughts then become the basis for actions. Positive statements uplift the spirits and help to convince you of your value.

4. **Visualize future successes.** Take a few moments during each day to picture yourself achieving a goal. Fantasize about the feelings associated with achievement, and think about the steps that lead to the goal. Picture yourself as a dynamic person and capable care provider; it will help to provide the blueprint for future growth. Besides, it is fun to do.

5. **Act the part.** Visualize yourself as a person with confidence and ability. You will find that your actual level of confidence grows each time you project an image of self-assurance. Developing a positive outlook will serve you well.

Nurturing Yourself

A critical first step in the development of self-awareness is to recognize and tend to your own needs. To **nurture** someone is to encourage their development. Care providers are expected

BOX 8.9 How to Nurture Yourself

1. Be knowledgeable.
2. Value each individual as a human presence.
3. Be responsible and accountable for your actions.
4. Be open to new ideas.
5. Connect with others. Support your colleagues.
6. Take pride in yourself.
7. Like what you do.
8. Recognize the moments of joy in the struggles of living. Take time to smell the roses.
9. Recognize and accept your own limitations, but strive to improve. At the end of the day, focus on your accomplishments rather than the things left undone.
10. Rest each day, and begin anew.

Data from Sherwood, G. (1992). The responses of caregivers to the experience of suffering. In P. L. Starck & J. P. McGovern, (Eds.), *The hidden dimension of illness: Human suffering.* National League for Nursing Press.

to work hard for the welfare of their patients, but they must also care for and nurture themselves. Energy cannot be continually spent without being renewed. Care providers function at a high level of wellness to provide the energy required by their patients. You have chosen to care for others. Part of the responsibility you accepted when making this decision was to care for yourself. To effectively care for your patients, you must first nurture yourself.

Health care providers seek to "instill hope, empower others, encourage independence, and help improve the other's condition. When we are unable to achieve that, unable to alleviate suffering, we often experience a sense of frustration and failure" (Sherwood, 1992). When this frustration occurs repeatedly, we become emotionally worn or burned out, as

many care providers call it. Somehow each of us must find the balance between the moral duty to care amid the stress of constant suffering and the concern for one's well-being. Box 8.9 offers basic principles for maintaining oneself when caring for others. Using these guidelines will assist you in finding the balance between giving and renewing. Remember them, because they are key to replenishing the energies that you so freely share with others.

To nurture yourself requires more than food, water, sleep, and activity. To nourish the part of the self from which one's therapeutic energies are drawn requires special renewal. Care providers nurture themselves in different ways. Some turn to a special source of comfort, whereas others find renewal in the adventure of trying new things. Spending time alone recharges some. Others need the challenge of physical activities, travel, or new relationships.

Research has pointed out the many benefits of daily meditation for stress reduction, relaxation, and renewal (Kabot-Zinn, 1994). Meditation, termed the *relaxation response* by Western medicine, is the practice of becoming still and quiet. Health care providers who practise meditation for as little as 15 minutes per day find it a valuable source of renewal and stress reduction.

In this busy world, it is easy to lose sight of one simple fact: Your ability to care for your patients depends on how well you care for yourself. How you choose to nurture and renew yourself is a matter of personal preference. The important thing is that you do it regularly and without guilt. A good diet, adequate exercise, and restful sleep must not be ignored, but the essence of caring must also be applied to the self. Care providers need to be willing to accept, love, and nourish themselves as much as they do their patients.

KEY POINTS

- A mentally healthy adult is a person who can cope with and adjust to the stresses of daily living in a socially acceptable way. Mentally healthy adults are content with themselves, able to love and express love, flexible, eager to learn, and unafraid of adversity.
- The main therapeutic tool of mental health care providers is the "self." Therapeutic use of self is used with the "do no harm" principle as a basis for practice.
- Understanding patients in relation to their work, family, and social environments encourages care providers to practise holistic health care.
- The seven principles of mental health care are as follows: do no harm, accept each patient as a whole person, develop mutual trust, explore behaviours and emotions, encourage responsibility, encourage effective adaptation, and provide consistency.
- Behaviour consists of perceptions, thoughts, feelings, and actions.
- In mental health terms, adaptation means sufficient improvement to carry out everyday activities.

- The goal of crisis intervention is to offer immediate emotional support. Procedures for crisis intervention focus on the concepts of immediacy, control, assessment, disposition, referral, and follow-up.
- Setting and enforcing limits can teach patients about the values of reliability, consistency, and stability.
- When used as a learning tool, the experience of failure can provide insight, encourage creativity, stimulate learning, and sharpen judgement.
- To prevent overinvolvement and co-dependency, care providers need to recognize the risk of a significantly greater level of concern for one patient than that for others, explore their feelings in relation to the patient, and discuss it with their supervisor.
- Care providers have the power to shape their patients' successes or failures based on their own personal values and beliefs.
- A commitment is a bond that moves an individual to action. Self-commitment involves a promise to do one's best in every situation. Professional commitment is

demonstrated by seeking out new knowledge, keeping up to date with the latest professional developments, and striving to improve one's therapeutic effectiveness.

- A positive mental attitude is developed by listening to your self-talk, changing recurrent negative themes, being your own cheerleader, visualizing future successes, and acting the part.

- Principles for nurturing yourself include being knowledgeable, valuing each individual, being responsible and accountable, being open to new ideas, connecting with others, supporting your colleagues, taking pride in yourself, enjoying what you do, recognizing the moments of joy in the struggles of living, recognizing and accepting your own limitations but striving to improve, and focusing on your accomplishments rather than the things left undone.

ADDITIONAL LEARNING RESOURCES

Go to your Evolve website (http://evolve.elsevier.com/Canada/Morrison-Valfre/) for additional online resources, including the online Study Guide for additional learning activities to help you master this chapter content.

CRITICAL THINKING QUESTIONS

1. Marion is a 43-year-old mother of three teenagers and is also caring for her 75-year-old mother who has Alzheimer's disease. Marion confides in you that she is having difficulty sleeping at night and always feels that something bad is going to happen because she has forgotten to do something. Marion states that she used to enjoy bowling with friends from work, but whenever she attends the weekly event, she just feels distracted and is constantly thinking about her children and her mother. Marion also describes feeling tired and worries that she is becoming irritable with her children as well as with her elderly mother. What is happening to Marion, and how might you respond to her about her concerns?

2. Carol is an RN and a work colleague whom you have known for several years. Recently, while you were working together on a night shift, Carol told you that she had enrolled in a masters (MScN) program but was finding the courses too difficult and had failed her most recent course. Considering Box 8.6 in the chapter, how might you respond to Carol and help her to reframe her feelings of disappointment and failure?

3. David is a new nurse on your community mental health support team. David excitedly shares the news that Mrs. Donovan, an older patient who has a history of depression, has given him a $100 gift card for Amazon because "David reminds me so much of my grandson…" What would be an appropriate response to David about the patient's gift?

REFERENCES

Chenevert, M. (1994). *Stat: Special techniques in assertiveness training* (4th ed.). Mosby [Seminal Reference].

Giger, J. N., & Haddad, L. G. (2020). *Transcultural nursing: Assessment and intervention* (8th ed.). Mosby.

Glasser, W. (1998). *Choice theory*. HarperCollins [Seminal Reference].

Kabot-Zinn, J. (1994). Meditate! . . . for stress reduction, inner peace . . . or whatever. *Psychology Today, 26*(4), 36.

Keltner, N. L., & Steele, D. (2019). *Psychiatric nursing* (8th ed.). Elsevier.

Morrison, M. W. (1993). *Professional skills for leadership: Foundations of a successful career*. Mosby.

Pilette, P. C., Berck, C. B., & Achber, L. C. (1995). Therapeutic management of helping boundaries. *Journal of Psychosocial Nursing and Mental Health Services, 33*, 40 [Seminal Reference].

Sherwood, G. (1992). The responses of caregivers to the experience of suffering. In P. L. Starck, & J. P. McGovern (Eds.), *The hidden dimension of illness: Human suffering*. National League for Nursing Press [Seminal Reference].

Stuart, G. W. (2013). *Principles and practice of psychiatric nursing* (10th ed.). Mosby.

Taylor, C. M. (1994). *Essentials of psychiatric nursing* (14th ed.). Mosby.

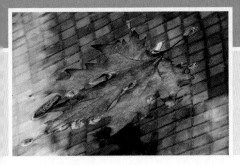

Mental Health Assessment Skills

KEY TERMS

affect (ĂF-ĕkt) (p. 102)
assessment (ă-SĔS-mĕnt) (p. 97)
calculation (KĂL-kyū-LĀ-shŭn) (p. 104)
data collection (DĂ-tă kă-lĕc-shŭn) (p. 98)
depersonalization (p. 103)
insight (p. 015)
interview (ĬN-tər-vyū) (p. 98)
judgement (JŬDJ-mĕnt) (p. 105)

memory (MĔM-ŏr-ē) (p. 104)
mood (p. 102)
nursing (therapeutic) process (NŬR-sǐng PRŎ-sĕs) (p. 96)
perceptions (pĕr-CĔP-shŭns) (p. 102)
risk factor assessment (p. 98)
sensorium (sĕn-SŌ-rē-ŭm) (p. 104)
thought content (p. 103)
thought processes (p. 103)

The ability to effectively obtain and use information about patients is a vital part of the multidisciplinary treatment plan and the foundation of the nursing (therapeutic) process. Uncovering patients' problems requires critical thinking abilities and exceptional assessment skills. Therapeutic communications, interactions, and assessment skills help care providers learn about all aspects of their patients. This chapter provides the starting point for making thorough mental health assessments. Good assessment skills are critical to quality health care. Care providers must first learn about the person before they can provide personalized care or judge the effectiveness of any therapeutic action.

MENTAL HEALTH TREATMENT PLAN

People enter the health care system because they are distressed, disabled, or suffering. The diagnosis and treatment of people living with mental health issues is challenging. Diagnoses of mental illness are not as easily identified and defined as physical disorders. According to the *Diagnostic and Statistical Manual of Mental Disorders,* fifth edition (*DSM-5*), "no definition adequately specifies precise boundaries for the concept of mental disorder" (American Psychiatric Association [APA], 2013). The relationship between the physical and psychological self is difficult to separate. It is important to

TABLE 9.1   World Health Organization Disability Assessment Schedule (WHODAS 2.0)

Domains of Functioning	Example
Cognition	Communication, understanding
Getting along	Interactions, meaningful relationships
Life activities	Responsibilities, home, work, school, etc.
Mobility	Moving, getting around
Participation	Social functioning, community activities
Self-care	Hygiene, dressing, eating, living situation

BOX 9.1   The Montreal Cognitive Assessment

The Montreal Cognitive Assessment (MoCA) is a brief, 30-question test that takes around 10 to 12 minutes to complete and helps assess people for dementia. It was published in 2005 by a group at McGill University working for several years at memory clinics in Montreal (Nasreddine, Phillips, Bédirian, V., et al., 2005).

The MoCA can be used to screen a variety of cognitive challenges associated with Alzheimer's disease, Lewy body dementia, brain metastasis, depression, head trauma, and many others.

BOX 9.2   Components of a Mental Status Exam

1. Appearance, physical activity, and behaviour
2. Speech, affect, and mood
3. Thought: form, content, and process
4. Perceptions
5. Conscious awareness
6. Insight
7. Judgement
8. Memory

Data from Muir-Cochrane, E., Barkway, P., & Nizette, D. (2014). *Mosby's pocketbook of mental health* (2nd ed.). Mosby Australia.

remember, however, that every psychological problem has physical effects, and each physical illness has psychological effects. The wise care provider is aware of both.

When individuals first enter the mental health care system, ideally they undergo a comprehensive assessment. Patients are interviewed by several members of the multidisciplinary health care team. Physical and psychological diagnostic testing is performed, and data (information) are gathered from as many sources as possible. The physician provides information regarding patients' physical state and need for medications. The social worker assesses the patient's family, work, and social interactions. The dietitian learns about the patient's nutritional status. The psychiatrist can prescribe medication in response to emotional and mental health challenges, the psychologist explores the patient's emotional and cognitive (intellectual) functioning, often over a prolonged period of time. The nurse assesses how the illness or disability affects the patient's activities of daily living. Other care providers contribute information through their observations and interactions with the patient.

Team members then meet to compare data, identify problems, and develop treatment approaches. When the team and the patient agree on the treatment goals, a course of action is planned. Usually medical treatments (medications) are combined with psychotherapies, behavioural therapies, and other therapeutic actions. The overall treatment plan is then developed for the individual patient. Therapeutic actions are implemented, and the patient's progress toward each goal is evaluated.

The mental health treatment plan serves several purposes. First, it is a *guide* for planning and implementing patient care. Nurses are guided by the treatment plan when they develop specific nursing care plans. Psychologists, social workers, and other therapists use the treatment plan as a framework for implementing their specialized therapeutic actions.

Second, the plan serves as a vehicle for *monitoring* the patient's progress and the effectiveness of therapeutic interventions. Patients meet often with treatment team members to discuss problems and attempts to meet their goals. Therapeutic interventions are evaluated, and the treatment plan is revised to include new information.

Third, the mental health treatment plan serves as a means for *communicating* and *coordinating* patient care. The plan prevents costly duplication of services and provides a focus for all therapeutic activities, regardless of specialty. This increases the effectiveness of each team member's efforts. Developing the mental health treatment plan is not a complex process, but it is always changing. Using the treatment plan, patients and care providers have the opportunity to work together to meet patient goals.

DSM-5 Diagnosis

Therapists who work with mentally or emotionally challenged individuals often use the *DSM-5* to aid in diagnosis and help guide clinical practice. One of the tools used in the *DSM-5* is the World Health Organization's Disability Assessment Schedule (WHODAS 2.0; Table 9.1). The diagnosis of mental health disorders remains the responsibility of the physician, but nurses and other care providers should be familiar with the multiaxial system of psychiatric assessment. Several tools are available for assessing mental status. A tool that is commonly used by health care providers in Canada is the Montreal Cognitive Assessment (MoCA) (Box 9.1; see https://www.mocatest.org/). An additional generic example of a mental health assessment tool is seen in Appendix A at the back of the text.

Nursing (Therapeutic) Process

Each step of the **nursing (therapeutic) process** is designed to support goal-directed care for patients (Stuart, 2013). The process is an organizational framework for effective care. It consists of five steps: assessment, diagnosis, planning, intervention, and evaluation. Use of this process encourages care providers to focus on the patient and to develop appropriate and effective care. The nursing process serves as a guideline that helps promote consistency in approach and use of language and terminology.

The first step, assessment, is the data-collection step. Bits of information relating to the patient are collected from every possible source. Medical records are reviewed, a history is obtained, and observations are made (Box 9.2). Through discussions with family members or friends, more information is added to the database. Soon a picture of the patient begins to emerge. Using the mass of collected information as a database, care providers plan care based on the needs, abilities, preferences, and concerns of the patient.

Next, data are organized into related areas, and problems are identified. Each problem is then examined in detail. Problem statements and nursing diagnoses are developed. Medical diagnoses and interventions relate to the patient's physical or mental dysfunctions. Nursing diagnoses and interventions focus on how the patient's problems affect their ability to carry out the activities of daily living. Patient needs are also considered when problem statements are being developed.

During the planning phase, specific short- and long-term goals are developed. The outcome of each problem is projected by identifying behaviours that would indicate that the problem is solved. These "expected outcomes" are then used to monitor the patient's progress. Therapeutic actions (interventions) are planned using goals and expected outcomes. Then a written care plan is developed.

The intervention phase includes the actual delivery of the planned actions. Therapeutic interventions, carried out by all mental health care team members, guide patients toward their goals. Patient responses to each intervention are monitored. As a care provider, work to keep an open mind when observing the patient's responses to care, and remember that many reactions are culturally determined.

CULTURAL CONSIDERATIONS

It is considered taboo in East Indian Hindu culture for a male to extend his hand when greeting a female. Initiating direct eye contact with a woman is seen as a seductive gesture. The proper way to introduce oneself to a female Hindu patient is to first greet the husband or oldest female companion. Many Hindu individuals are unwilling to give up speaking their native language, so a Hindu-English–speaking family member commonly accompanies the patient.

In the final phase of the process, evaluation, the effectiveness of care is determined. By comparing expected outcomes with actual results, care providers are able to note which actions met the goals and which did not. Those actions that did not result in meeting goals are reassessed, and the process is begun again.

In a patient-centred environment, patients are involved as partners in care. Patient-centred care includes promoting autonomy, providing privacy, ensuring comfort, honouring cultural preferences, and advocating for the patient and family (Stein & Hollen, 2020). Although some individuals are unable or too discouraged to make decisions, most patients are capable of participating in some part of their care. Care providers can help patients problem-solve by involving them in the care-planning process. Evaluations of both patients' and care providers' actions allow for adjustments in the dynamic

process known as *treatment*. Use of the nursing (therapeutic) process requires knowledge, experience, and the practice of good judgement. Experience grows with each application of the process, and sound judgement is gained by looking at every possible side of an issue before arriving at a decision. The nursing (therapeutic) process serves as a tool for defining and solving a wide range of patient presentations, but the tool is only as effective as the practitioner. The art of choosing the best course of action must be carefully practised. Let the "do no harm" principle guide you as you grow.

ABOUT ASSESSMENT

Assessment includes the "gathering, verifying and communicating of information relative to the patient" (*Mosby's Dictionary*, 2013). Patients are dynamic (changing) individuals who are affected by more than an illness or disorder. For this reason, the holistic assessment includes gathering information about the physical, intellectual, emotional, social, cultural, and spiritual aspects of each patient. The more complete the picture, the more effective the treatment approaches will be.

The process of assessing patients is ongoing. It begins with the patient's admission to the facility or service and ends only after the patient's relationship with the health care system has ended. To gain an understanding of patients, become observant and alert for any information that may have an effect on care.

Data Collection

Data (information) relating to patients are grouped into objective and subjective categories. *Objective data* refer to information that can be measured and shared. They are gathered through the senses of sight, smell, touch, and hearing. Blood pressure readings, pulse rates, and laboratory reports that are compared with "normal" illustrate objective data. When working with mental health patients, care providers obtain objective data through physical examinations, daily assessments, diagnostic testing results, and repeated observations of behaviours (see Box 9.2) (Potter, Perry, Stockert, et al., 2019).

Subjective data relate to patients' perceptions. These data include information that is abstract and difficult to measure or share. The experiences of pain, nausea, and anxiety, for example, cannot be measured by anyone but the individual experiencing them. Emotions and mental states are all subjective and difficult to measure. As a result, it is extremely important to document subjective information as descriptively and accurately as possible. Do not include interpretive statements (judgements). Document patient reactions and behaviours in exact terms. To say that the patient is angry (unless he states that he is angry) is an interpretive statement or judgement. It is better to state that the patient was pacing about the room while slamming his fist into the wall and swearing. When documenting subjective data, quote the patient as much as possible. Subjective information is collected during the initial health history interview and during every interaction with patients. The simple question "How do you feel?" can elicit much subjective information.

TABLE 9.2   Commonly Used Rating Scales for Assessing Mental Health

Diagnosis	Scale(s) Available	Notes
Alcohol withdrawal	The Clinical Institute Withdrawal Assessment for Alcohol Scale (CIWA-Ar)	A standardized clinical tool that facilitates assessment of alcohol withdrawal
Anxiety	Hamilton Rating Scale for Anxiety (HAM-A)	A rating scale that quantifies the severity of anxiety symptomatology. It is often used in psychotropic drug evaluation. The HAM-A contains 14 items, each defined by a series of symptoms.
Dementia	Mini Mental State Examination (MMSE)	Used to determine level of cognitive impairment, as well as changes to cognitive function over a period of time
	Montreal Cognitive Assessment (MoCA) (https://www.mocatest.org/)	Screening tool for detecting mild levels of cognitive impairment
Mood disorders	Mood Disorder Questionnaire	General questionnaire to assess presence of mood disorder

The term **data collection** refers to a variety of activities designed to gather information about a certain subject. Data-collecting tools and methods for care providers include interviews, observational techniques, and rating scales and inventories. An **interview** is a meeting of people with the purpose of obtaining or exchanging information (Keltner & Steele, 2019). Interviews can be formal and highly structured or informal and casual. Information gathered from formal interviews is usually documented on a standardized form. The interview is an excellent method for obtaining information. It also serves as the starting point for building the therapeutic relationship. Informal interviews usually occur casually and provide great opportunities to learn more about patients and their families. Care providers use informal interview techniques when they investigate patient issues or explore certain topics.

Data gathering through observational techniques is commonly used. Observation is the process of purposeful looking. When using observation as a data-gathering technique, care providers must be careful to be objective. Personal bias or attitudes can alter one's perceptions and affect the objectivity of the observations. The use of observation is an excellent method for gathering information when the caregiver can remain impartial and does not pass judgement.

Physical assessment skills are important to the data-gathering process. They are used to gather data, investigate changes in physical conditions, and evaluate the effectiveness of therapeutic interventions. Physical examination skills are special methods for obtaining information about the body's functioning. The technique of observation is called *inspection,* which means a purposeful examination of the body. With the skills of auscultation and percussion, the examiner uses their sense of hearing to detect sounds within the body. Finally, the technique of palpation requires the sense of touch to draw out information about temperature, texture, and pulsations of the body.

Social workers, psychologists, and other therapists frequently use rating scales and inventories. These are data-gathering tools specifically designed to bring out certain kinds of information. The results are then compared with standardized measurements. Rating scales and inventories can be very useful for focusing on specific aspects of patient issues.

There are several types of rating scales, typically focused on either determining a diagnosis or exploring an existing diagnosis. Examples of some rating scales that are currently in use are summarized in Table 9.2.

Assessment Process
Holistic Assessment

The physical, social, cultural, intellectual, emotional, and spiritual areas of a person's life have an effect on health. Without knowledge of these six aspects, health care providers become narrowed and limited in their effectiveness. The holistic assessment for those who work with mentally or emotionally troubled patients is the same as that used by care providers in any setting. In psychiatric treatment situations, however, the emphasis is on mental–emotional functioning. The psychiatric assessment tool focuses on obtaining data about the problems, coping behaviours, and resources of patients (Table 9.3). Information collected from assessment activities serves as part of the database from which medical, nursing, and other treatment decisions are made. An additional risk factor assessment is required for patients who may pose a risk of committing violence against themselves or others.

Risk Factor Assessment

A **risk factor assessment** helps "formulate a nursing diagnosis based on the identification of risk factors that potentially present an immediate threat to the patient" (Stuart, 2013) or others in the vicinity. With this assessment tool, five areas of potential risk for harm are identified (Box 9.3). Positive findings lead to more specific assessments and appropriate safety precautions (e.g., evaluation of lethality of a suicide plan, Box 9.4). A registered nurse completes the risk factor assessment, but other health care providers assist by gathering important information and making objective observations.

CASE STUDY

The police attend your hospital emergency department with a 55-year-old female named Bernice. They inform you that they received a 9-1-1 call from the sister of a female who was threatening to commit suicide by overdose. Police confirm that the female was mildly combative, resistant to attending the hospital, and was apprehended under the *Mental Health Act*. Police also state that the female does not appear to be intoxicated; however, they located 15–20 empty bottles of liquor in her apartment.

From outside the room, you hear a police officer negotiating for the removal of the handcuffs. Bernice confirms that she will not try to leave and will cooperate with the nurses and doctors. The police officer removes the handcuffs and steps out of the room. The triage nurse tells you that the bloodwork he drew when Bernice was first triaged appears relatively normal, and her ETOH (alcohol) level is not toxic; however, it suggests there was some alcohol consumption within the last 4 hours.

Bernice appears slightly older than her chronological age. She is dishevelled and appears to have worn the same clothes for several days. You can see that her eyes are red as she wipes tears away with a tissue given to her by the officer. You introduce yourself to Bernice and explain to her your role and intention to interview her, to determine how the team can best provide assistance. Bernice agrees to participate in the assessment.

You conduct a mental health and safety assessment. The following is a point-form representation of the information you've obtained from your assessments:

- Bernice is employed full-time as an administrative assistant with the local school board; however, she has been on leave for several months for the purpose of accessing treatment resources for a 2-year history of alcohol abuse.
- Bernice's 26-year-old daughter committed suicide exactly 2 years ago today, following the termination of a relationship.
- Bernice describes herself as a social drinker; however, she lost control of her drinking after her daughter's suicide.
- She was divorced 10 years ago and has had little to no contact with her former husband, who is the father of her deceased child. Bernice expresses considerable resentment at his lack of contact and support.
- Her employer has provided funding for a private alcohol abuse treatment program and has given her 8 months off work. As of yet, Bernice has not contacted the treatment facility.

- She confirms that her sister called her this morning and states, "She's a wonderful big sister; she calls me two or three times a day, but I never want to bother her with my problems."
- She does not recall telling her sister she planned to commit suicide by overdosing on her daughter's psychiatric medication and two full bottles of Tylenol #3's she found in her daughter's room; however, police have confirmed this from the text of the 9-1-1 call.
- Bernice discloses that she has had ongoing thoughts of ending her life since her daughter's death and that these thoughts have become more intense lately.
- Bernice states that the anniversary of her daughter's death is unbearable for her; she thinks the only solution is to be with her daughter.

Primary Concerns

- Bernice is currently endorsing a plan to commit suicide and has access to enough medications for an overdose. Police did not remove the medications from her home.
- Today is the anniversary of her daughter's death, causing an even higher level of anxiety and distress for Bernice.
- She has a 2-year history of alcohol abuse, triggered by the suicide.
- She is alone with no support from her former spouse and is not willing to utilize the support her sister is trying to provide.
- She feels estranged from her job and feels that co-workers think she is an alcoholic.

Points to Consider

- Bernice is at immediate risk for committing suicide.
- She has a plan to do so, and she has access to a means to do so.
- She has a history of alcohol abuse.
- She is not utilizing supports.
  As the crisis nurse, how would you respond to this situation?
- Based on safety concerns, recommend to the emergency department physician that Bernice be placed on a 72-hour *Mental Health Act* form that requires an assessment by a psychiatrist.
- Recommend involuntary admission to a mental health unit for stabilization and further assessment.

TABLE 9.3 Summary Psychiatric Assessment Tool

Area of Assessment	Example
Appraisal of health/illness	Events leading to problem, definition of problem, patient's goal, regular health care received
Previous psychiatric treatment	Diagnosis, type of treatment, medications, adherence, psychiatric history in family
Coping responses, physical status	Review of function in each body system, physical assessment, diet history, sleep patterns, exposure to toxic substances, activities of daily living
Coping responses, mental status	Appearance, speech, motor activity, mood, affect, interactions, perceptions, thought content and process, memory, concentration, calculations, intelligence, insight, judgement
Coping responses, discharge planning, needs	Patient's ability to provide for food, clothing, housing, safety, transportation, supportive relationships, work needs, financial needs
Coping mechanisms	Adaptive mechanisms, maladaptive mechanisms
Psychosocial and environmental problems	Educational, occupational, economic, housing problems; difficulties with support group, culture, access to health care services
Knowledge deficits	Understanding of psychiatric issue, coping skills, medications, stressors

Modified from Stuart, G. W. (2013). *Principles and practice of psychiatric nursing* (10th ed.). Mosby.

BOX 9.3 Risk Factor Assessment

The purpose is to identify threats to the patient. Remember "SAVES."

Risk Factor
Suicide/Self-Harm
Current or past suicidal thoughts or actions
History of self-harm or suicidal attempts

Alcohol or Drug Use
Frequency and amount
Interference with daily living activities
Past experiences with withdrawal

Violence
Current feelings of anger and/or aggression
History of assault, destructive behaviours, or striking out

Elopement
History of leaving against medical advice
Does patient wish to leave now?

Seizures
History of seizures
History of falls

BOX 9.4 Determining the Lethality of a Suicide Plan

The evaluation of a suicide plan is extremely important in determining the degree of suicidal risk. Five main elements must be considered when evaluating lethality (the degree of suicidal risk):
1. Presence of risk factors for suicide
2. Degree of suicidal ideation
3. Intent to carry out suicide plan
4. Means and availability of resources to carry out selected method of suicide
5. Degree of hope for improvement of psychological state

From Toth, M., Schwartz, R., & Kurka, S. (2007). Strategies for understanding and assessing suicide risk in psychotherapy. *Annals of the American Psychotherapy Association, 10*(4), 18–25. http://www.annalsofpsychotherapy.com/index.php

The Patient at Risk

Often in mental health, you will encounter patients who are a risk to themselves or to someone else. Typically, this risk is based on a mental health challenge, substance abuse, or a distressing life event (or sometimes a combination of these factors). When all crisis intervention efforts have failed, the only remaining option may be an involuntary admission to the hospital's mental health unit.

All provinces and territories have a provision for temporarily removing an individual's civil rights when they are unable to or incapable of caring for themselves or pose a risk to themselves or others (typically due to suicidal ideation or violent intentions toward another person). While this process can be distressing to the patient (and to the mental health workers involved), sometimes no other option is available to

ensure the patient's safety. Once the *Mental Health Act* form has been activated and the patient has been transferred to a secure inpatient setting, efforts can be made to stabilize the individual with counselling and therapy, along with pharmacological options.

OBTAINING A HISTORY

Each patient is interviewed on admission to the health care service. The purpose of the history interview is to obtain data about the unique individual who is the patient. It offers care providers an opportunity to introduce themselves and serves as a starting point for establishing the therapeutic relationship. During the interview, insight into patient concerns, worries, and expectations is gained. The interview also offers the opportunity to obtain clues that may require further investigation. When used appropriately, the interview is a powerful method for gathering important information and establishing the therapeutic relationship.

Effective Interviews

The success of any patient interview rests on the care provider's ability to listen objectively and respond appropriately. To enhance your interviewing skills, follow these guidelines:

- Remember that **personal values must not cloud professional judgements.** Reacting to a patient's personal appearance or behaviours can stereotype the patient and have a negative impact on the effectiveness of the therapeutic relationship.
- **Do not make assumptions** about how you think the patient feels. Discover what each event means to the patient and how they view the situation. The experience of losing a loved one, for example, depends on how an individual interprets or perceives an event.
- Always **take into account the patient's cultural and religious values and beliefs.** With mental health patients, this point cannot be emphasized enough. Care providers must learn about their patients' cultures if they are to understand their points of view. With patients from unfamiliar cultures, it is wise to research information about the culture and its religious practices before conducting the interview.
- **Pay particular attention to nonverbal communication.** Much can be learned if one is observant. Note which subjects are avoided or quickly passed over during the interview. These behaviours can be clues that indicate a need for further investigation. Observing methods of self-expression helps the care provider to focus on the patient's unspoken signals and the messages they communicate.
- **Have clearly set goals.** Know the purpose of the interview. Is this an initial assessment interview or the investigation of a specific condition? The assessment interview is not a random discussion; it is a purposefully planned interaction with the patient.
- **Monitor your own reactions** during the interview. Use self-awareness to signal when you are becoming too emotionally involved. While a care provider may identify

BOX 9.5 Health History for Mental Health Patients

Health Care History

General Health Care

Regular health care provider

Frequency of health care visits

Last medical examination and test results

Any unusual circumstances of pregnancy or births

Hospitalizations and surgeries: when, why indicated, treatments, outcome

Family history

Diagnosed brain problem

Head trauma: Details of accidents or periods of unconsciousness for any reason—blows to the head, electrical shocks, high fevers, seizures, fainting, dizziness, headaches, falls

Endocrine disturbances: Thyroid and adrenal function, particularly diabetes, stability of glucose levels

Lifestyle

Eating: Details of unusual or unsupervised diets, appetite, weight changes, cravings, caffeine intake

Medications: Full history of current and past psychiatric medications in self and first-degree relatives

Substance use: Alcohol and drug use

Toxins: Overcome by automobile exhaust or natural gas; exposure to lead, mercury, insecticides, herbicides, solvents, cleaning agents, lawn chemicals

Occupation (current and past): Chemicals in workplace (farming, painting)

Cancer: Full history, particularly consider metastases (lung, breast, melanoma, gastrointestinal tract, and kidney are most likely to be affected); results of treatment (chemotherapy and surgeries)

Lung problems: Details of anything that restricts flow of air to lungs for more than 2 minutes or adversely affects oxygen absorption (brain uses 20% of oxygen in body), such as with chronic obstructive pulmonary disease, near drowning, near strangulation, high-altitude oxygen deprivation, resuscitation

Cardiac problems: Childhood illnesses such as scarlet or rheumatic fever; history of heart attacks, strokes, or hypertension

Blood diseases: Anemia, arteriosclerotic conditions, HIV, work-related accidents, military experiences

Injury: Safe sex practices, contact sports and sports-related injuries, exposure to violence or abuse

Presenting symptoms and coping responses: Description—nature, frequency, and intensity; threats to safety of self or others; functional status; quality of life

HIV, human immunodeficiency virus.

From Stuart, G. W. (2009). *Handbook of psychiatric nursing* (9th ed.). Mosby.

with certain patients with similar interests or situations, self-awareness allows the care provider to understand the emotional responses generated by certain patients. Interviewing skills are used throughout the nursing (therapeutic) process. Work to develop and refine your interviewing skills because they are important tools.

Sociocultural Assessment

The health history includes information about both the physical and psychological functions of an individual. The sociocultural assessment focuses on the cultural, social, and spiritual aspects of an individual. During the history interview, the care provider obtains information about a patient's background and observes the patient's appearance, behaviours, and attitudes (these are also included in the mental status examination).

The sociocultural assessment focuses on six areas. Patients are asked questions about their age, ethnicity (culture), gender, education, income, and belief system. Risk factors and stressors are also defined during the sociocultural assessment (National Depressive and Manic-Depressive Association, 2014). This information helps care providers develop accurate and appropriate plans of care.

Review of Systems

The holistic assessment also includes a review of each body system and its functioning. Patients are first questioned about their general health care, past illnesses and hospitalizations, and family health history. Questions then focus on the function of each body system. Last, the lifestyle and activities of daily living are assessed. Box 9.5 lists the topics covered by the health history for patients living with mental health challenges. Data obtained from the health history, physical assessments, and various diagnostic examinations all help complete the picture of each individual patient.

PHYSICAL ASSESSMENT

Patients receive a physical examination on admission to a psychiatric service. The purpose of the examination is to discover physical problems that can be treated medically. Many alterations in behaviour are often traced to a physical cause. For example, low blood sugar levels can result in confused and uncooperative behaviour. Hormone imbalances, exposure to toxic substances, and severe pain can also affect behaviour.

A complete physical examination is performed by a physician or nurse practitioner. The patient's current health status is explored, and then each system is examined. Nurses have an obligation to assess each patient's health status on a routine basis. A complete physical assessment is not needed every day, but nurses must be alert to changes in their patients' conditions. Most nurses use a systems approach or head-to-toe assessment. Both take less than 5 minutes and can be performed any time information about physical functions is needed.

Diagnostic studies for patients with mental–emotional difficulties include standard laboratory tests (blood and urine tests, evaluation of electrolytes, and hormone function examinations). Many patients are screened for tuberculosis, human immunodeficiency virus (HIV), and sexually transmitted infections (STIs). Studies such as X-ray examinations, electrocardiograms (ECGs), electroencephalograms (EEGs), and brain imaging studies (computed tomography [CT], magnetic resonance imaging [MRI], positron emission tomography

TABLE 9.4	**The Mental Status Examination**
General description	Appearance; speech; motor activity; interaction during interview
Emotional state	Mood; affect
Experiences	Perceptions
Thinking	Thought content; thought processes
Sensorium (ability to sort information) and cognition	Level of consciousness; memory; level of concentration and calculation; information and intelligence; judgement

From Stuart, G. W. (2012). *Handbook of psychiatric nursing* (7th ed.). Mosby.

[PET] scans) may be ordered. To complete the picture, the patient's current mental and emotional state is assessed via a mental status examination.

MENTAL STATUS ASSESSMENT

The mental status examination allows care providers to observe and describe a patient's behaviour in an objective, nonjudgemental way. It is a tool for assessing mental health dysfunctions and identifying the causes of patients' problems. Understanding each part of the examination enables care providers to plan and deliver the most appropriate care for each patient.

The mental status examination explores five areas: general description, emotional state, experiences, thinking, and sensorium and cognition (Table 9.4).

General Description

Under the category of general description, the patient's general appearance, speech, motor activity, and behaviour during the interaction are assessed. This category includes everything that can be *readily observed* about a patient, such as physical characteristics, dress, facial expressions, motor activity, speech, and reactions. To assess a patient's physical characteristics, observe each part of the patient's body, noting anything unusual. Describe the person's build, skin colouring, cleanliness, and manner of dress. Does the person appear neat and tidy, or careless and unkempt? Note any body odours. If cosmetics are used, are they appropriately applied? Does the patient's appearance match their gender, age, and situation? People with depression, for example, may look unkempt and neglected. It is not uncommon for manic patients to dress in colourful but bizarre clothing and wear many cosmetics and jewellery. Document all findings. Facial expressions and eye contact should be noted. Do the patient's facial expressions match their emotions and actions? Is eye contact avoided or held for long periods? Note the size of the patient's pupils. Large, dilated pupils are seen in people with certain drug intoxications, whereas small pupils are associated with narcotic use.

Describe the rate, volume, and characteristics of the patient's speech. Note any abnormal speech patterns (see Chapter 10).

Next, turn your attention to the patient's motor activity, gestures, and posture. Observe the patient's physical movements for the level and type of activity. Note any unusual movements or mannerisms. Is the patient agitated, tense, restless, lethargic, or relaxed? Are there any tics, grimaces, repeated facial expressions, or tremors present? Excessive body movements are seen in individuals with anxiety or mania. They can also result from the use of stimulants or other drugs. Repeated movements or behaviours are seen in patients with obsessive-compulsive disorders, and picking at one's clothing is often seen in patients with delirium or toxic reactions.

To complete the general description, assess the patient's behaviour during the interaction. How did the patient relate to you? Was the patient cooperative, hostile, or overly friendly? Did the patient appear to trust you? Note if the verbal messages matched the behaviours. Patients who use unconnected gestures, for example, may be hallucinating.

CRITICAL THINKING

Cybil is being admitted to the clinic's day treatment program. She insists that she feels fine, but she will not speak, except to answer "yes" or "no" and refuses to make eye contact with her care provider.
• What messages is Cybil's behaviour sending?
• How do her verbal and nonverbal messages agree or disagree?

Emotional State

To assess the patient's emotional state, the care provider needs to consider the patient's mood and affect. **Mood** is defined as an individual's overall feelings. Mood is a subjective factor that can be explained only by the person experiencing it. Usually, people will have a basic mood, although it may change during the day. To illustrate, a basically relaxed and happy person may feel disappointed by an incident during the day but soon forgets it and returns to their commonly happy mood. **Affect** is the patient's emotional display of the mood being experienced. Table 9.5 explains several kinds of affect. A person's mood can range from overwhelming sadness to great elation and joy. These variations are referred to as one's range of emotion. Affect can be categorized as appropriate, inappropriate, pleasurable, or unpleasurable. To assess a patient's affect, ask what they are feeling and then observe the reactions. Do the responses to your questions match the subjects being discussed? Is the patient overreacting, not reacting at all, or responding inappropriately? Document objective descriptions of the patient's behaviours. Descriptions communicate much more information than does a single medical term.

Experiences

The category of experiences explores the patient's **perceptions**, the ways in which one experiences the world. An individual's perceptions are often called one's *frame of reference*. In short, a person's perceptions help determine their sense of reality.

TABLE 9.5   Common Emotional Responses (Affect)

Name of Affect	Description
Inappropriate Response	
Labile	Rapid, dramatic changes in emotions
Inconsistent	Affect and mood do not agree
Flat	Unresponsive emotions
Pleasurable Response	
Euphoria	Excessive feelings of well-being (feeling too good)
Exaltation	Intense happiness, often with feelings of grandeur
Unpleasurable (Dysphoric) Response	
Aggression	Anger, hostility, or rage that is out of keeping with situation
Agitation	Motor restlessness, often seen with anxiety
Ambivalence	Having both positive and negative feelings about the same subject
Anxiety	Vague, uneasy feeling, often from unknown cause
Depression	Sadness, hopelessness, loss that is present over time
Fear	Reaction to recognized danger

BOX 9.6   Assessing Illusions or Hallucinations

Ask the patient if they hear voices or see things when other people are not present. If the answer is yes, ask the patient to describe the experience. Questions can include the following:

- How many different voices (images) do you hear (see)?
- What do the voices say (images do)?
- Do you recognize any of the voices (images)?
- When did the voices (images) first begin? What was happening in your life at the time?
- How do you feel about the voices (images)?

TABLE 9.6   Disorders of Thinking

Disorder	Description
Thought Processes (How One Thinks)	
Blocking	Thoughts stop suddenly for no apparent reason
Flight of ideas	Rapid changes from one thought to another related thought
Loose associations	Poorly organized or connected thoughts
Perseveration	Repeating same word in response to different questions
Thought Content (What One Thinks)	
Delusions	False beliefs that cannot be corrected by reasoning or explanation
Obsession	Thought, action, or emotion that is unwelcome and difficult to resist
Phobias	Strong fears of certain things, places, or situations
Preoccupations	All experiences and actions are connected to central thought that is usually emotional in nature
Others	
Amnesia	Inability to remember past events
Confabulation	Using untrue statements to fill in gaps of memory loss

People who are experiencing mental health challenges may have difficulty perceiving the same reality as the rest of society. Hallucinations are perceptions that have no external stimulus. The patient may hear voices or see things that are not perceived by other people. Hallucinations involving taste, touch, or smell may indicate a physical problem. Visual and auditory hallucinations are associated with schizophrenia, the acute stage of alcohol or drug withdrawal, and organic brain disorders. Alterations in perceptions that have a basis in reality are called *illusions*. External stimuli are present, but the patient perceives them differently. For example, a patient perceives the person walking down the hall as a wolf. If a patient is having illusions or hallucinations, ask them to describe the experience. Box 9.6 lists several questions that can help explain the patient's experience.

Remember that hallucinations or illusions are very real to the person experiencing them. Care providers cannot "talk them out of it" or tell them to ignore what they perceive. However, because they are so real, patients usually are willing to describe them when asked.

Thinking

The "thinking" section of the mental status examination focuses on thought content and processes. **Thought content** relates to what an individual is thinking. Patients may be experiencing delusions, obsessions, phobias, preoccupations, amnesia, or confabulations. Disturbances in **thought processes** relate to how a person thinks—how they analyze the world, connect and organize information. Disorders of thought processes include blocking, flight of ideas, loose associations, and perseveration. Several disorders of thought processes are listed in Table 9.6.

Another problem of thinking is **depersonalization**, a feeling of unreality or detachment from oneself or one's environment. The unreal feelings produce a dreamlike atmosphere that overtakes the individual's consciousness. One's body does not feel like one's own. Events that are dramatic or important are seen with a detached calmness, as if the person were watching instead of participating in reality. Feelings of depersonalization can normally occur when a person is anxious, stressed, or very tired. Depersonalization disorders are often seen in patients with severe depression and in some forms of schizophrenia.

TABLE 9.7	**Levels of Consciousness**
Comatose/unconscious	Unresponsive to verbal or painful stimuli, may respond to deep painful stimuli
Stuporous	Responds only to strong physical stimuli; falls asleep if not stimulated
Drowsy/somnolent	Wakens with strong verbal stimuli; falls asleep if left undisturbed
Lethargic	Can be verbally aroused; shows decreased wakefulness; may have periods of excitability alternating with periods of drowsiness
Alert	Awake and responsive; oriented to time, place, and person
Hyperalertness	Increased state of alertness or watchfulness (hypervigilance)
Mania	State of extreme excitement, elation, and activity

TABLE 9.8	**Concrete Versus Abstract Thinking**
Concrete	**Abstract**
Obvious	Requires interpretation
Tangible	Conceptual
Superficial	More in-depth
Fact-based	Interpretation-based
What you can see and touch	The ideas you attach to what you can see and touch
Less complex	More complex

Assessment of the patient's thought content and process occurs throughout the entire mental status examination. Are the patient's thoughts based in reality? Are ideas communicated clearly? Do the patient's thoughts follow a logical order? Are there any unusual thoughts, preoccupations, or beliefs present? Does the patient have any suicidal, violent, or destructive thoughts (APA, n.d.)? Are there any persistent dreams? Does the patient believe that someone is intent on harming them (feelings of persecution)? Observe the patient closely, and listen intently. Much information will be revealed during the course of the interaction.

Sensorium and Cognition

The **sensorium** is that part of consciousness that perceives, sorts, and combines information. People with a clear sensorium are oriented to time, place, and person. They are able to use their memory to recall recent and long-term information. A person's level of consciousness and memory recall help in assessing a person's sensorium.

Level of consciousness can be determined by observing the amount of stimuli it takes to arouse the patient (Table 9.7). If the patient cannot be awakened by verbal stimuli, notify your supervisor immediately. If the patient is awake, note their responses to your questions, the degree of interaction, and the amount of eye contact that is being made.

Memory is the ability to recall past events, experiences, and perceptions. For the purpose of testing, memory is divided into three categories: short-term, intermediate-term, and long-term memory. Short-term memory is also referred to as *recall*. To assess short-term memory (recall), ask the patient to remember three things (e.g., a colour, an address, an object). Later in the conversation (at least 15 minutes), ask the patient to repeat the three items. Recall can also be tested by having the patient repeat a series of numbers within a 10-second period.

Intermediate-term memory includes events within the past 2 weeks. Care providers test recent memory by asking the patient to recall the events of the past 24 hours. Loss of recent memory is seen in people living with Alzheimer's disease or other diseases of dementia, anxiety, and depression.

Assessing long-term memory involves asking the patient questions about their place of birth, schools attended, ages of family members, and the person's background. This part of the mental status examination can easily be done during the nursing health history interview. It is sometimes difficult to tell whether the patient has accurate memories. Long-term memory loss is seen in patients living with organic (physical) problems, conversion disorders, and dissociative disorders.

Testing of concentration focuses on the patient's ability to pay attention during the conversation. **Calculation** is used to test the ability to do simple math problems. Have the person count rapidly from 1 to 20; perform simple addition, multiplication, and division problems; and subtract 7 from 100, then 7 from 93, and so on. Then ask practical questions such as the number of dimes in $1.90. Note how easily the patient becomes distracted during the tasks. People living with mental–emotional problems commonly have difficulty with concentration and calculations. These difficulties also occur in people with physical disorders, such as brain tumours, so it is important to assess the patient's ability to concentrate and do simple calculations.

During this phase of the mental status examination, the patient's education level, general knowledge, ability to read, use of vocabulary, and ability to think abstractly are also assessed. General knowledge can be tested by asking the person to name the past five Prime Ministers or five large cities. Ask the patient about the last grade completed in school.

To determine reading ability, print a command, such as "Close your eyes," on a piece of paper. Ask the patient to read it and follow the directions. During the conversation, also note the patient's choice of words and their use.

Assess the patient's ability to think abstractly (see Table 9.8) by having them explain the meaning of several well-known proverbs, such as "A stitch in time saves nine"; "A rolling stone gathers no moss"; "When it rains, it pours"; or "People in glass houses shouldn't throw stones." Many people with mental health challenges give concrete answers, such as "Moss only grows on the north sides of stones," or "People who live in glass houses shouldn't throw stones because it breaks the glass."

BOX 9.7   Mental Status Assessment at a Glance

1. Appearance
   _____ Manner of dress
   _____ Personal grooming
   _____ Facial expressions
   _____ Posture and gait
2. Speech
   _____ Manner of response (frank, evading)
   _____ Choice of words (to assess general intelligence, education, levels of function, thought)
   _____ Speech disorder
3. Level of consciousness
   _____ Level of alertness
   _____ Orientation (time, place, person)
4. Attention span
   _____ Ability to keep thoughts focused on one topic
   _____ Repeat a series of numbers
   _____ Serial sevens (ask patient to subtract 7 from 100, 7 from 93, etc.)
5. Memory
   _____ Short-term memory (ask patient to repeat words after 15 minutes)
   _____ Intermediate-term memory (ask patient about yesterday's activities)
   _____ Long-term memory (ask patient about dates of birth, marriage, schooling)
6. Understanding abstract relationships
   _____ Understanding of proverbs (concrete or abstract)
   _____ Ability to understand similarities (e.g., "How are a bicycle and an automobile alike?")
7. Arithmetic and reading ability
   _____ Simple addition, subtraction, multiplication, and division (ask patient to make change)
   _____ Ability to read newspaper, magazine
8. General information knowledge
   _____ Discuss newspaper or magazine article
   _____ General information questions (e.g., "How many days in a year?" "Where does the sun set?")
9. Judgement
   _____ Responses to family, work, financial problems
   _____ Responses to "What would you do if . . ." questions
10. Emotional status
   _____ Ask "How do you feel today?" or "How do you feel about . . ." questions
   _____ Affect
   _____ Current situation and coping behaviours

Modified from Jess, L. W. (1988). Investigating impaired mental status: an assessment guide you can use. *Nursing, 18*(6), 42–50.

Judgement refers to the ability to evaluate choices and make appropriate decisions. During the health history interview, observe how the patient explains personal relationships, their job, and economic responsibilities. Assess the patient's judgement by asking questions such as "What would you do if you

- found an addressed envelope on the ground?"
- ran out of medication before the next appointment?"
- won $25,000?"

Judgement is often impaired in people with chemical dependence, intoxication, schizophrenia, intellectual delay, and organic mental disorders. Document the patient's responses using the patient's own words whenever possible.

Insight refers to the patient's understanding of the situation. What is the patient's understanding of the disorder? Questions that help the care provider assess insight include "Have you noticed a change in yourself recently?" and "What do you think is the cause of your anxiety (discomfort)?" Expect patients to have different degrees of insight. For example, a person with an alcohol problem may realize that they drink too much but do not think that it is interfering with family life. Again, be sure to document the patient's statements rather than your opinions.

Although the mental status examination may appear to be a lengthy process, much of it can be performed during the history interview. Checklists that address each area of the examination are available (see Box 9.7 and Appendix A for a copy of Mental Status Assessment at a Glance).

Care providers often use parts of the mental status examination to assess patients whose mental state changes frequently. For example, the care provider may assess the hallucinating patient for thought content and process at intervals throughout the day.

Work to develop your powers of observation. Do not pass judgement or let your opinions interfere with data gathering. Remember, the results of the mental status examination can be affected by attitudes and beliefs. Learn to use assessment tools. Develop your observation and assessment skills, because they will serve you well in all practice settings.

KEY POINTS

- The ability to effectively obtain and use information about patients is a vital part of the multidisciplinary treatment plan.
- The mental health treatment plan is used as a guide for patient care, to monitor progress and assess the effectiveness of therapeutic interventions, communicate and coordinate patients' care, provide a focus for all therapeutic activities, and prevent duplication.
- Every psychological illness has physical effects, and psychological effects accompany every physical illness.
- Therapists who work with mentally and emotionally troubled individuals use the *Diagnostic and Statistical Manual of Mental Disorders*, fifth edition (*DSM-5*) to aid in diagnosis and help guide clinical practice.

- The nursing (therapeutic) process is a purposeful and organized approach to solving patient issues that requires knowledge, experience, and the use of sound judgement.
- Data-collecting methods for care providers include interviews, observational techniques, and rating scales and inventories.
- The process of assessing a patient is ongoing and begins with the patient's admission to the facility.
- Individuals' physical, social, cultural, intellectual, emotional, and spiritual areas of functioning are included in a holistic assessment.
- The psychiatric assessment tool includes an appraisal of the patient's health, previous psychiatric treatment, physical and mental coping responses, discharge planning needs, psychosocial and environmental problems, and needs for knowledge.
- The purpose of a risk factor assessment is to identify risk factors that may present an immediate threat to the patient or others.
- The history interview is an organized conversation with a patient that has the purpose of bringing out certain information about the patient's health status.
- Guidelines for conducting effective interviews relate to being nonjudgemental, considering cultural factors, having clear goals, and assessing communications.
- The sociocultural assessment focuses on cultural, social, and spiritual aspects.
- The mental status examination is a tool for assessing mental health dysfunction and identifying the causes of patients' problems.
- The mental status examination explores appearance, consciousness, behaviour, speech, mood, affect, thought content, intellectual performance, insight, judgement, and perception.
- Much of the mental status examination can be performed during the history interview using checklists. Care providers often use various parts of the mental status examination to assess patients whose mental state changes frequently.

ADDITIONAL LEARNING RESOURCES

Go to your Evolve website (http://evolve.elsevier.com/Canada/Morrison-Valfre/) for additional online resources, including the online Study Guide for additional learning activities to help you master this chapter content.

CRITICAL THINKING QUESTIONS

1. You attempt to assess a 25-year-old male who refuses to answer your questions. What other options might exist for you to gain insight into his current situation?
2. You are asked to conduct a mental status examination on a middle-aged male patient. When you introduce yourself, you cannot understand the patient because his words are slurred and nonsensical. He has obvious difficulty coordinating his movements and appears to be at risk for falling. You immediately direct him to lie down on an emergency room stretcher and raise both safety rails to prevent him from rolling off. You see on his chart that he has a history of drug and alcohol abuse. You also note that no bloodwork or toxicology screening has been ordered. What could you do at this point?
3. As you do rounds on the mental health unit where you work, you observe a patient pacing back and forth and appearing to speak to someone who is not there. The patient is becoming increasingly agitated and angry, and the volume of his voice is increasing. How might you approach this patient?

REFERENCES

American Psychiatric Association (APA). (n.d.) Mental status assessment. https://www.psychiatry.org/psychiatrists/practice/dsm/educational-resources/assessment-measures

American Psychiatric Association (APA). (2013). *Diagnostic and statistical manual of mental disorders* (5th ed.). American Psychiatric Publishing.

Keltner, N. L., & Steele, D. (2019). *Psychiatric nursing* (8th ed.). Mosby.

Mosby's dictionary of medicine, nursing, & health professions (9th ed.) (2013). Mosby.

Nasreddine, Z. S., Phillips, N. A., Bédirian, V., et al. (2005). The Montreal cognitive assessment (MoCA): A brief screening tool for mild cognitive impairment. *Journal of the American Geriatric Society, 53*(4), 695–699. https://doi.org/10.1111/j.1532-5415.2005.53221.x

National Depressive and Manic-Depressive Association. (2014). Patient's cultural background important in diagnosis and treatment. *DMDA Newsletter.*

Potter, P. A., Perry, A. G., Stockert, P., et al. (2019). *Essentials for nursing practice* (9th ed.). Mosby.

Stein, L., & Hollen, C. J. (2020). *Concept-based clinical nursing skills: Fundamental to advanced.* Elsevier.

Stuart, G. W. (2013). *Principles and practice of psychiatric nursing* (10th ed.). Mosby.

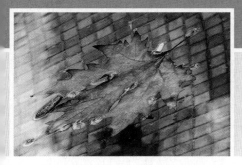

10

Therapeutic Communication

OBJECTIVES

Upon completion of this chapter, the student will be able to:
1. Examine two theories of communication.
2. Identify two types of communication.
3. List the five components or parts of any communication.
4. Compare the characteristics of verbal and nonverbal communications.
5. Identify three interventions for communicating with people who do not speak your language.
6. Explain eight principles of therapeutic communication.
7. Describe eight therapeutic communication skills.
8. Name three techniques for communicating with patients who have mental–emotional difficulties.

OUTLINE

KEY TERMS

active listening (p. 114)
aphasia (ə-FĀ-zhə) (p. 114)
communication (kŏ-MŪ-nĭ-CĀ-shŭn) (p. 107)
communication style (kŏ-MŪ-nĭ-CĀ-shŭn STĬL) (p. 111)
disturbed (də′stərbd) communications (p. 108)
dyslexia (dĭs-LĔK-sē-ə) (p. 114)
feedback (FĒD-băk) (p. 109)
incongruent (ĬN-kn-GROO-ent) communications (p. 114)
interpersonal (ĭn-tĕr-PĔR-sŭn-ăl) communications (p. 109)

intrapersonal (ĭn-trĂ-PĔR-sŭn-ăl) communications (p. 109)
nontherapeutic (nŏn-THĔR-ə-PYŪ-tĭk) communications (p. 114)
nonverbal (nŏn-VĔR-băl) communication (p. 111)
perception (pĕr-SĔP-shŭn) (p. 109)
responding strategies (p. 112)
speech cluttering (spēch CLŬ-tĕr-ēng) (p. 116)
therapeutic (THĔR-ə-PYŪ-tĭk) communications (p. 112)
verbal (VĔR-băl) communication (p. 110)

Communication is an essential component of survival for all creatures. Research has demonstrated that when insects attack a tree, it sends a chemical message to other trees in the area. Animals communicate in subtle and complex ways using both sound and movement, but the master communicator, the user of language, is the human being. Infants are born communicating with their first squall, and older persons die listening to a world they are about to leave.

The fulfillment of human needs requires interactions with others. To meet even the most basic needs for food and water requires the cooperative efforts of people, achieved through communication and understanding.

Communication is an interaction between two or more people that involves the exchange of information (Keltner & Steele, 2019). All people communicate, but members of the health care professions modify ordinary interactions. We practise therapeutic communications based on certain principles. Those who work with mentally or emotionally troubled individuals refine their therapeutic communication abilities to become highly skilled listeners who can plan and carry out interactions that are specifically designed to achieve patient outcomes. This chapter explores the elements and skills of therapeutically designed communication techniques.

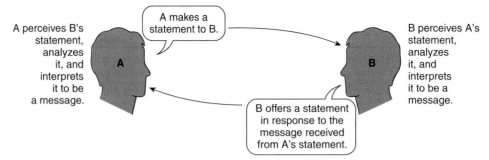

Fig. 10.1 Ruesch's feedback loop of communication. (Redrawn from Rawlins, R. P., Williams, S. R., & Beck, C. K. [1993]. *Mental health–psychiatric nursing: A holistic life-cycle approach* [3rd ed.]. Mosby.)

The study of interactions between human beings has been a source of interest for centuries. Paintings on walls of caves attest to early humans' desire for communication. The introduction of the printing press during the fifteenth century made mass production of the written word possible. As people learned to read and write, learning evolved from an oral form to a visual one. Communications became more complex and a step removed from face-to-face interpersonal contact.

The inventions of the telegraph, telephone, radio, television, and computer have made information available to everyone. Today, satellite communications, interactive computers, smartphones, and the Internet are transporting the exchange of information into new realms. Technological developments will continue, but the need for effective verbal and nonverbal communication skills will never be replaced by technology.

THEORIES OF COMMUNICATION

One of the earliest theorists on therapeutic communications was Florence Nightingale, whose book *Notes on Nursing* emphasized the need to effectively understand and communicate with patients. However, the rest of the medical world placed little focus on the value of interacting therapeutically until the 1950s, when the publication of several theories sparked an interest in patient–care provider communications.

Ruesch's Theory

A theory that considers communications as the social framework for health care was developed by J. Ruesch (1961) in the late 1950s. He saw communication as a circular process in which messages travelled from within one person to another person and back again (Fig. 10.1).

Events within the sender prompt the sending of a message. The message is then transmitted to another who receives it, processes it internally, and responds. Successful communications occur when agreement about the meaning of the message has been reached. Communications are unsuccessful when there is a lack of agreement or understanding about the message. Ruesch coined the term **disturbed communications** to describe unsuccessful interactions that result from an interference in the sending or receiving of messages, inadequate mastery of the language being used, insufficient information, or no opportunity for feedback.

Therapeutic communications are distinguished from ordinary communications by the intent of one of the participants to bring about a positive change. According to Ruesch's point of view, a

---

BOX 10.1   Transactional Analysis Communications

Parent: "I told you that was a foolish thing to do."
Child: "I just was trying to get what I wanted."
Adult: "In the past, this is what worked for me."

---

therapist is one who directs communications to bring about more satisfying social relations. Therapists seek to find the nature of patients' distress and problems. Then, with the use of therapeutic communication techniques, both patient and therapist agree on the nature of the problem and what should be done about it. Many of Ruesch's ideas are useful for interacting with patients.

Transactional Analysis

In 1964, Dr. Eric Berne, a physician with training in psychoanalysis, published *Games People Play,* which became a bestseller even though it was not intended for the general public (Berne, 1964a). In the book, Berne used the term *transactional analysis* to refer to the process of investigating what people say and do to each other. Berne also believed that three ego states exist within all of us: the parent (P), who focuses on rules and values; the child (C), who focuses on emotions and desires; and the adult (A), who bases their approach to the world on previous observations. These ego states make up one's individual personality, and Berne coined the term *structural analysis* to refer to the study of the personality. Box 10.1 gives an example of each communication type.

Many of the interactions in which people engage, Berne noted, have ulterior or hidden motives used to manipulate others. He labelled these manipulations *psychological games and rackets* and offered his game analysis to refer to the hidden interactions that lead to a payoff.

The main goal of transactional analysis, according to Berne, is to "establish the most open and authentic communication possible between the affective (feeling) and intellectual components of the personality" (Berne, 1964b). Analyzing one's structure, transactions, and games encourages people to gain insight and determine what changes are most desirable. Because Berne (like Maslow) believed that every person needs positive feedback or "strokes" to thrive, he encouraged communications that are positive in nature. This approach is particularly valuable for nurses and other health care providers. The focus on one's abilities fosters more effective and satisfying communications for everyone involved with the patient.

Neurolinguistic Programming

Much of the basis for neurolinguistic programming stems from the work of Milton H. Erickson, who, until his death in 1980, was considered a great medical hypnotist. To discover the keys to his success, Richard Bandler and John Grinder spent several years doing careful analyses of Erickson's extensive writings. Using their observations as a framework, they developed a method for analyzing an individual's system of communication based on the theory that communication involves a concentrated focus. Effective communications essentially alter a person's state of consciousness.

CRITICAL THINKING

Picture yourself in the forest, surrounded by tall, stately trees. You look up to see the sun filtering through the dense canopy of tree branches. Below you, the forest floor is dappled with sunlight, and shade patterns dance slowly across your shoes. The air is cool and musty, damp from the mist left from the night. The world is silent except for the chirping of a lone songbird.
- What did you experience when you were reading the preceding paragraph?
- Did you actually experience a moment in the forest?
- Do you wish that you could go there yourself?

If your answer is "yes" to any of these questions, then the communication was successful. The pattern of communication in the paragraph changed your awareness, which allowed you to share an experience. This is the "hypnosis" of neurolinguistic programming.

By learning an individual's communication patterns, one is able to achieve more effective and fulfilling interactions. Patterns include eye-accessing clues (ways in which people move their eyes while thinking), language patterns, and the pace and rhythm of speech. Health care providers are finding neurolinguistic programming to be a powerful tool for communicating.

Other theories of communication focus on the use of body language (kinesics), how people use their space (proxemics), and channels of communication. Becoming familiar with several theories allows care providers to expand and improve their communication skills and abilities.

CHARACTERISTICS OF COMMUNICATION

Communication is the act of sending and receiving information. When this definition is applied to a computer or some other mover of data, the interaction is simple. One machine contacts the other, data are exchanged, and the interaction is over. With people, however, the information exchange is much more complex. Human behaviours have strong influences on communications.

Types of Communication

People engage in two types of communications: intrapersonal and interpersonal. Each may occur singly or in combination, and each may be used in effective or maladaptive ways.

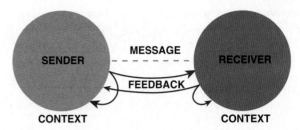

Fig. 10.2 Components of the communication process. (Source: Stuart, G. W. [2013]. *Principles and practice of psychiatric nursing* [10th ed.]. Mosby.)

Intrapersonal communications take place **within** oneself and are commonly referred to as our "self-talk" or "self-dialogue." They are conversations that we have with ourselves when solving problems, making plans, and reacting emotionally. Intrapersonal communications are adaptive when they help us cope or focus our energies. When dysfunctional, they can result in altered states of functioning, such as hallucinations or unusual thought content (also called *delusions*). Our intrapersonal communications affect our interactions with others. If your intrapersonal communications are upbeat and optimistic, then your interactions with patients will be too. If your self-talk is negative and glum, your communications will reflect this.

Interpersonal communications are interactions that occur *between* two or more persons—the verbal and nonverbal messages that are sent and received during every interaction. Symbols, language, culture, and behaviours have an impact on communications among people. As a result, interpersonal communications are complex and sophisticated. No matter what the communication, the importance of each message lies in its clarity. Clear communications offer a greater chance of success in every interaction.

Process of Communication

For a successful communication to occur, five elements must be in place (Fig. 10.2). There must be a *sender* who forms the message and transmits the message. A *receiver* is someone who accepts the *message* and responds. **Feedback** refers to the responses of each person when messages are being sent and received. Last, the *context* or setting in which the communication takes place must also be considered.

When a message is sent, a chain of events is triggered. First, perception is needed to recognize the presence of a message. **Perception** is the use of the senses to gain information. Vision, hearing, and touch are used to sense the meaning of the communication. A person's perceptions can be affected by many factors, including past experiences, emotional states, and physical problems.

The second step of the communication process is *evaluation*, the internal assessment of the message. All overt and hidden messages are considered and then compared with past experiences. The result is an emotional *reaction* to the message and preparation to return a message to the sender.

Transmission (a response) is the last step. It includes conscious and unconscious responses to the message received. As the receiver of the message responds with a message of their own, the cycle begins again and is repeated with every interaction. If a person has difficulty with any step of the

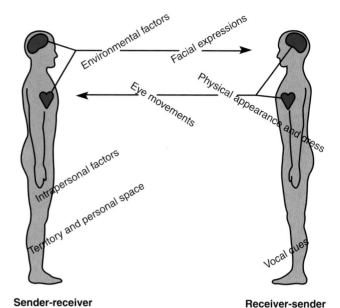

Sender-receiver   **Receiver-sender**

Fig. 10.3 Factors influencing communication. (Source: Balzer-Riley, J. [2017]. *Communication in nursing* [8th ed.]. Mosby.)

communication process—perceiving, evaluating, or transmitting messages—a communication problem may exist. Alert care providers are aware of each patient's process of communication and are prepared to intervene when patients are having communication difficulties.

Factors That Influence Communication

Interaction with others is influenced by many factors, but among the most important are culture (see Chapter 4), social class, relationships, perceptions, values, and parts of the message.

The social class to which one belongs has a profound influence on communications. People of various social classes interact using their own terminology, slang, clichés, speech patterns, gestures, and appearances. Variation in communication patterns can create problems for health care providers who interact with patients from social classes different from their own. Be careful not to label patients on the basis of their communications. Communicating with patients from different social classes requires effort and patience. Both the care provider and patient will feel misunderstood unless steps are taken to establish effective communication exchanges. Box 10.2 lists several therapeutic interventions for interacting with people from different social classes.

Relationships affect communications because of the level of relatedness of each person involved in the interaction. *Levels of relatedness* refer to the degree of intimacy, authority, and role status of the communicators. For example, people communicate differently with strangers than they do with family members.

Perceptions and *values* influence communications. One's internal experiences, when combined with personal values, result in a unique frame of reference for communicating. It is important for care providers to remember that it may be their perceptions that are impeding effective communication.

The content and context of a message have strong impacts on communications. The *content* of a message is the information being sent. The receiver is affected by the content and must choose an appropriate response—recognize the information, ignore the message, or change the subject. An awareness of the emotional effect related to the content of messages helps care providers communicate more effectively.

Communications are also affected by the *context,* or environment, in which they take place. If patients are expected to share personal information, an environment that fosters privacy is necessary. The dayroom or lounge is not a place for self-disclosure. Becoming aware of the context helps to send and receive messages with greater success. Many other factors, such as one's appearance, expressions, and body movements, also affect communications (Fig. 10.3).

LEVELS OF COMMUNICATION

Communicating is an energy exchange that takes place on several levels. Each person involved is a unique personality who interacts on verbal and nonverbal levels at one time. Communications at both levels occur with every person-to-person interaction.

Verbal Communication

Verbal communication relates to anything associated with the spoken word. Verbal communications include speaking, writing, the use of language and symbols, and the arrangement of words or phrases.

For many patients living with mental–emotional challenges, communicating with others can be difficult. Certain patients have difficulties in perceiving. The person who is experiencing hallucinations, for example, may be unable to understand a message is being sent because the communications within the inner world are drowning out the messages from the reality outside.

Understanding verbal messages involves the ability to form abstract ideas and concepts. People with schizophrenia often have great difficulty with abstraction and using words that are reality oriented. Transmitting messages is a problem for many depressed patients; messages that identify and verbalize what they feel are commonly stated in only one or two words.

Verbal communications are the most overt form of interaction. Words are only symbols that do not have the same meaning to all people. To complicate matters, the differences intensify as words become more abstract. Emotions are an excellent example of abstractions that cannot be easily communicated on the verbal level. This is an important point for care providers to remember. If communications are to be effective, you must understand the patient's meanings of their words.

Nonverbal Communication

Messages sent and received without the use of words define **nonverbal communication**. Nonverbal cues tend to be perceived and evaluated even before verbal cues, and can take on a greater significance in how others understand and interpret us. Messages sent at the nonverbal level are expressed in at least one of four ways: appearance, body motions, use of space, and nonlanguage sounds (verbalizations without words). One's appearance can convey strong nonverbal messages. Hygiene and personal grooming habits, choice of clothing and accessories, hairstyle, and jewellery all send messages. Facial expressions, gestures, posture, and use of the body can communicate one's emotions more easily than words. Care providers who are aware of this are careful to use their nonverbal behaviours therapeutically. To illustrate, note the position of your body when you are interacting with someone you find unpleasant. Are your arms crossed? Is your body position open and inviting communication, or closed with crossed legs or an angled stance? The use of space and distance (see Chapter 4) communicates concepts such as authority and intimacy.

In short, the nonverbal level of communication includes everything outside the realm of speaking, writing, or singing. It is a subtle world, filled with variation. The more care providers are able to recognize and use nonverbal levels, the more effective their interventions will become. Work to become alert to your own nonverbal behaviours. This self-awareness will help you avoid sending unintended or inappropriate messages to patients. Each level of communication, verbal and nonverbal, sends and receives messages during every interaction. If messages are successfully sent and received, the results are interactions rich in variety and complexity.

INTERCULTURAL COMMUNICATION

Communicating with people from other cultures requires special considerations. How people communicate is based on cultural backgrounds, language systems, and social patterns. Cultures are transmitted through communication, and cultures define how emotions are expressed and shared. The use of touch and other nonverbal forms of communication varies considerably with different cultures.

CULTURAL CONSIDERATIONS

Sidney Jourard (1971) studied the cultural differences relating to the use of touch by observing the behaviours of pairs of people in coffee shops throughout the world. Observations revealed that more touch occurred in certain cities.

City	Couples Touched (Times/hr)
San Juan, Puerto Rico	180
Paris, France	110
Gainesville, Florida	2
London, England	0

Cultures, and the social groups within them, vary in their use of verbal and nonverbal communications. Care providers who work with patients from culturally different backgrounds should resist the tendency to stereotype people and should work to learn the most culturally appropriate methods for communication.

Intercultural Differences

To fulfill basic needs, people must interact and communicate with one another. For people of differing cultures, this interacting with others can be a difficult process. Communication styles, nonverbal behaviours and values, as well as the use of the language, are areas in which cultural communications basically differ.

Communication style refers to the rituals connected with greeting and departure, the lines of conversation, and the directness of communication (Giger & Haddad, 2020). Assess greeting rituals by observing the greeting interaction, including the use of compliments and physical behaviours such as touching, handshaking, or kissing.

CASE STUDY

Sarah had been working with patients from a First Nations community for almost 6 months. During her interviews with her patients, she had great difficulty in obtaining information, although she knew she was practising good interviewing skills and attending behaviours.

One morning, she was discussing her problem with the community's primary care physician, who had been working with her patients for several years. He asked, "How is your eye contact?" "Good," she replied. "I always look patients in the eye when interviewing and express interest in what they say—when I can get them to talk to me." "That is your problem, then," the physician replied. "First Nations people believe that it is an invasion of privacy to give direct eye contact, especially if you are not a member of their group. Try looking at their feet. It will convey respect, and they may be more likely to communicate with you."

Sarah followed the suggestion, and soon her patients began sharing important health information.

How could Sarah have prevented this situation from occurring?

Are lines of communication linear or circular? *Linear* communication styles come directly to the point. *Circular* communication styles direct the conversation around the main point. Often, the main point is left unstated. Once the important information has been communicated, it is assumed that the receiver got the point. This style is sometimes found in Asian and Far Eastern cultures. "There's a fire in the wastebasket" is an example of a linear message, whereas "I saw someone drop a match in the wastebasket earlier; now it appears to be smoking" illustrates a circular style of communication.

The directness and openness with which people solve their problems influence communications. Are problems communicated directly, communicated in a circular manner, or denied and ignored? How appropriate is it to state an opinion or offer help?

BOX 10.3   **Improving Intercultural Communication**

To improve your intercultural communications:
1. Recognize what is different from your own cultural style.
2. Adapt your behaviour to accommodate the difference.
3. Call attention to the difference to explain the confusion in communication.
4. Accept the patient as a person with a willingness to work toward therapeutic goals of care.

Cultural differences affect the nonverbal tone of the receiver. Body language, such as eye contact, gestures, and distance, is culturally determined. Much of the message is lost when one does not understand the communications of the body.

Values guide many communications within cultures. They help determine whether the individual or the group is more important and how individuals of various statuses should be treated. For example, Inuit culture uses little verbal communication because each member of the group has a defined role. One's actions are known, especially in times of threat. Survival often depended on actions with few words. Silence is valued, so it is considered rude to engage in casual conversation or idle chatter.

How people from various cultures use time is an example of a cultural value that affects communications. North American culture tends to be fairly rigid in terms of how time is incorporated into daily life. Appointments are expected to be attended on time and much social disapproval is assigned to individuals who do not respect this. Other cultures take a less specific approach to time, seeing established times for meetings and activities as only a general guideline. For these cultures, arriving early or late, even significantly, is not cause for social disapproval.

Religious beliefs and practices can also affect communications. For example, some followers of Buddhism may not share that they are in pain because they believe their suffering is due to a failure of righteousness.

Cultures that place a high value on nonverbal communications practise "high-context" communications, in which nonverbal cues and sensitivity play a larger role than the actual verbal message. Cultures that practise **"low-context"** communications tend to focus more on the words than on the emotional tones of the message.

Another major cultural communication difference is the use of a society's language. Language use includes a culture's use of names and titles; the structure of grammar; the use of vocabulary, jargon, and slang; and vocal qualities such as tones, pronunciation, rhythm, and speed of communications. The meaning of silence also varies from culture to culture. Care providers must be aware of the meanings of culturally different communications; the effectiveness of the therapeutic relationship depends on this. Box 10.3 offers suggestions for improving intercultural communications.

THERAPEUTIC COMMUNICATION SKILLS

The goal of **therapeutic communications** is to focus on the patient and foster the therapeutic relationship. Therapeutic communication techniques are abilities that assist care providers in effectively interacting with patients. Each therapeutic communication skill is based on eight principles (Table 10.1) that serve as guidelines for effective interactions. Refer to them often because they will help you cope with the complexities of human communications.

Therapeutic communication techniques are divided into two equally important areas: listening skills and interacting skills. Each is vital if communications are to be clearly understood and therapeutic actions are to be successful.

Listening Skills

In our fast-paced world, people are so intent on sending their messages that they seldom take the time to listen—to truly hear what the other person is trying to communicate. The art of listening is a necessary ingredient for every health care provider, not just those who work in psychiatry. Effective listening improves one's abilities to meet patients' needs. In addition, effective listening can help to identify hidden messages and agendas, minimize misunderstandings, and clarify messages (Box 10.4). Although it may require time and practice to perfect your therapeutic listening skills, the rewards are worth the efforts (Box 10.5).

To polish your listening skills, first *concentrate on the speaker*. Next, *listen objectively*. Use appropriate eye contact and body language. Remember the speaker's cultural background. Maintaining a relaxed body position at eye level with the speaker communicates acceptance and interest. Make sure that your *nonverbal messages match the verbal messages*. Do not interrupt. Let the speaker be fully expressive. If you must interrupt, explain that the conversation is important but your time is limited. *Follow up* with telling the speaker when you will return to finish the conversation. The last and most important guideline for becoming an effective listener is to *clarify*. If you are uncertain about what was communicated, ask for clarification. Clarification is a primary therapeutic communication technique that, when used in combination with good listening skills, enhances every care provider's abilities to successfully interact with patients.

Interacting Skills

Therapeutic techniques that relate to the care provider's actions while communicating are called **responding strategies** or *interaction skills*. These are verbal and nonverbal responses that encourage patients to communicate in a way that encourages growth. To practise therapeutic interactions, use words that have meaning to the patient. Communicate directly, and relate to the situation. Messages with a clear meaning are more easily understood. Allow enough time for a response. Do not use the word *why* in a question because it requires a response that justifies one's actions or opinions.

Twelve commonly used therapeutic communication techniques (Stuart, 2013) encourage patients to continue communicating. Carefully study the information in Box 10.6. Practise these techniques and note the results. With patience and repeated use, these techniques will become important tools for effectively interacting with all patients.

TABLE 10.1 Principles of Therapeutic Communication

Principle	Illustration	Example
Acceptance	Communicate a favourable reception by implying, "You have a right to exist, to live your life, to have somebody care about you." One does not have to approve of another's behaviour to be accepting. It is only when people feel accepted for what they are that they will consider changing.	Patient: "I know it's been destructive for me to live with my parents, and I get irresponsible living there, but I feel like that's where I need to go after I leave the hospital." Care Provider: "I may not agree with your decision about where to live, but I accept your choice to do that and will work with you to evaluate how it works."
Interest	Communicate interest by expressing a desire to know another person. Interest is conveyed by asking about those aspects of a person's life that others often reject. Care providers communicate by their attitude that "everything can be talked about here."	Patient: "I'm so ashamed of what I've done, I can't tell you about it. You won't ever talk to me again!" Care Provider: "Sandy, I'm interested in everything about you, the good, the bad, the sad, the happy. This is not just a 'good times only' relationship. You and I have committed to working on a number of issues of importance, and I have a feeling that this is one of them. So why not go ahead and begin?"
Respect	Show consideration for another by communicating a willingness to work with the patient. Accept the patient's ideas, feelings, and rights. Listen attentively, express belief in the patient's ability to solve personal problems and assume responsibility for their own life, collaborate on shared goals, arrive and leave on time, and keep your word. False reassurance and critical judgement are to be avoided.	Patient: "I know it's silly for me to feel so frightened about living alone, but I'm terrified." Care Provider: "I could tell you that you have nothing to worry about, that you'll do just fine. But, I hear your terror, your voice is shaking, and you're sweating. It must be hard to imagine being able to survive on your own after being married for 30 years."
Honesty	Demonstrate honesty by being consistent, open, and frank. Communicate with the patient as an authentic person. Use tact and timing in judging the use of honesty so that patients are not burdened with information or feedback they are not ready to hear. Be honest and nondefensive about thoughts and feelings discovered through self-assessment.	Patient: "I hate the way he treats me; he takes me for granted, leaving and not telling me when he's coming home. It will never change." Care Provider: "Carol, we've discussed this pattern before and the alternative ways for dealing with the situation. Quite honestly, I think a major reason for Lou's not changing his behaviour is that you allow him to continue it." Patient: "What do you mean?" Care Provider: "I mean that unless or until you let him know that his behaviour is unacceptable, why should he change? This way he doesn't have to be accountable to anyone, even his wife."
Concreteness	Be specific, to the point, and clear. Use understandable language and avoid the use of jargon. Patients who speak in vague, general, unfocused ways are helped to be more specific and focused.	Patient: "I feel sort of uneasy, I get a feeling like... that every so often..." (perspiring, wringing hands, tapping feet). Care Provider: "Describe the feeling for me."
Assistance	Commit time and energy to therapeutic relationships. Convey that you are present and available and have tangible aid to offer that will help patients choose and develop more functional ways of living.	Care Provider: "While you're in the hospital, you and I will be meeting every day at 2 p.m. for 45 minutes. I am available to you to help you work out the problems that are bothering you. I'll also see you lots of other times since I work on the unit. I hope you'll feel free to approach me if you need something."
Permission	Communicate permission by conveying the message that it is acceptable to try new ways of behaving. Often patients are afraid to choose freely and act autonomously. They often need to be given permission and encouragement to see and do things in new ways.	Patient: "How can I suddenly trust people when I've been hurt so badly in the past?" Care Provider: "Clarify for me who hurt you." Patient: "Well, my brother, you know how he hurt me." Care Provider: "Yes, I do know that. What about other people? Can you tell me about them?" Patient: "Well, I can't tell you any others specifically. It's just the way I feel about people." Care Provider: "I think you may be looking at other people and seeing your brother in them. You might be bringing the past into the present."
Protection	Protect patients by ensuring safety. Work with patients to anticipate trouble spots with new behaviour and develop effective ways of dealing with anticipated or actual problems, thus maximizing the possibility of success.	Care Provider: "I hear that you're scared, and that's very natural for you to feel. Let's work together to try to anticipate what will happen over the weekend and see if, together, you and I can come up with some strategies for dealing with those hot spots."

From Haber, J., McMahon, A. L., & Krainovich-Miller, B. (1997). *Comprehensive psychiatric nursing* (5th ed.). Mosby.

BOX 10.4   Active Listening

Active listening is a communication concept that embodies an intentional empathetic form of listening for understanding collaboratively constructed meanings. There is a commitment to full attention on the patient, as well as on the topic. This means temporarily suspending your own reactions as you listen for understanding.

Active listening contributes to fewer incidents of misunderstanding, more accurate information, and stronger health-related relationships. Rather than listening to a one-sided narrative as a basis for problem exploration, the process of interactive dialogue represents a joint opportunity to consider new facts—leading to different possibilities, choices, and options. Active listening allows both communicators to offer presence and bear witness to one another in the telling of the patient's story

From Kagan, P. (2008). Feeling listened to: A lived experience of human becoming. *Nursing Science Quarterly, 21*(1), 59–67.

BOX 10.5   Therapeutic Listening Skills

- Concentrate on the speaker and the message.
- Keep distractions and interruptions to a minimum.
- Change the setting (environment), if necessary.
- Assess nonverbal communications.
- Listen objectively and without judgement.
- Discover which words trigger emotional responses in you.
- Use eye contact and body language that is culturally appropriate.
- Do not interrupt. Let the speaker finish delivering the message.
- Jot down notes if needed.
- Do not assume that you have understood another person's thoughts.
- Clarify any message about which you are unsure.

NONTHERAPEUTIC COMMUNICATION

Messages that hinder effective communication are called **nontherapeutic communications** because they are interactions that slow or halt the development of a helping relationship. Nontherapeutic communications include barriers that arise within the environment, the care provider, or the patient and the responses that block further communications.

Barriers to Communication

Barriers can arise during each step of the communication process. They are protective behaviours used when one feels threatened. The problem is that their use can increase the patient's insecurity and helplessness. If allowed to go unchecked, the use of barriers will smother the therapeutic relationship and prevent the patient from reaching the treatment goals.

Because the environment is difficult to control, it can often have a negative effect on communications. It may be too noisy or crowded for the sharing of personal information. Sometimes the patient will attempt to send an important message in an inappropriate setting—for example, while waiting in line at the lunchroom, your patient announces that he is leaving his wife. In this instance, the environment acts as a

barrier to further exploration because of the noise level and lack of privacy.

Problems with the individuals involved in the communication can arise. The care provider may be physically tired or prefer not to interact with the patient. Such feelings may lead to **incongruent communications**, in which the verbal messages do not match the nonverbal communications. Incongruent communications can be sent by either the patient or the care provider, but it is the care provider's responsibility to match the communication with the message.

On occasion, a patient will refuse to communicate or cooperate. This lack of cooperation erects a large barrier and prevents other people from attempting to interact. Such a patient requires extra patience and repeated messages of acceptance. With time and persistence, patients usually become more willing to interact because no person likes to remain cut off from their fellow human beings.

The following are methods for coping with the barriers to communications:

1. Recognize that a problem exists.
2. Identify what purpose or need the problem is filling.
3. Explore appropriate alternative behaviours.
4. Implement the alternative behaviours when interacting.
5. Evaluate whether communications have improved. If they have not, reassess and try another approach. Being aware of communication barriers allows you to intervene early and effectively.

Nontherapeutic Messages

Nontherapeutic communications can be classified as problems of omission or commission. Nontherapeutic communication techniques of *omission* relate to the care provider's failure to do something (e.g., to use a therapeutic technique) when the moment is right. Examples of communication acts of omission include failure to listen, probe, or explore the patient's point of view. Eliciting vague descriptions, giving inadequate answers, parroting, and following standard forms too closely are also in this category.

Those nontherapeutic techniques in which the care provider communicates in an undesirable manner fall into nontherapeutic communications of *commission*. They include giving advice or disapproval, being defensive, making judgements, challenging, making stereotyped responses, reassuring, or rejecting patient messages. Table 10.2 lists several nontherapeutic communication techniques. Become an observer of your own communications. See if your verbal and nonverbal communications send the same message. Evaluate your use of different techniques, and work to enhance your ability to effectively communicate.

PROBLEMS WITH COMMUNICATION

For many people, communicating with others can be a difficult process. Sensory-impaired patients have difficulty receiving or sending messages because of problems with sight, hearing, or understanding. Some people may have problems with sending messages. To illustrate, persons with **aphasia** (inability to speak), **dyslexia** (impaired ability to read sometimes accompanied by a mixing of letters or syllables in a

BOX 10.6   Therapeutic Communication Techniques

Listening
Definition: Active process of receiving information and examining reactions to messages received
Example: Maintaining eye contact and receptive nonverbal communication
Therapeutic value: Nonverbally communicates care provider's interest and acceptance
Nontherapeutic threat: Failure to listen

Broad Openings
Definition: Encouraging patient to select topics for discussion
Example: "What are you thinking about?"
Therapeutic value: Indicates acceptance by care provider and value of patient's initiative
Nontherapeutic threat: Care provider dominates interaction; rejecting responses

Restating
Definition: Repeating main thought expressed by patient
Example: "You say that your mother left you when you were 5 years old?"
Therapeutic value: Indicates that care provider is listening and validates, reinforces, or calls attention to something important that has been said
Nontherapeutic threat: Lack of validation of care provider's interpretation of message; being judgemental; reassuring; defending

Clarification
Definition: Attempting to put into words vague ideas or unclear thoughts of patient; asking patient to explain what they mean
Example: "I'm not sure what you mean. Could you tell me about that again?"
Therapeutic value: Helps to clarify feelings, ideas, and perceptions of patient and provides explicit correlation between them and patient's actions
Nontherapeutic threat: Failure to probe; assumed understanding

Reflection
Definition: Directing back patient's ideas, feelings, questions, and content
Example: "You're feeling tense and anxious, and it's related to a conversation you had with your husband last night?"
Therapeutic value: Validates care provider's understanding of what patient is saying and signifies empathy, interest, and respect for patient
Nontherapeutic threat: Stereotyping patient's responses; inappropriate timing of reflections; inappropriate depth of reflections; inappropriate responses to cultural experience and educational level of patient

Humour
Definition: Discharge of energy through comic enjoyment
Example: "That gives a whole new meaning to the word nervous," said with shared kidding between care provider and patient
Therapeutic value: Can promote insight by making conscious repressed material, resolving paradoxes, tempering aggression, and revealing new options; is socially acceptable form of sublimation
Nontherapeutic threat: Indiscriminate use; belittling patient; screen to avoid therapeutic intimacy

Informing
Definition: Skill of information giving
Example: "I think you need to know more about how your medication works."
Therapeutic value: Helpful in patient education about relevant aspects of well-being and self-care
Nontherapeutic threat: Giving advice

Focusing
Definition: Questions or statements that help patient expand topic
Example: "I think that we should talk more about your relationship with your father."
Therapeutic value: Allows patient to discuss central issues; keeps communication process goal directed
Nontherapeutic threat: Allowing abstractions and generalizations; changing topics

Sharing Perceptions
Definition: Asking patient to verify care provider's understanding of patient's message
Example: "You're smiling, but I sense that you are really very angry with me."
Therapeutic value: Conveys understanding to patient and can clear up confusing communication
Nontherapeutic threat: Challenging patient; accepting literal responses; reassuring; testing; defending

Theme Identification
Definition: Underlying patient issues or problems that emerge repeatedly during care provider–patient relationship
Example: "I've noticed that in all of the relationships you have described, you've been hurt or rejected by a man. Do you think this is an underlying issue?"
Therapeutic value: Allows care provider to promote patient's exploration and understanding of important problems
Nontherapeutic threat: Giving advice; reassuring; disapproving

Silence
Definition: Lack of verbal communication for therapeutic reason
Example: Sitting with patient and nonverbally communicating interest and involvement
Therapeutic value: Allows patient time to think and gain insights; slows pace of interaction and encourages patient to initiate conversation while conveying support, understanding, and acceptance
Nontherapeutic threat: Questioning patient; failure to break nontherapeutic silence

Suggesting
Definition: Presenting alternative ideas for patient's consideration relative to problem-solving
Example: "Have you thought about responding to your boss in a different way when he raises that issue with you? For example, you could ask him if a specific problem has occurred."
Therapeutic value: Increases patient's perceived options or choices
Nontherapeutic threat: Giving advice; inappropriate timing; being judgemental

Modified from Stuart, G. W. (2013). *Principles and practice of psychiatric nursing* (10th ed.). St. Louis: Mosby.

TABLE 10.2   Nontherapeutic Communications

Nontherapeutic Technique	Description	Example
Failure to listen	Placing own thoughts above patient; not being involved in communication	Yawning when patient is speaking, looking at watch frequently, missing patient's messages
Failure to explore patient's point of view	Does not ask patient to describe abstract words such as *pain, angry, sick*	*Patient:* "My head hurts." *Care Provider:* "You're just getting used to your new medication." *Better:* "Tell me more."
Failure to probe	Does not seek clarification or validation from patient	*Patient:* "I've had bad experiences with doctors." *Care Provider:* "That's too bad." *Better:* "Would you like to explain?"
Eliciting vague descriptions	Does not encourage patient to explain or expand on message	*Patient:* "I keep hearing voices." *Care Provider:* "OK." *Better:* "What do they say?"
Giving inadequate answers	Does not collect enough data to answer patient's question accurately	Instructs patient about medication and then finds out he is allergic to it
Parroting	Continuous repeating of patient's words	*Patient:* "I haven't slept in two nights." *Care Provider:* "You haven't slept in two nights?" *Better:* "What do you think is causing this?"
Following standard forms too closely	Using a question-and-answer format to elicit specific information	*Care Provider:* "Do you have any problems chewing?" *Patient:* "No, but I have this pain in my jaw at night." *Care Provider:* "Do you have any problems with indigestion or constipation?" *Better:* "Tell me about your jaw pain."
Being judgemental: giving approval or disapproval, agreeing or disagreeing	Many responses that tell patients that they must think as you do	*Patient:* "I saw my wife today." *Care Provider:* "You should be nicer to her." *Better:* "How did it go?"
Giving advice	Telling patients what to do; gives message that they are inferior and not able to make good decisions	*Patient:* "I'm nervous about meeting Dr. Dow." *Care Provider:* "You just march in there and say what you want, but don't raise your voice." *Better:* "I can understand that."
Being defensive	An attempt to protect something or someone; prevents patients from communicating	*Patient:* "That last nurse is a dope." *Care Provider:* "All of our nurses here are highly trained." *Better:* "What makes you think that?"
Challenging	Inviting or daring patient to explain, act, or compete	*Patient:* "I'm really dead, you know." *Care Provider:* "If you are really dead, then why is your heart still beating?" *Better:* "You're dead?"
Giving reassurance	Messages that negate feelings of patient	*Patient:* "I'll never get out of here." *Care Provider:* "Everything will turn out for the best." *Better:* "You feel that you have been here a long time?"
Rejecting	Refusal to discuss feelings or areas of concern	*Patient:* "You know that I raped my sister." *Care Provider:* "Let's not talk about that." *Better:* "Would you like to talk about it?"
Using stereotyped responses	Using clichés, popular sayings, or trite expressions	*Patient:* "I feel so depressed today." *Care Provider:* "Everyone gets the blues now and then." *Better:* "What's making you feel so blue?"

word when speaking), and **speech cluttering** (rapid, confused delivery of unrhythmic speech patterns) cannot focus on verbal communications as their main form of human interaction.

The first step in interacting is to achieve a successful introduction. If the patient knows your name and purpose, cooperation is more likely. If possible, learn how the patient communicates (signing, writing, touch) and then encourage them to become actively involved in the communication process. Maintain good eye contact (when appropriate) and attentive nonverbal behaviours. Tune in to the patient's nonverbal behaviours and become

extra alert for the messages being sent. Communicate directly with the patient. Do not try to finish the patient's sentence or fill in words. Allow extra time for the patient to think and form responses. Do not forget the importance of the use of appropriate touch. For people who have diminished sight or hearing, touch is a powerful communication tool. In addition, the speech therapist can be a valuable member of the multidisciplinary treatment team for patients with communication problems.

Developing communication systems for people with language problems is the goal of several research projects.

TABLE 10.3   Speech Patterns Associated With Some Mental Health Challenges

Speech Pattern	Description	Example
Blocking	Loses train of thought, stops speaking because of unconscious block	"Then my father…what was I saying?"
Circumstantiality	Describes in too much detail, cannot be selective	When asked "How are you?" replies, "My left hand aches a bit, my nose has been leaking, my hair won't stay in place…"
Echolalia	Repeats last word heard	"Please wait here" is responded to with "Here, here, here…"
Flight of ideas	Shifts rapidly between unrelated topics	"My cat is grey. The food here is good."
Loose associations	Speaks constantly, shifting between loosely related topics	"Martha married Jim, who is a cook. I can cook. Cows are something that we can cook."
Mutism	Able to speak but remains silent	
Neologism	Coins new words and definitions	"Zargleves are good to eat," referring to any candy snack.
Perseveration	Repeats single activity, cannot shift from one topic to another	Answers new question with previous question's answer.
Pressured speech	Speech becomes fast, loud, rushed, and emphatic	Persons with mania often move and speak very rapidly with great urgency.
Verbigeration	Repeats words, phrases, and sentences several times over	Nurse: "It's time to take your pill." Patient: "Take your pill, take your pill, take your pill . . ."

Computer devices now allow users to communicate by producing pre-prepared voice synthesized conversations at the touch of a button.

Communicating With Mentally Troubled Patients

Problems with communication are a common feature in many forms of mental illness. People living with mental–emotional difficulties often find it difficult to develop trust in other people. Loneliness is the companion of mental illness. Sincere, respectful caring of another person can help remove barriers that isolate the mentally ill individual from the world.

To communicate effectively with mentally and emotionally troubled patients, realize that *every interaction is a part of the total therapeutic process*. A climate of trust and respect must be established before patients feel safe enough to honestly share themselves. Establishing this trusting climate requires patience, persistence, and consistency. Mental health patients need *routine*, the security of a dependable environment, and care providers with calm, reliable temperaments. This consistency satisfies basic safety needs and enables patients to focus on communicating.

Begin your interactions with mental health patients by introducing yourself and explaining your purpose. Then introduce a neutral subject, such as weather, sports, or entertainment events. Wait quietly for the patient to comment, using the opportunity to assess nonverbal behaviours or barriers to communication. Once the patient is communicating, avoid a verbal assault of questions. Data may need to be obtained, but not at the expense of threatening the fragile communication line so recently established. As long as the patient is interacting, necessary data will eventually be revealed.

One of the most important tools for communicating with mentally ill patients is therapeutic listening. Attentive listening alone communicates acceptance and respect, messages not often received by mental health patients. Once the patient

believes that you sincerely care about them as a person, a flow of communications will come easily. Sample Patient Care Plan 10.1 is based on the use of therapeutic communication principles.

Assessing Communication

Because the flow of information between people usually occurs naturally, we seldom take the time to assess a patient's abilities to communicate. However, a communication assessment is an important component of the mental health workup.

First, assess the patient's ability to hear and speak. Then note the content, quality, and pace of the patient's speech. Is speech coherent, logical, or easy to follow? Is the pace fast or slow? Is the volume loud, too soft, or whispered? Are there any physical speech challenges, such as stuttering? Are the number of words used excessive or few? How much time lapses before the patient responds to your message? Can the patient read or write? Is a cultural communication assessment necessary? The answers to these questions provide a solid database and offer valuable information for the multidisciplinary treatment team in establishing appropriate therapeutic goals. Table 10.3 describes some of the more common abnormal speech patterns seen in patients with psychiatric conditions.

The ability to therapeutically communicate is an important skill. Good communication techniques must be practised daily and evaluated frequently. Assess each communication and evaluate your effectiveness by asking yourself, "Was the interaction appropriate to the goals of care? Was there enough communication and feedback to meet the goals? Was the interaction flexible enough to allow for a balance between spontaneity and control? Was the communication effective?" Practice, patience, and a continual willingness to evaluate your interactions are the keys to developing effective communication skills. Work hard to become a good communicator. Your patients' well-being depends on it, no matter what the diagnosis is.

SAMPLE PATIENT CARE PLAN 10.1   Communication

Assessment

History Amy, a 30-year-old married woman, is suffering from depression. Currently, she refuses to speak or acknowledge anyone, including her husband and children. Today she is being admitted for evaluation and treatment of her depression.

Current Findings An untidy woman who stares at the floor and does not respond to staff members' questions. Sighs frequently. Sits immobile in chair for long periods.

Multidisciplinary Diagnosis	Planning/Goals
Impaired verbal communications related to emotional state	Amy will communicate her wishes and feelings with at least one staff member by April 22.

THERAPEUTIC INTERVENTIONS

Interventions	Rationale	Team Member
1. Present a calm, patient attitude rather than attempting to make Amy speak.	Helps decrease fears and anxieties; demonstrates respect and acceptance	All
2. Actively listen, observe for verbal and nonverbal cues and behaviours.	Helps piece together communication methods in an effort to understand Amy's messages	All
3. Encourage other ways of communicating, such as drawing or writing.	Demonstrates empathy, helps develop trust, and encourages communication	All
4. Anticipate needs until Amy can communicate them.	Provides safety, comfort, and support; helps develop trust	Nsg
5. Spend time (at least 15 minutes twice each day) with Amy in a private, quiet setting.	Promotes trust and interest; helps promote self-esteem	Nsg
6. Praise any attempt to communicate.	Encourages communication and demonstrates interest	All

Evaluation The second day after admission, Amy began to draw. By the fourth day of hospitalization, she answered "yes" or "no" questions. On April 17, Amy was able to discuss her feelings with one nurse.

Critical Thinking Questions

1. Amy began to draw pictures on her second day of admission. How could the care provider encourage her to verbally communicate based on her drawings?

2. How do you think you would feel sitting in silence with another person for 10 minutes?

A complete patient care plan includes several other diagnoses and interventions.
Nsg, nursing staff.

KEY POINTS

- Communication is the exchange of information between two persons or among a group of persons.
- In the 1960s, Dr. Eric Berne coined the term *transactional analysis* to describe the process of investigating what people do and say to each other.
- Neurolinguistic programming focuses on patterns of an individual's communications, which include eye-accessing clues, different language patterns, and the pace and rhythm of speech.
- For communication to occur, there must be a sender, a message, a receiver, feedback, and a context.
- The process of communicating involves perception, evaluation, and transmission.
- Communications occur on both verbal and nonverbal levels at the same time.
- Health care providers who work with patients from culturally different backgrounds need to learn culturally appropriate methods for communication by recognizing different communication styles, adapting their own communications, and accepting the patient as a person.
- Therapeutic communication techniques are skills that assist in effectively interacting with patients.
- Principles of therapeutic communication include acceptance, interest, respect, honesty, concreteness, assistance, permission, and protection.
- The goals of therapeutic communications are to focus on the patient and foster the therapeutic relationship.
- The art of listening is a necessary ingredient for every health care provider.
- Therapeutic communication techniques (responding strategies) are verbal and nonverbal responses that encourage patients to communicate. They include listening, offering broad openings, restating, clarification, reflection, humour, offering information, focusing, sharing perceptions, identifying themes, suggesting, and silence.
- Messages that hinder effective communications are called nontherapeutic communications.
- Problems with communication are a common feature of many forms of mental illness.
- To communicate effectively with patients, remember that every interaction is a part of the total therapeutic process.
- A communication assessment focuses on the patient's ability to communicate, actual speech, and current or potential communication problems.

ADDITIONAL LEARNING RESOURCES

Go to your Evolve website (http://evolve.elsevier.com/Canada/Morrison-Valfre/) for additional online resources, including the online Study Guide for additional learning activities to help you master this chapter content.

CRITICAL THINKING QUESTION

1. Consider a time when you have interacted with a professional and you felt they were not actively listening to you. Can you recall when you first became aware of feeling frustrated or annoyed? How did this make you feel? What do you wish the professional person had done differently?

REFERENCES

Berne, E. (1964a). *Games people play: Psychology of human relationships*. Grove Press [Seminal Reference].

Berne, E. (1964b). *Principles of group treatment*. Oxford University Press [Seminal Reference].

Giger, J. N., & Haddad, L. G. (2020). *Transcultural nursing: Assessment and intervention* (8th ed.). Mosby.

Jourard, S. (1971). *The transparent self*. Van Nostrand Reinhold [Seminal Reference].

Keltner, N. L., & Steele, D. (2019). *Psychiatric nursing* (8th ed.). Mosby.

Ruesch, J. (1961). *Therapeutic communications*. Norton.

Stuart, G. W. (2013). *Principles and practice of psychiatric nursing* (10th ed.). Mosby.

11

The Therapeutic Relationship

KEY TERMS

autonomy (aw-TŎN-ə-mē) (p. 121)
congruence (p. 128)
countertransference (KOUN-tĕr-trăns-FĔR-ĕns) (p. 128)
dynamics (DĪ-nă-mĭks) (p. 120)
empathy (ĔM-pă-thē) (p. 121)
genuineness (JĔN-yū-ĭn-nĕs) (p. 123)
hope (HŌP) (p. 122)
limit (lĭ-mĭt) **setting** (p. 125)
mutuality (MŪ-tū-ĂL-ə-tē) (p. 122)
nonadherence (p. 128)

rapport (răh-PŎR) (p. 123)
resistance (rē-SĬS-tĕns) (p. 128)
secondary gain (SĔK-ŏn-dār-ē GĀN) (p. 128)
secondary resistance (SĔK-ŏn-dār-ē rē-SĬS-tĕns) (p. 128)
therapeutic relationship (THĔR-ə-PYŪ-tĭk rē-LĀ-shŭn-shĭp) (p. 120)
transference (trăns-FĔR-ĕns) (p. 128)
trust (trŭst) (p. 121)

The **therapeutic relationship** is a directed energy exchange between two people, a flow that moves patients toward more constructive ways of thinking and effective ways of coping. Care providers use their abundant energies to first balance or stabilize patients. Then they assist patients in mobilizing and directing their own energies into more life-fulfilling directions.

The art of helping others involves a dynamic energy exchange that takes place every time care providers interact with their patients. This chapter focuses on how health care providers use their energies to establish and direct the therapeutic relationship.

DYNAMICS OF THE THERAPEUTIC RELATIONSHIP

The term **dynamics** refers to the interactions that occur among various forces. A social relationship includes dynamics such as having fun together, supporting each other through difficult times, and enjoying each other's company. A *social relationship* is a two-way energy exchange based on the sharing of personal opinions, attitudes, and tastes.

A *work relationship* has the purpose of achieving certain goals. It includes the dynamics of motivation, performance, and evaluation. People within a work relationship are there to achieve a goal, produce a product, make a profit, or deliver a service.

The therapeutic relationship differs from other relationships. First, the focus of energies is primarily on the patient. Second, the therapeutic relationship is consciously directed. Friendships and other social relationships just happen. In therapeutic relationships, care providers consciously establish a connection with patients to help them cope with their life demands.

The dynamic components of the therapeutic relationship include the concepts of trust, empathy, autonomy, caring, and hope. Use these concepts as a framework to develop the skills and sensitivity necessary to direct your energies toward effective helping relationships.

Trust

Trust is defined as "a risk-taking process whereby an individual's situation depends on the future behaviour of another person" (*Mosby's Dictionary*, 2013). Attitudes regarding trust are based on experiences, which have the power to influence the present and future. Without trust, individuals become isolated and incapable of relying on other people. Within the therapeutic relationship, trust "implies a willingness to place oneself in a position of vulnerability, relying on health care providers to perform as expected" (Arnold & Boggs, 2011). Trust is an important part of any therapeutic relationship. Every person for whom we care needs to be able to trust that we will act in their best interests.

Illness or dysfunction of any kind requires energy. When patients arrive for care, their energies are usually very low. The role of "receiver of care" fosters a dependency on care providers and feelings of vulnerability. Learn to recognize this situation and work to establish a sense of trust in each patient.

Care providers direct their energies toward establishing trust with patients in several ways. They first *assess the patient's ability to trust* others. Each therapeutic behaviour is then designed to promote trust. For example, a care provider who says she will return in 10 minutes arrives at the appointed time. One simple action reassures patients that care providers will follow through on their verbal statements.

Second, care providers must *be honest* with their patients. To tell a child, for example, that the injection will not hurt makes them less likely to trust the next health care provider's explanations. If these experiences are repeated often enough, people develop a mistrust of the entire medical care system.

CRITICAL THINKING

Mary is a 42-year-old woman who has been treated for severe depression for 21 years. She has received several electroconvulsive therapy treatments that she was told would relieve her depression; they did not. Various psychotropic medications have had little success. Currently, you, as one of the staff at the community mental health centre, have been following Mary's care.

Although Mary is required to return to the clinic weekly for medication monitoring, she keeps her appointments only when she wants more medication. When questioned about her refusal to keep her appointments, she tells you that no one really cares about her so why go through the motions. "Just fill the prescription, keep your mouth shut, and let me go," she replies to your statement of concern.
• How could Mary be encouraged to return to treatment?

The third focus for establishing trust is *clear communication*. Give information to patients slowly, using terms that can be understood by the average person. Patients cannot learn to trust if they cannot understand what you are saying. Offer patients the time to share their feelings and apprehensions. As Sundeen and colleagues note, "Without the establishment of trust, the helping relationship will not progress beyond the level of mechanical provision for tending to superficial needs" (Sundeen, Rankin, Stuart, et al., 1998).

Empathy

Empathy is the ability to understand the emotions, viewpoints, and situations of another. Empathy allows one to "walk a mile in another person's shoes." It enables care providers to enter into the life of an individual and understand important emotions, meanings, and attitudes. Empathy is demonstrated verbally, nonverbally, and behaviourally. It is the *connection* between care provider and patient that increases the effectiveness of the therapeutic relationship. In short, empathy is the ability to understand without actually experiencing the patient's world.

Unfortunately, there are no specific directions for developing empathy. However, you can become more empathetic by focusing your attention (energies) on what patients are trying to communicate. Learn to listen with more than just your ears. Concentrate on the speaker and listen objectively, without passing judgement. Accept what is being said. You do not have to agree with what the patient says, but you need to demonstrate acceptance of the communications and the patient.

The development of empathy can also be nurtured by becoming secure in your therapeutic actions. When care providers are confident with their abilities, their energies can be devoted to patients and their situations, instead of being concerned about performance. The care provider's confidence sends a message that encourages patients to share of themselves.

Last, learn to consciously focus on your patient. Enter into each interaction expecting to learn something new. Become aware of the entire message the patient is sending. Observe body motions, gestures, eye movement, facial expressions, and vocal tones. Together, these small cues send powerful messages.

Autonomy

The concept of **autonomy** relates to the ability to direct and control one's activities and destiny. When people seek health care, they risk losing their autonomy because health care delivery is a specialized, complex world, full of the unknown.

People living with mental health difficulties have problems with autonomy because the nature of their illness often results in their making inappropriate decisions. However, autonomy is just as important for these individuals. Care providers commonly think that patients are incapable of making good health care decisions. They assume a controlling attitude and become the judge of what is best for the patient. This attitude limits the patient's ability to make decisions and increases dependency on others. Autonomy is encouraged by the care provider through use of the concept of mutuality.

The concept of **mutuality** relates to the process of sharing information and ideas with another person. When a therapeutic relationship has mutuality, both patient and care provider focus their unique strengths on fulfilling health care needs. The care provider has theoretical knowledge that can assist the patient in identifying specific problems and possible solutions, and the patient has the knowledge of self and needs that are important to the patient. All of these elements contribute to the plan of care.

Because patients are unique individuals, therapeutic interventions are modified to meet each person's needs. For example, patients who are unable to remember their appointments are reminded. Mutuality also helps both patients and care providers meet goals. When goals are based on the patient's needs, they are more apt to be achieved because patients have a role in establishing them.

Caring

Caring is a vital part of the therapeutic relationship; its thread is interwoven through every aspect and interaction. Caring is the energy that enables care providers to unconditionally accept all people, even when they are most unlovable.

Patients will often question care providers about their sincerity. Statements such as, "You are just doing this because it's your job" or "You don't really care—you're getting paid to be nice to me" express the need to be accepted, to be cared for and valued. People who have had negative experiences with the health care system become cautious and suspicious of the intentions of their care providers. They can tell when someone is sincere or merely concerned with the diagnosis, test, or function, rather than the person. Care providers who demonstrate high levels of caring are able to enjoy the uniqueness of each patient. They are able to give of themselves without losing their own identity. To develop and nurture your caring abilities, practise the behaviours listed in Box 11.1. Caring behaviours communicate concern, sensitivity, and compassion. Cherish and nurture your ability to care. It is the connection that enhances the therapeutic relationship.

Hope

The concept of hope involves the future. For many people, especially those who are ill or distressed, the future can appear bleak. Hope is not easily defined. From a therapeutic point of

view, we can say that **hope** is "a multidimensional dynamic life force characterized by a confident yet uncertain expectation of achieving a future good" (Dufault & Martocchio, 1985). For hope to be achievable, it must be realistic, possible, and personally significant. Hope is a highly personal concept, and it serves as an energy that motivates people toward health.

For care providers, hope is a therapeutic energy tool that can have a powerful effect on patient care outcomes. The emotions and behaviours relating to hope are many, ranging from feelings of despair to inspiration and determination. They are illustrated on a continuum or range (Fig. 11.1), with the behaviours of despair on one end and great hope on the other.

Dufault and Martocchio (1985) described six dimensions related to the concept of hope. The first is the *affective dimension*. It includes all the feelings that one has about hope, such as anticipation, the desirability attached to the outcome, and dread. It is the emotional aspect of hope.

The second area, the *affiliative dimension*, focuses on how hope is related or interwoven. It includes spirituality—how one relates to life and other people. Behaviours in this dimension include the seeking or receiving of help, using others as a source of hope, and seeking support and encouragement.

Third is the *behavioural dimension*, which consists of the actions or behaviours that may make the hoped-for situations come true. For example, people who begin an exercise program hoping that they will prevent heart problems are operating in the behavioural dimension.

Fourth is the *cognitive dimension*, or the thinking area. It is the process of thinking through and analyzing the hope. Some people operate within this dimension by defining their hopes. Others explore all the factors that relate to the hoped-for situation, whereas some compile facts to encourage a successful outcome. Acts associated with problem-solving are in the cognitive dimension.

Fifth is the *temporal dimension* of hope, the experience of time as it relates to hope. Because hope is accompanied by time, one's past, present, and future interact. One may hope to repeat the pleasant experiences of the past and use them as a frame of reference to avoid problems in the future.

Last is the *contextual dimension* of hope, which includes one's personal life situation as it relates to hope. It becomes much easier to have hope if one's environment is stable.

BOX 11.1 Developing Caring Abilities

To develop and nurture your ability to care, do the following:
1. Become aware of the patient as an individual.
2. Learn to respect the uniqueness of each person.
3. Increase your knowledge of the patient's needs.
4. Develop mutual sharing.

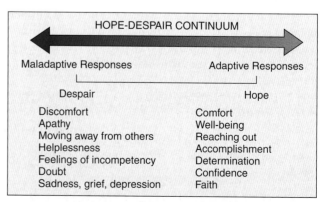

Fig. 11.1 The hope–despair continuum.

TABLE 11.1 Interventions Related to Hope

Dimension	Therapeutic Interventions
Affective	Provide an opportunity for expression of feelings Respond empathically Assist in coping with feelings
Affiliative	Support helpful relationships
Behavioural	Encourage appropriate actions Enhance self-esteem to decrease feelings of helplessness
Cognitive	Clarification Provide information
Temporal	Help to see the relationship between past experiences and hope
Contextual	Help to create a supportive, hopeful environment

Modified from Dufault, K., & Martocchio, B. C. (1985). Symposium on compassionate care and the dying experience. *Nursing Clinics of North America, 20*(2), 379–391.

BOX 11.2 Components of the Therapeutic Relationship

T = Trust
E = Empathy
A = Autonomy
C = Caring
H = Hope

Inadequate resources (physical, financial, emotional) provide a context in which hope may be difficult to summon. Hope conforms to an individual's point of view.

There are several therapeutic interventions relating to hope. Table 11.1 lists an intervention for each dimension of hope. The concept of hope is basic to the therapeutic relationship because without it, goals are meaningless.

The dynamics of the therapeutic relationship are not overt. They lie quietly, waiting to be energized by the therapeutic agent. Trust, empathy, autonomy, caring, and hope are the techniques with which care providers build the foundation of the therapeutic relationship. Look closely at the first letters of each word, which form the acronym *TEACH*. With these tools, care providers can guide the therapeutic relationship and move (teach) their patients toward their highest levels of wellness (Box 11.2).

CHARACTERISTICS OF THE THERAPEUTIC RELATIONSHIP

Therapeutic relationships vary in importance to patients. For patients who are hospitalized or institutionalized, the therapeutic relationship assumes a greater importance. People living with chronic conditions usually place a high degree of importance on their relationships with care providers. Those living with emotional or mental health challenges often need

the therapeutic relationship to serve as the bridge between mere existence and success. To establish a therapeutic relationship, the qualities of acceptance, rapport, and genuineness must be communicated to the patient.

Acceptance

The verb *accept* means to receive what is being offered. People entering the health care system arrive as complex individuals with histories, internal needs, and external realities. Every person must be accepted exactly as they are. Most people are cooperative and interested in working toward relieving the problems for which they sought care. However, some people are more difficult to accept, especially when their behaviours are unusual or not socially appropriate. As Vellenga and Christenson (1994) note, "it is difficult to fully understand the overwhelming experience of having to live with mental illness," but the importance of accepting these individuals cannot be stressed enough in the therapeutic relationship.

Care providers are concerned with the long-term aspects of a patient's mental illness, whereas distressed individuals are focused on their present pain and the need for relief. They must not only cope with the discomforts of their illness but also deal with the alienation forced on them by others. The stigma of being mentally ill follows them into their home and workplace and results in the loss of emotional relationships and vocational opportunities. Many individuals experience *distress,* which is described as feelings of hopelessness, fright, and an inability to function. For people living with emotional difficulties, acceptance is of prime importance.

Care providers can develop acceptance by remembering that it is the person (the individual) who must be accepted, not the behaviours or the attitudes. The very purpose of mental health care is to replace inappropriate behaviours with more effective actions. However, if the patient feels accepted for who they are, then treatment strategies will be far more effective.

Rapport

The second ingredient for an effective therapeutic relationship is **rapport**—the ability to establish a meaningful connection with patients. Rapport is a dynamic process, an energy exchange between care provider and patient that provides the background for all therapeutic actions. Rapport is a personal concept—the person of the care provider therapeutically interacting with the person of the patient.

Rapport is developed through a concern for others and an active interest in the well-being of one's patients. A belief in the worth and dignity of each individual, along with an accepting attitude, is essential for forming rapport. Every care provider has a certain degree of skill in establishing rapport with patients. Actively work to improve your abilities to establish meaningful connections with patients. Rapport is not a scientific tool but an application of our willingness to care.

Genuineness

Something that is genuine is real. **Genuineness** "implies that the nurse (care provider) is an open, honest, sincere person who is actively involved in the relationship" (Stuart, 2013).

TABLE 11.2   Phases of the Patient–Care Provider Relationship

Phase	Goals	Care Provider Behaviours
Preparation	Gather data	Reviews information and considers own reactions
Orientation	Develop mutual trust Establish care provider as significant other to patient	Establishes mutually acceptable contract Responds to testing behaviour of patient by adhering strictly to terms of contract
Working	Identify and address patient's problems	Highly individualized to nature of patient's problems Empathic, nonpunishing limit setting
Termination	Assist patient to review what was learned and to transfer this learning to interactions with others	Understands patient's sense of loss Helps patient express and cope with feelings Encourages patient to channel feelings into constructive activity, such as farewell party Recognizes own feelings of loss

The quality of honesty is a part of being genuine. However, the goal of the therapeutic relationship is to move the patient toward wellness. Sharing yourself must be done while remembering that the patient is the primary focus. In this way, you can be genuinely involved without using the therapeutic relationship to meet your own needs.

Therapeutic Use of Self

The most therapeutic tool of any care provider is the *self*—the ways in which we interact with, attend to, and encourage patients. Care providers are role models for health and coping, especially with people who are troubled. Our behaviours set examples for successful actions.

Care providers direct themselves therapeutically by focusing energies on the patient. Sometimes they share small bits of personal information, but that sharing always has a purpose that benefits the patient. For example, a patient asks how many children the care providers has. The care provider answers the question, and then focuses on the patient by asking him how many children he has. This technique allows you to maintain the focus on the patient.

To improve your skills in using "self" therapeutically, remember two important points. First, *feel good about yourself*. You cannot be therapeutically effective when your personal life is in turmoil. Patients can sense a care provider's emotional discomfort. Work to become aware of your own feelings and attitudes and how they affect your therapeutic relationships.

Second, work to develop an awareness of how your actions, gestures, and expressions *affect other people*. During each interaction, "step out" of the situation and consider how the patient may be reacting. With experience and effort, the majority of your actions will be therapeutic, regardless of the practice setting or patient you encounter.

PHASES OF THE THERAPEUTIC RELATIONSHIP

The therapeutic relationship is a patient-centred, time-limited, purposeful series of interactions. Every therapeutic relationship moves through four phases, and each phase

BOX 11.3   Stigma and Stereotype

Stigma is a negative stereotype, and *discrimination* is the behaviour or unfair treatment that results from this negative stereotype. Often, individuals living with a mental illness are faced with multiple, intersecting layers of discrimination as a result of their mental illness and their identity. For example, a woman with a mental illness may experience discrimination due to sexism as well as her illness, and a racialized individual may experience discrimination due to racism in addition to their mental illness. Living with discrimination can also have a negative impact on mental health.

From Canadian Mental Health Association. (2020). *Stigma and discrimination.* https://ontario.cmha.ca/documents/stigma-and-discrimination/

has identifiable tasks and goals (Table 11.2). As these tasks are accomplished, a readiness to move on to the next phase is experienced. Interventions are guided by the therapeutic goals of the patient's treatment plan throughout the relationship. The four stages or phases of the therapeutic relationship are the preparation, orientation, working, and termination phases.

Preparation Phase

The preparation phase is the data-gathering stage in which the care provider prepares for the relationship. Complete information about the patient is usually not available, but it is very important to learn as much as possible before the first meeting. The therapeutic goals for this phase are to establish a patient database and assess your own feelings regarding the patient.

To establish a database, *review all possible information* relating to the patient. Past medical records, current records, and interactions with significant others in the patient's life are excellent sources of information. Once information is gathered, look for the recurring patterns of behaviour to develop a picture of the patient. You can now begin to form ideas about the relationship and forecast possible problems. A word of caution: *Do not accept labels as fact* (see Box 11.3). Keep an open mind. Because a patient is labelled as psychotic, do not expect them to behave as other people with the same label. People are individuals with their own unique behaviours.

Because care providers are also unique individuals with attitudes and behaviours that affect the therapeutic relationship, the next step is to *look inward to your own reactions*. Identify your initial reactions to the patient. Is there anything that may block your ability to help? For example, a care provider's attendance at a support group for the spouses of alcoholics may have an influence on their ability to help a patient being treated for alcoholism.

Next, assess for *stereotyping*: If the patient is a member of a particular group or culture, will they behave in a certain way? The belief that people with mental illness cannot behave responsibly is a stereotype that can affect the therapeutic relationship. Be aware of any preconceived ideas or attitudes about the patient.

Finally, *recognize the anxiety* that is generally present in the care provider during this phase. Mild anxiety is common and sharpens the senses. High anxiety levels can affect one's judgement, so seeking assistance from a supervisor is advised when anxiety may affect the therapeutic relationship.

During this phase, care providers also begin to think about the termination phase. Because the therapeutic relationship is based on helping patients with their problems, it is time-limited, and care providers reinforce this throughout each phase of interaction.

The last step in the preparatory phase is to make plans for the first interaction with the patient. Find a quiet *setting*—free from interruptions. Plan for sufficient *time*, and identify what *information* must be obtained during the first interaction. Make a mental or written outline, and your preparations are complete.

Orientation Phase

During the orientation phase, care provider and patient become acquainted, agree to work with each other, and establish the purpose for the relationship. The first meeting establishes the tone and forms the impressions that both people carry with them throughout the entire relationship. The basic goals for this phase are to build trust and establish the care provider as significant in the life of the patient.

The most important step at this time is to identify each other. Introduce yourself by name and position. Establish how the patient wishes to be addressed. When the patient responds, an exchange begins. Next, explain your role as it relates to the patient. This gives the patient an idea of what may be expected in the relationship. Once patient and care provider are comfortable, an agreement to work with each other is established.

Establishing a working agreement (care provider–patient contract) is the next step in the orientation phase of the therapeutic relationship. Both patient and care provider discuss their expectations and then agree on the goals they want to meet. The contract, which includes a description of each person's roles and responsibilities, is then established in writing or verbally. The word *contract* may provoke anxiety in some persons, so it is seldom used when interacting with patients.

The term is less important than actually gaining the patient's agreement. Once arrangements are made, it is extremely important for the care provider to keep their end of the bargain and behave with consistency.

During the orientation phase, both the patient and care provider carry out assessments or "size up" each other. The care provider learns about the patient as a real person, unique and individual. The care provider must work to keep a nonjudgemental attitude. The label of "patient" will soon be replaced with a genuine person-to-person exchange that begins to evolve into a therapeutic relationship.

Patients will often test the reliability of their care providers. *Testing* is an important step in establishing trust in the therapeutic relationship. Although patients may not appear for scheduled appointments, use profane language, or resist sharing their feelings, the care provider must demonstrate a willingness to continue the therapeutic relationship by doing what was promised in the contract. This *reliability* is important because many troubled people have never had a consistent relationship. When the care provider has established reliability and the patient has developed enough trust to no longer test, the therapeutic relationship is ready for the next stage.

Working Phase

The focus of the working phase is to achieve the goals in the patient–care provider agreement. This is the time for solving problems and trying out new behaviours. During this phase, care providers are guided by their knowledge of human behaviour, the patient's plan of care, and the agreed-on goals.

The working phase consists of periods of growth and resistance. If the relationship is moving toward its goals, behavioural changes are seen in the patient. At this time, it is important to explore the meaning of the change with the patient and mutually decide whether the change is meeting the agreed-on goals. Periods of growth are accompanied by episodes of resistance. Changing one's behaviour is hard work. It requires energy and self-disclosure. Patients often feel self-conscious, shameful, and vulnerable during this time. The care provider's gentle acceptance and reliability can help patients move through their periods of resistance.

An important technique for care providers is knowing when to set limits. **Limit setting** is an intervention designed to prevent patients from harming themselves or others. The necessity for setting limits often occurs during the working phase as the patient may be experiencing many painful emotions. Setting limits requires a calm, nonthreatening manner. The patient is not being punished, just protected until self-control can be regained. Patients often feel a sense of relief and trust when they know that someone cares enough to protect them, even if the threat is from the self.

Patient and care provider continue to work on meeting the goals of the relationship. Other members of the treatment team may also be involved in specific areas of the patient's therapy. Therefore, it is important to understand how each member of the team functions and shares responsibility in relation to the patient. During the working stage, care providers frequently assess for behaviours that indicate the goals are

TABLE 11.3   Patient Responses to Termination

Regression	Withdrawal	Continuation
Return to previous maladaptive behaviour	Denial of caregiver's help	Tries to continue relationship
Increased anxiety	Demands to stop relationship now	Brings up new problems
Tardiness or absence from appointments	Absence from appointments	Becomes helpless
Expresses doubts about value of relationship	Superficially interacts with caregiver	Wants caregiver to solve their problems

Modified from Sundeen, S. J., Rankin, E. A. D., Stuart, G. W., & Cohen, S. A. (1998). *Nurse–patient interaction: Implementing the nursing process* (6th ed.). Mosby.

TABLE 11.4   Teaching Opportunities for Care Providers

Topic	Health Team Member
Activities of daily living	All members
Mental illness and its treatments	Nursing, therapists
Effects, adverse effects, adverse reactions of medications	Nursing
Early signs and symptoms of return to maladaptive functioning	All members
How to cope with stressors of daily living	All members
What to say to others about their mental illness	Nursing, therapists
Teaching the public about mental health and illness	All members

being met. Patients are educated about exploring community resources. Preparations are made for terminating the relationship. The time finally arrives when the goals are accomplished or one of the individuals is no longer able to maintain the relationship. It is the signal for the final phase, termination.

Termination Phase

When the goals of the therapeutic relationship are achieved, both the patient and care provider share a sense of accomplishment. However, this is balanced by the loss of a meaningful person in the patient's life. When the mutual goals have not been met, termination can be difficult. This is a major reason why it is important to set realistic goals at the beginning and to frequently monitor the patient's progress.

Steps toward termination should begin before the last meeting. Both parties need time to prepare the patient for independence. During this phase, the care provider reviews the steps taken toward achieving the goals. Patients feel a sense of pride and accomplishment when they can review their progress. This is also an opportunity to encourage patients to apply their new and more effective behaviours to other situations.

People respond to the loss of a therapeutic relationship as they would to any loss. Some may show signs of regression or withdrawal or engage in behaviours to continue the relationship (Table 11.3). The feelings underlying these behaviours should be identified and shared. Looking to the future and reminding patients of their progress can help ease the transition to independence. Saying goodbye is never easy, but a patient who is able to function more effectively as a result of your interventions is the reward of a successful therapeutic relationship.

ROLES OF THE CARE PROVIDER

Throughout the course of the therapeutic relationship, care provider's play several roles, each designed to assist patients in meeting specific therapeutic goals. Care providers who work with mental health patients assume the roles of therapeutic change agents, teachers, technicians, and therapists. Together, these roles help move patients toward more successful and adaptive coping behaviours.

Change Agent

The therapeutic environment is more than a physical space. The psychological atmosphere created by caregivers is one of the major contributions toward successful recovery. Caregivers provide an accepting atmosphere that values the contributions of each individual. They accept the fact that some patient behaviours may not be appropriate, but they never discredit the person. Individuals are encouraged to exchange their unsuccessful actions for more effective behaviours. Care providers' attitudes foster a climate that anticipates, expects, and promotes positive change. Each staff member acts as a role model for successful living, thus demonstrating to patients that there are other ways of behaving. When the atmosphere promotes change and provides the security to practise those changes, patients are more likely to improve.

Care providers also function as *socializing agents*. They assist patients in participating in group activities and various social interactions. They introduce patients to each other, encourage conversations, and help patients focus on the healthy aspects of their lives. Interactions with others are seen as opportunities to encourage successful social experiences for their patients.

Teacher

Members of the mental health care team are constantly alert for opportunities to teach. In the mental health care setting, teaching opportunities range from instructions about daily living activities to major lifestyle changes (Table 11.4).

While all patients must be taught about areas such as medications and diet, equally important opportunities for instruction exist with every patient interaction. Through these interactions, care providers are able to assess and monitor existing problems, plan for corrective learning opportunities, and forecast possible difficulties. Patients and their families learn to trust care providers, and they often confide in them. Times of sharing become great teaching opportunities. Teaching is an important part of care because it provides a solid bridge for the passage to effective adaptation and independence.

Technician

The technical roles of the mental health team members focus on holistic care; attention is paid to the whole patient. The providers involved with the patient's care sometimes focus on the mental–emotional status of the patient and exclude the physical status. For this reason, care providers must remain alert to the physical problems that may be present with mental health patients. Remember Maslow's hierarchy of needs—physical needs must be satisfied first. Many mental health patients experience physical problems, just as many medical patients experience psychological problems. The technical role for nurses in the mental health setting includes administering, monitoring, and evaluating medications; managing medical problems within the mental health environment; assessing the difference between physical and psychiatric conditions; maintaining safety; and managing environmental factors. Other team members have technical roles related to their specialties.

Therapist

Care providers use every opportunity to assist patients in developing more effective behaviours. In this sense, all care providers are mental health therapists. However, some care providers are specifically trained as therapists. Nurses, social workers, occupational therapists, physicians, registered psychotherapists, and psychologists are entitled to practise psychotherapy in most provinces in Canada (Colleges of Nurses of Ontario [CNO], 2020).

Care providers function in many roles when working with mental health patients. Through "practised awareness," they are able to use a variety of roles to assist patients in working toward their goals. The therapeutic use of self is applied each time care providers interact with their patients, and every interaction is seen as a teaching/learning opportunity.

PROBLEMS ENCOUNTERED IN THE THERAPEUTIC RELATIONSHIP

Throughout the therapeutic relationship, care providers continually assist their patients in achieving more effective functioning. However, problems or barriers can arise and challenge care providers to devise creative solutions. The most common problems fall into three broad areas: the environment, the care provider, and the patient. By remaining alert for these potential areas of difficulty, care providers are able to prevent larger problems and increase their therapeutic effectiveness.

Environmental Problems

Problems with the environment include things such as a lack of privacy, an inappropriate meeting place, or uncomfortable furniture, lighting, or temperature. Noise and frequent interruptions disrupt interactions and can become troublesome, especially if patients are attempting to share personal information.

CASE STUDY

It took 3 weeks for Marguerite's patient to engage in a meaningful conversation with her. Today, as the discussion progressed, Marguerite could see that her patient was about to share something important. Suddenly three people entered the room and began to demand that the patient join them for coffee. The moment was lost; the patient mumbled something about later and left.

• How could Marguerite have prevented this interruption from happening?

To minimize environmental barriers to communication, make appropriate arrangements for interactions with the patient. Find an area where interruptions and distractions will be minimal. Being interrupted stops the communication flow between care provider and patient and does little to foster the relationship. Be alert to how the environment affects the therapeutic relationship and problems will be easier to prevent.

Problems With Care Providers

The barriers relating to care providers in the therapeutic relationship include difficulties with attitude, setting helping boundaries, and countertransference.

Care providers are human beings with attitudes, opinions, and problems of their own. Working within a therapeutic relationship requires energy, time, and persistence. If the care provider is expending energies in coping with personal difficulties, there can be little left for the patient. Historically, health care providers were taught to leave their personal lives at the door and ignore them during working hours. Now we know that it is not possible to separate the care provider from the person. They are one, and it is the "person" aspect of the caregiver that is so effective in helping patients.

Personal health (physical and mental) is a primary ingredient of effective patient care. Several studies have found that workers in the personal care and service category have high rates of depression (Hoben, Knopp-Sihota, Nesari, et al., 2017; Office of Applied Studies, 2007; Pun, 2019). To prevent this, care providers must renew themselves routinely if they are to be effective with their patients.

Attitude is also important in how the care provider views the patient. Care providers who are skeptical about the patient's willingness or ability to change are already dooming the relationship to failure. Discomfort with the feelings expressed by the patient can also impair the relationship. To be effective, one must know oneself and be comfortable with one's beliefs and values.

Modified from Pilette, P. C., Berck, C. B., & Achber, L. C. (1995). Therapeutic management of helping boundaries. *Journal of Psychosocial Nursing and Mental Health Services, 33*(1), 40–47.

BOX 11.4   Self-Assessment of Helping Boundaries

1. Have you ever felt too involved with a patient?
2. Have you ever received feedback that you are overly intrusive or involved with patients or their families?
3. Do you have difficulty setting and enforcing limits?
4. Do you spend more than the allotted time with the patient or arrive early or stay late for appointments?
5. Do you relate to patients as you do family members?
6. Do you feel that you are the only one who "really understands" the patient?
7. Do you feel that other staff members are too critical of "your" patient or jealous of the relationship you have with the patient?
8. Do you find it difficult to handle the patient's unreasonable requests or behaviours?
9. Do you look forward to the patient's praise, appreciation, or affection?

   A "yes" answer to any of these questions indicates a need to identify the behaviours that are blurring the boundaries of the therapeutic relationship.

Compassion is a key quality, but when that compassion leads one to "rescue" patients, the care provider is becoming too involved. "Owning" patient problems wears out the care provider and does nothing to promote the patient's abilities to cope. To prevent this situation, establish your own professional boundaries that define the limits of the patient–care provider relationship. The focus of the therapeutic relationship is the *patient*. Patients must be allowed to own their problems or the therapeutic relationship loses its effectiveness. care provider actions must be designed to move patients toward the goals of therapy. Box 11.4 offers a tool for assessing your helping boundaries.

Congruence is the agreement between verbal and nonverbal messages. Sitting with crossed arms and legs while inviting a patient to share sensitive information sends a double or *incongruent* message. Usually the patient will react to the nonverbal message first. Become aware of how your verbal and nonverbal communications match (or may not match).

Countertransference is a barrier in the therapeutic relationship that is based on the care provider's inappropriate emotional responses to the patient. The caregiver's personal needs or reactions begin to inhibit the effectiveness of the therapeutic relationship. Common responses include intense feelings of caring, involvement, disgust, hostility, or anxiety. To prevent countertransference, remember that the focus of the relationship is the patient. Recognizing when one's personal needs are beginning to overshadow the patient's needs is a good way to prevent countertransference.

Problems With Patients

Progress in the therapeutic relationship can also be slowed or blocked by the patient. Frequently, patients engage in various behaviours to stall the effectiveness of therapeutic actions.

Patient behaviours that block progress fall into three basic categories: resistance, transference, and nonadherence.

Resistance was first defined by Freud as a patient's attempts to avoid recognizing or exploring anxiety-provoking material. Behaviours are classified into primary and secondary types of resistance. Patients who demonstrate *primary resistance* are unwilling to change, even when they are aware of the need for change. Behaviours include attempts to thwart the therapeutic process, a refusal to work toward the therapeutic goals, and attempts to manipulate the situation. Patients may also resist in reaction to the care provider's interventions. In addition, if the caregiver is not an appropriate role model for therapeutic behaviour, primary resistance may occur.

Secondary resistance occurs when the patient is motivated by drives other than the need to regain health. Many times the payoff for remaining ill outweighs the advantages of recovery.

Secondary gain occurs when patients profit or avoid unpleasant situations by remaining ill. For example, the patient who is facing legal problems on discharge attempts to remain in the therapeutic environment because he does not want to go to jail. Secondary gain can be a powerful motivation for resisting the treatment team's therapeutic efforts.

Transference is a patient's emotional response, based on earlier relationships, to the caregiver. The most outstanding characteristic of transference is the inappropriateness of the patient's responses. Because the patient is transferring emotions associated with one person to another (the caregiver), little opportunity for self-awareness exists. Patients may become hostile, express their feelings by demanding an end to the relationship, or show no interest in therapeutic interventions. Other patients can become dependent, submissive, and passive or overvalue the care provider's characteristics and place unreachable expectations on the relationship.

To prevent or cope with transference, first listen. Hear what the patient is trying to communicate. Recognize areas of resistance, and then clarify them with the patient. Explore behaviours and try to identify possible reasons for their use. With time and experience, you will become adept at working with the unique behaviours of transference.

Nonadherence is not following the prescribed treatment regimen. For individuals with mental–emotional difficulties, nonadherence is high. Reasons for nonadherence can include poor insight, substance abuse, a negative attitude toward medication, and cognitive impairment (Velligan, Sajatovic, Hatch, et al., 2016). According to Forman (1993), the main reasons for nonadherence are a lack of knowledge, medication adverse effects, and the care provider–patient relationship. Throughout the therapeutic relationship, care providers are continually assessing and monitoring the progress of their patients. Identifying and sharing problems of adherence with the patient can help to remove another barrier from recovery.

When patients are prescribed medications for the control of their symptoms, every care provider must remain especially alert for adverse effects. Many patients stop taking their psychotropic medications because of distressing adverse effects. Others simply feel that they do not need their medications. Whatever the reasons, care providers are in an excellent position to monitor and encourage their patients' adherence during the therapeutic relationship.

Health care providers have powerful tools for patient care within the therapeutic relationship. Throughout each phase, patients are encouraged to focus their energies toward more effective and adaptive ways of living. Sample Patient Care Plan 11.1 describes several interventions for establishing a therapeutic relationship. Learn to work with the dynamics of the therapeutic relationship. These are the tools that promote the patient's movement toward self-awareness and independent functioning.

SAMPLE PATIENT CARE PLAN 11.1   Therapeutic Relationship

Assessment
History Heather is a 14-year-old girl who is being treated for an eating disorder. She and the members of the treatment team have set a goal for a weight gain of 0.9 kg (2 lb) per month. Sue, the treatment team's nurse, has assumed responsibility for seeing Heather weekly and monitoring her weight gain.

Current Findings Heather keeps her appointments but tends to display negative reactions to every suggestion offered by the treatment team. Discussions with other care providers are superficial with little meaning. When interacting, Heather assumes a challenging attitude. Her weight has remained stable for the past 3 weeks.

Multidisciplinary Diagnosis	Planning/Goals
Ineffective coping related to a disturbance in self-concept	Heather will establish a trusting relationship as evidenced by a meaningful communication with a member of the treatment team by September 23.

THERAPEUTIC INTERVENTIONS

Interventions	Rationale	Team Member
1. Prepare for first meeting by researching data about Heather, her family, and her past history.	Helps define the patient as an individual with particular strengths and problems	All
2. Plan time, setting, and outline of goals for each meeting.	Helps to define and focus on the goals of the relationship	All
3. Establish an atmosphere of warmth and acceptance during first meeting.	Communicates respect and a willingness to become involved with Heather	All
4. Help Heather define her problems.	Helps reduce emotional reactions and break her problems into smaller, more manageable units	Psy, Nsg
5. Develop a contract (working agreement) for a self-motivated weight gain of 0.9 kg (2 lb) per month.	Defines limits, expectations of goals; helps to plan steps for meeting goals	Psy, Nsg
6. Assist Heather in learning positive thinking techniques.	Helps replace self-defeating thoughts and actions with more effective ways of coping	All

Evaluation Heather remained silent during the first two interactions with Sue. By September 10, she was willing to talk to Sue. By September 19, Heather began the interaction and stated that she would be willing to work on gaining weight and discussing her problems.

Critical Thinking Questions
1. How does a working agreement (contract) allow Heather to retain some control over her situation?
2. What would Sue (the nurse) do to encourage the relationship when Heather begins to initiate conversation?

A complete patient care plan includes several other diagnoses and interventions.
Nsg, nursing staff; *Psy*, psychologist.

KEY POINTS

- The therapeutic relationship is a directed energy exchange between two people that guides patients toward more effective behaviours. A social relationship is an energy exchange based on the sharing of personal opinions, attitudes, and tastes.
- The dynamic components of the therapeutic relationship include trust, empathy, autonomy, caring, and hope. Remember the acronym *TEACH*.
- Characteristics of rapport include a concern for others, an active interest in the well-being of the patient, a belief in the worth and dignity of each individual, and an accepting attitude.

- Therapeutic use of self relates to the ways in which care providers interact with, attend to, and encourage patients. Care providers act as role models for health and coping by using behaviours that set examples for successful actions.
- Care providers direct themselves therapeutically by focusing energies on the patient.
- To use the "self" therapeutically, feel good about yourself and work to develop an awareness of how your actions, gestures, and expressions affect other people.
- The four stages or phases of the therapeutic relationship are the preparation, orientation, working, and termination phases.

- To successfully establish a therapeutic relationship, the care provider communicates the qualities of acceptance, rapport, and genuineness to the patient.
- Care providers who work with mental health patients function as therapeutic change agents, teachers, technicians, and therapists.

- The most common problems in the therapeutic relationship relate to the environment, the care provider, and the patient.

ADDITIONAL LEARNING RESOURCES

Go to your Evolve website (http://evolve.elsevier.com/Canada/Morrison-Valfre/) for additional online resources, including the online Study Guide for additional learning activities to help you master this chapter content.

CRITICAL THINKING QUESTIONS

1. Stigma or stereotype? Discuss the following scenarios and decide if they represent a stigma or a stereotype:
   a. A primary school teacher tells an Asian student that he should focus on math and science because "Asians are always good at those subjects."
   b. A woman calls about a rental listing for a basement apartment. During their brief conversation, the landlord asks, "And where do you and your family come from? Were you born in Canada or did you immigrate here?" When told the caller is from Trinidad, the landlord says that she is very sorry, but the apartment has been rented and hangs up the phone.
2. You suspect that a patient is not demonstrating adherence to their prescribed medication. When you ask the patient to open their mouth and show that they have swallowed the pill, the patient becomes upset and accuses you of not trusting them. How might you respond to this patient?

REFERENCES

Arnold, E. C., & Boggs, K. U. (2011). *Interpersonal relationships: Professional communication skills for nurses* (6th ed.). Saunders.

College of Nurses of Ontario (CNO). (2020). *Legislation and regulation: Rhpa: Scope of practice, controlled acts model.* Author. http://www.cno.org/globalassets/docs/policy/41052_rhpascope.pdf

Dufault, K., & Martocchio, B. C. (1985). Hope: Its spheres and dimensions. *Nursing Clinics of North America, 20*(2), 379–391.

Forman, L. (1993). Medication: Reasons and interventions for noncompliance. *Journal of Psychosocial Nursing and Mental Health Services, 31*(10), 23–25.

Hoben, M., Knopp-Sihota, J. A., Nesari, M., et al. (2017). Health of health care workers in Canadian nursing homes and pediatric hospitals: A cross-sectional study. *CMAJ Open, 5*(4), E791–E799. https://doi.org/10.9778/cmajo.20170080

Mosby's dictionary of medicine, nursing, & health professions (9th ed.) (2013). Mosby.

Office of Applied Studies. (2007, October 2011). Depression among adults employed full-time, by occupational category. National Survey on Drug Use and Health Report (2007). Substance Abuse and Mental Health Data Archive. https://www.datafiles.samhsa.gov/study-publication/depression-among-adults-employed-full-time-occupational-category-nid15024

Pun, J. (2019, July 25). *The state of mental health in Canada's health care workers [Blog].* Starling Minds. https://www.starlingminds.com/resources/blogs/the-state-of-mental-health-in-canadas-healthcare-workers/

Stuart, G. W. (2013). *Principles and practice of psychiatric nursing* (10th ed.). Mosby.

Sundeen, S. J., Rankin, E. A. D., Stuart, G. W., et al. (1998). *Nurse-client interaction: Implementing the nursing process* (6th ed.). Mosby.

Vellenga, B. A., & Christenson, J. (1994). Persistent and severely mentally ill clients' perceptions of their mental illness. *Issues in Mental Health Nursing, 15*(4), 359–371.

Velligan, D. I., Sajatovic, M., Hatch, A., et al. (2016). Why do psychiatric patients stop antipsychotic medication? A systematic review of reasons for nonadherence to medication in patients with serious mental illness. *Patient Preference and Adherence, 2017*(11), 449–468. https://doi.org/10.2147/PPA.S124658. https://www.dovepress.com/why-do-psychiatric-patients-stop-antipsychotic-medication-a-systematic-peer-reviewed-fulltext-article-PPA

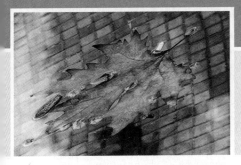

12

The Therapeutic Environment

OBJECTIVES

Upon completion of this chapter, the student will be able to:

1. List two situations that indicate a need for hospitalization.
2. Describe three types of patients treated in the inpatient therapeutic environment.
3. State two goals of the therapeutic environment.
4. Discuss five environmental factors that are assessed daily.
5. Explain the importance of setting limits on patients' behaviours.
6. Identify three ways the therapeutic environment helps patients meet their needs for love and belonging.
7. Examine how care providers' expectations influence patients' behaviours.
8. List three techniques to improve patient adherence to treatment.

OUTLINE

KEY TERMS

acceptance (p. 137)
chronicity (krō-NĬS-ĭ-tē) (p. 132)
involvement (ĭn-VŎLV-měnt) (p. 137)
limit setting (p. 136)

nonadherence (p. 138)
recidivism (rē-SĬD-ĭ-vĭz-m) (p. 133)
therapeutic (THĔR-ə-PYŪ-tĭk) **environment (milieu)** (mil-YOO) (p. 131)

The history of treating individuals with mental health challenges has been unkind. Historically, governments tended to establish custodial care institutions designed for housing and treating the mentally ill. Once people were admitted, they usually stayed for months or years, regardless of their ability to function in the community. Currently, mental health services are available in community hospitals, clinics, and institutions that specialize in providing mental health–related services. Although many people living with mental health challenges are treated on an outpatient basis, admission to a therapeutic environment remains an important component of psychiatric and mental health care.

In 1953, Maxwell Jones published a small book in England that described the value of the environment as a therapeutic tool. It was later published in Canada and the United States under the title *The Therapeutic Community*. The publication soon sparked the development of treatment settings that promoted personal worth and dignity (Jones, 1953). The therapeutic environment has become an important part of patient treatment plans.

The term **therapeutic environment (milieu)** describes certain settings or environments designed to help patients replace inappropriate behaviours with more effective personal and psychosocial skills (Stuart, 2013) (see Box 12.1). Principles of treatment are based on the concept that every interaction within the patient's environment has therapeutic potential. Physical surroundings are pleasant but safe. Activities are structured. Patients are expected to participate in their treatments. Therapeutic milieus can exist within hospital, home, or community settings. Because most therapeutic environments require certain limits and controls, they are most often located in inpatient settings, as part of a community hospital, for example.

Most people living with mental–emotional challenges manage within their communities. However, there are times when a more secure and stable environment is required. Admission to an inpatient facility can be on a voluntary or an involuntary basis. Box 12.2 lists the most common reasons for admission. Once patients are in the facility, treatment plans are designed to return them to their communities as soon as possible.

> #### BOX 12.1   The Therapeutic Milieu
>
> A therapeutic environment is a vital ingredient in facilitating the journey of recovery for patients within health care settings. Attention to the therapeutic environment ensures protection of patients from potentially harmful effects and maximizes opportunities for patients to learn something about themselves and their difficulties in everyday living. The terms *therapeutic environment* and *therapeutic milieu* are sometimes used interchangeably to describe the atmosphere of a psychiatric setting. Regardless of the term used, all treatment environments have an impact on patient outcomes.

From Keltner, N. L., & Steele, D. (2019). *Psychiatric nursing* (8th ed.). Elsevier.

> #### BOX 12.2   Criteria for Inpatient Admission
>
> Admission to a psychiatric inpatient facility occurs when any of the following are true:
> 1. A person's behaviour becomes a threat to the safety of themselves or others.
> 2. People within the environment are not able or willing to support the mentally troubled person.
> 3. The person perceives themselves as unable to cope or maintain behavioural control.

Care providers in inpatient settings provide the framework for the quality of the environment. Without a staff that possesses insight, understanding, personal warmth, and skill, the concept of a therapeutic community could not be a reality. The ways in which mental health care providers communicate, interact, behave, and use therapeutic techniques require study and practice to learn. Therapeutic tools include the use of eye contact, facial expressions, body movement, and other nonverbal behaviours. Other techniques are developed through experience and interactions with people from various cultures and backgrounds.

Psychiatric nursing practice has moved from custodial care to the management of complex therapeutic environments. Nurses in psychiatric facilities are now required to manage patients' environments, implement therapeutic interventions, coordinate and integrate multidisciplinary care delivery, and evaluate the outcomes of treatment for each patient with whom they work.

USE OF THE INPATIENT SETTING

Today's psychiatric facilities offer shorter stays, more intensive therapies, and support during the transition from institution to community. Inpatient services are provided for three main groups of people: those experiencing crises, those with acute mental or emotional challenges, and those with chronic mental illness.

Crisis Stabilization

People experiencing a crisis seek help when their discomfort becomes greater than their ability to resolve their problems privately. In many cases, *crisis stabilization* interventions are provided by placing patients in 1- or 2-days treatment settings in which balance (homeostasis) can be re-established.

Patients undergo counselling designed to resolve their immediate problems and concerns. Medications, such as antidepressants or sedatives, may be prescribed. Stress-management techniques are frequently taught to help modify stressful behaviours. Cognitive, relaxation, and behavioural therapies are often used to assist patients. The goal of inpatient crisis therapy is to help patients successfully cope with crisis. After patients are discharged from a crisis stabilization unit, they may be referred for assertiveness training; time, anger, or conflict management; other types of lifestyle supports; or problem-solving education.

Acute Care and Treatment

The inpatient environment is also necessary when people cannot function sufficiently to satisfy their basic needs or they pose a danger to self or others. By the time people seek voluntary admission to a treatment facility, they typically feel weakened and hopeless (Cohen, 1994). Patients may be drug-impaired or intoxicated. Some have experienced severe stress, such as a job layoff, illness, or loss of support systems.

For most people, admission to an inpatient psychiatric unit is a highly emotional experience. Those who are admitted involuntarily may experience intense discomfort during their first hospital experience and a sense of failure on subsequent admissions. Hospitalization can "dehumanize" an individual. Personal items, including clothing, are often taken away and, unfortunately, staff members sometimes remember the patient's diagnosis before the name of the patient. Care providers should try to "humanize" the hospital experience because the foundation of the patient's success or failure lies with the first experiences in the therapeutic environment. Most people with acute psychiatric problems can be successfully treated if interventions are vigorous and well coordinated. Even with the best of therapies, however, some individuals progress to chronic maladaptive responses and cycles of repeated admissions.

The Chronically Mentally Ill Population

Many mental health disorders are associated with a degree of **chronicity**. These are *long-term, persistent difficulties*. People living with chronic mental disorders may have periods of relative comfort and then fall rapidly into acute psychiatric states. For these people, life evolves into a seesaw existence between two worlds.

Often people with chronic mental health challenges know when they are beginning to decompensate (or "lose it," as some say) and will voluntarily admit themselves to an inpatient facility. Many more, however, do not have the insight or judgement to know when they are acting in maladaptive ways. Others experience paranoia (suspicious, afraid of others) and do not seek help or will refuse treatment when it is offered. Last, there is a growing number of mentally troubled individuals who have never sought assistance or received treatment. They live with their distresses as best they can.

The inpatient therapeutic environment fills many needs for troubled individuals. The physical necessities of clean water, wholesome food, clean clothing, and a comfortable bed are available. It also provides protection, safety, and security from a harsh world, along with a staff of care providers who offer attention and emotional support. From the chronically troubled person's point of view, life in the inpatient facility actually may be better than a lonely existence in the community.

CRITICAL THINKING

Many patients who have chronic mental challenges will admit themselves to an inpatient unit because they are looking for "three hots and a cot."
- What is the meaning of the statement?
- How does this statement relate to Maslow's hierarchy of needs theory? (Hint: see Chapter 5.)
- How do you think the statement affects the patient's attitude toward the therapeutic treatment plan?

Recidivism (repeated inpatient admissions) has become a way of life for many chronically troubled individuals. This is especially true for patients with cycles of assaultive behaviours. Recidivism is a frustrating aspect of inpatient mental health care for both patients and care providers. Patients feel like failures, and care providers become frustrated that their efforts during past admissions were not successful. Several suggestions for managing feelings associated with return patients are listed in Box 12.3. Recidivism, also called the *revolving-door syndrome*, continues to be a problem, especially for individuals with schizophrenia and chemical use. The primary reason that patients return to the inpatient environment is their refusal to take their prescribed psychotropic medications (adherence) or they do not engage with other supportive community-based resources.

GOALS OF A THERAPEUTIC ENVIRONMENT

Dr. Peter Breggin, author of *Toxic Psychiatry* (1991), defines mental illness as "overwhelm" and believes that people should be offered mental health care in small, local "sanctuaries" (rather than in psychiatric institutions) until they are able to cope with the demands of everyday life once again. Effective therapeutic environments provide the safety, security, and time to cope with difficulties. Members of the health care team offer therapeutic human contact designed to assist patients in learning about themselves and how they relate to others.

The goals of a therapeutic environment (milieu) are to provide protection, support, and education. A treatment team, composed of several specialists, is assigned to work with each patient. On admission, a thorough assessment is performed and a therapeutic plan of care is developed with the patient. Figure 12.1 illustrates the roles of the mental health team members. Nurses are more involved with direct care and management; however, all care team members communicate, collaborate, and teach.

BOX 12.3 Coping With Recidivism

Relating to Patients
Accept patients for themselves. They are doing the best they can at this time.
Learn about their lives outside the inpatient setting.
Explore after-discharge resources in the community.
Maintain a positive attitude. Patients do better when they are encouraged, rather than discouraged.

Relating to Care Providers
Remember who "owns" the problem. Care provider roles are to support, educate, and assist.
Attend a support group regularly. Discuss ways to stay positive.
Keep patient problems "at the office."

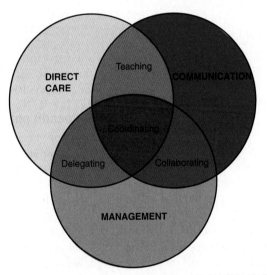

Fig. 12.1 Mental health practice. (From Stuart, G. W. [2013]. *Principles and practice of psychiatric nursing* [10th ed.]. Mosby.)

Help Patients Meet Needs

People are often admitted to supportive environments because the challenges of managing their mental health needs become so demanding that their ability to function independently is severely impaired. Care providers assist inpatient patients in meeting their most basic needs first. Food, shelter, safety, and security are provided. Socialization needs are met during therapy and interactions with staff and other patients. Treatment plans provide opportunities for satisfying self-esteem needs through vocational training.

Teach Psychosocial (Adaptive) Skills

People use behaviours that tend to work. When actions result in success, behaviours are more likely to be repeated, regardless of whether or not they are socially acceptable. Admission to an inpatient therapeutic treatment environment gives people with maladaptive actions the opportunity to learn more acceptable ways of behaving. With the help of the treatment team, patients can learn to replace their usual ways of behaving with more effective and adaptive actions.

TABLE 12.1   Mental Health Challenges and Interventions Associated With Food

Challenge	Nursing Intervention
Patient believes food is poisoned or tainted.	Serve each food item in single-serving, disposable containers. Allow patient to casually observe other people eating same food items.
Patient has no interest in food or eating.	Serve meals at regular intervals. Leave food within easy reach of the patient. Offer frequent snacks. Use aromas of certain foods to encourage patient to eat.
Patient uses food as an emotional substitute.	Provide opportunities for interaction with people who do not relate to eating. Work with patient to discover which needs are being met through use of food.

THE THERAPEUTIC ENVIRONMENT AND PATIENT NEEDS

Maslow's theory of a hierarchy of needs (see Chapter 5, Fig. 5.1) states that if a basic physical need goes unmet, it will be fulfilled before other, higher-level needs. People who are experiencing mental and emotional troubles frequently are unable to obtain even the most basic of life's requirements.

We all feel hunger and thirst, but the person with a mental illness may not be able to recognize or act on the body's signals. Sometimes that person's reality makes no provisions for the care of the body. For example, some people may believe that it is inappropriate to eat or practise good hygiene, some do not care about the condition of their bodies, and others are just not aware of their bodies. The therapeutic environment offers a constructive setting for people to learn how to meet their own needs, as well as the support and encouragement to practise effective physical care behaviours.

Remember that a change in one area of functioning will bring about a response within the whole person. Therefore, assisting patients in satisfying their more basic needs prepares the way for changes in other areas of life. Using Maslow's hierarchy as a guide, consider how the therapeutic environment relates to meeting human needs.

Physiological Needs

The first and most basic need is to *breathe*. Breathing enables us to exchange oxygen and carbon dioxide to maintain homeostasis.

The second basic need is for *nourishment*. Many patients have had little to eat before admission and welcome the opportunity to receive wholesome food and clean drinking water. Others may require special diets because of their medical conditions or medications. Some medications have adverse effects that alter the ability to taste foods. Changes in

appetite can also occur. Frequently, patients who are experiencing hallucinations or paranoid (suspicious) thoughts will refuse to eat or drink for fear of being poisoned, drugged, or controlled.

> **! MEDICATION ALERT**
>
> Remember that patients who are taking monoamine oxidase inhibitors (MAOIs) are not allowed to eat certain meats (bologna, liver), dairy products (aged cheeses, sour cream, yogourt), vegetables (fava beans, avocados), fruits (bananas, figs), and alcoholic beverages (beer, ale, red wines, sherry). Patients should not eat chocolate and should avoid taking in caffeine in large amounts.
>
> Monitor patients' food and fluid intake daily. Also routinely monitor vital signs, especially pulse and blood pressure. Report any complaints of chest tightness, stiff neck, or throbbing headache to the physician immediately because these symptoms may herald the onset of hypertensive crisis.

The act of eating and sharing food is a social event in many cultures. Numerous customs have evolved around obtaining, preparing, and consuming food and drink. Learn about patients' perceptions associated with food. How does the cultural background influence the foods they consume? What are their food preferences? How do their mental health issues involve food? Are they bothered by eating in front of others, especially strangers? Assessing patient behaviours associated with food enables care providers to intervene at a basic level, prevent further problems, and evaluate the effectiveness of therapeutic actions. Table 12.1 lists several patient issues and therapeutic actions related to food.

Hygiene needs are important in the therapeutic environment. Patients are frequently admitted in various states of cleanliness, ranging from obsessively tidy to extreme neglect. People who are experiencing acute episodes of schizophrenia, for example, seldom relate to their state of hygiene. Some individuals will dress inappropriately, putting on several shirts at one time or wearing undergarments over their clothing.

Encourage good hygiene habits. Discover whether the patient has a preference or ritual for bathing or dressing. Compliment patients on their appearance when efforts are made. Good hygiene practices help fill more than one basic physical need; they also communicate a willingness for social contact.

The *physical surroundings* of the therapeutic environment are important. Today the architecture of the old asylum has been replaced by environments that include provisions for personal space and privacy. Physical properties of an environment have an effect on the people who live within that space. The physical properties of a therapeutic environment include temperature, lighting, sound, cleanliness, and aesthetics. Care providers are responsible for monitoring how each aspect of the physical environment affects patients.

The *temperature, air circulation,* and *humidity* of the unit all have an effect on patients. People respond in highly individual ways. For example, an agitated or hyperactive

TABLE 12.2	**A "Sound" Exercise**
Action	**Evaluation**
Listen to a short composition of classical music.	Record your feelings as soon as the piece is finished.
Listen to a hard rock musical selection.	Record your feelings as soon as the piece is finished.
Compare your immediate feelings associated with both musical selections.	Does one composition make you feel more excited, calmer? How do you think different types of music affect your mental health patients?

individual may find the environmental temperature too high and react by becoming even more distressed. Hot days and high humidity can increase aggression or make patients lethargic. People who are depressed and hypoactive may be more adversely affected by cooler temperatures. Care providers must be aware that the environmental temperatures and humidity levels have an impact on behaviour. The daily assessment of the therapeutic environment should include temperature and humidity.

Next, the environment's *lighting* must be assessed. This assessment includes the amount of light, its diffusion, and the reflection of light waves off environmental surfaces, combined with the impact of surface colours (Haber, McMahon, & Krainovich-Miller, 1997). Lighting should be constant and of the right intensity. Flickering lights can trigger delusions or hallucinations, whereas lighting that is too bright can result in overstimulation and aggressive behaviours. Lighting that is too low can present inaccurate stimuli, resulting in misperceptions of actual objects. For example, particularly for those who experience hallucinations, it becomes easier to perceive an animal where a chair is located when the room's lighting distorts environmental cues. Sunlight has an increased effect on patients who are receiving certain psychotherapeutic medications. While outdoors, patients must protect themselves from the sun by wearing protective clothing, sunscreen lotion, and a large-brimmed hat. They may also need extra fluids.

Some patients experience hypersensitivity to *colour*, especially if they are confused, agitated, or hyperactive. Colours are very symbolic. Bright colours are stimulating, whereas dark colours are depressing. Neutral colours tend to calm emotions and behaviours. Certain colours hold meaning for some patients. Care providers should assess the effects of colour and lighting for each patient and observe patient behaviours in various settings.

The acoustical or *sound* environment is composed of noises generated by people and equipment. Walls, floors, and objects within the environment have sound-absorbing or acoustical qualities. Floors with carpeting, for example, absorb sound waves and quiet the environment, whereas hard tile floors tend to magnify sounds. Upholstered furniture absorbs more sound than does wooden or plastic furniture.

Environmental noise can have a calming or agitating effect on patients. High noise levels can lead to distorted perceptions, altered thinking, and sensory overload. High noise levels in inpatient environments are common and result in "negative physical effects because of increased physiological stress on the body. Excessive sound also interferes with cognitive functioning" (Holmberg, 1999). Calm music, the sound of ocean waves, or a light rain can produce relaxation.

People experiencing mental illness are commonly hypersensitive to sounds. When noise levels become too intense, patients tend to become overstimulated, which can lead to distraction and agitation. This does not imply, however, that each staff member must walk around in silence, but it should alert one to the important role that sound plays in the therapeutic environment (Table 12.2).

Hygiene associated with the environment refers to the state of *cleanliness* of the physical space and the objects within it. Because many patients live close to one another, the likelihood of infection is increased. The stresses of mental illness can also decrease resistance to infection. In addition, the potential for nuisances such as mice, cockroaches, and other vermin is increased if the physical surroundings are not kept clean.

People experiencing mental or emotional difficulties can have little regard for the cleanliness of their surroundings. Sometimes people with lice, scabies, or crabs are admitted to the therapeutic environment, and if these problems are allowed to continue unchecked, every patient within the area will require treatment. Nurses and direct care providers need to assess the state of the unit's cleanliness on a daily basis. Patients should be protected from communicable health problems. Small assessments today prevent large problems from developing tomorrow.

Last is the issue of *aesthetics*. Does the environment make one want to stay and relax or leave quickly? Is the space pleasing to the eye? The condition of the furniture and other objects within a setting leaves people with a certain impression. An environment that is orderly and in good condition sends a message of caring and pride. The careful use of colour and texture can also produce an environment that communicates a sense of hospitality and belonging.

It is important for health care providers to remember that we go home every night to our own homes. Patients who are living within the therapeutic setting do not. They are there 24 hours of every day. If you were in this situation, you would appreciate the efforts of others to make the physical environment as pleasant as possible.

Safety and Security Needs

The safety and security of the therapeutic environment are the most important factors in mental health care. Safety and security needs within the therapeutic environment include the feeling of physical safety, the security of a limited setting, and the ability to feel secure with others. For patients who are depressed or suicidal, the therapeutic environment offers special protection from self-harm. Patients with aggressive behaviours are protected from themselves and assured that limits will be placed on their actions.

Safety also includes a freedom from hazards. Objects that have the potential for harm are removed from the environment, and the design of electrical fixtures, doors, and other equipment helps to promote safety. Paging systems with identification codes allow help to be summoned quickly when needed. Often a patient will "act out" or behave impulsively. When this occurs, members of the treatment team set limits on the maladaptive actions and then attempt to identify the feelings that motivated the behaviours.

People also need to feel secure within their environments. The inpatient therapeutic environment provides the comfort of order and organization in the form of a daily routine, a set of rules, schedules, and activities. For many psychiatric patients, knowing what is going to happen tomorrow adds to their sense of security today.

The use of *space* is important in maintaining a therapeutic environment. The design of the building has an influence on how space is used for daily activities. Factors such as the location of the recreation room, medication area, and patients' sleeping areas define how physical space is used. Care providers are also concerned with the concepts of space that relate directly to patient care: territory and distance.

Chapter 4 discusses distance and territory in detail, but the importance of these two concepts to the therapeutic environment is emphasized here. Each person needs personal space with defined boundaries (Goren & Orion, 1994). Mental health patients in an inpatient setting establish a territory that "belongs to them." Usually patients claim their rooms, dressers, and sleeping areas as their own. Every person who works with patients or their environments (e.g., housekeepers) must be aware of potentially invading patients' territories. Behaviours such as knocking or announcing oneself before entering a patient's room demonstrate respect for personal space.

The physical *distance* between people affects patients. People with feelings of suspicion usually feel more comfortable when care providers and others are outside their intimate space. Depressed persons may need touch and physical contact—an excellent opportunity for therapeutic touch. Aggressive patients may interpret the close presence of a care provider as threatening. Touch must be used cautiously as a therapeutic tool and with the patient's best interest in mind. Inappropriate use of touch can lead to charges of sexual harassment and possible litigation (legal proceedings). When patients are observed carefully, it is usually possible to tell which distances are most comfortable for interacting.

Limit setting helps keep the therapeutic environment consistent and predictable. Every human being must function within certain limits established by their culture, social group, and laws. Many patients with mental health challenges have difficulty behaving within these limits. Patients know that care providers will enforce the external controls that keep everyone within the environment safe. Knowing that aggressive actions will be contained fosters a sense of safety and security. Two important therapeutic interventions for setting limits are to reinforce the established structure (rules,

routine) of the therapeutic setting and to be consistent. When the environment is controlled, patients have an opportunity to safely explore their feelings and learn new, more effective behaviours.

CASE STUDY

Ned was admitted 4 days ago and proved to be manipulative and deceptive when interacting with staff and peers. When other patients were involved with therapy or other group activities, Ned would be found lying on his bed, reading comic books. He often offered the excuse that another care provider had given him permission to be in his room. The staff agreed to limit his behaviour by keeping him involved in physical activities. By 10 a.m., Ned was complaining of a headache and wanted to lie down. He pleaded with three different care providers, and they all tried to refocus him into an activity. His request to the fourth staff member was feeble, and by noon he was no longer complaining of a headache.

- What message(s) did the staff's behaviour toward Ned send?
- How did Ned react to the situation?

The concept of *time* is impaired for many psychiatric patients. This causes various degrees of disorientation and insecurity about the environment. The perception of the passage of time may be altered, and time may pass very quickly or too slowly. Some individuals do not pay attention to time. As a result, patients have problems with appointments, scheduled events, and tasks—anything that involves the concept of time (Table 12.3). Interventions focus on routinely orienting patients to time with clocks, written schedules, and diaries.

Love and Belonging Needs

The fact that a person is struggling with a mental health challenge does not dismiss the need to be accepted and find one's place within a group. Life in the community can be a lonely existence when there are no friends, few acquaintances, and fewer resources. The isolation of mental illness is intense. Sometimes, the lack of human contact, combined with an existing psychiatric problem and the roadblocks created by stigma, overwhelms the individual and results in more intense or frequent psychotic episodes. The therapeutic environment offers patients many opportunities to appropriately meet their needs for companionship and group identification. Patients' love and belonging needs are fulfilled within the therapeutic setting through exposure to communication, social interactions, and relationships.

Communication takes place on several levels, and not all aspects of every communication are obvious. In the inpatient setting, patients are respected as individuals who have the right to express themselves, as long as their behaviours are appropriate. Care providers communicate respect by encouraging patients to interact. Through caring, sensitive communications, and interest in each person, care providers help their patients fulfill their needs for human companionship.

TABLE 12.3 Examples of Impaired Time Concepts

Disorder	Change in Concept of Time
Organic mental disorders (Alzheimer's disease and others)	Difficulty understanding passage of time. *Example:* Patients ask frequently about date, day, schedules. Patients think they were just admitted when they have been there for several days. Patients are poor historians.
Substance abuse Hallucinogenics	Time passes quickly, space is smaller. *Example:* Patients arrive early, write larger than usual.
Tranquilizers	Time passes slowly, space is larger. *Example:* Patients arrive late, writing is small, cramped. Patients tend to ignore past, focus on present, and are unrealistic about the future.
Depression	Time passes slowly. Patients tend to focus on the past, ignore the present, and show little interest in the future.

Needs for love and belonging are also met through the social group to which one belongs. Whenever people are together, they tend to form groups. Patients with mental health challenges are no different in this respect. Patients will attempt to form relationships with others. Activities as simple as walking together to an appointment can help patients meet their belonging needs.

Social relationships can contribute greatly to meeting patients' needs for belonging, but the potential for abuse does exist. Care providers need to be alert to the social relationships that form among patients within the therapeutic environment. They must observe, monitor, and evaluate the appropriateness of certain relationships and discuss their concerns with the treatment team. Social relationships within the therapeutic environment have the same potential for positive or negative outcomes as any other relationship, and patients can become too dependent on other patients for social support. Many inpatient units have visiting regulations for patients after they are discharged. Care providers must protect the more vulnerable and easily led patients from becoming dependent or being taken advantage of by more aggressive or manipulative people. The initiation of an intimate or sexual relationship in an inpatient setting can serve as a distraction to a patient's recovery.

The care provider–patient relationship is another major tool for meeting patients' needs for love and belonging. All members of the treatment team interact therapeutically with patients, but direct care providers assist patients with the activities of daily living. They are in the special position of always being there, demonstrating consistency, reliability, and acceptance. It is the energy exchange of the therapeutic relationship that helps patients move from the overwhelming aspect of their illness to the dependency of the therapeutic environment and then to the independence of autonomy.

Self-Esteem Needs

Respect, esteem, and recognition must be granted first to oneself. Self-respect, self-esteem, and self-recognition must be realized first. You must love and respect yourself before others can love and respect you. In the therapeutic setting, care providers assist patients in meeting self-esteem needs through acceptance, expectations, and involvement.

Acceptance, in the mental health context, means that care providers acknowledge patients as human beings worthy of respect and dignity. Although patients may behave in maladaptive or unacceptable ways, they are still worthy of respect. It is very important to *separate the behaviour from the person.* As a care provider you may not approve of the patient's actions, behaviours, or attitudes, but you do accept the person. If a patient is to be corrected or reminded, focus on the behaviour rather than on the person. For example, the statement "I have trouble following your thoughts when you speak so loudly" communicates more acceptance than "Stop yelling." Correcting or refocusing the behaviour instead of the person spares self-esteem.

Expectations play a role in the development of patients' abilities to meet self-esteem needs. When care providers communicate what is expected, patients commonly meet those expectations. This can work both ways. There is a valuable lesson here: do not limit patients with your own expectations. Assume that they will succeed, but keep observations and assessments based in reality. You may be surprised at what patients are capable of achieving.

Patients also need involvement to meet their self-esteem needs. **Involvement** is the process of actively interacting with the environment and those persons within it. When patients are involved, they are actively sharing. These experiences foster ego strength and feelings of worth and importance. Involvement also offers opportunities to modify ineffective behaviours and try out new ones. Therapeutic settings that focus on patient involvement exhibit cooperation, compromise, and therapeutic confrontation to bring about behavioural control, effective social interactions, and a sense of self-worth in each patient.

Self-Actualization Needs

The need to achieve one's full potential lies within all of us. However, not all people will become self-actualized. Remember Maslow's basic point: lower-order needs must be fulfilled first before the person can take steps to meet higher-order needs. Consequently, people who cannot meet their basic physical needs will have little success in addressing self-esteem or self-actualization needs.

As patients in the therapeutic environment begin to stabilize, they become better able to cope. With the treatment team's assistance, new ways of behaving are developed and tried. The process of trying and of becoming actively engaged leads patients in the direction of self-actualization. Living up to one's full potential means being the best one can be. People living with mental–emotional challenges deserve the opportunity to strive for this goal no less than the rest of us.

VARIABLES OF THE THERAPEUTIC ENVIRONMENT

Psychiatric hospitalization is a traumatic experience for most patients. Before admission, people often experience intense discomfort with the activities and details of their lives. Individuals who are being admitted for the first time report a sense of panic and lack of control over their situation. Those patients who are facing readmission often express a sense of failure and worthlessness (Joseph-Kinzelman, Taynor, Rubin, et al., 1994). Health care providers can do much to relieve the discomforts that patients face. The mental health treatment team develops the therapeutic treatment plan, and each member has a special role in caring for the patient. However, every staff member assists patients with the activities of daily living and monitors each step made toward the treatment goals.

Admission and Discharge

The process of admitting a patient to a health care facility is straightforward. However, when patients are admitted to a psychiatric setting, their emotional state plays a large role in the actual admission process. Care providers try to explain the rules, routines, and rituals of the unit, but patients are usually too anxious to understand or remember anything in detail. They are then expected to follow the rules and engage in the appropriate activities, even though the memory of the first few days at the facility is absent or blurred.

People with high anxiety levels seldom remember what was said, especially when they are in an unfamiliar setting. Therefore, it is important to approach patients in a calm and respectful manner. Give simple but clear explanations, and patiently repeat them as necessary. Provide simple, written instructions that allow patients to read about the rules after their anxiety decreases. Answer any questions the patient may have. Make sure that the patient is more important than the admission form you must complete. Take the time to behaviourally communicate that you are concerned for their welfare. Make efforts to support the patient in becoming familiar with the therapeutic environment.

Most inpatient facilities have an established procedure for admitting patients and standard forms for data collection (see Chapter 9). During the admission process a person may be interviewed by several members of the treatment team, with all of them asking the same questions. This situation causes unnecessary anxiety for patients and is a poor use of therapist time. Having one person perform the initial admission interview prevents confusion and added stress for the patient. Once the patient is emotionally stabilized, additional information can be obtained. The admission process establishes the tone for the patient's entire stay. This experience with the therapeutic environment often leaves long-lasting impressions.

The process of preparing for discharge begins on admission. The length of stay for mental health patients has decreased dramatically. Because of this, discharge planning has assumed an important role in treatment as the bridge from the sheltered therapeutic environment to the reality of life in the community. Little research has been done to discover how well patients reintegrate into their communities. Care providers are in an excellent position to assist patients in applying the new behaviours learned within the therapeutic setting to the less predictable world of the community.

By the time most patients are ready for discharge, they are actively participating in their treatment program. Decisions about housing, employment, treatment, and management of their mental health challenges are made with the treatment team's assistance. A multidisciplinary discharge care plan is developed. Appropriate referrals to various agencies are arranged, and follow-up care in the community is planned. Patients are assigned a case manager to work with them after discharge.

Returning to the community is a hopeful but demanding time. The support of the treatment team, as well as family and friends, helps to ease the transition. As one researcher has stated, the mentally ill "have no formal ceremonies to transform them back to 'normal' status" (Herman, 1993). The activities of the treatment team are vital in reinforcing and strengthening patients' adaptive abilities throughout the discharge process.

Adherence

Patients who follow prescribed treatments are said to be "in adherence." The term **nonadherence** refers to not cooperating with the treatment plan. Assisting patients to adhere to treatment can be care providers' biggest challenge, especially when working with troubled people. Estimates indicate that "40% to 80% of all patients don't comply with their prescribed therapeutic course" (Wichowski & Kubsch, 1995). To improve patients' adherence, care providers must understand the reasons for patients' unwillingness to follow the treatment plan (Table 12.4).

TABLE 12.4	Reasons for Nonadherence
Problem	**Intervention**
Lack of One or More:	
Understanding	Education, support
Finances to pay for treatment	Refer to social services
Access to treatment services	Refer to social services
Support from family and significant others	Involve family, support groups
Ability to understand or follow treatment plan	Education, involve family
Patient Suffering From:	
Physical adverse effects	Refer to physician; monitor patient's response to medication
Mental–emotional side effects	Communication, therapy, support

A complete assessment of patients, their daily activities, their attitudes toward treatment, and their coping resources will help to identify the overt (outward) causes of nonadherence. However, many times the reasons for nonadherence lie within patients' negative attitudes toward treatment and recovery. Alert care providers can help their patients recognize and change many self-defeating attitudes that bind them to their problems.

Challenging patients to expect more from themselves is one technique for increasing adherence. Helping patients to remove self-imposed boundaries offers them the hope that improvement is possible and attainable. Other techniques involve using a positive outlook and redirecting negative attitudes into more constructive ones. A genuine concern for patients is a powerful tool. These techniques are designed to help patients improve their outlook on life. When one believes that success is attainable, it becomes easier to adhere to the therapies and medications prescribed in the plan of care. Sample Patient Care Plan 12.1 offers some specific interventions to improve adherence.

SAMPLE PATIENT CARE PLAN 12.1   Nonadherence

Assessment

History Tom is a 24-year-old man with a history of paranoid schizophrenia and several admissions to the unit. After his last discharge, he refused to take his medications or seek follow-up therapy and, consequently, began to hallucinate and behave inappropriately. He is being admitted today to adjust his medications and devise a plan of treatment.

Current Findings A dishevelled young adult who refuses to eat or drink because people "are trying to poison my brain."

Multidisciplinary Diagnosis	Planning/Goals
Nonadherence related to suspiciousness	Tom will eat three meals per day by June 22.

THERAPEUTIC INTERVENTIONS

Interventions	Rationale	Team Member
1. Offer prepackaged foods every 3 hours while awake.	Tom may think there is less likelihood that food is poisoned	Nsg, Diet
2. Monitor food and fluid intake.	Prevents malnutrition and dehydration; to find which foods and fluids Tom is willing to consume	Nsg
3. Offer fluids (prepackaged) every 2 hours.	Prevents fluid imbalance; to gain trust	Nsg, Diet
4. Leave snacks within reach.	Tom may eat when he thinks that he is not being watched	Nsg, Diet
5. Allow Tom to see what other patients are eating and drinking.	Helps lessen suspiciousness	Nsg

Evaluation By the fifth day of hospitalization, Tom was drinking 1 000 mL of prepackaged liquids. He was still refusing to eat but would occasionally take a bite of bread if someone else started eating bread from the same source first.

Critical Thinking Question
1. How can care providers structure (change) the environment to encourage Tom to eat solid food?

A complete patient care plan includes several other diagnoses and interventions.
Diet, dietitian; *Nsg*, nursing staff.

KEY POINTS

- The therapeutic milieu is an environment that is structured to assist patients in controlling inappropriate behaviours and learning effective coping skills.
- Therapeutic environments provide services for people experiencing crises, acute mental or emotional challenges, and chronic mental illnesses.
- The basic goals of a therapeutic environment are to protect the patient and others during periods of maladaptive behaviours, help individuals develop self-worth and confidence, and teach more effective adaptive skills.
- The physical properties of a therapeutic environment should be assessed daily; these include temperature, lighting, sound, cleanliness, and aesthetics.
- Setting limits allows the therapeutic environment to be consistent and predictable; patients know that external controls will be enforced.
- Patients' needs for love and belonging are fulfilled within the therapeutic setting through communication, social interactions, and care provider–patient relationships.
- In the therapeutic setting, care providers assist patients in meeting their self-esteem needs through practising acceptance, setting expectations, and showing involvement.
- When care providers communicate what is expected, patients usually live up to those expectations.
- To improve patients' adherence to treatment, care providers need to understand the reasons for patients' unwillingness

to follow the treatment plan; perform a complete assessment; challenge patients' expectations; help remove self-imposed boundaries; offer a positive outlook; redirect negative behaviours or attitudes into more constructive ones; and offer genuine concern.

- Discharge planning is the bridge from the sheltered therapeutic environment to life in the community.
- An important responsibility of the inpatient staff is to educate and encourage patients to play an active and responsible role in their own care.

ADDITIONAL LEARNING RESOURCES

Go to your Evolve website (http://evolve.elsevier.com/Canada/Morrison-Valfre/) for additional online resources, including the online Study Guide for additional learning activities to help you master this chapter content.

CRITICAL THINKING QUESTIONS

1. How does maintaining consistency contribute to a therapeutic milieu for patients?
2. During the night shift, several staff members are being loud at the nurses' station of an inpatient mental health unit. The nurse asks them to "hold down the noise." Why is it important to address excessive noise in a therapeutic milieu?
3. We often hear that plans for patient discharge begin on admission. What is meant by this, and how does this concept support a therapeutic milieu?

REFERENCES

Breggin, P. R. (1991). *Toxic psychiatry*. St. Martin's Press [Seminal Reference].

Cohen, L. J. (1994). Psychiatric hospitalization as experience of trauma. *Archives of Psychiatric Nursing, 8*(2), 78–81 [Seminal Reference].

Goren, S., & Orion, R. (1994). Space and sanity. *Archives of Psychiatric Nursing, 8*(4), 237–244 [Seminal Reference].

Haber, J., McMahon, A. L., & Krainovich-Miller, B. (1997). *Comprehensive psychiatric nursing* (5th ed.). Mosby.

Herman, N. J. (1993). Return to sender: Reintegrative stigma-management strategies of ex-psychiatric patients. *Journal of Contemporary Ethnography, 22*(3), 295–330 [Seminal Reference].

Holmberg, S. K. (1999). Ambient sound levels in a state psychiatric hospital. *Archives of Psychiatric Nursing, 13*(3), 117–126 [Seminal Reference].

Jones, M. (1953). *The therapeutic community*. Basic Books [Seminal Reference].

Joseph-Kinzelman, A., Taynor, J., Rubin, W. V., et al. (1994). Clients' perceptions of involuntary hospitalization. *Journal of Psychosocial Nursing and Mental Health Services, 32*(6), 28–32 [Seminal Reference].

Stuart, G. W. (2013). *Principles and practice of psychiatric nursing* (10th ed.). Mosby.

Wichowski, H. C., & Kubsch, S. (1995). Improving your patient's compliance. *Nursing 95, 25*(1), 66–69 [Seminal Reference]. https://journals.lww.com/nursing/Citation/1995/01000/IMPROVING_YOUR_PATIENTS_S_.29.aspx

Mental Health Challenges
Across the Lifespan

13

Challenges of Childhood

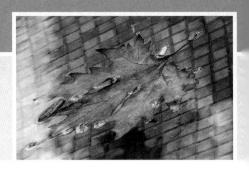

OBJECTIVES

Upon completion of this chapter, the student will be able to:

1. Identify three common challenges of childhood and list two therapeutic interventions for each.
2. Describe the effects of homelessness, abuse, and neglect on children.
3. Identify two therapeutic interventions for the child with anxiety.
4. Name four behaviours that are seen in children with attention-deficit/hyperactivity disorder.
5. Explain the importance of early diagnosis of disruptive behavioural (conduct) disorders.
6. State three therapeutic actions for children with intellectual delay.
7. Identify three types of learning disorders.
8. Describe the behaviours seen in children with pervasive developmental disorders.
9. List three general interventions for children with mental health challenges.

OUTLINE

KEY TERMS

abuse (ə-BŪS) (p. 147)
anxiety (ăng-ZĪ-ĭ-tē) (p. 158)
attention-deficit/hyperactivity disorder (ADHD) (p. 150)
autism (AW-tĭzm) (p. 154)
bullying (p. 150)
cephalocaudal (SĔF-ă-lō-KAW-dəl) (p. 143)
communication (kŏ-MŪ-nĭ-CĀ-shŭn) disorders (p. 154)
conduct disorders (kŏn-DŬKT DĬS-ŏr-dĕrz) (p. 151)
development (dəˈveləpmənt) (p. 143)
dyslexia (dĭs-LĔK-sē-ə) (p. 153)
encopresis (ĕn-kō-PRĒ-sĭs) (p. 153)
enuresis (ĕn-ū-RĒ-sĭs) (p. 152)
growth (GRŌTH) (p. 143)
intellectual development disorder (p. 153)

learning (LĔR-nēng) disorder (p. 153)
neglect (nĭ-glĕkt) (p. 147)
pervasive developmental (pŭr-VĀ-sĭv dĕ-vĕl-ŭp-MĒN-tăl) disorders (p. 154)
pica (PĪ-k ă) (p. 152)
post-traumatic stress (PŌST-trĂ-mĂ-tĬc strĕs) disorder (PTSD) (p. 149)
proximal-distal (PRŎK-sĭ-məl DĬS təl) (p. 143)
rumination disorder (p. 152)
schizophrenia (SKĬ-sō-FRĒ-nē-ə) (p. 155)
sensitive period (p. 143)
somatoform (sō-MĂT-ō-form) disorder (p. 149)
victimization (VĬK-tĭ-mī-ZĀ-shən) (p. 147)

TABLE 13.1 Theories of Childhood Growth and Development

Theory	Explanation
Freud—psychosexual development	Individuals grow and develop by taming their primitive libidinal (sexual, pleasurable) energies as they move through the stages of childhood.
Piaget—intellectual (cognitive) development	Growth is the ability to organize and integrate experiences.
Erikson—psychosocial development	Each person has a core task or problem that must be resolved before they can successfully move on to the next stage.

From Hockenberry, M. J., & Wilson, D. (Eds.). (2010). *Wong's nursing care of infants and children* (9th ed.). Mosby.

Growth and development are a vital part of life. We are all involved in a lifelong process of learning and mastering life's tasks. Children grow with great speed and constantly changing mental, social, and emotional abilities. Each child develops at an individual rate and may master the skills in one area of development while lagging in another. Behaviours considered normal in one age group become worrisome when they occur at another age. Health care providers who work with children must have an understanding of normal growth and development, as well as an awareness of each child's individual pace.

This chapter presents an overview of developmental patterns considered normal for children, the mental health challenges that can arise during childhood, and therapeutic actions for the care of mentally, emotionally, and developmentally troubled children.

Many theories about the growth and development of children exist. Table 13.1 lists the most common theories of childhood development. Chapter 5 provides a more thorough explanation of each theory.

Maslow's hierarchy of needs (see Fig. 5.1), although not a developmental theory, is also important to consider when working with children. Basically, Maslow states that a child's most basic physical needs (air, water, food, elimination, sleep) must be met before higher-level needs (e.g., security, love, belonging, esteem) are considered. Children must master skills that move them from complete dependence to independent functioning in only a few short years. Health care providers have a responsibility to nurture and foster the development of our youngest patients—children.

NORMAL CHILDHOOD DEVELOPMENT

Growth is the increase in physical size. It is measured in kilograms or centimetres. **Development** refers to the increased ability in skills or functions. Although each child moves at an individual pace, all follow organized and orderly patterns throughout the growth process. Children grow in a **cephalocaudal** direction, where growth occurs from head to toe. Infants learn to control head movements before those of the trunk and arms. Growth also occurs in a **proximal-distal** (near-far) pattern. For example, the child's central nervous system develops before the peripheral nervous system. Last, growth moves from simple to complex (*differentiation*). Children learn to control the body's large muscle groups, such as walking, before mastering the fine motor skills of writing or building.

Growth is a continuing process. Recognizing the general patterns and principles of growth and development allows us to accurately assess, assist, and guide young patients (Box 13.1).

Development is the result of growth, learning, and the ability to combine the two. Development proceeds from simple to complex, from gross to fine, and from large to small. To illustrate, a child's reasoning is simple and uncomplicated until the nervous system develops the more complex organization required for abstract thinking. Children with growth or learning problems often mature later than other children.

Social and emotional development also moves from simple to complex. Younger children have simpler emotions and communication abilities. Emotional development is an ongoing process. During each stage, the child must learn to solve a central problem or task, which lays the basis for the next stage of development. If the child is unable to cope with the task or central problem, then mental health difficulties may arise (Table 13.2).

The process of growth includes **sensitive periods**—certain times in which children are more affected by influences (positive or negative) within the environment. For example, according to the developmental psychologist Erik Erikson, without a consistent adult caregiver during infancy, the child could develop problems trusting other people. Without nurturing, a child is ripe for developing mental health challenges that may last a lifetime. Children who were raised in institutional settings often have difficulties bonding with significant others as adults. Nurses and other care providers often provide the only consistency in these children's young lives.

Common Behavioural Challenges of Childhood

Children may experience challenges during each developmental stage. The most common behavioural difficulties during the early years of childhood are colic, problems with feeding and sleeping, temper tantrums, and breath-holding spells.

Colic is a set of behaviours most commonly seen in middle-class infants. Severe periods of late-afternoon crying begin when the infant is about 2 weeks old. The infant cries with clenched fists and pained looks and refuses attempts to soothe them. Behaviours usually peak around 2 or 3 months, but they can persist until the infant is 4 or 5 months old. A *colicky infant* is defined as a healthy and well-fed child who cries for more than 3 hours every day for more than 3 weeks (Hockenberry & Wilson, 2014). Interventions designed to calm both the parents and child appear to help. Teach parents to manage colic by helping them learn about the normal characteristics of crying and recognize their infant's cues. Changing feeding procedures and allowing adequate time

BOX 13.1   Developmental Periods

Prenatal Period: Conception to Birth
Germinal: Conception to approximately 2 weeks
Embryonic: 2 to 8 weeks
Fetal: 8 to 40 weeks (birth)

A rapid growth rate and total dependency make this one of the most crucial periods in the developmental process. Adequate prenatal care is extremely important for a healthy child.

Infancy Period: Birth to 12 Months
Newborn: Birth to 28 days
Infancy: 1 to approximately 12 months

The infancy period is one of rapid motor, cognitive, and social development. Through bonding with the caregiver (parent), the infant establishes a basic trust in the world and the foundation for future interpersonal relationships. The critical first month of life is filled with major physical adjustments to life outside the womb and psychological adjustment of the parents.

Early Childhood: 1 to 6 Years
Toddler: 1 to 3 years
Preschool: 3 to 6 years

This period, which extends from the time the child attains upright locomotion until they enter school, is characterized by intense activity and discovery. It is a time of marked physical and personality development. Motor development advances steadily. Children acquire language and social relationships, learn role standards, gain self-control, develop increasing awareness of dependence and independence, and begin to develop a self-concept.

Middle Childhood: 6 to 10 Years
Frequently referred to as the "school age," this period is one in which the child is directed away from the family group and is centred on the wider world of peer relationships. There is steady advancement in physical, mental, and social development, with emphasis on developing skill competencies. Social cooperation and moral development take on more importance. This is a critical period in the development of a self-concept, as peers' and teachers' evaluations become part of the child's self-assessments.

Later Childhood: 10 to 19 Years
Prepubertal: 10 to 13 years
Adolescence: 13 to approximately 19 years

The period of rapid maturation and change known as adolescence is considered to be a transitional period that begins at the onset of puberty and extends to the point of entry into the adult world. Biological and personality maturation are accompanied by physical and emotional turmoil, and there is a redefining of self-concept. In the late adolescent period, the child begins to internalize all previously learned values and begins to focus on an individual identity.

---

for burping and cuddling can help control symptoms. Other effective measures include creating a quiet, restful environment, aromatherapy with lavender, and avoiding over handling the infant. Massage can soothe, relax, and calm some infants. Most children outgrow colicky behaviour by age 5 months, but parents need a great deal of emotional support and encouragement during this stressful time.

Feeding disorders range from overeating (which leads to obesity) to undereating (which leads to malnutrition). Approximately 15%, or one in seven children are considered to be obese. Several studies suggest that this number has remained relatively unchanged over a period of more than 10 years, which is encouraging. The impact of sociodemographic factors such as age, sex, socioeconomic status, and place of residence on development and levels of obesity requires further study (Rao, Kropac, Do, et al., 2016). In addition, early intervention and education are needed to prevent the long-term complications that result from childhood obesity.

Infants may not feed if the experience is not satisfying. Young children may refuse to eat if they have had an unpleasant experience with food (being force-fed or choking) or are engaged in a conflict (power play) with caregivers. Physical problems, such as poor oral motor control or swallowing problems, can cause unpleasant experiences with food. Children suffering from depression often refuse to eat, and adolescents may engage in self-destructive behaviours such as anorexia or bulimia.

Problems with sleep are common to many children. They include night terrors, problems falling asleep, and nighttime awakenings. In the past, the usual course of action was for the parents to let children "cry it out" until they fell asleep. Today, each child's sleeping characteristics are assessed and parents' expectations and fears are addressed. Treatments are then designed to assist both the parents and child in establishing restful sleep patterns. Following bedtime rituals, such as reading a book or limiting television viewing, is often helpful. The Canadian Paediatric Society (CPS) recommends no screen media and screen time for children under 2 years of age, and recommends less than 1 hour of total screen time per day for children aged 2–5 years (CPS, 2017).

Temper tantrums are a common expression of anger and frustration for children between 1 and 4 years of age. In fact, temper tantrums occur in 50 to 80% of children in this age group (Hagerman, 2014). In the young child, temper tantrums are seen as normal behaviour. Children are attempting to master their environments and become frustrated when they are unable to achieve control. Temper tantrums are the result of a *loss of control*. Most children feel a blow to their self-image, and some children are quite upset about the experience. Tantrums only become a problem when children use them to express more emotions than just frustration or when they occur so frequently that they disturb family functioning. Adults in the environment should remain calm during the tantrum. Therapeutic interventions for temper tantrums are listed in Box 13.2.

Breath-holding spells rarely occur before 6 months of age and can last until the child is about 5 years of age. Typically,

TABLE 13.2   Emotional Developmental Tasks of Childhood

Stage	Age	Core Task
Infancy	Birth–1 year	Trust vs. mistrust
Early childhood	1–3 years	Autonomy vs. shame and doubt
Preschool years	3–6 years	Initiative vs. guilt
School age	6–12 years	Industry vs. inferiority
Puberty	12–18 years	Identity vs. diffusion

the child becomes frustrated or upset in some way and begins to cry, but no sound emerges. They stop breathing, begin to turn blue, go limp, and become unresponsive. Seizure-like behaviours, in which the child arches the back and jerks uncontrollably, may occur. Fortunately, the spell resolves within 30 to 60 seconds when the child catches their breath and begins to cry or scream. A physician should examine the child after the first episode to rule out any medical problems. Thereafter, the treatment is to not reinforce the breath-holding behaviours. This must be done consistently. After ensuring that the child has not choked on something, parents should ensure that the child is in a safe place and then ignore the behaviours. Behaviours that are not rewarded or reinforced soon fade because they are no longer useful to the child.

Mental Health Challenges of Childhood

Each stage of life flows into the next. In reality, there are no clear divisions in the process of growth and development. Many mental–emotional conditions diagnosed in adulthood find their roots in the experiences of childhood. Health care providers play an important role in the recognition and treatment of children's mental health issues, because without this assistance such problems can follow a person into adulthood and compromise personal well-being. The major mental health challenges of childhood are grouped into eight categories (Table 13.3). Patients may be labelled with one diagnosis yet engage in behaviours that belong to another category. Remember, each child is an individual; the diagnosis is less important than the person.

Many children have "mental health challenges" at some time during the journey from infancy to adulthood. Emotional difficulties arise more frequently during periods of change. The birth of a sibling or moving to a new city can disrupt a routine, create new demands, or make children more vulnerable. Stresses can push children to behave in worrisome ways. Peers can have influences that are not always desirable. How do parents know when their children's problems are a part of the normal process of growing up and when they are serious enough to require professional assistance? When a child demonstrates an *absence of growth,* an inability or *refusal to change,* or a *failure to achieve the developmental tasks* of their age group, mental health assistance should be sought.

BOX 13.2   Interventions for Temper Tantrums

Prevent Tantrums

1. Childproof the environment: Remove anything that the child is not allowed to touch. Fewer restrictions lessen the chances for conflict.
2. Present choices and options: Allow the child to choose (within acceptable limits). Offer the opportunity to practise autonomy and mastery skills.

Control Tantrums

1. When frustration increases, use distraction. Focus the child's attention on calmer activities, and reward positive behaviours.
2. Protect the child during the tantrum. Do not allow a child to hurt themselves or others.
3. Do not abandon the child during the tantrum. Stay close, but do not intrude on their space.
4. Point out to the child that they are out of control. Do not react negatively or try to discipline the child. Praise when control is regained.
5. Fight only those battles that must be won. The conflicts that serve no important purpose should be avoided. However, do not give in to the demands that led to the tantrum.

After the Tantrum

1. Do not hold a grudge or hold on to negative emotions. Recognize that the child probably feels worse than you do.
2. Praise the child for gaining control.
3. Keep reinforcing desired behaviours. Do not overreact to undesirable actions.

Environmental Issues

Many children must cope with more than just developmental tasks. Growing up is a difficult process for children who are poor, homeless, abused, or neglected, as well as for children in foster care. Issues associated with the environment can have a strong impact on mental health. In Canada in 2017, 622 000 children under 18 years of age, or 9%, lived below the poverty line, down from 11% in 2016. The child poverty rate has declined fairly steadily since reaching its most recent peak of 15% in 2010 (Statistics Canada, 2019a).

Homelessness

The lack of a permanent residence (*homelessness*) affects children in many ways (Fig. 13.1). Many studies have revealed that homeless children have very high infant mortality rates, twice the normal incidence of illness and disease, and elevated lead levels in the blood. They also experience hunger; behavioural problems, developmental delays, speech delays, sleep disorders, and immature motor actions; short attention spans, withdrawal, aggression, and return to toddler behaviours; inappropriate social interactions with adults; and immature peer interactions. According to the American Psychological Association (2018), "schooling for homeless children is often interrupted and delayed, with homeless children twice as likely to have a learning disability, repeat a grade, or to be suspended from school." The scenario described in the Case Study on page 147 is unfortunately all too common.

TABLE 13.3 Mental Health Challenges in Childhood

Category	Examples/Symptoms
Anxiety	• Being very afraid when away from parents (separation anxiety) • Having extreme fear about a specific thing or situation, such as dogs, insects, or going to the doctor (phobias) • Being very afraid of school and other places where there are people (social anxiety) • Being very worried about the future and about bad things happening (general anxiety) • Having repeated episodes of sudden, unexpected, intense fear that come with symptoms like heart pounding, having trouble breathing, or feeling dizzy, shaky, or sweaty (panic disorder)
Depression	• Feeling sad, hopeless, or irritable a lot of the time • Not wanting to do or not enjoying doing fun things • Showing changes in eating patterns—eating a lot more or a lot less than usual • Showing changes in sleep patterns—sleeping a lot more or a lot less than normal • Showing changes in energy—being tired and sluggish or tense and restless a lot of the time • Having a hard time paying attention • Feeling worthless, useless, or guilty • Showing self-injury and self-destructive behaviour
Oppositional defiant disorder (ODD)	• Often being angry or losing one's temper • Often arguing with adults or refusing to comply with adults' rules or requests • Often resentful or spiteful • Deliberately annoying others or becoming annoyed with others • Often blaming other people for one's own mistakes or misbehaviour
Conduct disorder (CD)	• Breaking serious rules, such as running away, staying out at night when told not to, or skipping school • Being aggressive in a way that causes harm, such as bullying, fighting, or being cruel to animals • Lying, stealing, or deliberately damaging other people's property
Attention-deficit/hyperactivity disorder (ADHD)	• Daydreaming a lot • Forgetting or losing things a lot • Squirming or fidgeting • Talking too much • Making careless mistakes or taking unnecessary risks • Having a hard time resisting temptation • Having trouble taking turns • Having difficulty getting along with others
Tourette syndrome (TS)	• The main symptoms of TS are tics • Symptoms usually begin when a child is 5 to 10 years of age • The first symptoms often are motor tics that occur in the head and neck area • Tics usually are worse during times that are stressful or exciting; they tend to improve when a person is calm or focused on an activity
Obsessive-compulsive disorder (OCD)	• Having unwanted thoughts, impulses, or images that occur over and over and which cause anxiety or distress • Having to think about or say something over and over (e.g., counting or repeating words over and over silently or out loud) • Having to do something over and over (e.g., handwashing, placing things in a specific order, or checking the same things over and over, like whether a door is locked) • Having to do something over and over according to certain rules that must be followed exactly in order to make an obsession go away
Post-traumatic stress disorder (PTSD)	• Reliving a traumatic event over and over in thought or in play • Having nightmares and sleep problems • Becoming very upset when something causes memories of the event • Experiencing a lack of positive emotions • Intense ongoing fear or sadness • Irritability and angry outbursts • Constantly looking for possible threats, being easily startled • Acting helpless, hopeless, or withdrawn • Denying that the event happened or feeling numb • Avoiding places or people associated with the event

Data from Centers for Disease Control and Prevention (CDC). (2019). *Children's mental disorders.* Retrieved from https://www.cdc.gov/childrensmentalhealth/symptoms.html; American Psychiatric Association (APA). (2013). *Diagnostic and statistical manual of mental disorders* (5th ed.). Author.

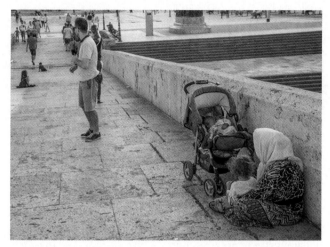

Fig. 13.1 Many of the homeless are young mothers with young children. (iStockphoto/Neil Bussey)

CASE STUDY

Carol had come to us as a very lost, exhausted, young girl, dressed in tattered jeans and with sad, red eyes that seemed to cry every time she opened her mouth to talk to us.

For her first few weeks at Covenant House, we could not really get her to talk about herself—who she was, why she was here, where she came from, how we could help her. The only words she spoke were cried out unconsciously in her nightmares, which crept up on her while she was vulnerable and alone at night, unable to run away.

"You don't want to know about me." "It hurts too much," she would say. "I . . . I can't talk about it."

Finally, one night after another nightmare, her lonely pain became unbearable, and she began to open up. She was born in Winnipeg but ran away because her parents beat her. "They were on drugs," she shrugged. "I guess they couldn't help it," she said. Frightened for her life and unable to stand the abuse any longer, she had run away to the city. Penniless and alone, she soon began to sell the only worldly possession she had—her body.

Then one night she met "him." He was 70, like a grandfather. "He said he would take care of me. I was so alone. And those first few days were great. He gave me everything—money, clothes. He made me feel good. Then he started crawling in bed with me at night . . . and doing terrible things. He began to give me cocaine and stuff to make it easier. He . . . I had no place to go. And then he started to hit me for no reason. I ran away, but I am so afraid he will find me."

- In which behaviours did Carol engage to fulfill her basic needs?
- How do you think Carol can be helped?

Modified from McGeady, M.,R. (1995). *"Does God still love me?" Letters from the street.* Author.

TABLE 13.4	Therapeutic Actions for Patients Who Are Homeless
Topic	**Nursing Actions**
Psychological	Know your own feelings about homeless people. Approach patients with a positive attitude. Greet patients and communicate that they will be treated with care and respect.
Patient interview	Delay asking questions about occupation, address, next of kin, educational level until later in the interview. Promise that information is confidential. Ask simple, concrete questions: Where do you get your money? When did you have your last drink? Relate to homelessness in a matter-of-fact way.
Health assessment	Educate as you assess. Assess children for signs of malnutrition, abuse, or neglect.
Discharge planning	Ask these questions: Do you understand what your problem is? How will you get your prescriptions filled? Where will you sleep tonight? Help patient to keep follow-up appointments. Write down all instructions.

Data from Hunter, J. K. (1992). Making a difference for homeless patients. *RN, 55*(12), 48–54.

Abuse and Neglect

Victimization is the process of causing an individual harm. **Abuse** is defined as causing harm to or maltreating another. **Neglect** is not meeting a child's basic needs for food, clothing, shelter, love, and belonging. Child abuse and neglect are reaching crisis levels in not only Canada; the problems of abuse and neglect are becoming threats to the lives of infants and small children throughout our world.

Studies reveal that 32% of Canadians have experienced some form of abuse before the age of 16 (26% physical abuse, 10% sexual abuse, and 8% exposure to intimate partner violence) (Public Health Agency of Canada [PHAC], 2018; Statistics Canada, 2019b). Of significance, rates of childhood abuse among Indigenous people have now reached 40%. According to the Canadian Incidence Study of Reported Child Abuse and Neglect, types of childhood trauma include exposure to intimate partner violence (34%), neglect (20%), physical abuse (20%), emotional abuse (9%), and sexual abuse (3%) (PHAC, 2010).

The victimization of children comes in many forms. Physical abuse is commonly associated with burns, bruises, fractures, and head and abdominal injuries. Sexually abused children have been violated with inappropriate sexual activities. Emotional or psychological abuse erodes children's self-esteem through rejection, criticism, isolation,

Care providers must learn about the lifestyles of their patients and families. It is important to practise good communication skills and remain nonjudgemental. Table 13.4 offers other special guidelines for care providers who work with homeless patients of all ages.

or terrorism. Children also suffer from neglect, in which their physical, emotional, and medical needs are not met. Childhood abuse and neglect also have long-term effects. Today, a wide variety of behavioural and physical disorders are seen in adulthood, such as chronic anxiety and depression, that are thought to be associated with childhood abuse.

Factors that influence the potential for abuse and neglect include parental characteristics, such as social isolation, teenage motherhood, and difficulty controlling aggressive impulses. Children who are unwanted or disabled are at a higher risk for abuse and neglect. Environments filled with chronic stress may lead to child mistreatment. Researchers have found that family or parental stress is a significant precipitating factor in child maltreatment, especially physical abuse and chronic neglect (Feiring & Zielinski, 2011). By recognizing these problems and referring families to appropriate services, health care providers may prevent abuse and neglect from occurring. Preventing and treating child abuse and neglect are the responsibility of every health care provider, no matter what their training or title. Education is a powerful first step.

Helping the victims of child abuse also requires care providers to look at their own feelings about abuse. Being objective and supportive can be difficult in these situations, but it is vitally important. Health care providers are in positions to recognize abuse and to help provide early intervention. Care providers need to recognize that the problems of our children are the problems of us all.

Every province and territory has child abuse legislation that requires health care providers, such as nurses and doctors, to report witnessed or suspected child abuse or neglect directly to their local child protection agency. To encourage reports of suspected cases, the laws offer legal immunity for the reporter if the report is made in good faith. Health care providers who do not report suspected child abuse or neglect may be held liable for civil or criminal action (Astle, Duggleby, Potter, et al., 2019).

PROBLEMS WITH PARENT–CHILD INTERACTION

A healthy family is able to cope with most of its emotional challenges and knows when to seek help. Every child faces difficult emotional adjustments throughout childhood as change creates many new demands for children and their parents. One of the most common parent–child problems is conflict.

Parent–Child Conflicts

Children require consistent guidance and unconditional acceptance. Relationships with their caregivers serve as a testing ground for learning right from wrong and which behaviours result in reward or punishment. Parents who *set limits* and *enforce them consistently* provide the stability for children to test their limits in healthy ways. Conflicts between children and parents frequently occur and can take the form of verbal arguments or silent power struggles. No child or parent escapes childhood without conflict; however, when conflicts are constant and worsen over time, mental health assistance should be sought.

Primary Caregiver Dysfunction

When a parent is unable to meet the needs of a child, a disturbance in the parent–child interaction exists. The parent is often a person who has had difficult times in the past with personal relationships, psychiatric disorders, or behavioural problems. Perhaps the pregnancy was unwanted, or the child seems unresponsive. In these situations, the child is frequently described by the caretaker as difficult, defective, or disappointing.

The signs and symptoms seen in the child that suggest primary caregiver dysfunction include feeding and sleeping problems, delays in development, failure to thrive, signs of inadequate physical care or abuse, frequent visits to the physician, and excessive parental worry. Treatment focuses on supporting and educating the parents and helping them develop more effective and appropriate childcare skills. With aggressive intervention, the long-term outlook for the children of these parents can improve.

EMOTIONAL CHALLENGES

Emotional challenges may occur in children when they cannot successfully cope with their situations. Such challenges can range from anxiety to severe depression and suicide. Fortunately, most children are able to cope successfully with life's anxieties when they are nurtured and supported. This section focuses on the emotional challenges of children that are most likely to be encountered in everyday treatment settings: anxiety, depression, somatoform disorders, and post-traumatic stress disorders.

Anxiety

Anxiety is a vague, uneasy feeling that occurs in response to a threat. Most children experience fear and anxiety as a part of growing up. One of the most frequent anxieties of infants and toddlers is *separation anxiety,* a fear of being apart from their parents. Eventually, the fear decreases as children broaden their world to include others. However, if a child older than 4 years of age has separation anxieties lasting for more than a few weeks, a problem may exist. Severe levels of anxiety in children may result in obsessive-compulsive behaviour, a condition that is discussed in Chapter 18.

Anxiety-based school refusal, or *school avoidance,* is a behavioural pattern in which the child refuses to attend school. Causes include anxiety or fear of leaving home (separation anxiety). Fear of being ridiculed or embarrassed at school (*social phobia*) or great concern about some aspect of school (*school phobia*) can also result in avoidance behaviours. The main goals of treatment are to help the child identify the source of the anxiety. Then the child is assisted in confronting and overcoming the anxiety so they can return to school. Many times, health care providers work with school personnel and parents to develop a plan for returning the child to school in a supportive manner. Antidepressants may be prescribed for severe symptoms of anxiety or depression.

> ## CRITICAL THINKING
>
> Bullying is becoming a problem in many countries.
>
> In Canada, 47% of Canadian parents report having a child who is a victim of bullying (Canadian Institutes of Health Research [CIHR], 2012). At least one in three adolescent students in Canada have reported being bullied recently (Molcho, Craig, Due, et al., 2009).
>
> In Great Britain, "8 out of 10 children with a learning disability are bullied or scared to go out due to fear of being bullied" (Mencap, n.d.).
>
> A Finnish study revealed that bullying behaviours in childhood predicted antisocial personality, substance abuse, and depressive and anxiety disorders among children who bullied. Victim behaviours "predicted anxiety disorders, and mixed bully–victim status predicted antisocial personality and anxiety disorder" (Sourander, Jenson, Rönning, et al., 2007).
>
> In the United States, studies reveal that "6 out of every 10 students witness bullying in school at least once a day" (National Center for Education Statistics, 2017).

Depression

The number of children being diagnosed with mood disorders such as depression is increasing. The term *depression* describes a symptom, an emotional state, and a clinical syndrome. Depression occurs in children and adolescents, but symptoms often go unnoticed and untreated. Children who have one or more depressed parents are more likely to be depressed themselves. Depression is seen more frequently as children grow older, and it occurs equally in boys and girls.

The clinical findings of depression arise from a persistent state of unhappiness that interferes with pleasure or productivity. Hazel (2002) notes: "Children with depressive disorders lack interest in activities they previously enjoyed, criticize themselves, and are pessimistic or hopeless about the future." School-age children often "act out" their depression by becoming disruptive or failing academically. Older children and adolescents may become withdrawn. The clinical signs and symptoms of depression are discussed in Chapter 21. Treatment is designed to relieve the child's discomforting symptoms and help those in the child's environment to respond to the child's needs. Therapeutic interventions focus on reducing the problems that are causing the depression and providing the child with emotional support to cope effectively.

Somatoform Disorders

A **somatoform disorder** is one in which the afflicted person has the signs or symptoms of illness without a traceable physical cause. The individual does not consciously take on the signs or symptoms, but they truly feel ill. Children often complain of headaches, upset stomachs, or pain.

Somatic symptoms are common in school-age children. Such symptoms are thought to be expressions of stress, anxiety, or underlying conflict. Sometimes the child's signs or symptoms resemble those seen in another family member. In most cases, when the stress is relieved, the child returns to a healthy level of functioning. Somatoform disorders are covered in greater depth in Chapter 22. Here, it is important to remember that children with somatoform disorders need understanding and reassurance.

Post-Traumatic Stress Disorder

When children are repeatedly exposed to or participate in acts of violence, their psyches take steps to emotionally protect them. **Post-traumatic stress disorder** (PTSD) may develop following an extremely traumatic event that involves injury or threat to the child. Examples include experiencing a fire or witnessing a shooting death. The child feels intense helplessness, fear, and horror. In younger children, behaviours become agitated and disorganized. Traumatic events are relived repeatedly, and the child goes to great lengths to avoid anything associated with the trauma. Eventually, the traumatic event becomes generalized into nightmares of monsters or threats to the self. The past is relived through the playing out of events related to the trauma. Somatic complaints, such as an upset stomach and other discomforts, may occur. Treatment focuses on early recognition and emotionally supportive care.

BEHAVIOURAL CHALLENGES

Children experiment with various behaviours to test the limits of their environments and the people within them. Every child goes through periods of misconduct: refusing to do as told, lying, cheating, stealing, or bullying others. Most often, these behaviours decrease with time and consistent guidance. However, we all need to become aware of the influence that everyday violence has on children.

Children and Violence

According to the Canadian Radio-television and Telecommunications Commission (CRTC), Canadian children between the ages of 2 and 11 watch an average of 17.8 hours of television per week (CRTC, 2019). Studies reveal that greater aggressiveness and less sensitivity to others are seen in children who view TV violence. Acts of aggression are common in schools, where children may be bullied or intimidated. Children may witness violence in the home and adopt it as a method for solving problems or resolving conflict.

BOX 13.3   Warning Signs of Violence in Children

Loss of temper on a daily basis
Frequent physical fighting
Vandalism or damage to property
Carries a weapon
Announces threats or plans to hurt others
Use of drugs, alcohol, or both
Enjoys hurting animals
Engages in risk-taking behaviours
Details plans to commit acts of violence

Modified from Hockenberry, M. J., & Wilson, D. (Eds.). (2010). *Wong's nursing care of infants and children* (9th ed.). Mosby.

Young children engage in violent behaviour, but it is often dismissed as just a "phase" the child is going through; however, aggressive behaviour should always be taken seriously. Children can engage in a wide range of aggressive behaviours ranging from explosive temper tantrums to bullying, cruelty, and destruction of property.

Bullying, which is the repeated use of aggressive behaviours to intentionally intimidate another, is very common in schools today. Children who bully others often behave aggressively toward parents, teachers, and other authorities. They tend to have strong self-esteem and little ability to relate to the emotions of others. Bullies use violence, manipulation, and intimidation to achieve control over their victims.

The victims of bullying tend to be smaller, quieter, and more sensitive than their peers. Often they are different, physically or behaviourally. Many have poor self-worth, believing they are stupid, ugly, or unwanted. If allowed to continue, bullying can result in serious academic, behavioural, legal, and social problems for both bullies and their victims.

As behaviours become more difficult to manage, these bullying children clash with friends and classmates. They may develop a reputation for being unruly bullies or, worse yet, dangerous. The American Psychological Association has developed a checklist for the warning signs of violence in children (Box 13.3). Children who demonstrate these behaviours are at risk for engaging in violent behaviours.

When a child's conduct becomes inappropriate over time, a *disruptive behavioural disorder* is usually diagnosed. Sometimes behavioural problems are linked to a physical cause, such as a lack of neurotransmitter production in the brain. The two disruptive behavioural disorders most commonly encountered by nurses are attention-deficit/hyperactivity disorder and conduct disorder.

Children and Electronic Media

The effects of the computer and its resulting social media platforms on children is an important new area of study. Media psychologists are researching the effects of media technologies on the growth and development of children. According to the website *Techaddiction.ca*, the time spent with on-screen media dramatically increases from the toddler to preschool to school-age years. Children under age 2 have a screen time average of 53 minutes per day. This increases to almost 2.5 hours per day among 2- to 4-year-olds and to almost 3 hours per day for children in the 5- to 8-year-old range (Conrad, 2020). Middle-school children now spend more time with their devices than they do with their parents, school, or social activities.

Because children are inexperienced, they have difficulty distinguishing reality from fantasy. They lack the ability to self-regulate, to tell good from harmful. As children grow, they become increasingly influenced by peer pressure. Cyberbullying is a real concern for many children.

Studies are showing that increased, unsupervised exposure to media can result in hyperactivity disorders, stress, anxiety, eating disorders, and impulse control disorders. Children who are exposed to media violence tend to behave in more aggressive ways. Attention spans are decreasing because of increased use of fast-paced media. Physical and social activities are decreased as children spend more time in the digital world. Without guidance from concerned adults, some children will develop mental health issues, and many more are at risk for developing such issues.

Attention-Deficit/Hyperactivity Disorder

Attention-deficit/hyperactivity disorder, commonly called **ADHD**, is now the most commonly diagnosed mental health condition in childhood. It affects approximately 4.8% of Canadian children (Centre for ADHD Awareness Canada; 2020; Waddell, Offord, Shepherd, et al., 2002), and its symptoms can persist into adulthood. ADHD occurs more frequently in boys, with a ratio of about seven boys to one girl. Although ADHD was thought to be primarily a problem of childhood, it is often seen in adolescents and adults. It is a syndrome—a cluster of behaviours relating to inattention and impulsive actions. Within the ADHD category, a variety of subgroups exist: ADHD with learning disabilities, ADHD without hyperactivity, ADHD with speech disorders, ADHD with other psychiatric disorders, and ADHD with disorders of brain function. Box 13.4 lists the diagnostic criteria for ADHD.

There are two common clinical histories for children with ADHD. The first is the child who has been "fussy" or "a difficult child" from birth. As infants, they were difficult to soothe, and they have behaved impulsively as far back as family members can recollect. They are remembered as being "a handful." The second type of child is referred to as an immature child who displays silliness, distractibility (short attention span), restlessness, and clumsiness. Both types of children have problems with self-control, hyperactivity, relating to others, and focusing their attention. On entry into school, children with ADHD have difficulty completing their schoolwork because they are easily distracted. They are usually academic underachievers, although they may have normal or above-average intelligence. They may also have problems making friends because of their excitable

BOX 13.4 Attention-Deficit/Hyperactivity Disorder

A. A disturbance of at least 6 months during which at least eight of the following are present:
1. Often fidgets with hands or feet or squirms in seat (feelings of restlessness in adolescents)
2. Has difficulty remaining seated when required to do so
3. Is easily distracted by outside stimuli
4. Has difficulty awaiting turn in games or group situations
5. Often blurts out answers to questions before they have been completed
6. Has difficulty following through on instructions from others (e.g., fails to finish chores)
7. Has difficulty sustaining attention in tasks or play activities
8. Often shifts from one uncompleted activity to another
9. Has difficulty playing quietly
10. Often talks excessively
11. Often interrupts or intrudes on others (e.g., butts into other children's games)
12. Often does not seem to listen to what is being said to them
13. Often loses things necessary for tasks or activities at school or at home (e.g., toys, pencils, books, assignments)
14. Often engages in physically dangerous activities without considering possible consequences (e.g., runs into street without looking)
B. Onset before age 7 years
C. Does not meet the criteria for a pervasive developmental disorder

! MEDICATION ALERT

Psychotherapeutic medications are powerful chemicals. When these medications are prescribed for children, parents must be taught to routinely monitor for adverse effects, adverse reactions, and interactions with over-the-counter medications, such as cold medications (see Chapter 7). Nurses have an important responsibility to provide parents with written information about the medication(s) the child is receiving, how to monitor the child's response to the medication, and what adverse effects to report. They should be willing to monitor the child throughout the period their child is receiving psychotherapeutic medications.

TABLE 13.5 Medications for Children With ADHD

Medication Examples	Patient Teaching
Long-Acting Stimulants	
lisdexamfetamine (Vyvanse)	Monitor mental status, growth rate
dextroamphetamine (Adderall)	Avoid caffeine, alcohol, OTC drugs
methylphenidate (Ritalin, Concerta, Daytrana (Ritalin patch)	Watch for effects on growth; behaviour deteriorates when medications are stopped abruptly. Watch for skin irritation with patches.
Nonstimulants	
atomoxetine (Strattera)	Take dose in morning, avoid OTC medications
Antidepressants	
imipramine (Tofranil) clomipramine (Anafranil)	May cause dry mouth, blurred vision, constipation, insomnia
chlorpromazine (Thorazine) haloperidol (Haldol)	May cause dry mouth, blurred vision, weight gain, low blood pressure. Report any abnormal muscle and body movements to physician.

ADHD, attention-deficit/hyperactivity disorder; *OTC*, over-the-counter.

and impulsive behaviours. Almost half the children with ADHD show symptoms of anxiety, aggression, depression, and resistance to any authority.

Treatment for children with ADHD requires a multidisciplinary approach. Families are educated about the condition, and many children receive special education. Positive reinforcement programs help children choose more socially appropriate behaviours and reduce impulsive actions. Therapeutic interventions for children with ADHD focus on providing a consistent and structured therapeutic approach. Caregivers must be prepared to set limits on patients' behaviours and then be consistently willing to enforce them. They should also strive to acknowledge and reward the child for appropriate behaviours.

Medication therapies include long- and short-acting stimulants, Strattera (a nonstimulant), and some antidepressants. Antipsychotics may infrequently be prescribed. An alternative medication prescribed by homeopathic practitioners is called Synaptol. Refer to Table 13.5 for a list of commonly used medications for treating ADHD. In cases where the child is receiving any drug therapy, care providers must carefully monitor the child's response to the medications.

Disruptive Behavioural (Conduct) Disorder

Misconduct is common in every child, but when a persistent pattern of unacceptable behaviours is present, a conduct or disruptive behavioural disorder is established. Children with **conduct disorders** are defiant of authority. They engage in aggressive actions toward other people, refuse to follow society's rules and norms, and violate the rights of others. Many come from broken homes and backgrounds of violence, drug abuse, alcoholism, poverty, and lack of consistent caregivers.

The typical picture of a child with a conduct disorder is a boy with social and academic problems, truancy, and failure in school. He is defiant to authority and often engages in temper tantrums, running away, and fighting. Treatment focuses on providing a stable environment and consistently enforced limits. Associated neurological, educational, or psychiatric problems are also treated. The long-term outlook for children with conduct disorders is poor if the problems are present before the child is 10 years old or the adults in the environment engage in antisocial behaviours. Nearly half these children grow up to have antisocial or conduct disorders in adulthood. This makes early diagnosis and treatment especially important if these children are to become productive members of society.

Oppositional Defiant Disorder

Oppositional defiant disorder is a recurring pattern of disobedient, hostile behaviour toward authority figures. Children with this disorder frequently lose their temper, argue with adults, deliberately annoy other people, and refuse to compromise. They blame others for their misbehaviour and continually test their limits by arguing, ignoring, or becoming aggressive. Treatment includes family therapy that stresses limit setting and consistency.

CHALLENGES WITH EATING AND ELIMINATION

The most common mental health issues seen in children that relate to eating are feeding disorders, pica, anorexia nervosa, and bulimia. Disorders of elimination include encopresis and enuresis. Eating disorders are most often encountered in adolescents, but young children can also use food inappropriately to cope with their emotions. Early recognition and treatment help prevent greater problems later in life. Anorexia nervosa (a severe disturbance in eating behaviour that results in a reduction in body weight to much lower than what is ideal) and bulimia (uncontrolled ingestion of large amounts of food, followed by inappropriate methods to prevent weight gain) are discussed in Chapters 14 and 23.

Eating Disorders

Children with eating disorders either do not eat enough or eat the wrong things. The diagnostic category of *feeding and eating disorders of infancy or early childhood* describes children who routinely fail to eat adequately. Weight loss or a failure to gain weight for at least 1 month in a child with no gastrointestinal tract symptoms is the most significant sign. Food is available, but the child does not eat. Most feeding disorders occur in children under 1 year of age, but they can occur in some 2- and 3-year-olds. The long-term complications are malnutrition and delays in development.

Feeding disorders can result from repeated unsuccessful attempts to feed an irritable infant. Infants may be difficult to console, apathetic, or withdrawn during feedings. Some infants may have difficulty regulating their nervous system, resulting in altered periods of alertness. Other factors associated with feeding disorders are parental mental health difficulties, abuse, and neglect. Treatment focuses on ruling out a physical cause, teaching parents appropriate feeding techniques, and monitoring the child's weight and developmental gains. In some cases, family therapy is helpful.

Pica is the persistent eating of nonfood items for more than 1 month. The nonfood items chosen seem to vary with age. Infants and younger children will typically eat paint, hair, string, plaster, or cloth. Older children may eat sand, pebbles, insects, animal droppings, or leaves; adults may consume clay, soil, or laundry starch. Pica is often seen in children with developmental delays and pervasive developmental disorders (e.g., autism). Treatment includes ruling out any physical problems, such as vitamin or mineral deficiencies, removing the item from the child, and helping the child to replace the unacceptable item with more acceptable foods.

Rumination disorder is an uncommon feeding disorder in which the infant regurgitates (brings up) and rechews food. It is most often seen in infants from 3 to 12 months old but may occur in older children or adults with intellectual delays. Characteristically, the infant will arch the back, hold the head back, make sucking movements with the tongue, and give the impression of receiving satisfaction when the food is regurgitated. Malnutrition may occur because the food is brought back to the mouth soon after it is eaten. The disorder often disappears as the child grows older, but if the behaviours continue, erosion of the esophagus from exposure to stomach acids may result.

Elimination Disorders

The two most common elimination problems of childhood are enuresis and encopresis.

Enuresis is involuntary urination of a child age 5 years or older. Enuresis is divided into three categories: *primary* nocturnal enuresis (wetting the bed at night), *diurnal* enuresis (daytime wetting), and *secondary* enuresis (develops after child has achieved bladder control). This disorder is often familiar.

Primary nocturnal enuresis is common in children. It occurs three times more frequently in boys and often disappears without intervention. The actual cause of nighttime wetting is not known, but it is believed that a developmental delay in the sleep–wake mechanism or bladder capacity of the child may be a factor. Daytime wetting (*diurnal enuresis*) is less common. It is usually seen in shy children or those who have ADHD. Daytime wetting occurs equally in boys and girls. Approximately 60 to 80% also wet the bed at night.

Secondary enuresis develops when a bladder-trained child becomes incontinent. Usually it follows a stressful event, such as the birth of a sibling or a divorce. Both diurnal enuresis and secondary enuresis are associated with high levels of emotional stress and anxiety.

Once any physical cause is ruled out, treatment for children with enuresis ranges from simple reassurance to various mental health therapies. Medications (desmopressin, imipramine) may be prescribed. Nurses can help parents cope by obtaining an accurate history of the child's problems, helping parents to establish a bedtime routine for the child, and providing emotional support. When mental health therapy is required, the focus is on helping the child verbally express the feelings associated with the symptoms.

TABLE 13.6   Classification of Intellectual Disability Levels

Mild (85% Incidence)	Moderate (10% Incidence)	Severe (3–4% Incidence)	Profound (2% Incidence)
Develops social and communication skills; has academic skills to grade 6 level; has skills adequate for self-support; may need supervision and guidance but is able to successfully live in community	Develops communication skills; has academic skills to grade 2 level; profits from vocational training; can attend to personal care with supervision; can work in sheltered setting or work in community under supervision; adapts well to community life in supervised environments	May learn to talk and do basic self-care skills; can learn key "survival" words (e.g., *stop, bus, police*); performs simple tasks with close supervision; adapts well to life with families or group homes	Exhibits associated neurological conditions, delays in development; has impaired sensorimotor function; is unable to care for self independently; may improve in highly structured environment; will always require sheltered environment with close supervision

Encopresis is defined as the repeated, usually voluntary, passage of feces in inappropriate places carried out by a child over 4 years of age with no physical abnormalities. It affects boys four times more frequently than girls and is rarely seen in adolescence. Treatment focuses on establishing a routine bowel care program. Praising the child for continent periods and having them assume the responsibility for rinsing the soiled clothing is often effective. Children who show little concern or distress about their incontinence are more difficult to treat.

DEVELOPMENTAL CHALLENGES

Children develop by mastering increasingly more difficult and complex tasks. Because each child is unique, some lags in certain areas of development are common and to be expected. However, if the child persistently falls behind in a developmental area, a disorder of intellectual functioning, learning, or communication is suspected. The developmental challenges most often seen by health care providers include developmental delays, various learning disorders, and several types of communication disorders.

Intellectual Development Disorder

Children who function significantly below the average intellectual level for their age group and are limited in their abilities to function are said to be *intellectually delayed*. The American Psychiatric Association now identifies the condition with the diagnosis of **intellectual development disorder**. This diagnosis is a powerful label and too often applied in haste. For a child to be considered to have an intellectual development disorder, they must exhibit difficulties in general intellectual and adaptive functioning.

The degree of intellectual functioning is established by having the child complete one or more standard intelligence (IQ) tests. Children who repeatedly score lower than 70 are defined as intellectually delayed. The more important measure is the child's adaptive functioning: how well the child copes with the demands of life. It includes the skill areas relating to self-care, home living, communication, social skills, use of community resources, academic skills, self-direction, and the child's work, leisure, safety, and health activities. Table 13.6 describes the various levels of intellectual delay.

Fetal alcohol spectrum disorder (FASD) is the leading known cause of intellectual delay in children. Inborn errors of metabolism, Down syndrome, birth injuries, shaken baby syndrome, high fevers, hormonal imbalances, poisonings, accidents, and falls are known causes of intellectual delay. Heredity; problems with fetal development, pregnancy, or infancy; and environmental influences are thought to be related factors. However, no clear cause of intellectual delays can be found for 30 to 40% of all occurrences. Treatment is individually developed and focuses on encouraging the child to function at the highest levels possible. Therapeutic actions focus on meeting the child's basic needs, providing a safe environment, and encouraging the development of life skills.

Learning Disorders

Formally called *academic skills disorders,* the category for problems with learning is broad. A **learning disorder** is diagnosed when a child with normal intelligence routinely falls below the results of other children in the same age and grade groups on standard reading, mathematics, or written tests. Learning disorders can affect the child's thinking, reading, writing, calculation, spelling, and listening abilities. Many children in the public school system have learning disabilities.

Children with learning disabilities often feel low self-esteem and lack the social skills of other children. Many become discouraged and drop out of school early. Although no specific cause has been found for learning disorders, they have been associated with conditions such as fetal alcohol syndrome, lead poisoning, and fragile X syndrome (a genetic problem). Learning disorders are diagnosed only after physical disorders such as hearing, speech, and visual problems are ruled out. Cultural influences are also considered. A child is said to have a learning disorder only if the specific problem interferes with academic achievement or the activities of daily living.

Children with a reading disorder may have problems reading, understanding the written word, reading aloud, or writing. Individuals with **dyslexia** have problems with reading because although they can see and recognize letters, they have difficulty integrating visual information and thus tend to twist, substitute, distort, or omit many words. Children are seldom diagnosed before they have received several years of reading instruction in school. Early intervention is important because special education often results in great improvement in their skill level and confidence. Reading disorders, if not addressed, may follow the child into adult life.

Many learning disorders are seen in children with ADHD. Other children with learning disabilities are quiet, with low activity levels. They are frequently overlooked because of their quiet manners or are mistaken for being intellectually delayed. Most children with learning disabilities respond well to special education classes and encouragement.

Communication Disorders

In children, the most common **communication disorders** are problems with expression, receiving messages, the pronunciation of words, and stuttering. Communication disorders may be the result of neurological or other medical conditions, but the cause is often unknown.

Problems with language usually begin in children around age 3 years. The child may fail to use expected speech sounds for their age group (*phonological disorder*); speak at a rapid or slow rate, with strange rhythms and word use (*expressive language disorder*); or have a disturbance in the pattern of speech in which sounds are frequently repeated (*stuttering*). Each is considered a disorder only if the problem interferes with the child's activities of daily living or ability to academically achieve.

Children with developmental challenges must struggle for their learning more than other children. They need love, patience, and encouragement on a daily basis. Too often, adults fall into the "label trap" and condemn these children to performing at levels far below their actual abilities. Care providers must remember that working with developmentally different children comes with a commitment to help them achieve to the best of their abilities.

PERVASIVE DEVELOPMENTAL DISORDERS

The word *pervasive* is defined as a tendency to spread throughout. When applied to mental health, the word means that a problem is severe enough to affect several areas of functioning. Children with **pervasive developmental disorders** have difficulty with social interaction skills, communication skills, and learning. Their behaviour is definitely different from that of other children of the same age and developmental level. Actual causes for these disorders remain unknown, but they are often seen with intellectual delays, congenital infections, and abnormal central nervous system functions.

Pervasive developmental disorders include the following:

- **Autism**: A disorder of communication, social interactions, and behaviour.
- Asperger's syndrome: A specific cluster of autistic symptoms, typically occurring in people with normal or near-normal intelligence (Klauber, 2018).
- Rett syndrome: The development of motor, language, and social problems and loss of previous skills that occur between 5 months and 4 years of age; head growth declines, hand movements resemble hand wringing, and loss of social interest and severe speech impairments occur.

- Childhood disintegrative disorder: A period of severe regression in many areas after 2 years of normal development.

Rett syndrome and childhood disintegrative disorder appear after a period of normal functioning, whereas autism and Asperger's syndrome are present in infancy. Autism is the most often encountered pervasive developmental disorder of childhood. It shares many of the same characteristics with the other listed disorders and serves as an example for learning about the behaviours of children with pervasive developmental disorders.

Autism

Autism is not a disease but a syndrome of associated behaviours. It results from some condition that affects the development of the nervous system, and it can remain with the individual throughout life. Autism is diagnosed when the child has serious problems with social interactions, communication, and use of imagination and demonstrates a markedly restricted scope of activities and interests.

The onset of autistic signs and symptoms begins in infancy or early childhood. Autistic disorders affect children from all classes and groups. Typically, autism is seen four times more frequently in boys. The majority of autistic children measure low on IQ tests. Motor skill development may be good, but the child's use of motor skills is inappropriate. Many autistic children become functioning adults, whereas others are totally dependent for care. Children who are able to develop language skills before the age of 5 years have better outcomes. If the child has seizures around puberty, the outlook for improvement is generally poor.

No single behaviour or symptom is diagnostic of autism. Behaviours must be considered in relation to the whole child and their functioning. Monitoring children's early social responses, communication skills, and behaviours allows health care providers to intervene early when a problem is suspected.

The outstanding feature of autism is its *different behaviours*. Autistic children tend to use people in the environment like objects; they are unable to imitate others or make social contact. Other characteristics of autistic disorder include abnormal speech and communications, abnormal play activities, preoccupation with certain objects and routines, restricted body movements, and a very narrow range of interests.

Care providers who work with children must become keen observers and careful history takers. Parents are questioned about the child's birth, developmental history, social responses, and communications. The picture of an autistic child begins to emerge when it is learned that the child does not act appropriately for their mental age, even with family members and other familiar people. Once the disorder is suspected, the child receives a complete physical examination to rule out central nervous system problems. The child is then referred to a treatment team that specializes in children with autistic challenges. Parents are encouraged to work with physicians, nurses, therapists, and special educators. Programs are designed to meet the individual child's unique needs. Then the parents, child, and treatment team work together for each small gain in functioning.

TABLE 13.7 Pediatric Mental Health Screening Tool

Assessment	Subject
Childhood history	Ambulation, behavioural problems, bowel and bladder training/habits, communication (difficulties with speech or learning), discipline, eating habits, playmates (social interactions), psychiatric history (treatments, medications, suicide potential), school (reactions, experiences), computer/social media use, sleep habits, unusual illnesses or injuries, current problem (with description of events that led to current situation)
Family history	Current household (members, relationship to child), parents, type of family (birth, blended, adopted, foster), mental health history of family (e.g., drug, alcohol use; arguments; violence; suicide attempts)
Mental status examination	General appearance, communication, emotion (mood, affect), intellectual level, orientation, thought processes

BOX 13.5 Mental Health Nursing Diagnoses for Children

Anxiety
Risk-prone health **behaviour**
Reduced self-concept
Reduced verbal **communication**
Ineffective coping: family, individual

Denial
Ineffective **environmental** interpretation syndrome
Interrupted family process

Fear
Delayed growth and development
Ineffective health maintenance

Hopelessness
Disorganized infant behaviour
Ineffective infant feeding pattern
Potential for injury
Deficient knowledge
Potential for loneliness
Imbalanced nutrition (inadequate nutrition [malnutrition]; excessive nutrition [obesity])
Impaired parent–child attachment
Parental role conflict
At risk for ineffective parenting
Disturbed personal identity
Post-trauma syndrome
Powerlessness
Inadequate protection
Rape-trauma syndrome
Deficient self-care

SCHIZOPHRENIA

Schizophrenia is a condition associated with disturbing thought patterns and a distorted reality. Considerable disagreement exists concerning the onset of schizophrenia in childhood. Schizophrenia usually develops during late adolescence or early adulthood, but it has been seen in children. Recent research has demonstrated that schizophrenic children may have attention and memory problems that interfere with their ability to carry information into the short-term or working memory. As a result, many are unable to monitor the responses of other people, or they interact and respond with illogical or disconnected statements (Frazier, McClellan, Findling, et al., 2007).

The signs, symptoms, and behaviours of children with schizophrenia vary widely, but the core disturbance lies in a lack of contact with reality and the child's retreat into their own world. Common behaviours include bizarre movements; alternating periods of hypoactivity and hyperactivity; inappropriate emotions, language, and use of the body; distorted sense of time; treating self and others as nonhuman; compulsions; phobias; and temper tantrums. Early recognition and treatment are important because schizophrenia is often a long-term disorder.

THERAPEUTIC ACTIONS

Therapeutic interventions for children with mental health challenges are first directed toward early identification and treatment. Health care providers play a valuable role by performing health screening and routine examinations for healthy children in a variety of settings (Table 13.7).

Once a disorder is diagnosed, special treatment programs and specific goals are developed for the child. Nurses routinely assess and monitor the child's progress toward meeting each goal. All care providers can provide the emotional support and encouragement that are much needed by the parents and other family members.

The care for each child is special and based on individual needs. Nursing diagnoses for children with mental health challenges are listed in Box 13.5. Therapeutic actions are focused on providing holistic care within an environment that fosters growth and development. The Sample Patient Care Plan 13.1 offers an example of a care plan for a child with intellectual delays. General interventions are focused on meeting basic needs, providing opportunities, and encouraging self-care activities.

Meet Basic Needs

Meeting the child's basic physical needs can range from a gentle reminder to providing total personal care. Caregivers are responsible for making sure the child adequately eats, sleeps, eliminates, and maintains personal cleanliness. Helping a child to meet basic needs includes the provision of love and acceptance, no matter how unusual or odd the behaviours. Many children with mental health challenges have a special need to be nurtured. Often the child's caregivers are the only persons in the environment who provide that energy.

Provide Opportunities

Even the most profoundly intellectually delayed or mentally troubled child will achieve something if given the opportunity, instruction, and support. Assessment tools, such as those listed in Table 13.8, allow care providers to screen for developmental levels, school readiness, and potential problems.

Each child is capable of something. As a care provider, encourage young patients to grow and to reach for higher levels of function. Provide opportunities for small successes, which encourage everyone (especially the child) to strive for more.

Encourage Self-Care and Independence

Mentally troubled children grow and develop just as do ordinary children. Despite their problems, many become productive adults who live successfully within their communities. Health care providers who work with these children can help them learn the important skills of daily living. Daily hygiene skills, such as how to dress, bathe, brush teeth, and comb hair, are taught and reinforced. Caregivers coordinate with teachers, occupational therapists, and physiotherapists to help teach the more complex skills of living, such as how to take a bus, spend money, or pay bills. Many of these children will not be able to engage in the more complicated activities of daily life, but each child deserves the encouragement to function as independently as possible.

Caring for children with mental health difficulties is challenging work, but the rewards are many and worth the efforts. Our children are our priceless gifts to the future, and even the most troubled deserve our best efforts.

SAMPLE PATIENT CARE PLAN 13.1 Intellectual Delay

Assessment

History BJ is a 6-year-old boy who has moderate intellectual delays. His birth and the first 6 months of life were uneventful. At 7 months, BJ contracted "a virus" and since then has shown little developmental progress.

Current Findings A slightly overweight 6-year-old boy who is screaming uncontrollably at the time of interview. Mother reports that BJ is able to speak but prefers to communicate by pointing at the desired object and grunting. When needs are not immediately met, BJ begins to scream in a shrill voice. He feeds himself finger foods and refuses to use a spoon. He is not bowel or bladder trained and follows no daily routine at home. He has no eating and sleeping routines.

Multidisciplinary Diagnosis

Altered growth and development related to physical dysfunctions as evidenced by impaired developmental abilities

Planning/Goals

BJ will develop a daily routine for eating, sleeping, and activities by October 2.

THERAPEUTIC INTERVENTIONS

Interventions	Rationale	Team Member
1. Supervise closely for first 7 days on unit.	To assess strengths, abilities, and needed interventions	All
2. Approach BJ in a calm, peaceful manner.	Promotes self-esteem, decreases anxieties	All
3. Introduce no more than two new people into the environment per week.	Decreases anxiety, provides security	All
4. Establish a daily routine for food, naps, activity.	Prevents anxiety, provides security	Nsg
5. Name each object that BJ points to, and encourage him to repeat the name.	Encourages the use of speech and control over environment	All
6. Assist with personal care as needed; praise any attempt at self-care.	Promotes comfort, acceptance. Praise encourages further attempts at self-care	Nsg, OT

Evaluation By the 10th day in the unit, BJ was able to follow a simple daily routine with frequent coaching. Sleep at night progressed from 3 to 9-hour periods.

Critical Thinking Questions
1. How can the health care team ensure that BJ will maintain his new routine at home?
2. What information should be included in the family teaching plan?

A complete patient care plan includes several other diagnoses and interventions.
Nsg, nursing staff; *OT,* occupational therapist.

TABLE 13.8	**Behavioural and General Developmental Screening Tools**				
Screening Tool	**Age Group(s)**	**Completed by**	**Time Required to Complete**	**Availability**	**Additional Comments**
Ages and Stages Questionnaires (ASQ)	4 months to 5 years	Parent	10–20 minutes	Available for purchase. Available in French.	These questionnaires assess a child's global development: gross motor, fine motor, language functions and social-emotional development, and adaptive skills. Screening tool for developmental delay and to identify specific strengths and weaknesses a child may present.
Child Developmental Inventory (CDI)	15 months to 6 years		30–50 minutes	Requires permission for use	Used for children 15 months to 6 years of age to assess development in eight areas of functioning including cognitive and language. Reliability: Author reports internal consistency alphas, categorized by age range and by scale, ranging from .43 to .92. Validity: Author reports evidence of convergent and construct validity, as well as age discriminative validity.
Conners Early Childhood	2–6 years	Parent, teacher, care provider	5–25 minutes depending on type of assessment	For purchase	To assess a child's social, emotional, behavioural development
HEADSS for Adolescents	12–18 years	Physician with patient	5–10 minutes	Free	Provides questions to ask of adolescents that may point out areas of concern. This tool may be used to identify risky behaviours, as well as for health promotion (seat belt, helmet, protective gear use).
Nipissing District Developmental Screen (NDDS)	Up to 6 years	Parent	Under 5 minutes	Available for purchase in several languages. The NDDS is currently offered free to health care providers in Ontario.	Examines 13 key developmental stages.

Continued

TABLE 13.8   Behavioural and General Developmental Screening Tools—cont'd

Screening Tool	Age Group(s)	Completed by	Time Required to Complete	Availability	Additional Comments
PEDS: Parents' Evaluation of Developmental Status	Birth to 11 years	Parent		Permission required to use. Available in French.	Used to screen for developmental delays in children. **Reliability:** Author reports an internal consistency reliability (alpha) of 0.81, test-retest reliabilities of 0.80–1.00, and inter-rater reliabilities of 0.80–1.00 as well. **Validity:** Author reports evidence of good sensitivity and specificity, discriminative validity, and convergent/concurrent validity.
Youth Resiliency: Assessing Development Strengths (YR:ADS)	13–18 years	Self-report		Permission required for use	Assesses factors associated with adolescent resilience, such as parental support/expectations, peer relationships, community cohesiveness, commitment to learning, school culture, cultural sensitivity, self-control, empowerment, self-concept, social sensitivity.

From Canadian Paediatric Society (CPS). (2019). *Behavioural and general developmental screening tools.* https://www.cps.ca/en/tools-outils/behavioural-and-general-developmental-screening-tools

KEY POINTS

- Health care providers who work with children must have an understanding of normal development and an awareness of the child's individual pace of growth and development.
- Common behavioural difficulties during the early years of childhood are colic, problems with feeding and sleeping, temper tantrums, and breath-holding spells.
- Many children must cope with mental health challenges that are a result of poverty, homelessness, abuse, or neglect.
- Behavioural problems, developmental delays, speech delays, sleep disorders, immature motor actions, and short attention span are common in homeless children.
- The most common emotional problems of children include anxiety, depression, somatoform disorders, and post-traumatic stress disorder (PTSD).
- Most children's anxieties are relieved when they receive reassurance and emotional support from significant others.
- The two disruptive behavioural disorders most commonly encountered by care providers are attention-deficit/hyperactivity disorder (ADHD) and conduct disorder.
- Children with ADHD have problems with behavioural self-control, hyperactivity, relating to others, and focusing their attention.
- The long-term outlook for children with conduct disorders is poor if the behavioural problems are present before the child is 10 years old. This makes early diagnosis and treatment very important to prevent antisocial or conduct disorders in adulthood.
- The most common pediatric mental health conditions that relate to eating are feeding disorders, pica, anorexia nervosa, and bulimia.
- Disorders of elimination include encopresis and enuresis.
- The developmental challenges most often seen in children include intellectual delays, various learning disorders, and several types of communication disorders.
- Interventions for intellectually delayed children focus on meeting the child's basic needs, providing a safe environment, and encouraging the development of life skills.
- Children with pervasive developmental disorders have serious problems with social interaction skills, communication skills, and learning.
- Autism is characterized by few social interactions, a lack of communication, little use of imagination, and a restricted scope of activities and interests.
- The signs, symptoms, and behaviours of children with schizophrenia vary widely, but the core disturbance is a lack of contact with reality and the child's retreat into their own world.
- General therapeutic interventions include meeting basic physical and emotional needs, providing opportunities for each child to grow and develop, and encouraging self-care activities.

ADDITIONAL LEARNING RESOURCES

Go to your Evolve website (http://evolve.elsevier.com/ Canada/Morrison-Valfre/) for additional online resources, including the online Study Guide for additional learning activities to help you master this chapter content.

CRITICAL THINKING QUESTIONS

1. You are a home care nurse visiting an older man just after dinner to provide an assessment and a postoperative dressing change. You attend later in the day than you usually do, because of bad weather. While you are changing the patient's dressing, you see the man's grandson, approximately 8 years old, walk to the kitchen. He is not wearing a shirt, and you notice red marks on his back. The patient says, "His mother punishes him sometimes … too much, but what can I do?" The man appears to be upset when he shares this information with you. What obligations do you have in a circumstance like this? What sort of information would you take note of?

2. A friend tells you that she is upset because her family physician told her that her 6-year-old son is overweight. She wonders if it is because the babysitter lets him watch too much TV. How might you address your friend's concerns?

3. Your patient discloses to you that her 9-year-old has suddenly refused to go to school. He has made up excuses and pretends to be ill to avoid going. She states that he used to love school and is considered to be academically gifted. She asks if you have any ideas why a bright 9-year-old would suddenly hate school so much. What would you tell her?

REFERENCES

American Psychological Association. (2018). *Effects of poverty, hunger, and homelessness on children.* https://www.apa.org/pi/families/poverty

Astle, B. J., Duggleby, W., Potter, P. A., et al. (Eds.). (2019). *Canadian fundamentals of nursing* (6th ed.). Elsevier Canada.

Canadian Institutes of Health Research (CIHR). (2012). *Canadian bullying statistics.* Author. https://cihr-irsc.gc.ca/e/45838.html

Canadian Paediatric Society (CPS). (2017). *Screen time and young children.* https://www.caringforkids.cps.ca/handouts/screen-time-and-young-children

Canadian Radio-television and Telecommunications Commission (CRTC). (2019). *Communications monitoring report, 2018.* Government of Canada. https://crtc.gc.ca/eng/publications/reports/policymonitoring/2018/cmr4c.htm

Centre for ADHD Awareness Canada (CADDAC). (2020). *ADHD facts—dispelling the myths.* Author. https://caddac.ca/adhd/understanding-adhd/in-general/facts-stats-myths/

Conrad, B. (2020). *Media statistics—children's use of TV, Internet, and video games.* http://www.techaddiction.ca/media-statistics.html

Feiring, C., & Zielinski, M. (2011). Looking back and looking forward: A review and reflection on research articles published in child maltreatment from 1996 through 2010. *Child Maltreatment, 18*(1), 3–5.

Frazier, J., McClellan, J., Findling, R. L., et al. (2007). Treatment of early-onset schizophrenia spectrum disorders (TEOSS): Demographics and clinical characteristics. *Journal of the American Academy of Child & Adolescent Psychiatry, 46*(8), 979–988.

Hagerman, R. J. (2014). Growth and development. In W. H. Hay, M. J. Levin, R. R. Deterding, & M. J. Abzug (Eds.), *Current pediatric diagnosis and treatment* (22nd ed.). Appleton & Lange.

Hazel, P. (2002). Depression in children. *British Medical Journal, 325*(30), 229.

Hockenberry, M., & Wilson, D. (2014). *Wong's nursing care of infants and children* (10th ed.). Mosby.

Klauber, T. (2018). *The many faces of Asperger's.* Routledge.

Mencap. (n.d.). Bullying wrecks lives: The experiences of children and young people with a learning disability. https://www.mencap.org.uk/sites/default/files/2016-07/Bullying%20wrecks%20lives.pdf

Molcho, M., Craig, W., Due, P., & HBSC Bullying Writing Group, et al. (2009). Cross-national time trends in bullying behaviour 1994–2006: Findings from Europe and North America. *International Journal of Public Health, 54*(S2), 225–234.

National Center for Education Statistics. (2017). *Fast facts: Bullying.* https://nces.ed.gov/fastfacts/display.asp?id=719

Public Health Agency of Canada (PHAC). (2010). *Canadian incidence study of reported child abuse and neglect—2008: Major findings* Author [Seminal Reference].

Public Health Agency of Canada (PHAC). (2018). *Family violence: How big is the problem in Canada?* Author. https://www.canada.ca/en/public-health/services/health-promotion/stop-family-violence/problem-canada.html

Rao, D. P., Kropac, E., Do, M. T., et al. (2016). Childhood overweight and obesity trends in Canada. *Health Promotion & Chronic Disease Prevention Canada, 36*(9), 194–198. https://doi.org/10.24095/hpcdp.36.9.03

Sourander, A., Jensen, P., Rönning, J. A., et al. (2007). What is the early childhood outcome of boys who bully or are bullied in childhood? *Pediatrics, 120*(2), 397–404.

Statistics Canada. (2019a). *Canadian income survey, 2017.* The Daily. February 26. https://www150.statcan.gc.ca/n1/daily-quotidien/190226/dq190226b-eng.htm

Statistics Canada. (2019b). *Family violence in Canada: A statistical profile, 2018.* The Daily. December 12. https://www150.statcan.gc.ca/n1/daily-quotidien/191212/dq191212b-eng.htm

Waddell, C., Offord, D. R., Shepherd, C. A., et al. (2002). Child psychiatric epidemiology and Canadian public policy-making: The state of the science and the art of the possible. *Canadian Journal of Psychiatry, 47*(9), 825–832.

14

Challenges of Adolescence

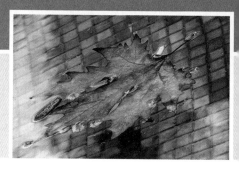

OBJECTIVES

Upon completion of this chapter, the student will be able to:
1. Describe three common challenges of adolescence.
2. Discuss three challenges faced by adolescents with troubled family lives.
3. Identify the diagnostic criteria for behavioural disorders.
4. Explain how the signs and symptoms of adolescent depression differ from those seen in adult depression.
5. Define two eating disorders that may begin during adolescence, and describe the associated signs and symptoms and behaviours.
6. Describe the stages of chemical dependency in adolescence.
7. List four signs or symptoms indicating a potentially suicidal teen.
8. Identify four therapeutic interventions designed specifically for adolescent patients.
9. Explain how health care providers help adolescents develop effective coping skills.

OUTLINE

KEY TERMS

adolescence (ăd-ō-LĔS-ĕns) (p. 160)
anorexia nervosa (ăn-ŏ-RĔK-sē-a nĕr-VŌ-să) (p. 167)
anxiety disorders (p. 167)
bulimia (bŭ-LĔM-ē-ă) (p. 167)
chemical dependency (KĔM-ĭ-kăl dē-PĔN-dĕn-sē) (p. 168)
conduct disorders (p. 166)
cyber-bullying (p. 164)
eating disorders (p. 167)
gangs (găngz) (p. 164)
gender dysphoria (p. 169)
harm reduction (p. 169)

maturation (MĂCH-ū-RĀ-shən) (p. 161)
mood disorders (p. 167)
neurotic behaviours (p. 170)
obesity (ō-BĒS-ĭ-t ē) (p. 167)
peer groups (pēr groops) (p. 162)
personality disorder (DĬS-ŏr-dĕr) (p. 169)
psychotic behaviours (p. 170)
puberty (PYOO-bĕr-tē) (p. 161)
sexual disorder (sĕk-shū-ĂL DĬS-ŏr-dĕr) (p. 169)
suicide (SOO-ĭ-sīd) (p. 170)
surveillance (sĭr-VĀL-ĕnts) (p. 171)

Adolescence is a time of great change. Generally, **adolescence** begins at age 11 to 12 years and ends between ages 18 and 21 years. Physical and sexual growth are usually complete by age 16 to 18 years, but in Western societies, "the adolescence period is prolonged to allow for further psychosocial development

before the young person assumes adult responsibilities" (Kaplan & Mammel, 2014). Adolescents are also called teenagers or teens. All adolescents share the same growth and developmental processes, but each person's society and culture strongly influence that process of "growing up."

Researchers at the University of Michigan (Crystal, Chen, Fuligni, et al., 1994) studied the frequency of stressed and anxious feelings in more than 4 000 US, Taiwanese, and Japanese teenagers. They found some interesting results. Japanese adolescents were found to have the fewest reports of physical problems and depressed moods, whereas Taiwanese teens displayed more physical complaints and depressed moods. Students in the United States and Taiwan thought of school as a source of stress, but only US teens mentioned out-of-school activities and sports as sources of stress. Japanese teens felt that peers were a greater source of stress.

Parents in the United States expected lower academic performance of their teens than the parents of Japanese and Taiwanese adolescents. Doing well in school was more supported and encouraged by the families of Asian teenagers. High achievers in the United States reported that they were frequently torn between their desires to put extra time into their studies and to follow other activities, such as dating, working, playing sports, and socializing.

ADOLESCENT GROWTH AND DEVELOPMENT

The journey from child to adult is a time of physical and psychosocial growth. Adolescents undergo great changes in the physical, intellectual, emotional, social, and spiritual areas of their lives. Care providers should understand how adolescents grow and change if they are to assist them through this important developmental stage. Many adult challenges find their roots in adolescence.

Physical Development

Changes in the body during adolescence occur in two general areas: physical maturation and sexual development. **Maturation** is the process of attaining complete development (Hockenberry & Wilson, 2014). Physical maturation is the process of developing an adult body. Many physical changes occur during adolescence. Weight and height increase, and muscles grow. The major organs of the body double in size, and one's voice and appearance change.

Adolescence is also a time for sexual development. As changing bodies begin to secrete certain hormones called *gonadotropins,* the process of puberty begins. **Puberty** is defined as the stage during which an individual becomes physically capable of reproduction. With girls, puberty begins between 8 and 14 years of age. Today, the average girl in Canada experiences the 24- to 36-month puberty growth spurt around 9 years of age and begins to menstruate (menarche) at about 12 years and 9 months. Menarche begins as early as 10 years or as late as 16 years of age. Breast development, body fat distribution, and the other physical changes that prepare the teen's body for adulthood are usually complete by age 16 to 18 years.

Boys develop more slowly. The first signs of puberty in boys occur around age 10 to 12 years. The testicles enlarge, pubic hair develops, and the penis increases in length and width. The male growth spurt begins at age 11 years and continues

until about 14 years. Puberty lasts until about 18 years of age, but most male adolescents as young as 12 years old are capable of fathering children. Puberty is a time of change for both boys and girls. For a more thorough review of the growth and development of adolescents, you are encouraged to consult a text on pediatric nursing.

Psychosocial Development

The term *psychosocial* refers to the nonphysical realms of functioning. There are periods in teens' lives when they feel awkward, inadequate, and unworthy. Adults who are aware of these changes are better able to offer the emotional support and acceptance so needed by an adolescent. This section briefly explores the major developmental tasks for each psychosocial area of functioning.

Intellectual changes (*cognitive development*) involve learning to use abstract thinking. Children's thinking is *concrete*, based on what is observed or experienced in the present time. Young adolescents (10–13 years) have trouble thinking realistically about the future. As teens mature, thinking moves from the present and concrete to the future and what is possible. To illustrate, an 8-year-old makes a judgement based on what they see; a 17-year-old makes a judgement based on reasoning. Teens begin to look at the world in new and exciting ways, think beyond the present time, consider a sequence of events or relationships, and solve problems through scientific reasoning and logic.

By the middle teens (14–17 years), *abstract thinking* (adaptable, flexible thinking that uses concepts, generalizations, and problem-solving) is well entrenched, along with a feeling of power and self-centredness. Many believe that they can change the world by just thinking about it. At about 17, teens' abstract thinking becomes more realistic, and they become able to plan reachable actions, goals, and careers.

Emotional development during adolescence is marked by rapid periods of change and adjustment. By age 10 to 13 years, the emotional stability of childhood is replaced with a preoccupation with body changes. This brings about changes in self-esteem, body image, and self-concept. Coping with all these changes becomes confusing to the adolescent. Behaviours swing rapidly from the pleasant, cooperative child to the moody, unpredictable, emotional teen. Early adolescence is marked by rapid shifts between disturbed behaviour and relative calm. Moods swing from upbeat and happy to withdrawn and depressed. Reactions to small events can trigger outbursts and aggressive behaviours.

Adolescents also *daydream* much of the time. Daydreaming is important for adolescents because it allows them to try out new roles and place themselves in "what if" situations. Consequently, they often miss many messages from other people and may become labelled as sullen or withdrawn.

The emotions and mood swings of puberty become intense when teens are between 14 and 17 years old. At this age, many adolescents tend to stay alone, looking within themselves and at how they fit into the world. For some teens, this is a troubled, lonely time. By about 18 years of age, most adolescents are in control of their emotions and have an established self-concept.

Social development is an important area for adolescents. Younger teens struggle to establish a group identity, as well as a personal identity. Most teenagers feel the need to belong to a group. At this age, many needs are fulfilled by **peer groups**. The most important function of the group is to help adolescents define the differences between themselves and their parents. Dress, music, dancing, and language are all designed to display differences and to show how unique the group really is. Unless the standards set by the peer group place teens in danger, they should be tolerated by adults. Belonging to a group serves as a stepping stone in the process of establishing an individual identity and separating from the family.

Middle teens establish their identities by experimenting with different images of themselves. By this time, the peer group determines new standards for dress, behaviour, and activities. Teens at this stage begin to see themselves as others might see them. The social relationships of 14- to 16-year-olds are usually self-centred. Sexuality becomes more important, and by age 18 years, the majority of adolescents have engaged in sexual intercourse. Social relationships for adolescents over 17 years shift from the group to the individual. Caring more about others than oneself begins, and dating becomes more personal and intimate.

Spiritual development for adolescents begins with questioning family values and beliefs. Some teens cling furiously to family values during periods of conflict, whereas others completely disregard them. Adolescents also use their new abstract-thinking abilities to question their childhood religious and spiritual practices. Often they will stop attending religious services, change place of worship, or choose to worship within the privacy of their rooms or other special space. Many teens are attracted to new religious groups or movements that suggest promises of unconditional acceptance and love during a time when adults are seen as critical and intolerant. Most teenagers experience great inner emotional turmoil. Because teens fear that nobody will understand, they may become extremely private. Most adolescents have deep spiritual concerns and require acceptance, understanding, and patience as they struggle to develop spiritual meaning that can support them into adulthood.

Adolescence is a time of rapid and uncontrollable change. Between the ages of 10 and 20 years, adolescents grow, develop, and mature within each area of functioning. Table 14.1 offers a brief outline of the major changes experienced throughout adolescence. As adolescents mature, they begin to move away from the family and function independently. Society welcomes them as adults, with all the rewards and obligations of the adult role.

COMMON CHALLENGES OF ADOLESCENCE

The world is large and complex. Even the most successful people feel overwhelmed by the sheer amount of information and experiences that are currently available. Adolescents, who are just beginning to emerge from the security of childhood, must gain understanding and control of themselves. At the same time, they must learn to cope with living in an uncertain world. Most of the common challenges of adolescence fall into two categories: problems that arise from within oneself (internal sources) and those that are rooted outside the teen's sphere of control (external sources).

Internal (Developmental) Challenges

Most difficulties of early adolescence arise from within the individual. Physical changes are taking place, and new sensations are experienced. One's own body ceases to cooperate at times, and floods of intense emotions bring on dramatic, emotional ups and downs. An important developmental issue of adolescence is defining oneself—establishing an identity separate from one's family. At this stage, teens begin to look into themselves. They engage in *introspection* (the process of examining one's own thoughts, emotions, reactions, attitudes, opinions, values, and behaviours by looking at the inner self). They consider who they are, how they see themselves, how they think others may see them, and how relationships with various people affect them. This process of looking inward helps teens to define themselves, but it also brings about many changes in mood, attitude, and behaviour. Challenges that can threaten self-esteem or confidence routinely arise during the journey to adulthood. It is important for teens to feel secure and emotionally supported by adults during these confusing periods. Just knowing that someone accepts and cares about them goes a long way toward helping teens through troubled times.

External (Environmental) Challenges

Problems that arise outside the teen are called *external challenges*. They fall into three basic areas: family, social, and environmental. Even teens who are blessed with the best of everything experience difficulties in these areas of functioning.

A growing concern with children, especially adolescents, is *sleep deprivation*. The majority of adults in Western society function on inadequate sleep. Teens require 8 to 10 hours of restful sleep each night to function well during the day. It is estimated that more than 30% of children between the ages of 6 and 13 years have issues with sleep. Adolescents aged 14 to 17 years fare even worse, with the number having sleep issues climbing to 42%. That "percentage rises to 50% to 75% in children with mental health and neurological/developmental disorders" (Gerber, 2014; Michaud & Chaput, 2016). See Chapter 23 for a more detailed discussion of sleep disorders.

Family problems change as the adolescent develops independence. During early adolescence (age 11–14 years), teens experience the pull between wanting to stay dependent and moving toward independence. They begin to seek their freedom but still require the emotional ties provided by the family structure.

By mid-adolescence (age 14–17 years), the push for independence is in full swing, and major conflicts relating to control motivate the teen to detach from the family. Conflicts slowly fade as the adolescent matures into an independently functioning adult. Separating from the family and establishing independence are processes faced by every teen, but

TABLE 14.1 Growth and Development During Adolescence

Early Adolescence (11–14 Years)	Middle Adolescence (14–17 Years)	Late Adolescence (17–20 Years)
Growth		
Rapid growth	Growth slowing in girls	Physically mature
Reaches peak	Reaches 95% of adult height	Structure and reproductive growth almost
Sexual growth begins	Sexual growth well advanced	complete
Cognition (Intellect)		
Explores ability for limited abstract thought	Developing abstract thinking	Established abstract thought
Groping for new values and energies	Enjoys intellectual powers, often in idealistic terms	Can perceive and act on long-range operations
Compares "normal" with peers of same gender	Concern with philosophical, political, and social problems	Able to view problems comprehensively
		Intellectual and functional identity established
Identity		
Preoccupied with rapid body changes	Modifies body image	Body image and gender role definition nearly secured
Trying out various roles	Very self-centred	Mature sexual identity
Measures attractiveness by acceptance or rejection of peers	Tendency toward inner experience and self-discovery	Brings together identity
Conformity to group norms	Has rich fantasy life	Stability of self-esteem
	Idealistic	Comfortable with physical growth
	Able to perceive future implications of current behaviour and decisions	Social roles defined
Relationships With Parents		
Defining independence–dependence boundaries	Major conflicts over independence and control	Emotional and physical separation from parents completed
Strong desire to remain dependent on parents while trying to detach	Low point in parent–child relationship	Independence from family with less conflict
No major conflicts over parental control	Greatest push for emancipation; disengagement	Emancipation nearly secured
	Final and irreversible emotional detachment from parents; mourning	
Relationships With Peers		
Seeks peers to counter instability generated by rapid change	Strong need for identity; self-image	Peer group fades in importance in favour of individual friendships
Close idealized friendships with members of the same gender	Behavioural standards set by peer group	Testing of male–female or same-sex relationships; possibility of permanent alliance
Struggles for mastery within peer group	Acceptance by peers extremely important—fear of rejection	Relationships characterized by giving and sharing
	Explores ability to attract persons of gender they feel drawn toward (opposite or same sex)	
Sexuality		
Self-exploration and evaluation	Multiple relationships	Forms stable relationships and attachments
Limited dating, usually group	Decisive turn toward heterosexuality (if is gay, lesbian, or bisexual, knows by this time)	Able to give and take
Limited intimacy	Exploration of "self-appeal"	Dating as a pair
	Feeling of "being in love"	Intimacy involves commitment rather than exploration and romanticism
	Begins to establish relationships	
Psychological Health		
Wide mood swings	Tendency toward inner experiences; more introspective	More constant with emotions
Intense daydreaming	Tendency to withdraw when upset	Anger more apt to be concealed
Anger outwardly expressed with moodiness, temper outburst, verbal insults, and name-calling	Wide emotion swings in time and range	
	Feelings of inadequacy common; difficulty in asking for help	

Modified from Hockenberry, M., & Wilson, D. (2014). *Wong's nursing care of infants and children* (10th ed.). Mosby.

difficulties often arise from within the family that are not related to the adolescent's developmental stage. Families can range from the overprotective parents who limit their children's experiences and thus do not allow them to make decisions to those whose children grow up on the streets with little or no sense of belonging.

Children have no control over the child-rearing methods chosen by their parents, living conditions, or the environment in which they must grow. Many adolescents must cope with physical violence, sexual abuse, neglect, or parents who abuse alcohol or drugs. Approximately 357 000 Canadian children (or 4.6% of those who are 19 years of age or younger) have a parent who is incarcerated (Withers & Folsom, 2008). These types of problems cannot be solved simply by waiting for the adolescent to outgrow them. They must be coped with every day, and they require energy that should be spent in self-discovery.

Adolescents who are not fortunate enough to have a caring, supportive family are at risk because the conditions to which they are currently exposed may threaten further development (see Case Study). Every adolescent has some family problems because that is the nature of the maturing process. Those teens who are not blessed with a nurturing family can face problems that would test the strongest adult.

CASE STUDY

Carol was a bright, energetic 5-year-old when her parents divorced, which forced her mother to live on a welfare income. Between the ages of 6 and 13 years, Carol experienced a series of "fathers" who lived with them for various periods of time. Some were kind to Carol, but one physically and sexually abused her. Her mother was usually away from home or with other adults, and Carol soon learned to fend for herself. By age 12, Carol had already experimented with different drugs and found alcohol most to her liking. By the time she was 14 years old, Carol was uncontrollable. She had learned to drive and would often steal her mother's car after her mother was asleep for the night. Unprotected sex happened frequently. Soon Carol dropped out of school because "it really doesn't matter."

- List the factors in Carol's life that put her at risk.
- Identify two of her problems.
- What do you think could help Carol?

Adolescents are also challenged with numerous social issues. Early teens seek out their peers and form intense bonds with certain groups. Peer groups are important for the social growth of adolescents. They serve many purposes and help teens cope with their life changes (Box 14.1).

Peer groups and gangs both consist of adolescents of about the same age and circumstances. The difference between the two groups lies in the behaviours or actions of the members. **Gangs** are usually associated with negative behaviours or destructive actions. Peer groups focus their energies in constructive ways, such as volunteer work and projects that benefit their communities. Peer groups are often influenced by

BOX 14.1   Peer Groups and Adolescents

Functions of Peer Groups

- Help to loosen family ties
- Provide stability during times of change
- Help adolescents define present and future social roles; test their views of themselves; learn to trust their own choices; learn to make and stand by their commitments
- Establish behavioural and dress standards

Positive Aspects	**Negative Aspects**
• Provide emotional support, a sense of belonging	• Rules and standards of the group may be too rigid
• Help teens establish values and behavioural standards	• Values and behaviours may not be in keeping with society's definitions
• Provide protection, safety	• May encourage self-destructive behaviours and disregard for others outside the group
• Allow teens to test and try out new behaviours	

adults. Examples include coaches for sports teams or leaders for youth religious groups. Adolescents choose to join groups. Concerned parents should support their teen's choices but remain aware of the powerful influences that groups exert on a developing individual.

Teens are commonly the focus of bullying. In the past, bullies were confined to the school setting. Today, we have **cyber-bullying,** in which the intimidation occurs via Internet communications. Teens have dropped out of school and some have even committed suicide as a result of the remarks made by bullies. Parents need to be alert to changes in their teen's behaviours, particularly if they are due to bullying.

Other social challenges encountered by most adolescents relate to exploring and establishing their sexuality. Intimacy (emotional closeness) is limited in early adolescence and same-gender friends are still of primary importance. As time passes, for most adolescents, interest in people of the opposite sex begins to increase, and for approximately 4% of the population, interest in the same gender increases. By age 14 years, teens explore the concepts of "sex appeal" and "being in love." More than 50% of them have experienced sexual intercourse by this age. Dating may be limited to one person at a time, but many relationships are experienced as adolescents struggle to define themselves, both socially and sexually. Around 20 years of age, people begin to form stable, attached relationships based on a sense of giving rather than just receiving.

Finally, environmental conditions affect adolescent development because problems in the environment can threaten basic needs. The dirty air of so many cities, the quality and quantity of foods eaten, and the purity of the water influence, however subtly, developing human beings. While becoming the face of the climate movement, many young people develop considerable anxiety when confronted with the dangers and potential outcomes of climate change. Exposures to drugs, crime, prostitution, corruption, and violence are also very real environmental problems for many teens. Activities that glamorize sex and violence through music, television, and the movies have a strong impact on the developing teen psyche. Adults who push children into becoming adults too soon are also environmental influences with which teens must cope.

Teens and Electronic Media

The statistics about teens and their use of electronic media are surprising: 54% send text messages daily, and one third send more than 100 each day: teens average more than 7 hours every day using media (more than any other daily activity), and many teens "multitask," doing homework while instant messaging and listening to music (Chauhan, Amin, & Khullar, 2013; Rogers, 2019).

Social media and electronic entertainment have a strong influence on developing adolescents. According to the psychologist Carl Pickhardt (2009), "problems of short attention span, increased distractibility, and high need for stimulation . . . make it much more difficult for young people to accommodate to the traditional demands for consistency of effort, concentration, and compliance that family and school make upon them." Delayed maturity is also seen in teens with excessive electronic use when they are unable or unwilling to develop the behaviours and habits of successful adults.

Most adolescents, however, are concerned with more immediate problems of learning to function effectively within their physical and social environments—the problems that "come with the territory" and are a part of daily life. Environments that foster growth offer fewer problems than

TABLE 14.2	Adolescent Mental Health Disorders
Classification of Disorders	**Examples**
Behavioural disorders	Conduct disorder, attention-deficit/hyperactivity disorder
Emotional disorders	Anxiety disorder, mood disorders (e.g., depression, post-traumatic stress disorder, suicidal thoughts and attempts)
Eating disorders	Anorexia nervosa, bulimia
Chemical dependency	Abuse of alcohol, amphetamines ("Molly"), caffeine, cocaine, marijuana, nicotine, hallucinogens, inhalants, opiates, prescription medications
Personality disorders	Antisocial disorder, borderline personality disorder, dependent disorder, obsessive-compulsive disorder, paranoid personality disorder
Schizophrenia	Paranoid-type schizophrenia, disorganized-type schizophrenia, delusional disorder
Sexual disorders	Gender dysphoria, inappropriate sexual behaviours
Other disorders of adolescence	Adjustment disorder, impulse-control disorders, problems related to abuse or neglect

surroundings that require a constant state of awareness or vigilance just to get through the day. Health care providers must recognize the environmental conditions and challenges that accompany teens if we are to provide teenagers with the tools for a successful transition to adulthood.

MENTAL HEALTH CHALLENGES OF ADOLESCENCE

Adolescence is the time for teens to develop the personal strengths and social skills that promote effective functioning in the adult world. It is a period involving great emotional swings, focus on oneself, and increasingly active sexual and aggressive drives. In an effort to cope with these changes, adolescents engage in a wide variety of behaviours. Some actions help teens to successfully adapt, whereas others result in negative outcomes. This is a period of "trying out" new behaviours, and adults need to consider this fact.

Adolescent mental health also includes the concept of well-being, the inner strengths that promote optimal functioning. Well-being includes the ability to function well socially (*social competence*), have positive interactions with others, cope with stress and troubled times, and become involved in activities and relationships with others.

The word *dysfunction* is defined as impairment in everyday life. It means that the problems faced by the teen are so severe that they cannot or will not partake in the activities of daily living. When an adolescent's problems or emotions impair performance (school, social, or work) or threaten physical well-being, a mental health challenge exists. Table 14.2 lists several categories of mental health disorders that affect adolescents.

Mental health services for adolescents focus on promoting positive life skills, prevention, and treatment of dysfunctions. Nursing interventions focus on health education, assisting with group and individual therapy, medication management, setting limits, and providing emotional support.

Behavioural Disorders

Every child goes through periods of misconduct, of refusing to do as told, of "being bad." However, for some teens, the misconduct continues to occur. Behaviours begin to disrupt their families, social interactions, and performance at school. These teens may clash with classmates, developing a reputation for being unruly, mean, or even dangerous. When a persistent pattern of disruptive behaviours is present, mental health interventions are usually necessary. Disruptive behavioural disorders consist of two basic diagnoses: attention-deficit/hyperactivity disorder and conduct disorders.

Attention-deficit/hyperactivity disorder (ADHD) is usually diagnosed earlier in childhood (see Chapter 13), but its effect lasts through adolescence and into adulthood (Box 14.2). ADHD is a persistent pattern of the following three key features: inattention, hyperactivity, and impulsiveness. Teens with ADHD experience problems in focusing their attention, behavioural self-control, and relating to others. Because of these difficulties, many of these teens become chronically unhappy. They may begin to abuse chemicals or go on to develop conduct disorders.

Treatment for adolescents with ADHD requires a multidisciplinary approach. Small, structured classes and firm, but nonjudgemental, teachers are needed in the school environment. Positive reinforcement programs that reward appropriate behaviours are helpful at home and at school. Behavioural therapy can assist both teens and their parents. Parents are taught how to structure and enforce limits on the teen's behaviours without becoming overly harsh, inconsistent, or angry. If the adolescent has specific learning disabilities, special education may be necessary. Medications to treat ADHD include stimulants, tricyclic antidepressants, and antipsychotics (Table 14.3; see Medication Alert). Adolescents who are taking prescribed medications may also be using various other substances; serious drug interactions can occur when street and pharmaceutical drugs are mixed. As the teen's care provider, it is important not to judge them. Be sure to obtain a complete history of past and current use of chemically active substances.

Conduct disorders are characterized by a defiance of authority and aggressive behaviours toward others (see

> ### ! MEDICATION ALERT
>
> When conducting a teen's medication history, be sure to obtain a complete history of all drugs, herbs, vitamins, or tonics taken by the patient. Write the names of each substance as they are given by the patient. Many different names are used for the same item. Remember to ask about over-the-counter items as well. Assess the teen's understanding of the prescribed medication, especially the adverse effects.

> ### BOX 14.2   Adolescents With ADHD
>
> Only about one third of children with ADHD reach mid-adolescence with no diagnosable psychiatric disorder (Clark, 2014). Teens with ADHD often have low self-esteem and poor socialization skills. Impulse control is usually a problem.

ADHD, attention-deficit/hyperactivity disorder.

Chapter 13). Often teens with conduct disorders violate the rights of other people or defy society's norms and standards. A common factor in the development of conduct disorders appears to be harsh parental discipline with physical punishment. Early harsh discipline tends to foster aggressive behaviours later in a child's life.

The typical adolescent with a conduct disorder is a boy with a history of social and academic problems. Common symptoms include fighting, temper tantrums, running away from home, destroying property, problems with authorities, and failure in school. Stealing and fire setting may occur. Truancy, vandalism, and substance abuse are frequently encountered. Many teens with conduct disorders, especially those with violent histories, also have various physical and mental health challenges, such as anxiety disorders and depression.

Treatment for adolescents with conduct disorders focuses on first stabilizing the teen's home environment and then working to improve family interactions and disciplinary techniques. Individual therapy and family therapy can help the family learn to communicate and problem-solve effectively. A combination of behavioural, emotional, and cognitive therapies can help the teen learn self-control. Success hinges on including the family, teachers, and other adults who are involved with the teen. Efforts are made to treat the adolescent within the home environment; however, residential (inpatient) treatment may be necessary when the teen becomes a danger to themselves or others.

The outlook for adolescents with conduct disorders is poor. Nearly half the children with antisocial behaviours or conduct disorders go on to develop antisocial personality disorder as adults (Clark, 2014). These teens need care providers with patience, a willingness to set limits, and the courage to enforce them.

Emotional Disorders

Disturbed feelings or moods are a normal part of everyday living. Adolescents, because of their many developmental tasks, experience frequent emotional changes. Periods of feeling "down" or "blue" are common with teens. However, when

TABLE 14.3   Medications for Teens With ADHD

Medication Examples	Dosage	Patient Teaching
Stimulants		
dextroamphetamine (Adderall)	5–60 mg/day, divided doses	Avoid caffeine, alcohol, OTC medications
methylphenidate (Ritalin, Concerta)	0.3–1.5 mg/kg, 1–3 doses daily	Watch for effects on growth; behaviour deteriorates when medications are stopped abruptly
Antidepressants		
imipramine (Tofranil)	No more than 5 mg/kg/day	May cause dry mouth, blurred vision, constipation, insomnia
clomipramine (Anafranil)	No more than 5 mg/kg/day	
Nonstimulants		
atomoxetine (Strattera)	0.5–1.2 mg/kg/day	Higher risk for suicide, liver dysfunction, low blood pressure, nausea, decreased appetite, mood swings
guanfacine HCL (Intuniv)	1 mg/day	Sedation, headache, abdominal pain
clonidine HCL (Kapvay)	0.1 mg at bedtime	Fatigue, constipation, dry mouth, insomnia, hallucinations

ADHD, attention-deficit/hyperactivity disorder; *OTC,* over-the-counter.

moods or feelings disrupt the teen's daily activities, mental health care may be needed.

Problems that affect the emotional realm of human functioning include anxiety disorders and mood disorders. While a more detailed discussion is presented in later chapters, a brief description of how these disorders affect adolescents is important here.

Anxiety disorders result when an adolescent's ability to adapt is overwhelmed. When teens are overstressed, anxiety may balloon into an ever-present emotional state that triggers physical changes as the body attempts to adapt. The combination of physical and emotional symptoms can result in conditions such as panic disorder, phobias, obsessive-compulsive disorder (OCD), and post-traumatic stress disorder (PTSD). Anxiety is also associated with the development of depression and substance abuse. It is important to recognize and treat anxiety in children as early as possible, because long-standing problems become difficult to change.

Mood Disorders

Adolescents with *affective* or **mood disorders** display a wide range of behaviours, from profound depression to racing hyperactivity. Mood is the ever-present emotional state that colours one's perception of the world. Moods change rapidly as adolescents struggle with issues of self-image and confidence. Most teens have short periods of "the blues," but when sad moods are prolonged or the teen's behaviour alternates between extreme highs and lows, an emotional disorder is suspected.

According to the Canadian Mental Health Association (CMHA), approximately 5% of male youth and 12% of female youth, aged 12 to 19 years, have experienced a major depressive episode (CMHA, 2013). Many exhibit the primary signs and symptoms of depression listed in Box 14.3. Many, however, suffer in silence, with their symptoms going unnoticed.

Other interpersonal difficulties are often present, such as problems with parents and siblings, drug use, and fighting. Acting out depression through antisocial behaviours, such as theft, vandalism, and truancy, may result in involvement with the law and its criminal justice system. Sexual acting out is also common. Depression in adolescence is "characterized by irritable moods and acting-out behaviours, in contrast to the classic 'depressed mood' and 'loss of interest' characteristic of adults" (Hogarth, 1991). In short, depressed adults lose interest; depressed teens act out.

BOX 14.3 Signs and Symptoms of Depression in Adolescents

Moodiness: irritable moods, acting-out behaviours, gloomy, sad
Decreased social activity
Decreased school performance
Hopelessness
Difficulty thinking
Inability to concentrate, make decisions, or solve problems
Physical complaints: loss of energy, headache, stomachache, eating, and sleeping problems

Severe anxiety and depression are not average adolescent conditions. The majority of teens negotiate this developmental period without major problems. They develop positive personal identities, manage healthy peer relationships, and maintain close family ties. The best prevention for emotional disorders in teens is early recognition. Emotional problems left untreated in adolescence frequently develop into serious mental health disorders in adulthood.

Eating Disorders

Teens' eating patterns and food behaviours may follow the latest trend or change to reflect the preferences of the peer group, but as long as the teen is well nourished, there is little cause for concern. **Eating disorders** are severe disturbances in eating behaviours that can result in a body weight that is far below or above its ideal.

The weight-control practices of adolescents have become a cause for concern in today's society. According to the CMHA, between 1 and 2% of adolescents and young adults have an eating disorder (CMHA Ontario, 2020). The message of "slim equals attractive" bombards individuals throughout childhood, especially females, and weight control can become an important concern.

Childhood obesity rates have tripled in Canada over the last 25 years, with rates among Indigenous children and youth being two to three times higher than the Canadian average. The World Health Organization (WHO) defines overweight as a body mass index (BMI) greater than 25, and obesity as a BMI greater than 30 (Perry, Hockenberry, Lowdermilk, et al., 2018). **Obesity** is defined as a body weight that is 20% or more above the average weight for a person of the same height and build. Because the eating patterns of obese teens do not pose an immediate threat to their health, chronic overeating is not considered a mental health disorder. However, many overweight teens use food to help themselves through troubled times. In these cases, mental health interventions may help individuals find more effective ways of satisfying their needs. Eating disorders are on the rise. While about 90 to 95% of teens with eating disorders are girls, eating disorders do occur in male teenagers, usually athletes. The mortality rate for eating disorders is about 9%—a mental health disorder that can lead to death.

Common eating disorders in adolescence are anorexia nervosa and bulimia. **Anorexia nervosa** is a prolonged refusal to eat in order to keep body weight at a minimum. It is characterized by an intense fear of becoming fat and a relentless pursuit of thinness. **Bulimia** is a cycle of binge eating followed by purging. Anorexia is seen from about age 12 years, with peaks around 13 to 14 years and again at 17 to 18 years. Bulimia often may not occur until age 17 years or so. Both disorders also occur in adults, but the incidence decreases sharply after the mid-30s.

The typical picture of an anorectic teen is one of an overly cooperative, achievement-oriented girl who sees herself as overweight and begins to diet. There may be a history of eating or mood disorders in the family. Over a period of months, her concern with dieting evolves into an obsessive need to be thin. All her behaviours soon focus on remaining thin. She

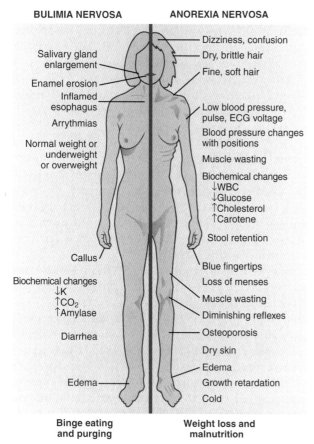

Fig. 14.1 Physical and clinical signs and symptoms of bulimia nervosa and anorexia nervosa. *ECG*, electrocardiogram; *WBC*, white blood cell count.

may restrict calories, exercise excessively, induce vomiting, or use laxatives, diuretics, diet pills, or street drugs to prevent even the smallest weight gain.

As the disorder progresses, the teen cuts back on her social activities and begins to avoid friends. She becomes increasingly anxious, irritable, and depressed. Now all her thoughts focus on food and weight loss. Although it is glaringly apparent to others that she is too thin, the anorexic teen will deny that a problem exists. Soon the physical and psychological effects of starvation begin to appear (Fig. 14.1). Long-term, even life-threatening complications can result unless medical and mental health interventions are undertaken.

Bulimia is more difficult to detect because of the secretive nature of the problem. However, it is estimated that as many as 20% of university-age women are bulimic. The road to bulimia begins with an intense interest in dieting. Struggles with food result in secret binge-eating episodes in which the person consumes 5 000 to 20 000 calories of high-carbohydrate foods. Feelings of intense guilt or depression follow bingeing. The teen then makes extreme attempts to control weight gain through vomiting, exercise, or the use of drugs. Self-imposed starvation may occur between binges. Some weight loss may occur, but body weight usually remains within 20% of normal. The medical complications of bulimia include erosion of tooth enamel, gastric dilation, inflammation of the pancreas, and electrolyte abnormalities. Most people with bulimia are

aware of their behaviour, but they are ashamed and afraid to admit that they are out of control. Binge episodes frequently follow a stressful life event.

Treatment for eating disorders has three goals: to manage the medical dangers, such as metabolic disturbances, cardiac problems, and dehydration; to restore normal nutrition and eating patterns; and to meet the psychiatric treatment needs of the patient and family.

Nursing (care team) diagnoses for eating disorders include activity intolerance, imbalanced nutrition (more or less than body requirements), disturbed thought processes, disturbed body image, chronic low self-esteem, defensive coping, denial, and disabled family coping. Attempts are made to treat the teen within the family setting, but if the condition is severe, the teen is hospitalized. A plan to gradually improve the teen's nutritional intake (a refeeding program) is developed by the dietitian and other team members. Therapeutic interventions are designed to stabilize the patient's physical condition. Force-feeding is discouraged because the goal is to help the teen choose to eat.

As the teen begins to feel better, she is encouraged to express her feelings. With both types of eating disorders, the primary issue is one of control, not food. Psychotherapy can help the teen to recognize underlying depression that is often present and develop more effective coping skills.

Chemical Dependency

For adolescents, the temptation to "find out what it is like" is a strong motivator. Most teens who experiment with alcohol and drugs do not become dependent or addicted. However, for a growing number of teens, the use of chemicals is becoming a way of coping with the difficulties of life. The problems associated with substance abuse are many: accidents caused by lack of judgement, interpersonal violence, depression, and worsening relationships with others. Young adolescents who use chemical substances usually become sexually active at an earlier age. Perhaps the most critical fact is that the use of chemicals interferes with normal adolescent growth and development.

All adolescents are at risk for developing substance abuse problems, especially those who were abused as young children. Teens from families who approve of, use, or promote the use of chemicals and teens with other mental health issues, are also at high risk.

Chemical dependency is a state in which one physically and psychologically requires a drug. Identifying teens with substance abuse or chemical dependency problems is difficult. Many of the signs and symptoms of long-term abuse are absent.

Teens who become chemically dependent progress through four general stages: experimentation, active seeking, preoccupation, and burnout (Box 14.4). Frequently, the most important clues to substance abuse in teens are small ones. A change in habits, mood, or personality often hints at a problem. Sometimes a teen suddenly becomes rebellious. The adolescent disappears with friends and avoids contact with family members. The teen who becomes chemically

BOX 14.4 Stages of Chemical Dependency

1. *Experimentation:* Pleasant moods and social belonging associated with drugs are experienced; drugs are used for the first time within the comfort of the peer or other social group.
2. *Actively seeking:* Teen looks forward to and actively seeks out the mood changes brought about by the chemicals; becomes expert in the use of chemicals to regulate moods; schoolwork and relationships with family erode; friends become limited to other teens who "use."
3. *Preoccupation:* Teen believes that they cannot cope without chemicals; has lost control over the use of the drug; develops a tolerance and may begin to use other substances; chemical is now used to prevent withdrawal symptoms; psychosocial functioning begins to fail; friends are lost and may be replaced with antisocial, illegal, or violent behaviours.
4. *Burnout:* Focus of drug use now is to prevent negative feelings; if the teen attempts to stop using the chemical, withdrawal symptoms appear; those who progress to this level of addiction are usually no longer able to function productively in society; most are late adolescents or young adults.

BOX 14.5 Personality Disorders

According to the American Psychiatric Association, a **personality disorder** is "an enduring pattern of inner experience and behaviour that:
1. Deviates markedly from the expectations of the individual's culture
2. Is universal and inflexible
3. Has an onset in adolescence or early adulthood
4. Is stable over time
5. Leads to distress or impairment"

Data from American Psychiatric Association. (2013). *Diagnostic and statistical manual of mental disorders* (5th ed.). Author.

with a personality disorder. Box 14.5 lists the common behaviours associated with these problems.

A major characteristic of a personality disorder is *impulsivity*—the temptation to engage in acts harmful to oneself or others. Spur-of-the-moment decisions lead to inappropriate actions, such as overeating, casual sexual practices, shoplifting, and thrill seeking. Intense emotional changes lead to anger and depression. Self-esteem and self-confidence are low. The ability to look inward (introspection) is minimal.

These teens tend to develop "all-or-nothing" relationships, in which others are either idealized or considered worthless. They flip between distance and closeness within their relationships and harbour deep fears of being abandoned. Some become suspicious. Many attempt suicide. Frequently a personality disorder will coexist with another mental health challenge.

Treatment for teens with personality disorders involves the use of psychotherapy and various medications. Recent studies have shown that personality disorders may be related to problems with the neurotransmitter serotonin. Treatment with selective serotonin reuptake inhibitors (SSRIs), such as fluoxetine hydrochloride (Prozac), has been successful. Long-term individual therapy, in combination with selective medications, provides a promising outlook for teens with personality disorders.

Sexual Disorders

One of the tasks during adolescence is to establish a sexual identity and role. To do this, many teens experiment with various sexual attitudes, outlooks, and behaviours.

A **sexual disorder** is characterized by significant distress and impaired ability to function. Adolescents with sexual disorders relating to gender identity are still struggling with conflicts that began in childhood. Individuals with **gender dysphoria** have a continual discomfort with their assigned gender. There is a strong and persistent need to identify with the other gender. The individual often insists on wearing clothing designed for the other gender. During play, they identify with or role-play the opposite gender. Playmates and activities are limited to those associated with the desired gender. For example, a boy might like to wear dresses, play house acting as the mother, and choose only girls as friends.

dependent needs mental health intervention. Underneath a hardened exterior lies an individual who has few friends and little or no self-esteem.

Treatment focuses on helping the teen replace the use of chemicals with more effective coping skills. Many treatment programs in Canada, the United States, and Great Britain are modelled on the principles of Alcoholics Anonymous, whose goal is a chemical-free lifestyle. While still controversial, some programs provide a **harm reduction** approach, which is an evidence-based, client-centred approach that seeks to reduce the health and social harms associated with addiction and substance use, without necessarily requiring people who use substances from abstaining or stopping (Thomas, 2005).

Settings for treating teens range from outpatient counselling to residential treatment programs and therapeutic communities. Individual psychotherapy and group psychotherapy are often combined with behavioural and cognitive therapies. Therapeutic inpatient care provides a safe environment; many of these teens are suicidal.

Drug and alcohol abuse is a complex problem affecting all aspects of an adolescent's life. Few teens seek treatment, and therapies for chemical dependency vary in their effectiveness. Prevention and early recognition remain the most effective tools for coping with adolescent substance abuse.

Personality Disorders

Personality is the combination of behavioural patterns that each of us develops to cope with living. Our personalities are important parts of our identities. They characterize us as unique individuals and allow us to function effectively within society. However, adolescents who have long histories of inappropriate or maladaptive behaviours may be diagnosed

As these teens grow older, they become preoccupied with ridding themselves of their sexual characteristics and assuming those of the desired gender. They may request hormonal therapy, surgery, or other procedures that may produce characteristics of the desired gender. Treatment consists of medical and mental health therapies to relieve distress and help teens resolve their challenges related to gender identity.

Sexually acting out is common for teens. However, if their behaviours result in discomfort or harm to themselves or others, the behaviours are considered to be inappropriate. Many sexual challenges faced by adolescents can be solved with good communication skills. Replacing ignorance with accurate knowledge can assist a teen along the road toward healthy sexual maturity.

Psychosis

The defining feature of *schizophrenia* and other psychoses is a grossly impaired ability to function because of not being in touch with reality. Psychotic disorders are discussed in detail in Chapter 31; here, it is important to know that the onset of schizophrenia usually takes place in adolescence. The adolescent who suffers from schizophrenia is typically a good child who begins to develop a whole new set of (sometimes bizarre) behaviours and activities.

CRITICAL THINKING

Neurotic behaviours are recognized by the person as unacceptable, recurring, and persistent. Behaviours may be odd or unusual, but they are within socially acceptable limits. The individual is in contact with reality and able to carry out activities of daily living.

Psychotic behaviours are characterized by personality disintegration, reduced awareness, and an inability to function within socially acceptable limits. The individual is not in contact with reality and is unable to carry out activities of daily living.

• When do neurotic behaviours become psychotic?

The major characteristic of adolescent psychosis is *loss of contact with reality*. The teen may have hallucinations, delusions, and feelings of paranoia. The person lacks judgement, behaves impulsively, and shows little insight. Behaviours may become inappropriate, ritualistic, or repetitive. Disordered thought patterns lead to communication problems and difficulties with relationships. As a result of this loss of contact with reality, personal hygiene (even eating and drinking) may be neglected. The teen usually requires hospitalization and close supervision.

Treatment for psychosis includes a combination of psychotherapy and medication. Antipsychotics, antidepressants, and lithium may be ordered. Care is focused on providing basic physical needs, including feeding, bathing, and exercise; providing a safe environment; and developing skills for successful living. As the adolescent begins to respond to treatment, education about the nature and control of the disorder is begun. Schizophrenia is a lifelong disorder, and the major problem with management is poor adherence to taking the

---

BOX 14.6   Warning Signs of Teen Suicide

Change in grades at school
Loss of interest, initiative
Rapidly changing emotional highs and lows
Defies rules, regulations; pushes limits
May become secretive
Withdraws from family interactions
Changes in personal hygiene
Nightmares
Isolates self from others
Discusses suicide with peers, close friends
Gives away prized possessions
Hints about intentions (e.g., "After I'm gone . . .")

---

prescribed medications. Both adolescents and their families need ongoing support. Family members are often encouraged to join a support group for the emotional assistance needed to cope with a teen who has a psychosis.

Suicide

In Canada, **suicide** is the second highest cause of death for youth aged 10 to 24 years. Each year, on average, 294 youths die from suicide (Canadian Children's Rights Council, 2020). Adolescent girls attempt suicide three times more often than their male counterparts, but boys are more successful in their attempts because they choose more lethal methods. Teens who are hospitalized for injuries or motor vehicle (especially single-car) accidents may actually be attempting suicide.

A suicide attempt by an adolescent is a *call for help*. Today's society is complex and has many stresses on a developing adolescent. Factors that may influence suicidal behaviour include more competition for fewer resources, exposure to abuse and neglect, instability within the family, the presence of depression or other illness, the availability of handguns or other weapons, and an increased use of alcohol and drugs. Box 14.6 lists the warning signs of suicide.

Teenagers who attempt suicide usually fall into one of three groups: the teen with depression, the teen who is trying to influence others, and the teen with a serious mental health problem. When a teen cannot keep up with school and social activities, withdraws from others, has problems eating or sleeping, and feels hopeless, then they are at risk for suicide resulting from depression.

The teen who uses a suicidal gesture as a way to get back at someone (usually a parent, boyfriend, or girlfriend) is attempting to influence someone. Often there is little or no depression and no real wish to die. The teen is angry, and the gesture has the goal of gaining attention or scaring another person. Teenage girls engage in this type of suicidal behaviour more often than do boys.

Adolescents who attempt suicide in the third group are seriously ill. They can see no other way out of their discomfort and actually welcome the relief they expect death to bring.

The group at highest risk for suicide is white adolescent males who have expressed their intention to die. Previous attempts, written plans, and available tools for committing

BOX 14.7	Therapeutic Interventions for Suicidal Teens

Surveillance
Limit setting
Building self-esteem and confidence
Role modelling
Skill development

BOX 14.8 Interventions to Build Self-Esteem

Use *eye contact* (consider the cultural background).
Address each individual by their *name*.
Actively *listen* (use the therapeutic communications in Chapter 10).
Convey *respect*—ask, do not order.
Help teens to assume *responsibility* for their behaviours and their consequences.
Praise each effort at changing behaviours, and point out their progress and successes.
Teach *problem-solving,* and help them apply it to their own behaviours and problems.
Enforce limits respectfully; focus on the behaviours that need to be changed.
The goal is to *encourage responsibility* for one's own actions and self-development.

suicide all heighten the risk for future attempts. Increases in suicidal attempts are often seen after a schoolmate has committed suicide. Teens who are overweight, gay, or bisexual are at higher risk for suicide. Those who are bullied are also at high risk. Health care providers who work with adolescents must assess every teen for suicidal risk. Chapter 27 takes a more in-depth look at this problem.

The goals of treatment for suicidal adolescents are to protect them from harm, build trusting therapeutic relationships, and assist them in developing self-awareness and alternate coping skills. Sample Patient Care Plan 14.1 illustrates a patient care plan designed for an adolescent who is suicidal.

THERAPEUTIC INTERVENTIONS

Adolescents require special mental health care because they are developing and maturing at the same time they are experiencing problems. Although each adolescent is unique, several therapeutic interventions can serve as strategies for all teens. The relationship between patient and care provider serves as an instrument for understanding and helping each teen. Therapeutic communication skills help adolescents define their problems and then develop new and more effective ways of solving them. Specific interventions for adolescents centre around five basic strategies (Box 14.7).

Surveillance and Limit Setting

Surveillance is the process of watching over patients to determine whether they are safe, following their rules, making good decisions, or need adult intervention. The severity of the problem determines the amount of surveillance. Some adolescents need only minimal supervision, whereas others may require 24-hour-a-day observation. The goal of surveillance is to assist teens in developing new skills and coping methods, as well as to protect them from harm. The alert care provider can turn a potential crisis situation into an opportunity for growth.

Setting limits is also essential for adolescents. Part of the process of growing up is to test the limits of authority. Teens are struggling with learning to control their emotions. Care providers working with teens aim to change the focus of control from external to internal (self-control). Situations in which the teen attempts to exceed the limits are treated as learning experiences. When limits are set on behaviours, it is important that the teen understand what is acceptable behaviour and the consequences of inappropriate behaviours. The goal of setting limits is to encourage responsibility.

Quite often, adolescents do well with the problem-solving approach. Here, the teen is asked what they are feeling and doing. The teen is encouraged to see whether the behaviour

is helping to get what they want. The teen then develops a plan for meeting the goal or coping with the feelings and follows it through. This process helps adolescents learn to solve problems and gain some control over their situations. Positive actions are praised and reinforced, and the teen is encouraged to apply the process to other situations.

Building Self-Esteem

Adolescents, even the best-adjusted ones, experience the discomfort of low self-esteem at some time or another; but for the teen with mental health challenges, this discomfort can be great. Teenagers are masters at reading nonverbal behaviours. Care providers who use eye contact, address each teen by name, and actively listen can make them feel accepted and valued. It is important not to lecture or give advice. Instead, direct teens toward problem-solving and assuming responsibility for their feelings. Convey respect by requesting rather than ordering, and thank them for their help. Praise each small effort, and point out the adolescent's progress (Box 14.8). If limits must be enforced, then do so without anger or embarrassment for the teen.

Self-esteem is also fostered through *role models*. The impression that care providers present will influence the effectiveness of therapeutic actions. Adolescents watch how their therapists and care providers interact with one another and solve problems; it is important to remember that as a care provider you are always being watched and evaluated. If teens feel that your behaviours are effective, they will often adopt them for use in similar situations. Acting as a role model for healthy behaviour requires a lot of energy, but it is a highly effective way of helping teens learn how to cope.

Skill Development

One of the most important therapeutic interventions involves assisting adolescents in developing the skills that are essential for functional living. Care providers can help their teen patients with cognitive (intellectual) skills, such as applying the problem-solving process to actual problems. They help young patients practise appropriate social skills. Working cooperatively within a group, learning how to listen to other people, and exploring new methods for controlling anger or

SAMPLE PATIENT CARE PLAN 14.1   Suicidal Adolescent

Assessment

History Rita is a 15-year-old girl admitted to the medical unit of the local hospital for suicidal attempts. About 4 hours ago, she consumed approximately 35 tablets of diazepam (Valium) and had her stomach pumped in the emergency department. Three earlier suicidal attempts have involved drug overdoses and slashed wrists.

Current Findings A sleepy teenage girl in no acute distress. Answers questions with one-word statements. States she attempted suicide to "get everyone off my back." Skin on wrists and forearms has numerous jagged scars. Rita has refused further physical assessment.

Multidisciplinary Diagnosis

Risk for self-directed violence related to family behaviours, developmental conflict

Planning/Goals

Rita will contract with staff for no suicidal attempts.
Rita will verbalize an awareness of her pattern of self-harm by May 7.

THERAPEUTIC INTERVENTIONS

Interventions	Rationale	Team Member
1. Assess potential for self-harm.	Helps prevent harm or injury; helps determine level of surveillance needed	All
2. Ensure safety; place on suicidal precautions.	Prevents impulsive reactions to stressful situations	All
3. Monitor activities continually for first 24 hours.	Helps assess level of suicidal intention, effectiveness of behaviours	Nsg
4. Establish a verbal or written contract not to harm self; renew every 24 hours.	Prevents suicidal behaviours, demonstrates respect	Nsg
5. Establish rapport; offer support; be available to listen; ensure confidentiality.	Acceptance of Rita's feelings shows respect and encourages self-worth even though her behaviour is unacceptable	All
6. Encourage Rita to keep a diary and write in it daily.	Helps Rita identify her reactions and behaviours	Psy

Evaluation Rita willingly contracted each day for no self-harm. By May 1, Rita was seeking Mary P., a nurse, for interaction. By May 7, Rita was able to identify one area in which she was having problems.

Critical Thinking Questions
1. Given her history of past suicide attempts, what can be done to change Rita's harmful coping behaviours?
2. How important is therapeutic rapport in this case?

A complete patient care plan includes several other diagnoses and interventions.
Nsg, nursing staff; *Psy*, psychologist.

aggression are other therapeutic actions designed to help adolescents develop *effective living skills*. Working with adolescent patients is demanding and rewarding. Effective mental health interventions at this stage of life are extremely important in order to prevent future problems.

KEY POINTS

- The passage from child to adult is a time of physical, sexual, and psychosocial growth.
- Many common challenges of adolescence arise from internal and external sources.
- A mental health problem exists when an adolescent's problems impair performance or threaten physical well-being.
- The category of disruptive behavioural disorders is divided into attention-deficit/hyperactivity disorder (ADHD) and conduct disorders.
- Emotional ups and downs are a normal part of adolescence, but many teens suffer from anxiety and mood disorders, such as depression.
- Anorexia nervosa and bulimia are eating disorders characterized by severe disturbances in eating behaviour, which can result in body weight that is far below its ideal.
- Teens who become chemically dependent or addicted move through four general stages: experimentation, active seeking, preoccupation, and burnout.

- Adolescents with long histories of inappropriate or maladaptive behaviours may be diagnosed with a personality disorder.
- A sexual disorder is diagnosed when problems cause the teen significant distress and impair their ability to function.
- The major characteristic of adolescent psychosis, such as schizophrenia, is a loss of contact with reality.
- Teenagers who attempt suicide are usually depressed, trying to influence others, or suffer from a serious mental health condition.
- In addition to the use of therapeutic relationships and communications, interventions for adolescents centre around five basic strategies: surveillance, limit setting, building self-esteem and confidence, role modelling, and skill development.

ADDITIONAL LEARNING RESOURCES

Go to your Evolve website (http://evolve.elsevier.com/Canada/Morrison-Valfre/) for additional online resources, including the online Study Guide for additional learning activities to help you master this chapter content.

CRITICAL THINKING QUESTIONS

1. While attending a family event, you observe your sister's teenage children text messaging extensively during dinner. Your sister has asked them several times to put their phones away; however, after placing their phones in their pockets for a brief period of time, they resume texting. You also learn that they text late into the night, often until 2 or 3 a.m. Your sister appears frustrated and discloses that she doesn't know what to do. What could you tell her?

2. Your 14-year-old patient hasn't attended the LGBTQ2 support group for the second week, and has called and cancelled his weekly counselling appointment. Some of his peers tell you that he has been talking a lot about suicide. Based on your knowledge of the challenges facing LGBTQ2 adolescents, what would be your primary concern? What would you do to reach out to this patient?

3. You observe your daughter's best friend eating ravenously at an "all you can eat" buffet. Your daughter notes that her friend "eats like this constantly" but never seems to gain any weight. In fact, she appears to be slightly underweight for her height. What eating disorder would you suspect is a potential risk for your daughter's friend?

REFERENCES

Canadian Children's Rights Council. (2020). *Youth suicides in Canada and elsewhere.* http://www.canadiancrc.com/Youth_Suicide_in_Canada.aspx

Canadian Mental Health Association (CMHA). (2013). *Fast facts about mental illness.* https://cmha.ca/fast-facts-about-mental-illness

Canadian Mental Health Association (CMHA) Ontario. (2020). *Understanding and finding help for eating disorders.* Author https://ontario.cmha.ca/documents/understanding-and-finding-help-for-eating-disorders/

Chauhan, A., Amin, G., & Khullar, R. (2013). *Social media and the future of childhood.* https://www.slideshare.net/ratna1958/impact-of-social-media-on-the-future-of-childhood

Clark, R. B. (2014). Psychosocial aspects of pediatrics and psychiatric disorders. In W. W. Hay, M. J. Levin, D. T. Deterding, et al. (Eds.), *Current pediatric diagnosis and treatment* (22nd ed.). Appleton & Lange.

Crystal, D. S., Chen, C., Fuligni, A. J., et al. (1994). Psychological maladjustment and academic achievement: A cross-cultural study of Japanese, Chinese, and American high school students. *Child Development, 65*(3), 738–753. https://doi.org/10.2307/1131415 [Seminal Reference]; https://www.jstor.org/stable/1131415

Gerber, L. (2014). Sleep deprivation in children. *Nursing, 44*(4), 50.

Hockenberry, M., & Wilson, D. (2014). *Wong's nursing care of infants and children* (10th ed.). Mosby.

Hogarth, C. R. (1991). *Adolescent psychiatric nursing.* Mosby.

Kaplan, D. W., & Mammel, K. A. (2014). Adolescence. In W. W. Hay, M. J. Levin, R. R. Deterding, et al. (Eds.), *Current diagnosis and treatment pediatrics* (22nd ed.). Appleton & Lange.

Michaud, L., & Chaput, J. (2016). Are Canadian children and adolescents sleep deprived? *Public Health, 141,* 126–129. https://doi.org/10.1016/j.puhe.2016.09.009

Perry, S. E., Hockenberry, M. J., Lowdermilk, D. L., et al. (2018). *Maternal child nursing care in Canada* (2nd ed.). Elsevier Canada.

Pickhardt, C. (2009). Adolescence in the age of electronic entertainment [blog]. *Psychology Today.* November 29. https://www.psychologytoday.com/intl/blog/surviving-your-childs-adolescence/200911/adolescence-in-the-age-electronic-entertainment

Rogers, K. (2019). *US teens use screens more than seven hours a day on average—and that's not including school work.* CNN Health. October 29. https://www.cnn.com/2019/10/29/health/common-sense-kids-media-use-report-wellness/index.html

Thomas, G. (2005). *Harm reduction policies and programs for persons involved in the criminal justice system.* Canadian Centre on Substance Use.

Withers, L., & Folsom, J. (2008). *Incarcerated fathers: A descriptive analysis.* Correctional services Canada. https://www.csc-scc.gc.ca/research/r186-eng.shtml

15

Challenges of Adulthood

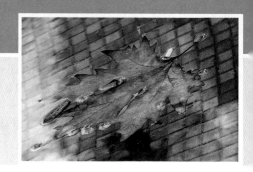

OBJECTIVES

Upon completion of this chapter, the student will be able to:
1. List two developmental tasks of young adults.
2. Explain the importance of having a strong sense of personal identity.
3. Identify three characteristics of a successful adult.
4. Discuss three internal (developmental) challenges faced by most adults.
5. Name four stresses associated with parenting or guiding the next generation.
6. Describe how environmental challenges can limit an adult's ability to function effectively.
7. Identify two effects of a lack of social support for adults.
8. Explain how the fear of human immunodeficiency virus (HIV) and acquired immunodeficiency syndrome (AIDS) is affecting young adults.
9. Name three therapeutic interventions to help the psychosocial functioning of adults with challenges.

OUTLINE

KEY TERMS

acquired immunodeficiency syndrome (AIDS) (p. 179)
adulthood (ă-dŭlt-hood) (p. 174)
marriage (MĂR-ăj) (p. 177)
maturity (mă-CHOOR-ĭ-tē) (p. 174)

mortality (mŏ-TĂL-ĭ-tē) (p. 176)
poverty (PŎV-ĕr-tē) (p. 178)
social isolation (SŌ-shəl Ĭ-sō-lā-shŭn) (p. 179)
spiritual dimension (SPĬR-Ĭ-choo-ăl dĭ-mƒĭn-shŭn) (p. 176)

For many years, adulthood was thought of as the end of growth and development. Once adolescents reached the age of 21 years or so, they were viewed as adults, completely mature and ready to assume their full places in society. Adulthood was once considered a time of stability with little or no change. Today, however, we see adulthood as dynamic, filled with learning, struggle, rewards, and change. Adulthood is a time of personal, professional, and social development. It is the time to nurture and guide the next generation. This is a time for individuals to move beyond themselves and direct their energies for the benefit of others.

The period of life labelled **adulthood** includes ages (approximately) 18 to 65 years. **Maturity** is the ability to accept responsibility for one's actions, delay gratification, and make priorities. Remember, these divisions are for the sake of discussion. In reality, each adult is an individual who ages at their own particular pace.

Adulthood, like every other age, is filled with tasks, challenges, and opportunities for learning. Refer back to Chapter 5, and review Erikson's developmental theory and Maslow's hierarchy of needs (Fig. 5.1). All young adults are faced with the developmental tasks of establishing their careers, their identities, and the relationships that will emotionally support them throughout their lives. As they age, adults must learn to cope with changes in families, careers, and relationships. All of this is accomplished within a society so complex and interconnected that no single person is able to comprehend all its workings and effects.

ADULT GROWTH AND DEVELOPMENT

Physical growth for men is complete by about 21 years of age. Women mature earlier, reaching their full growth at around 17 years. Physical abilities are at their peak efficiency in young adulthood. Body systems have a remarkable ability to compensate, so the young adult is able to maintain a healthy state with little interruption, even during periods of illness (Edelman & Mandle, 2013). Because of this remarkable ability, young adults usually have few, if any, physical health concerns. Although many adults begin to show signs of aging after 30 years, a healthy lifestyle and the absence of any chronic conditions usually allow them to enjoy good health well into later life.

Physical growth may be complete, but adults continue to develop in other dimensions. The emotional, intellectual, sociocultural, and spiritual areas of one's character begin to receive attention. The developmental tasks of young adulthood centre on becoming fully functional and capable of living independently. Other core tasks include choosing a career or vocation, establishing long-term goals, and committing oneself to personal relationships.

For many, adulthood is also a time of change, marriage, family, and parenting. Middle adulthood sees the growth and maturity of one's family and profession. As individuals encounter each life change, they rely on previously learned behaviours to help them cope. If one has learned to solve problems effectively as a child, then adulthood will pose fewer crises. However, problems of childhood, if not resolved, can follow one through life.

Emotional development of young adults centres on learning to function within a stressful environment. Work and school offer many opportunities to cope with stress. When used positively, stress motivates young adults to achieve their goals, some of which are long term. When ignored, stress can lead to many problems. Young adults still have occasional emotional outbursts, but they attempt to find new ways of coping with the many feelings experienced during this time. Those providers who care for young adults must be willing to explore inappropriate or troublesome feelings with them. Assessments of the emotional status for all adults should include "the patient's perception of how his emotions affect his ability to develop satisfactory relationships or achieve professional goals" (Rawlins, Williams, & Beck, 1993).

Later in adulthood, emotional development deals with the struggle of seeing oneself age. Individuals who have successfully coped with life's challenges may gracefully accept and adapt to the fact that they are growing older. The anxiety generated by the prospect of a limited time on this earth motivates many middle-age adults to make the best of the benefits of middle age.

Fear of poor health, death, and loss of financial security can cause anxiety in many adults, which can result in stress-related illness and behavioural challenges. Feelings of anger can arise when interactions with work and family members are not as expected. Guilt over parents, children, and the failure to meet personal goals is often experienced. Health care providers should always assess their adult patients for signs of stress, anxiety, and depression. According to the National Alliance on Mental Illness (2019), "one in four adults . . . experiences mental illness in a given year."

Intellectual development focuses on the young adult's ability to solve intellectual and abstract problems. Young adults must process large amounts of information and learn many

---

BOX 15.1 Social Tasks of Adults

Commitment—to significant other, to career
Communications—with significant other, with children, with co-workers
Compromise—with significant other, with children, with co-workers

---

new skills to become successful in education or employment. As young adults effectively cope with their situations, their horizons broaden and they develop *flexibility*—the ability to adapt to change. This flexibility, combined with the willingness to take risks, encourages them to respond to available personal and career opportunities.

Adults continue to grow intellectually if they use their abilities to think. People who exercise their intellect have few losses of mental ability. Those who do not engage in productive mental activities may experience a decline in intellectual performance as they age. The "use it or lose it" principle associated with physical fitness also applies to the use of intellectual abilities.

Social development for young adults focuses on interactions and relationships with others (Box 15.1). If the sense of personal identity is strong and well established, individuals learn to form close personal relationships and become willing to make lasting commitments. Habits learned in childhood are likely to become lifelong. Patterns of communicating and interacting with others help to establish young adults' interactional styles, which have a strong influence on employment, relationships, and choice of goals. For example, low self-esteem and withdrawal from social situations may result from an ineffective interactional style with inadequate social or communication skills.

Establishing intimacy is an important task for young adults. Those who have a strong sense of personal identity are able to merge themselves with another in marriage or a long-term relationship. Individuals still struggling with their identities may seek serial relationships to fill their unmet psychosocial needs.

Parenting is a major challenge for most adults. The responsibilities of parenthood force an individual to shift their energies from being self-focused to caring for others. Parenthood is a 24-hour-per-day career. Its demands can create anxiety, feelings of inadequacy, and a sense of isolation and helplessness. Parents who manage both parenting and working outside the home are especially vulnerable to feeling stress. As the family unit gradually stabilizes and children begin to gain independence, parents often expand their focus beyond the immediate family or work situation and become involved in community activities.

Social tasks for adults also relate to the change from parent back to the role of partner. As children prepare for their own careers and move out of the home, the middle-age couple has the opportunity to redefine their marriage relationship. With the responsibilities of parenting over, the couple is able to re-explore their relationship with each other.

Marriages that have weathered the challenges of career and parenting are based on a solid foundation. Each partner recognizes the individuality of the other and the other's need to achieve personal growth. Couples who have *effective communication* can freely share their attitudes, opinions, and emotions. They reaffirm their commitment to each other and the relationship. Couples who are unable to communicate are frequently faced with the possibility of divorce or separation.

Compromise involves a willingness to negotiate and enter into interactions in which neither person wins nor loses. Conflicts are resolved by defining and solving the problem. The focus is kept on the issue. Couples who compromise, communicate openly, listen carefully, and try to understand their partner's point of view find that their relationship is respected and cherished.

Development within the **spiritual dimension** focuses on defining one's value system and belief system. Young adults often challenge their current religious practices by changing their place of worship (if they have one) or refusing to attend services. A re-examination of values occurs as individuals become established within the community and begin to raise families. Children offer many opportunities for parents to reflect on their values, beliefs, and ethics.

The spiritual tasks of adults are also concerned with finding meaning in life. Religious and spiritual beliefs tend to be re-examined in light of one's own **mortality** (eventually having to die). Religious, social, and community activities may become important. Volunteering to help others enriches adults' lives and provides many opportunities for socialization.

Frequently, middle-aged adults will dramatically change their lifestyles. The 40-year-old wealthy businessperson who sells everything and volunteers at a homeless shelter and the mother who begins to study for a post-secondary degree are examples. Adults who do not find meaning in their lives can become emotionally stagnant, self-absorbed, and isolated. The potential for serious mental health challenges is greater for the unhappy, self-focused adult, no matter what their age.

To summarize, adults with good mental health are able to adapt to life's changes. Once their personal identities have been established, they are capable of using life experiences as lessons in personal growth. They develop the abilities to solve problems, set priorities, and identify reasonable expectations for themselves. They form bonds with other people and become willing to devote their energies to guiding the next generation or making the world a better place in which to live. They are able to give of themselves in both intimate and social situations, and their self-confidence remains unaffected by the opinions of others. There is a balance between give and take. In short, successful adults have developed the inner strength to carry them through the joys, sorrows, and everyday activities of daily living (Box 15.2).

COMMON CHALLENGES OF ADULTHOOD

Diagnosable mental health disorders that affect adults are described in detail in later chapters. Here we consider some of the risk factors and difficulties facing every adult in today's society.

All adults cope with situations that produce anxiety. The stresses that accompany everyday life are many. Physical and psychological stress-related challenges can develop when

---

> **BOX 15.2**   **Characteristics of a Successful Adult**
>
> Accepts self
> Adapts to changes, is flexible
> Establishes priorities
> Sets realistic goals and expectations
> Learns from past experiences
> Functions in stressful circumstances
> Has achieved emotional control
> Solves problems and thinks abstractly
> Makes sound decisions
> Establishes and maintains intimate and social relationships
> Guides next generation
> Finds meaning in life
> Finds balance between give and take
> Has inner strength to effectively adapt to new situations

---

individuals become too anxious. Common difficulties that challenge adults are divided into internal and external types of problems. One's personal outlook (internal) defines stressful or anxious situations, and the environment (external) plays an important role in determining the opportunities for jobs, education, and living conditions.

Internal (Developmental) Challenges

Because life is a dynamic process, everyone must cope with change. As we do, we learn and, hopefully, develop more effective ways of living. As children, our developmental challenges are clear. As adolescents, we discover that we are unique individuals within a seemingly ever-changing body. Adults experience developmental challenges too, but theirs are not so obvious. They must cope with decisions about themselves and about relationships, education, occupation, marriage, and family. Choices made affect one's life. When adults feel they have made the right choices, they develop the inner strength to weather future storms. When they allow anxiety, anger, or other emotions to be the focus, effective adaptation does not occur as easily. Those who provide health care for adults should be aware of patients' problems and coping skills. Intervening early is a good form of preventive mental health care.

Personal Identity

Problems with establishing a strong *personal identity* begin in childhood. People who were not guided, nurtured, or accepted in childhood find it more difficult to feel good about themselves as adults. Overcoming a childhood filled with negative examples is a difficult task. It requires the willingness to look at one's behaviours and learn new methods of handling complex situations. With the support and examples of effectively functioning people, many adults are able to overcome the difficulties of their childhood. They mature into capable individuals with strong senses of personal identity and self-worth.

Care providers have many opportunities to assist individuals by offering the emotional support and encouragement to problem-solve. They can act as valued resources, directing their patients to support groups and other community

BOX 15.3 Therapeutic Interventions for a Positive Personal Identity

Assist the individual to:

Define a life dream.

Develop occupational choices and goals.

Differentiate self from the nuclear family by sorting through the beliefs and values of childhood to establish a belief system that is one's own.

Decide about relationship choices and levels of commitment, such as marriage, cohabitation, remaining single.

Assess how one's emotions influence the ability to achieve professional goals and develop healthy interpersonal relationships.

Data from Haber, J., Krainovich-Miller, B., & Leach McMahon, A. (Eds.). (1997). *Comprehensive psychiatric nursing* (5th ed.). Mosby.

resources. Helping a young adult develop a positive personal identity will lessen the possibility of future mental health challenges. Box 15.3 lists several interventions designed to help young adults establish a positive personal identity.

Problems of personal identity can also relate to a person's intellectual abilities: how one solves problems, makes decisions, and interprets stress. When an individual's ability to solve problems in effective ways is limited, behavioural and personality difficulties are much more common.

Emotional challenges are faced by all adults, but those who are able to put things into perspective usually cope with fewer stress-related effects. Mentally healthy adults can identify and accept their emotions without acting inappropriately on them. Unfortunately, anger-control problems plague many adults, especially those who were exposed to aggressive acts as children. Drug and alcohol abuse may also result from a person's need to deal with emotional difficulties, such as feelings of inadequacy, anxiety, or depression.

Cultural Identity

Cultural identity is the identification or feeling of belonging to a cultural group. It is part of a person's self-conception and self-perception and is related to nationality, ethnicity, religion, social class, generation, locality, or any kind of social group that has its own distinct culture. In this way, cultural identity is both characteristic of the individual but also of the group of people who share the same cultural identity or upbringing. Cultural identity is often a protective factor for individuals, mitigating the severity of such mental health diseases like anxiety, depression, addiction, and adjustment disorder (Gopalkrishanan, 2018). Because it provides the expectation of acceptable behavioural rules and the meaning of life, a solid cultural identity may also help with a recovery from many mental health conditions.

Interpersonal Relationships

Human beings are always changing and adapting. Young adults, who are still discovering their unique nature, also search for relationships that will fulfill their needs and encourage their personal growth. Adulthood is a time for commitment to others, be it through marriage or partnership,

family, or career. The need for intimacy and belonging is great throughout life, and adults usually form many relationships. Young adults may seek relationships in an attempt to fill a personal void or escape an unhappy situation. Sometimes errors in judgement have enormous consequences for their future.

Many adults commit themselves solely to another in marriage. In Canada, **marriage** is a legal state that bonds two people as a family unit. Most often, children are produced, and the responsibilities of life focus on nurturing and providing for the offspring. As children mature and leave home, the marriage relationship is re-evaluated and decisions are made to continue or end the relationship. Other adults choose to cohabitate (live together) in opposite-gender or same-gender relationships. LGBTQ2 families fill the same needs and engage in the same tasks as heterosexual families, but they are at greater risk for mental health challenges because of the stigma and discrimination that still exist.

Many adults (especially women) are caught in the cycle of violence that comes with abusive relationships. Despite more frequent health care visits, most women still are not screened for intimate partner violence. Chapters 25 and 26 discuss these issues in depth.

Caring for one's aging parents is fast becoming an additional role, and sometimes a challenge, for many adults. Today, members of the "sandwich generation" face the dual responsibilities of caring for their children and their aging parents at the same time. Providing care for both adds many new stresses to the family as adults work to balance the requirements of career, children, and parents.

Conflict relating to gender roles and their stereotypes can arise when adults wish to engage in activities, behaviours, or career choices that have traditionally been associated with one gender. To illustrate, a woman who wants to become a heavy equipment operator faces greater social resistance than a woman who works as a beautician.

Problems with interpersonal relationships can extend to work and social environments. Individuals who have little or no ability to see how their attitudes and behaviours affect other people often have difficulties with long-term relationships. They become superficial and unwilling to consider the feelings of others. Small problems with social relationships can balloon into serious mental health problems. Learning effective communication and interpersonal skills can spell the difference between a functional adult and an unhappy, unfulfilled adult. Nurses and other care providers can play an important role in preventing mental illness by identifying those patients with interpersonal problems and offering them support, education, and resources.

Guiding the Next Generation

Most adults have children, and children are not isolated events. They arrive as package deals, along with responsibility, fatigue, self-doubt, love, and joy. If pregnancies are planned, children are eagerly anticipated. Unplanned pregnancies, however, are stressful and sometimes unwanted. Choices about terminating the pregnancy, single parenting, or marrying for the sake of the child are decisions faced by unmarried adults that will influence the rest of their lives.

BOX 15.4 Factors That Influence Child-Rearing Practices

Family relationships
Financial status
Health practices
Housing, living environment, safety
Parenting styles
Socialization with others
Spiritual beliefs
Type of discipline

The child-rearing practices of adults vary considerably. Most parents raise their offspring based on how they were treated as children. Parents who were strongly disciplined as children tend to use physical discipline when correcting their children. Likewise, adults who were disciplined in nonphysical ways will likely continue these practices with their offspring. Other factors such as money, family relationships, safety, housing, health practices, and spiritual beliefs all affect the family, parenting practices, and children. For example, relationships between individuals and with extended family members, as well as social interactions, can support or discourage certain child-rearing habits. Box 15.4 lists several factors that influence child-rearing practices.

The rise of the lone-parent family also needs consideration here. Today, more households in Canada are headed by women alone (Statistics Canada, 2015). In these families, the single parent must function as parent and as provider. The joys of children can be overshadowed by the work and stress of providing for them. Without support and intervention, these families have a high potential for developing several mental health challenges.

Single parenthood can also be a positive experience. The conflict of different outlooks about child-rearing practices is not present. Providing the guidance that allows children to experience life in positive ways and securing environments free from adult conflicts are other rewards of single parenthood.

With remarriages (blended families) and some adoptive families, children and adults who were once strangers instantly become relatives "without the shared experience of developing their parent–child relationship over time" (Stanhope & Lancaster, 2016). These families must establish new relationships, roles, and family boundaries. Sometimes they must cope with a biological parent living outside the family.

Childless adults can contribute to the next generation through devotion to a career or volunteer activities. The need to share and leave one's mark increases by middle adulthood.

Economics

One of the greatest stressors for adults of all ages is financial security. Young adults must choose a vocation or profession that offers an opportunity to provide the necessities of life. Food, shelter, and clothing cost money, a fact that many young adults fail to learn until they leave the security of the

family. Decisions about education and training, made young in life, will affect the quality of living far into the future.

Unemployment is a multisided problem. A parent who does not work becomes unable to financially provide for their children. Loss of self-esteem and self-worth can accompany loss of employment. This absence of a regular income along with its associated stresses can start the family on a downward spiral that may include poverty, physical illness, and psychosocial disorders. A stressful family environment with an unemployed head of household is sometimes associated with child neglect, maltreatment, and abuse. Care providers can play an important role in assisting families in finding support and retraining services.

Although adults experience many challenges, most learn to cope with each problem and apply lessons learned to the next difficulty they face. As time passes, the inner strength built through experience becomes a part of who we are. This inner strength provides encouragement to grow and expand beyond the limits of who we are today.

External (Environmental) Challenges

The environment plays a strong role in the development of an individual during childhood. In adulthood, one's environment can limit or encourage further development. Some of the major environmental problems affecting adults today include a lack of education, poverty, homelessness, substance abuse, infection with human immunodeficiency virus (HIV) or the coronavirus, living with acquired immunodeficiency syndrome (AIDS) or some other chronic illness, the effects of climate change, and lack of social support. Each of these conditions can have a strong influence on the mental health of adults. Health care providers should be aware of these problems.

Education

An individual's training or education is closely associated with their economic status. Less educated people tend to be poorer, with little savings or financial reserves. Many families live from paycheque to paycheque, where one small demand (e.g., the car breaking down or a sick child) can throw the family into financial turmoil. Adults who are vocationally trained or educated tend to have more financial and health care resources and are better able to cope with everyday problems. As a care provider, you can encourage your patients to seek further education or training by referring them to various community agencies that offer help or training. A lack of education can limit opportunities and thus foster more stress.

The result of unemployment (or underemployment) is poverty. **Poverty** is the lack of resources necessary for reasonable and comfortable living. Poverty means unstable housing, poor educational opportunities, work problems, and an increased risk for becoming a victim. Adults who survive below the poverty line often have children who suffer because of their parents' misfortune. Poverty, homelessness, and a lack of education often go hand in hand. Adults who must cope with this three-pronged dilemma usually need support and intervention.

People who are homeless in Canada are a diverse group. Many are single men, but 27.3% are homeless women and children, 18.7% are youth, and 28 to 34% are Indigenous (Gaetz, Dej, Richter, et al., 2016). Many chronically mentally ill people inhabit the streets because they are unable to use their resources wisely. Discouraged by their prospects and living with the social stigma of being homeless, homeless individuals run a much greater risk for depression, drug abuse, and other mental health disorders. Homeless people have special health care needs. Health care interventions must consider each individual's situation and lifestyle. Therapeutic actions are effective when they are realistic and attainable.

CASE STUDY

Joan is a nurse in a centre for homeless people located in a large Canadian city. She describes the qualifications necessary for her position: patience, persistence, and the ability to apply creative approaches to patient care challenges. Her role is one of facilitator and advocate who helps patients gain access to other services in the community. She ensures that each person is clean and presentable when requesting services. Although the shelter provides shower and laundry facilities, Joan makes sure everyone uses the toothbrushes, deodorant, soap, and razors.

She reschedules missed appointments for her homeless patients, providing for transportation if necessary. Clarifying instructions from other agencies and helping patients with job applications are also on her list of caregiving interventions. Every opportunity to provide patient education is taken. Joan instructs her homeless patients on the importance of good nutrition, safer sexual practices, communicable diseases, and other health-related subjects. She works with each individual to set and reach realistic goals. She sees every person as worthy of respect and dignity. Although her successes may be small, "hearing someone express that since he was able to get help for his problems, he now feels better about himself and is motivated to change his lifestyle provides this nurse's personal reward and professional satisfaction in working with the homeless" (Foster, 1992).

- According to Maslow, what needs is Joan helping her patients fulfill? (Refer to Chapter 5.)
- What resources are available for homeless people in your community?

Lack of Social Support

Perhaps one of the most distressing problems for adults is **social isolation**—a lack of meaningful interactions with others. Before the time of rapid transportation, families tended to remain in one geographic area for generations. Small communities were often composed of relatives and extended family members who could provide strong emotional and social support during difficult times. People shared their anxieties, hopes, and difficulties with one another and received the emotional support and energy to cope with their problems.

Today, families live physically apart from one another—surviving as isolated, single units. The social interconnectedness that bonded people together in the past is no longer intact. Adults must establish new connections, new relationships, and new support systems each time they move

to a different community. When these new connections are not made, people can feel socially isolated and disconnected from their fellow human beings. The recent requirement to maintain physical distancing and isolation in response to the COVID-19 (coronavirus disease 2019) threat risks instilling or exasperating feelings of social disconnection from others within our society.

Social support is the friendship from others that helps carry individuals through life's more difficult moments. With trusted friends, adults can share their problems, concerns, and stresses. These interactions can make the difference between mental health and illness. As a health care provider, be sure to assess patients' social support systems (ask about friendships, and help them identify possible support people, such as neighbors or co-workers). Refer them to various support or community groups as needed. Remember that social isolation is not healthy for human beings. Acknowledging this fact can help prevent many future mental health difficulties.

Acquired Immunodeficiency Syndrome

Acquired immunodeficiency syndrome (AIDS) was first recognized in the United States in 1981. Since then, millions of people, especially adolescents and young adults, have been exposed to this devastating disease. It is spread through sexual activities, the sharing of needles, or exposure to blood and body fluids. AIDS prevents the body from fighting off infectious diseases, and its signs and symptoms are not apparent for many years in some cases.

People with AIDS often have vague physical issues, such as night sweats, cough, weight loss, or fever. Other problems can include ear, nose, throat, or stomach complaints or skin changes. About one third suffer from anxiety, depression, or lapses in memory.

While AIDS has an impact on all members of society, it is especially felt among sexually active young adults. People this age are more vulnerable to contracting the disease because they lack the emotional maturity and judgement to make sound decisions and they feel the invulnerability of youth—the attitude that "it will never happen to me." Only when a friend or loved one contracts the disease does its reality strike home. Adults who can appreciate the seriousness of the disease have made changes in their lifestyles or suffer the anxieties associated with high-risk behaviours.

Fear of AIDS has spread to persons whose lifestyles offer little likelihood of contracting the disease. The acronym *AFRAIDS* (acute fear regarding AIDS) has been coined to describe an anxiety-related condition caused by a fear of AIDS. Individuals with poor or marginal coping skills may find it difficult to deal with the emotional aspects of this epidemic.

Every health care provider has a responsibility to educate patients about AIDS. The most important tool for the prevention of this devastating disease is education. Knowledge can be a powerful weapon if it leads individuals toward making health-promoting decisions. Knowledge can also decrease fear and anxiety. When patients know the symptoms of a

BOX 15.5   Common Adult Mental Health Disorders

Adjustment disorders
Anxiety disorders
Cognitive disorders: delirium, dementia, amnesia
Dissociative disorders
Eating disorders
Factitious disorders
Impulse-control disorders
Mental disorders resulting from a general medical condition
Mood disorders
Personality disorders
Schizophrenia and other psychotic disorders
Sexual and gender identity disorders
Sleep disorders
Somatoform disorders
Substance-related disorders

disease and how it is transmitted they are better able to discern the need for diagnosis and treatment. AIDS has many physical consequences, but its psychosocial and emotional effects can be equally devastating. This also holds for the more recent pandemic of COVID-19.

There are many potential health problems, both physical and mental, in the adult world. Decisions made regarding oneself and one's environment have greater consequences than they did during earlier years. Health care providers working with adult patients can find many opportunities to encourage and teach healthy living practices, which in turn can prevent future problems from developing.

MENTAL HEALTH CHALLENGES OF ADULTS

A great number of the mental health disorders experienced by adults have their roots in childhood. Adults who were diagnosed in childhood with attention deficit/hyperactivity disorder (ADHD), conduct disorders, or learning disorders must now learn to cope with the responsibilities of adulthood. Many become substance abusers, others become members of the prison system, and a few progress toward successful adulthood.

It is sobering to think that 25% of the adult population has some diagnosable mental disorder (Centre for Addiction and Mental Health [CAMH], 2020), and one in three Canadians experience mental illness at some point during their lifetime (Government of Canada, 2017). Millions of adults are struggling with depression or addictions (alcohol, drugs, gambling, shopping). Box 15.5 lists the most common adult mental health challenges.

All adults must cope with the problems and crises of everyday living. Health care providers have countless opportunities to provide the psychosocial care so needed by so many. Remember that beyond the diagnostic label lies an individual. If care providers are willing to put aside their biases and values, they will do much to encourage higher levels of functioning in each patient.

Therapeutic Interventions

Although specific interventions for each mental health disorder are described in later chapters, a look at the interventions available in every practice setting may be helpful. The focus of most therapeutic mental health interventions relates to prevention and assisting patients to cope.

Health Care Interventions

When working with adults, nurses can use their assessment skills to enable patients' descriptions of their difficulties. Frequently, the physician or nurse will actively intervene with a problem that is not as important to a patient as it is to the health care provider. Make sure patients are allowed to define their problems, which may include using their own words and terminology to express their understanding of it. Therapeutic actions will have greater results if the goals of care are as important to the patient as they are to the health care provider. Sample Patient Care Plan 15.1 for an adult with situational problems offers some suggestions for interventions.

It is important to work within the patient's reality. Learn about the patient's living conditions. Assess the cultural influences relating to the patient. It does no good to instruct a patient to take medication four times daily if they have no watch or other means of telling time. Too many therapeutic interventions fail because the patient's total situation is not considered.

CULTURAL CONSIDERATIONS

Culture has a powerful influence on one's outlook relating to health and illness, especially mental illness. Some Inuit people, for example, explain bizarre behaviour by spirit possession. People in Burundi define illness as having insufficient food and poor hygiene. In the Dominican Republic, it is believed that people with the "evil eye" can cause illness in others, especially children. Health care providers must consider each patient's cultural beliefs if treatment is to be effective.

Give patients *written instructions* if you expect educational efforts to be effective. Everyone experiences anxiety when interacting with the health care system. People do not remember information when they are under stress. Written instructions allow them to refer back to the information when they are less anxious and more willing to follow instructions.

Preventing Mental Illness

Health care providers in every setting can do much to prevent mental–emotional disorders. Always remember it is the whole person who receives our care. We may separate the human being into parts, but we must consider and treat the entire person.

Each physical illness has emotional components, and each mental disorder is accompanied by physical changes. Therapeutic interventions need to include all aspects of the patient's problems. A positive step toward preventing mental illness is to recognize the need for making mental health interventions available for all individuals, not just those people who are "diagnosed" with a mental disorder.

SAMPLE PATIENT CARE PLAN 15.1   Ineffective Coping

Assessment

History Abdul is a 33-year-old man who has recently lost his job and his wife and is now being sued. Last night, he had several drinks before driving home. His car ran off an embankment and rolled into an irrigation ditch. Abdul was found uninjured, sleeping in the car early this morning. He has been referred to the clinic for evaluation.

Current Findings In no acute distress; several bruises on arms and face; odour of alcohol. Abdul states that 6 months ago his business as a roofer failed. After 4 months of trying to find employment, Abdul began to drink. One evening, he and his wife had an argument. When he returned later that night, she had moved her personal belongings out of the house and left a note saying that his drinking was becoming more than she could tolerate. For the past 2 months, Abdul has been spending his time "getting drunk."

Multidisciplinary Diagnosis

Alcohol use disorder related to loss of support systems

Planning/Goals

Abdul will remain sober throughout treatment.
Abdul will attend Alcoholics Anonymous meetings every evening.
Abdul will recognize his maladaptive behaviours and take action to solve his identified problems by July 10.

THERAPEUTIC INTERVENTIONS

Interventions	Rationale	Team Member
1. Establish a trusting relationship with Abdul.	Trust must be present if problems are to be solved.	All
2. Assess for degree of anxiety, depression, and intent to do self-harm.	To determine interventions needed; to understand Abdul's viewpoint.	All
3. Help Abdul identify each of his problems and current coping mechanisms.	Problems must be defined before they can be solved.	Psy, Nsg
4. Have Abdul make a list of his available resources and support systems.	Use of previously successful coping mechanism helps develop multiple skills.	Soc Svc
5. Replace the use of alcohol with crisis support person and phone number to call at any time.	Abdul knows his drinking is an excuse to forget about his problems and is willing to call his support person when he wants a drink.	Nsg, Soc Svc
6. Help Abdul devise new, more effective coping responses.	Builds on Abdul's current abilities to solve problems.	All
7. Refer to social services for placement in the employment program.	Provides new resources for exploring job availability and opportunities.	

Evaluation During the first 3 weeks of clinic visits, Abdul had been drinking. By the fourth week, he had decided to quit drinking so that he could concentrate on "getting his life back together." By the sixth week, Abdul was able to identify two of his most pressing problems.

Critical Thinking Questions

1. What strategies should Abdul and his care providers devise to keep him from using alcohol as a coping mechanism?
2. How does establishing a trusting relationship with Abdul help him solve his problems?

A complete patient care plan includes several other diagnoses and interventions.
Nsg, nursing staff; *Psy*, psychologist; *Soc Svc*, social services.

KEY POINTS

- Adults continue to develop the emotional, intellectual, sociocultural, and spiritual dimensions of their character long after physical growth is completed.
- Developmental tasks of young adults include choosing a career or vocation, establishing long-term goals, and committing to personal relationships with others.
- Parenting provides many challenges for most adults.
- Adults who are responsible for their behaviour, use effective communications, are willing to make commitments, and cooperate with others successfully adapt to life's changes.
- If an individual's sense of personal identity is strong and well established, they learn to form close personal relationships.
- Developmental challenges faced by most adults include decisions about themselves, their relationships, education, occupation, marriage, and family.
- The family, parenting practices, and children are affected by factors such as money, family relationships, safety, housing, health practices, and spiritual beliefs.
- Some of the major environmental problems affecting adults today include a lack of education, poverty, homelessness, substance abuse, and minimal social support.

- People feel socially isolated and disconnected without social support. Without trusted friends, adults cannot share their problems, concerns, and stresses.
- The acronym AFRAIDS (acute fear regarding AIDS) has been coined to describe an anxiety-related condition caused by fear of AIDS.
- Each physical illness has emotional components, and each mental disorder is accompanied by physical changes.

- Basic therapeutic interventions allow care providers to elicit the patient's definitions of their problems, work within the patient's reality, and provide written instructions during educational efforts.
- Health care providers must recognize the need for making mental health interventions available for all patients.

ADDITIONAL LEARNING RESOURCES

Go to your Evolve website (http://evolve.elsevier.com/Canada/Morrison-Valfre/) for additional online resources, including the online Study Guide for additional learning activities to help you master this chapter content.

CRITICAL THINKING QUESTIONS

1. Your cousin is 28 and still lives at home with his parents. His room is in the basement. He spends most of his time in his room, reading or engaging in online role-playing games. He is currently unemployed and doesn't express much interest in securing employment. You are aware that his mother provides him with an "allowance," but she disclosed to you that she is beginning to resent doing so. According to Erikson's theory of psychosocial development, what developmental task(s) is your cousin not meeting? What possible repercussions could this have for him?

2. How would elements such as culture, financial status, occupation, religion, and ethnicity contribute to a person's self-concept? Which of these elements are more important at different stages of life?

3. You and a friend pass by a homeless man on the street. He is asking passersby for spare change. You observe that he looks clean and that his clothing is also clean. Your friend comments, "There's no way that guy is homeless, he looks too hygienic!" Based on what you know about the homeless, do you think your friend's statement is correct?

REFERENCES

Centre for Addiction and Mental Health (CAMH). (2020). *Mental illness and addiction: Facts and statistics.* https://www.camh.ca/en/driving-change/the-crisis-is-real/mental-health-statistics

Edelman, C. L., & Mandle, C. L. (2013). *Health promotion throughout the lifespan* (8th ed.). Mosby.

Foster, J. (1992). The nurse in a center for the homeless. *Nursing Management, 23*(4), 38–39 [Seminal Reference].

Gaetz, S., Dej, E., Richter, T., et al. (2016). *The state of homelessness in Canada 2016.* Canadian Observatory on Homelessness Press. https://homelesshub.ca/sites/default/files/SOHC16_final_20Oct2016.pdf

Gopalkrishanan, N. (2018). Cultural diversity and mental health: Considerations for policy and practice. *Frontiers in Public Health, 6,* 179–195. https://doi.org/10.3389/fpubh.2018.00179

Government of Canada. (2017). About mental illness. https://www.canada.ca/en/public-health/services/about-mental-illness.html

National Alliance on Mental Illness. (2019). Mental health by the numbers. https://www.nami.org/mhstats

Rawlins, R. P., Williams, S. R., & Beck, C. K. (1993). *Mental health–psychiatric nursing: A holistic life-cycle approach* (3rd ed.). Mosby [Seminal Reference].

Stanhope, M., & Lancaster, J. (2016). *Public health nursing: Population-centered health care in the community* (9th ed.). Mosby.

Statistics Canada. (2015). Lone-parent families. Insights on Canadian Society (Cat. No. 75-006-X). Author. https://www150.statcan.gc.ca/n1/pub/75-006-x/2015001/article/14202/parent-eng.htm

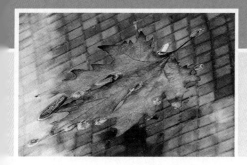

16

Challenges of Late Adulthood

OBJECTIVES

Upon completion of this chapter, the student will be able to:

1. Examine the facts relating to three myths associated with aging.
2. Identify three mental and behavioural changes seen in older persons.
3. Explain how a lack of finances or access to health care affects the mental health of older persons.
4. Describe the drug misuse (abuse) patterns of older persons.
5. Define the term *elder abuse* and describe a typical victim.
6. Explain how depression can affect older persons' abilities to function.
7. Identify three interventions that help older persons learn.
8. Identify three therapeutic interventions that promote mental health in older persons.

OUTLINE

KEY TERMS

ageism (ĀJ-ĭsm) (p. 185)
aging (Ā-jēng) (p. 183)
delirium (p. 191)
dementia (p. 191)
depression (p. 191)
elder abuse (ĕl-dər ă-BŪS) (p. 191)
functional assessment (FŬNK-shŭn-əl ă-SĔS-mĕnt) (p. 192)

gerontophobia (GĔR-ŏn-tō-FŌ-bē-ə) (p. 185)
hoarding (HŌR-dēng) (p. 189)
integrity (ĭn-TĔG-rĭ-tē) (p. 185)
memory loss (MĔM-ŏr-ē lŏs) (p. 192)
neuroplasticity (noo r-oh-PLA-stici-tee) (p. 185)
polypharmacy (pol-ee-FAHR-muh-see) (p. 189)

Aging is the process of growing older. Older adulthood, or *maturity,* is the period in life from 65 years of age until death. Until recently, people older than 65 years were seen as "old," but our ideas of aging have changed. We now consider more than the number of years an individual has been alive. There are several theories or ideas about the aging process. Biological theories attempt to explain why we age physically, including what changes happen in our brains. These changes, among other things, impact the formation of new stimuli and functioning of old conditional stimuli, and, as a result, our psychosocial health. This chapter focuses on the psychosocial

adaptations made by us all as we age and the mental health disorders that commonly affect older persons.

OVERVIEW OF AGING

The aging process begins at birth, but few signs are noted until well into middle age. With the passage of time, however, changes become apparent. Physical maturity is replaced by the aging process. These are the senior citizen, geriatric, or elderly years. This is a time when outlooks can range from deep satisfaction and happiness to despair and sadness (Fig. 16.1).

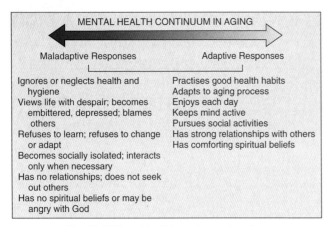

MENTAL HEALTH CONTINUUM IN AGING

Maladaptive Responses | Adaptive Responses

Maladaptive Responses	Adaptive Responses
Ignores or neglects health and hygiene	Practises good health habits
Views life with despair; becomes embittered, depressed; blames others	Adapts to aging process
	Enjoys each day
Refuses to learn; refuses to change or adapt	Keeps mind active
	Pursues social activities
Becomes socially isolated; interacts only when necessary	Has strong relationships with others
	Has comforting spiritual beliefs
Has no relationships; does not seek out others	
Has no spiritual beliefs or may be angry with God	

Fig. 16.1 Mental health continuum in aging.

BOX 16.1 Changing Statistics for Older Persons in Canada

There are now 5.9 million older Canadians, compared to 5.8 million Canadians aged 14 and under.

By 2031, about 23% of the Canadian population will be older persons, similar to Japan, which has the world's largest percentage of older persons.

By 2061, there could be 12 million older persons, compared to only 8 million children in Canada.

In 1966, there were twice as many people entering the labour market as there were heading for retirement. Today, there are just 4.3 million Canadians between the ages of 15 and 24, compared to 4.9 million Canadians aged 55–64.

Data from Grenier, E. (2017). Canadian older persons now outnumber children for 1st time, 2016 census shows. *CBC News,* May 7. https://www.cbc.ca/news/politics/2016-census-age-gender-1.4095360

Canadians aged 65 and older represent 16.9% of the population. One in five Canadians aged 65 and older (or nearly 1.1 million older persons) reported working during the past year. Highly educated older persons were more likely to work longer than their less educated counterparts: 3 in 10 older persons with a bachelor's degree or higher worked in 2015, twice the percentage of those with a high school diploma or less (Statistics Canada, 2019). It is estimated that the percentage of older persons (aged 65 and older) will almost double in Canada within the next 25 years: from 14.1% in 2010 to 23 to 25% by 2036 (Statistics Canada, 2019) (Box 16.1).

Today, because of scientific, medical, and technological advances, we are living longer and enjoying better health than our ancestors did (Fig. 16.2).

Facts and Myths of Aging

Many people carry mental pictures or myths of older persons as people who are wearing out, biding their time until the inescapable end arrives. These are myths—beliefs based on little or no fact. In reality, the majority of older persons are dynamic individuals, living within their homes, and functioning successfully within their communities (Edelman & Kudzma, 2018).

Another myth is that elders live in nursing homes. In reality, the majority of older persons live outside institutions. More than half of adults over 65 years of age are still living at home with a spouse. Many maintain their households alone.

"The majority of the elderly are poor" and "the majority of the elderly are rich" are two myths that explode on further examination. The economic status of older persons is as varied as that of any other age group. Perhaps the cruellest myth, however, is that the ideals of the young and attractive are "good," whereas the old and imperfect are "bad." Today's modern society places little value on its elders. Other cultures hold older persons in high esteem and value their wisdom and experience (Giger & Haddad, 2020).

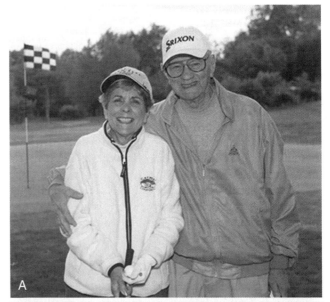

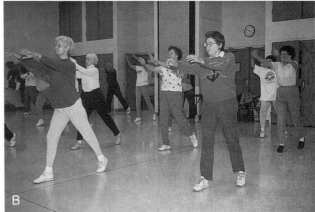

Fig. 16.2 Older adulthood can be a rewarding time. (A, B, from Sorrentino, S. A. [2011]. *Long-term care assistants* [6th ed.]. Mosby.)

CULTURAL CONSIDERATIONS

In traditional Korean families, elders hold a high place of honour. The responsibility of caring for them in old age falls to the firstborn son, who inherits the family leadership and most of the property.

The Japanese have close ties between the generations. Care of older individuals traditionally falls to the oldest son or an unmarried adult in the family. Until recently, there were few long-term care facilities for aged people in Japan.

Indigenous people often turn to their Elders for traditional, historical, and cultural knowledge. Indigenous older persons have lived through many changes in their communities, and they are considered an important link to the teachings of the past.

The Chinese value the family and consider it their responsibility to care for their elders. Older Chinese family members are respected and obeyed. Decisions are made through agreement of family members.

Black Canadians have large support groups that offer help and comfort for their older members.

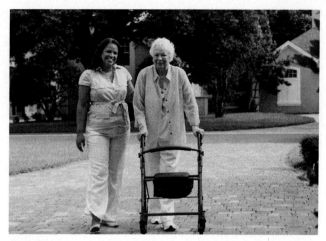

Fig. 16.3 Decreased sensory abilities and function. (iStockphoto/kali9)

It is difficult for young people to imagine growing old. As they mature, adults and children alike are routinely exposed to the negative aspects of aging. Through the years, a fear of growing old develops and anything associated with aging becomes something to avoid. The fear of aging and refusal to accept older persons into the mainstream of society is known as **gerontophobia** (Williams, 2019). This attitude leads to **ageism**, a practice of stereotyping older persons as feeble, dependent, and nonproductive. It is important for health care providers to look at their own attitudes and values about aging. For example, a Canadian study found that patients older than 65 often have to wait for their spinal surgery twice as long as younger Canadians (Ahn, Bailey, Rivers, et al., 2015).

The journey through life is, for the most part, taken as an adult, swimming through the currents of change.

Physical Health Changes

As an individual ages, so too does every body system. The physical changes of aging are not noticeable until the late 30s. By the 50s, one cannot deny the effects of time. Signs of aging continue to show themselves until around 85 years of age. After that, people appear to age little.

The physical aging process varies greatly. It is affected by genetics, early physical and mental health care, current lifestyle practices, and attitude. Refer to a basic text for a discussion of the physical changes that are associated with normal aging. Figure 16.3 shows one effect of decreasing sensory abilities in an older woman.

Mental Health Changes

Older adulthood is a time for adjusting to change, or adaptation. Developmental tasks at this stage are challenging. According to Erikson, older persons who have developed a sense of personal **integrity** (state of wholeness) accept the worth and uniqueness of their lifestyles. They are able to find order and meaning in their lives. A sense of the flow of time (past, present, future) allows them to face life's challenges with grace and inner strength. They know they will survive because they have so many times in the past. If relationships with their children have been positive, they tend to experience love and respect from their offspring. In short, the older person is able to accept their life (as it actually was and is) and value the contributions that they have made.

For older persons who have not reached a sense of wholeness, life can be filled with despair. Individuals may become unhappy and feel that life has been a waste. They focus on what might have been. They blame others for life's misfortunes. A sense of loss and contempt for other people can lead these older persons to a sad and lonely lifestyle.

Mental health changes in older persons have been the subject of much recent study. The popular belief was that mental abilities decrease slowly with advancing age. The truth, we are learning, is not so simple. Some mental functions peak in childhood and others in adolescence. Although short-term memory and mental speed begin to decline in the 40s, mental capabilities, such as judgement and wisdom, continue to improve as one grows older. Research over the past decades shows that the mind constantly adjusts its way of doing things and compensates nicely for any losses in efficiency. Table 16.1 lists several mental changes associated with aging and their resultant behaviours.

Research and Aging

Recent research findings are changing our knowledge about the aging process. Aging is no longer considered a natural decline in health and abilities. One exciting new view in science is that the brain is "actually neuroplastic (**neuroplasticity**)—meaning that its circuits are constantly changing in response to what we actually do out in the world. As we

TABLE 16.1   Mental Changes Associated With Aging

Area of Function	Behaviours Associated With Aging
Attention: Alertness, maintaining focus, noticing	Attention declines slowly after age 70 but remains intact with practice; becomes easy to distract
Cognitive style: Ability to adapt, to roll with punches	Mental decline is more rapid in people who are rigid; adaptability in midlife reduces risk for mental decline
Crystallized intelligence: Specialized accumulated knowledge (nursing, engineering, technical skills)	Remains intact until 75 years or older; may possibly remain intact until death; learning abilities remain intact, especially with physical exercise
Episodic memory: Ability to register and store memories of events in time and space, to retrieve memories	Retains memories of recent events when able to anchor them to own experiences, knowledge base; long-term memory better than short-term memory
Information processing: Ability to relate to, store, and retrieve information	Processing speed decreases with age; may take longer to retrieve information; needs time to process information
Learning new tasks	Learning enhances many mental functions; people who do not continue to learn experience slowing and decline in many areas (which is reversible when one resumes learning)
Memory: Names and faces	Decreases fairly rapidly in middle age; often considered worse than truly is; like people of all ages, older persons process information by associating it to related data
Metamemory: Judgement of one's ability to monitor and control one's own mental processes	After age 40, older persons make conscious efforts to learn, manage, store, and remember new information; metamemory remains active in older persons who use their intelligence and lead active lives
Mood: Emotions, feelings	People with frequent negative emotions have a higher incidence of depression; depression caused by loss is common in older persons
Perceptual speed: Ability to become alert and respond	Perceptual speed slows after age 50, but may not be noticed; older persons score lower on timed tests but better on others
Personality: Behavioural traits that make one a unique individual	Personality is established in childhood and remains stable throughout life; if one was a happy child, one is usually a happy older person
Reasoning: Ability to solve problems and make choices, comparisons, and judgements	Great individual differences between 60 and 80 years; after age 80, some loss is noticed; people with active mental lives decline more slowly
Retrieval of information: Ability to bring stored information into active consciousness	Takes longer after age 50; more errors in retrieving; as persons age, there are more data to match up; slower information retrieval is sign of rich, well-stocked memory
Working memory: Random access memory; memory to which one refers	Increases through childhood and peaks during early adulthood; because the brain is neuroplastic, it strengthens with use

think, perceive, form memories or learn new skills, the connections between brain cells also change and strengthen" (Doidge, 2015). Other studies have found that regular physical and mental exercise lowers the risk for developing dementia and slows the aging process. Regular meditation has also been found to improve well-being. Socializing with others has been found to be effective for both physical and psychological health. As new discoveries are made, our ideas about and journeys into aging will be filled with new learning.

COMMON CHALLENGES OF OLDER PERSONS

Older persons cope with many changes. They must adjust to physical changes that accompany the passage of time. They learn to cope with losses through the deaths of a spouse, family, and friends. Retirement can bring a loss of income and opportunities for socialization. Living arrangements may need to be changed, and relationships with adult children are often redefined. Sometimes, several losses occur at the same time. For example, the individual who has just suffered a stroke (brain attack, cerebrovascular accident [CVA]) faces losses of function, physical health, mobility, body image, and independence at the same time. Losses that occur at the same time can seriously decrease the older person's ability to cope effectively. For some older persons, adaptation to change comes easily and without discomfort. For others, however, each life change is stormy and produces major stresses.

Health care providers, especially those in the nursing profession, play a major role in caring for older persons. As the population ages, health care providers will be called on to assist many patients in coping with the changes of growing older.

One common occurrence among older persons is falls; it is estimated that 10% of all falls among older persons result in a serious injury (Abraham & Cimino-Fiallos, 2019). There are many conditions that may contribute to an elevated risk of falls. Often, older patients take medications that can cause orthostatic hypotension (a rapid drop in blood pressure). Teaching older patients about making gradual, slow position changes can be helpful. Ensuring that they have an uncluttered, wireless, and even floor surface can help prevent falls, too.

Older male patients frequently experience micturition syncope (the temporary loss of consciousness upon urinating). Teaching older males about the need to sit while urinating, especially at night, can prevent that condition.

Physical Adaptations

Because of normal changes associated with aging, many people believe that an inability to perform physical activity is the natural result of growing older. However, much research has pointed to the importance of remaining physically active throughout life. Aerobic and muscle-strengthening exercises can prevent many of the physical problems associated with aging. Although a 70-year-old man cannot perform the same amount of physical labour in the same time a 30-year-old man does, he can perform the same amount if given extra time. The task will be done—it just takes longer. It is important to encourage daily physical activity in every patient. A sound physical body has a better chance of housing a sound psychosocial "body."

Besides changes in endurance and the ability to do physical work, older persons must cope with a body that wants to adjust itself to a new routine. Changes in eating and sleeping patterns take place as one ages. Once, one was able to sleep through the night. Now, some need or another often awakens the older person. One used to be able to eat anything, and now antacids are placed at strategic locations throughout the house. The volume on the television creeps up; lights are adjusted to decrease the glare; and the odours drifting from the kitchen while awaiting dinner seem to be less inviting. Even without the problems of a chronic illness, older persons must adjust to the small, everyday physical changes of aging.

Older persons face many alterations in their lifestyles that may affect them physically. Individuals who live alone, for example, tend to neglect their nutritional needs. They may eat too much or not enough. Too often, they use their limited finances to buy costly, empty-calorie foods. Many older persons are not physically able to prepare their meals. Others suffer from sensory, dental, or digestive problems. Over time, the lack of adequate food intake results in chronic malnutrition. Resistance to the effects of stress and disease drops, and the risk for serious health problems increases.

Canada's Dietary Guidelines are helpful for ensuring a healthy diet. They recommend a healthy diet that is based on vegetables, fruit, whole grains, and protein foods, which should be consumed regularly. Among protein foods, plant-based foods should be consumed more often. Foods that contain mostly unsaturated fat should replace foods that contain mostly saturated fat (Government of Canada, 2019a).

CASE STUDY

Stefan was 70 years old when he lost his beloved Christina, his wife of 52 years. They met while they were still in high school, married soon after the war, and vowed never to be apart again. Four children filled the years with joy and hard work, and retirement was packed with new friends and experiences. But once Christina was gone, life for Stefan became filled with gloom. He no longer sought out his longtime friends and stopped playing golf or horseshoes. He sold the motor home and retired into his darkened living room. Well-meaning friends often stopped by, but by the time they departed, they had taken on Stefan's gloom instead of cheering him up.

Soon Stefan stopped eating. Christina had always prepared his meals, and he felt lost and unhappy every time he walked into the kitchen where Christina had spent so many hours. By the time his daughter visited Stefan, he was confused and unable to care for himself. Assuming he had suffered a stroke, Stefan's children admitted him to a long-term care facility.
- Describe early interventions that could have prevented Stefan from being removed from his home.

Sexuality remains important for many older persons. The focus shifts from having children to an expression of caring, intimate communication, and sharing. Adaptations may be needed in the expression of sexuality because of physical limits or chronic health problems. A decrease in hormone levels leads to physical changes in the reproductive systems of older persons, but both men and women are capable of remaining sexually active well into their 90s.

Physical adaptations to aging include the loss of ability to move about freely. Losing a driver's license has a strong effect on one's independence and ability to provide for the necessities of living. Without private or public transportation, many older people are severely restricted in their abilities to move freely about the community.

Adapting to the physical changes of aging can pose many problems that place an individual at higher risk for mental health disorders. Physical problems can lead to changes in mental status. Older persons commonly have vague, nonspecific physical signs and symptoms that may mask a mental health disorder. Medication–medication interactions, food–medication interactions, or medication adverse effects can cause both physical and psychological problems. Every health care provider who works with older persons must be alert for the existence of physical problems. Early assessment and intervention are essential for keeping older persons' minor problems from becoming major ones.

Health Care Services

The availability of health care is an important factor in maintaining the health of older persons. In Canada, all provinces and territories have publicly funded medical health insurance, but it does not include prescription drugs; however, all of them have some form of drug coverage program for their older citizens (Government of Canada, 2017).

Provincial medical insurance recipients are required to cover some out-of-pocket expenses, such as some medication costs and associated deductible and coinsurance costs. Many older individuals place their health care needs in the background when they are unable to afford the costs.

Health services may be available and affordable, but without transportation, visits to health care providers are few. Older persons who live alone or have sensory impairments can find it difficult to obtain health services because of the obstacles they must overcome. Periods of confusion and forgetfulness may cloud an older person's ability to follow therapeutic instructions, and many confused people attempt to disguise their problem by being cooperative and voicing understanding.

Psychosocial Adaptations

In today's world, growing old has become more impersonal. The comforts of family and friends may be miles away. Older persons may have difficulties relating to money, adequate food and housing, or health care. The loss of loved ones, social status, and earning power withers social support systems, and decreasing sensory abilities leave many older persons questioning the soundness of their judgements.

Scientists have found loneliness to be a major issue that negatively affects adults during all stages of life. Yet, for persons aged 80 and older, loneliness is the most dangerous risk factor for poor health. The exact connection is still unclear, but the assumption is that loneliness impacts our capacity to deal with stress, which leads to elevated levels of stress hormones that negatively affect all body functions and tissues. Fortunately, research has also found that increased intelligence contributes to older persons' ability to cope with loneliness. The belief is that high intelligence helps with self-reflection and with building new social connections (Lee, Depp, Palmer, et al., 2018).

Health care providers who work with older persons can help fill the gap for missing family members by providing emotional and social support. The following sections discuss a few of the most important problems faced by the older population and some basic therapeutic interventions.

Economics

The financial outlook of older persons differs greatly from that of young adults. Many can remember their parents sacrificing food from their own mouths to feed their offspring.

Because of inflation, the value of a country's currency (e.g., dollar, pound, euro) changes, sometimes dramatically. During this time, many older persons have followed savings plans or invested for their later years. Some are now financially comfortable. Others, not having realized the change in the actual value of a currency, are coping with fewer resources than they had expected. People who made no preparations for later life often find themselves at the mercy of an impersonal system, living on meager resources with a poor quality of life.

Older individuals are also challenged with the problem of being financially vulnerable. Older persons trust other people and take them "at their word." This background, combined with diminishing senses or understanding, can leave older persons vulnerable to the scams, deceptions, exploitations, and threats of con artists and criminals. Many older persons have lost their life's savings because they could not understand the language on a contract. Many allowed themselves to be charmed or intimidated out of their money.

Care providers can assess for indications of financial problems and refer patients to the appropriate resource. Remember to monitor older patients for such indications because worries about money can lead to mental health challenges such as depression, anxiety, or paranoia.

Housing

Problems with housing for older persons range from having "too much house" to having none at all. The 2011 Canadian Census of population counted nearly 5 million (4 945 000) older persons aged 65 and over in Canada. Of these individuals, 92.1% lived in private households or dwellings (as part of couples, alone, or with others), while 7.9% lived in collective dwellings, such as seniors' residences or health care and related facilities (Statistics Canada, 2018).

The problems of "too much house" usually arise when one spouse passes away and the remaining person is unable to care for the property. Because women tend to outlive men, the most common scenario is that of a newly widowed woman faced with the care of a house with maintenance she knows nothing about. She may live there for many years of widowhood, but eventually she will be forced to move to a safer environment with less responsibility and upkeep.

The problems of "too little house" (inadequate housing) include homelessness and despair. Others have been forced out of their homes because they were unable to afford the expenses associated with them. Although older persons represent a small proportion of the Canadian homeless population, that proportion is growing. There is a high prevalence of mental illness and cognitive impairment among homeless older persons, with a greater proportion of older women than men having severe mental illness (Stergiopoulos & Herrmann, 2003).

As the older population increases, new arrangements in housing are being developed. Inventive new plans and living arrangements for older persons are evolving. Independent living centers, life contract facilities, foster homes, subsidized housing, and assisted living situations are all being explored as housing options for older persons.

Loss and Death

We travel life's paths with companions, friends, relatives, and people who have become important in our lives. With the passage of time, many older persons lose the individuals who are important for their emotional support and well-being. When a spouse of many years is lost, the remaining partner is left to cope alone. Depression often becomes one's companion after the death of a spouse or significant other. Frequently, couples who have been together for many years will die within months of each other. It seems the will to carry on without the loved one is lost, and for some, death becomes an opportunity to be reunited.

Losses during the older years also arrive in various other forms. The loss of physical stamina and endurance and the loss of sharp senses with which to enjoy the world present challenges for older persons. Although the concept of loss is described in Chapter 20, it is important to remember here that coping with loss is one of the most difficult experiences of older persons. Compassion, understanding, and support can help them re-establish the psychosocial connections that bind us together.

CRITICAL THINKING

- How do you picture yourself at 80 years of age?
- How physically active do you expect to be?
- Have you thought about or made any plans for retirement?
- At what age do you feel a person should think about retirement?

Substance Abuse

The use, misuse, and abuse of medications is a complex issue for older persons. Older people tend to have a great number of prescription medications to treat multiple and chronic health problems (Box 16.2). Plus, older persons are the largest group of over-the-counter (OTC) medication consumers (Centre for Addiction and Mental Health [CAMH], 2020). Although the predisposition for addiction is genetic, some studies have shown that certain organic changes in older persons' brains may lead to this same predisposition (Roussotte, Jahanshad, Hibar, et al., 2015). Many *use* their medications correctly by understanding the purpose for the medication and taking the correct dose at the specified times in the safest manner (example: two pills, with food, at 8 a.m., 12 noon, 4 p.m., and 8 p.m.). The *misuse* of medications, related to taking more than one medication for the same condition, occurs when the individual is taking a medication for no therapeutic reason, or is taking medications to treat adverse effects of other medications being taken. Drug/medication abuse occurs when one is addicted to the medication and suffers withdrawal when the medication is no longer taken. Mixing medications with alcohol is another example of drug abuse.

Many older persons mix OTC medications with their prescription medications. The term **polypharmacy** describes the use of five or more medications a day or unnecessary or excessive use of medications. Therapeutic polypharmacy is necessary in some complex medical conditions, and the medications are carefully monitored by clinicians. Nontherapeutic or contratherapeutic polypharmacy occurs when an individual is taking multiple medications without frequent, routine monitoring. The individual may see and receive prescriptions from several providers, then have the prescriptions filled at different pharmacies. Many times,

---

BOX 16.2 Medication Facts for People Older Than 45 Years

- 75% use some kind of medication.
- More than 30% of over-the-counter medication sales are to older persons.
- 30% of all prescriptions are written for persons over age 65 years.
- The average 65-year-old takes three to five medications daily.
- Many older persons share medications or skip their medications to help keep costs down.
- Many do not know the purpose of the medications they are taking.
- Few older individuals have knowledge about adverse effects or medication interactions.

---

older persons will continue to take a medication that was prescribed for an acute, short-term episode of illness. OTC medications are often considered harmless, but some adverse effects and mixtures of prescription medications and OTC medications can result in serious problems, especially in older persons.

Older persons also metabolize and excrete medications more slowly. The kidneys and liver function less effectively. Most drug studies are conducted on young or middle-aged adults. In older persons, there is a decreased tolerance for most medications that can result in overdoses and severe interactions with other medications and foods. Many medications cause sedation and confusion in older people. Sight and memory impairments also contribute to the misuse of medications by older persons.

Older persons with several health problems may visit many specialists, with each one prescribing a different medication. In one study, only 15% of older persons on medications could recall the medication names, dosages, or reasons for taking them ("Can your patient name her drugs?," 2002). The use of OTC medications compounds the situation by increasing the potential for adverse reactions. In addition, many older persons use several pharmacies, share their prescriptions with friends, and follow the recommendations of anyone offering relief from their discomfort. **Hoarding** medications is common because of the expense and possible need for them in the future. Many individuals will underdose themselves to save money and make medications last longer. Outdated medications are seldom thrown away.

Nurses have a special responsibility to ensure that their older patients are using their medications correctly. This responsibility includes a thorough assessment of a patient's medication history, current medication use (prescribed, OTC, and recreational), and an understanding of the medications currently being taken. The following Medication Alert offers a tool for assessing an older person's medication and substance use.

! MEDICATION ALERT

Nursing Process

Assessment

1. Obtain a complete medication history: name of medication, reason prescribed, amount taken, how often taken. Is medication taken with other medications, on an empty or full stomach, at a certain time? What is your patient's knowledge about the medication's use, adverse effects, medication–food interactions? Is the patient sharing prescription or nonprescription drugs with friends?

2. Instruct the patient to put every medication bottle they have into a paper bag and bring them to you. Check each medication for its expiration date. Be alert for several bottles of the same medication. Include all over-the-counter products, vitamins, and herbal or natural remedies.

3. Assess the patient's ability to follow verbal and written instructions and willingness to learn about each medication.

Planning

1. On the basis of the patient's abilities to understand and cooperate, develop a plan for teaching and monitoring the patient's use of each medication.

2. Arrange for the patient to show you the steps in identifying and taking the medication if necessary. Include family members in the teaching process when possible.

Nursing Diagnoses

Possible nursing diagnoses include the following:

- Insufficient knowledge related to use, administration, and monitoring of prescribed medications

- Ineffective therapeutic regimen management because of sensory loss
- Nonadherence related to altered thought processes
- Polypharmacy

Therapeutic Interventions

1. Teach the patient and significant others about the proper use and dosage of each medication, adverse effects and what to do about them, and expected therapeutic actions.

2. Devise a system for taking daily medications. Pill dispensers are available at most pharmacies. These multiboxed units can hold up to 1 week's medications. They usually consist of a series of small compartments, which are filled with all the medication that must be taken at a certain time. The patient opens the compartment at the prescribed time and takes every medication in the box. Having the patient return weekly with their medications and pill dispenser allows the nurse and other care providers to monitor the medications taken.

Evaluation

1. Assess the patient's therapeutic response to the medications. Did the medication do what it was intended to do?

2. Evaluate the patient's willingness and ability to cooperate. Has there been any change in the patient's alertness, level of understanding, or memory?

3. Routinely evaluate the number and kinds of medications taken on a daily basis.

Although the use of recreational or street drugs decreases with age, some drugs, especially alcohol, still cause problems for many older persons. Alcohol use helps provide a substitute for social interactions. Many older people drink to dull the discomforts associated with isolation. Older persons who were heavy drinkers in the past often show the results of long-term alcohol abuse.

As with many addictions, it is not enough to have a predisposition for a particular addiction. To became addicted, exposure is also important. Older persons who are retired have time for such exposure. Pathological gambling is less prevalent among people aged 60 and over than it is among younger adults: In Ontario, the prevalence is 2.1% for people over 60 compared to 4.6% for people below 60. Yet, due to limited financial resources for the majority of people over 60, this problem has greater consequences (CAMH, 2006). For older persons across the globe, gambling is a very popular way to spend time. Some researchers have identified strategies for older persons to use to ensure responsible gambling. These include delayed gratification, perception of futility of gambling, setting limits, maintaining balance, seeking help, and having an awareness of disordered gambling in self or in others. Family interventions include pleading and threatening, compelling help-seeking, as well as a family exclusion order (Subramaniam, 2017).

The use of opiates (heroin, opium) is even more invisible than that of alcohol. Older Asian Canadians with opium addiction or retired white-collar workers addicted to cocaine

seldom reach the attention of health care providers unless their habits result in serious medical complications. In Canada, as of October 17, 2018, the *Cannabis Act* has made it legal to use marijuana and edible cannabis for people older than 18 years of age (Government of Canada, 2019b).

All health care providers need to assess and monitor older persons for signs of substance abuse, especially when an unusual accident or event occurs. Often a history of minor accidents and injuries signals a problem with drugs. If problems with drug or alcohol use are suspected, the patient is referred to a physician for a medical assessment.

MENTAL HEALTH CHALLENGES OF OLDER PERSONS

People over age 65 experience the same mental health disorders as adolescents and younger adults do. They also face the challenges of vulnerability, abuse, memory loss, dementia, and Alzheimer's disease (discussed in Chapter 17). Mental health difficulties can result from physical or biochemical disorders, such as diabetes or medication imbalances. Many mental health threats arise from loneliness and social isolation. Psychological issues with which individuals have struggled throughout their lives often follow them into old age. Although all major mental health disorders can occur in older persons, by far the most common disorders relate to loss, depression, abuse, and dementia.

TABLE 16.2 Forms of Elder Abuse

Type of Abuse	Description and Examples
Abandonment	Leaving another who is unable to care for themselves alone without basic resources.
Exploitation (financial)	Improper use of a person for one's own profit. *Examples:* theft of objects, diversion of an older person's money, use of legal power assigned by the older person for own gain. An estimated 10% of older persons are exploited.
Neglect	Refusing to meet basic physical and mental health needs. *Examples:* depriving food, drink, clothing, shelter, hygiene, corrective, and remedial devices (e.g., glasses, hearing aids); refusal to seek medical care, even when urgently needed; refusing to interact, to provide for love, belonging, social needs. About 65% of abused older persons are neglected.
Physical abuse	Physical harm caused by the actions of another person. *Examples:* beating, whipping, scalding, cigarette burns, bruises, fractures.
Psychological abuse	Threats to mental health caused by another person. *Examples:* poor personal hygiene, grooming, environmental conditions; threats of nursing home placement; being humiliated, threatened, or socially isolated; verbal assaults, name calling; being treated like a child; being placed in seclusion.
Self-neglect	Refusal or inability to provide for one's basic needs.
Sexual abuse	Unwanted physical and verbal sexual behaviours.
Violation of rights	The refusal to allow another the exercise of individual rights, including the right to consent for medical treatment or surgery, to refuse treatment, to live in a safe environment of choice, to privacy, and to use personal financial resources as desired.

Elder Abuse

Elder abuse is defined as any action that takes advantage of an older person, their emotional well-being, or property. The three basic categories of elder abuse are domestic abuse, where the abuser has a special relationship with the elder; institutional abuse, where caregivers who are legally obligated to provide protective care fail to do so; and self-neglect or self-abuse. Acts of elder abuse appear in various forms, ranging from physical neglect to stealing money and exploiting the older person's resources. Table 16.2 lists several ways in which elder abuse occurs.

The victims of elder abuse are divided into two groups: one in which the older person lives with physical or mental impairment and depends on the family for daily care needs, and one in which the older person's care needs are overshadowed by the abusive behaviour of the caregiver. The typical abused older person is a woman, 77 years of age, with physical or mental challenges, who is living with a relative. Often the responsibilities of care can lead even well-intentioned family members or caregivers to lose their tempers when they feel stressed or pressured. Older persons who are exploited by family members often refuse to report the problem because they do not want to see a relative in jail.

One in five Canadians believes they know of an older person who might be experiencing some form of abuse. Older persons from all walks of life are vulnerable to elder abuse, and it is happening in communities across Canada (Government of Canada, 2016). In 2015, more than 9 900 seniors (65 years and older) were victims of police-reported violent crime in Canada. Of these victims, one-third (33%) were victimized by a grown child, spouse, sibling, or extended family member (a rate of 60 per 100 000 population) (Conroy, 2017). Every care provider must be alert for the indications of abuse in every older patient. If abuse is suspected, it should be reported to

the police. Most Canadian jurisdictions have laws that require health care providers to report abuse when the victim lives in a retirement home or a long-term care facility.

Chapter 26 focuses on the recognition, prevention, and treatment of elder abuse.

Dementia, Depression, and Delirium

Dementia, depression, and delirium are three conditions that often share similar symptoms but have a very different etiology and therefore require different treatments, with different degrees of urgency.

Dementia is a progressive cognitive disorder that interferes with memory, communication, attention, judgement, the ability to think clearly, behaviour, and activities of daily living. People who have dementia have a predisposition to delirium and depression. **Delirium** is a medical emergency with a sudden onset, fluctuating course, confusion, altered consciousness, and disturbance in attention, thinking, perception, and language.

Depression is a treatable mental illness that negatively affects one's thoughts, feelings, memory, behaviour, self-esteem, and physical health. Depression is probably the most common mental health disorder of late adulthood. It is estimated that more than 15% of older persons in the community have depressive signs and symptoms. Along with the losses experienced through death, retirement, and relocation, many older persons are faced with losing their social supports. Individuals feel hopeless and powerless to do anything about it. The future holds no joy, only the possibility of suffering more tomorrow than today. This is the face of depression in older persons (see Chapter 21). Older persons in long-term care institutions or hospitals have even higher rates of depression.

Depression is commonly underdiagnosed and undertreated. Sometimes vague complaints are the only clue. Other times, depression will mask itself as a physical illness.

BOX 16.3   Validation Therapy

Older individuals must justify having lived, resolve old con-flicts, and make peace with themselves. *Validation therapy* acknowledges the truth of patients' feelings by using a com-bination of the following:

- Eye contact
- Touch
- Mirroring the patient's body movement
- Matching the patient's voice and rhythm patterns
- Empathy
- Putting the patient's cues about feelings into words
- Accepting the patient without passing judgement
- Genuine, total listening

Knowing patients' lifestyles, preferences, social habits, and attitudes toward life is important. With this know-ledge, nurses can assess for the behaviours that signal the onset of depression. Frequently the signs and symptoms of depression can mimic dementia (loss of multiple abilities, including memory, language, and understanding). Careful assessments are required to distinguish the difference. Many medications, such as cardiovascular medications, antican-cer medications, psychotropic medications, hormones, and anti-inflammatory agents, are associated with depression in older persons.

Memory impairment is often responsible for the genera-tion of some confabulations (made-up stories to fill in mem-ory gaps) by older persons. These stories may generate an emotional reaction and even distress. An acceptable approach that staff should use to deal with such confabulation is *valida-tion therapy* (rather than reality orientation [Erdmann & Schnepp, 2016]; see Box 16.3).

THERAPEUTIC INTERVENTIONS

Therapeutic care for older persons is not effectively accom-plished unless a special ingredient is present. That special ingredient is respect: the courtesy, consideration, and esteem due each individual who has reached this stage of life. Every older person, alert or not, cooperative or not, deserves respect. Respect is demonstrated by each action and each interaction we perform. Treat patients as you would like to be treated if you were in their situation.

When assessing an older patient, remember to perform a **functional assessment,** which is an analysis of the patient's ability to perform the activities of daily living. This assess-ment is usually performed by an occupational therapist to assess a patient's fragility and determine necessary supports. There are many different types and complexities of this assessment. It can be done in the hospital emergency room following medical evaluation, or it can be done in a patient's house or at a long-term care facility. The environment in which the patient lives, as well as cultural and social patterns, should also be assessed. Proper functional assessment may identify a patient's strengths that were underutilized or that staff or family members were not aware of. This may enable the patient to stay home in a familiar environment and avoid placement in a long-term care facility.

Age-Related Interventions

Therapeutic interventions for older persons differ from those for younger people in several ways. The normal process of aging slows the older person's mental functions.

Memory loss is a natural part of the aging process relating to the inability to recall certain details or events. Therapeutic interventions need to account for this by allowing more time for completion of tasks. More time is also needed to recover from physical exertion.

The "capacity of the brain to process, store, and retrieve information begins to function less efficiently" (Burke & Laramie, 2004) in older persons, so finding the right word in conversation can become difficult. Allow extra time for the older person to communicate, and listen carefully. Face the patient, and speak slowly and clearly. Use nonverbal com-munications to help convey your message. It is best not to overload the patient with information. One simple yet under-stood message is more effective than a lengthy discourse.

Music therapy is proving to be "a powerful tool for main-taining and restoring health and is particularly suited to elder care" (Kramer, 2001). Music can alter moods and provide relaxation or distraction. For older persons, music provides an opportunity to remember and enjoy.

When teaching older persons, there are several things to keep in mind. First, assess for any physical or sensory chan-ges that may interfere with their learning (and your teaching). Patients who have cataracts usually cannot make out the dif-ferent colours of their pills, especially blue, green, and violet (Ruholl, 2003). Therefore, refer to the medications by name and shape rather than colour. If patients are hard of hearing, be sure their hearing aids are working at the proper settings. Face patients. Speak slowly and clearly in lower tones. Ask them to repeat your message.

Draw on patients' wisdom and knowledge. Find out what they already know. Break down a complex task into small, key steps. Be patient and respectful. Write out important points. Your patients' willingness and ability to learn will greatly improve with this approach.

Mentally Ill Older Persons

With a stable environment and daily routine, adults with serious mental illness can continue to function well into old age. However, many will be coping with the complications of long-term antipsychotic medications. The most common complications are movement disorders, such as tardive dysk-inesia (medication-induced movements of the muscles of the face, trunk, arms, and legs), and cognitive deficits. Cognitive deficits can also significantly impair activities of daily living. These patients may require assistance with grooming and other activities of daily living.

A decrease in intellectual function (cognitive impairment) is common in older persons with a long history of mental ill-ness. Patients should be assessed for their level of impairment so that therapeutic interventions can be individually tailored to promote the highest level of functioning.

SAMPLE PATIENT CARE PLAN 16.1 **Polypharmacy**

Assessment

History Senedu is a 77-year-old, overweight female who is having difficulty with her daily activities. She complains of dry mouth, dizziness, daytime drowsiness, and forgetfulness. She has "several different doctors" and is currently taking 12 different medications a day. Her friend recently shared her new medication with Senedu, and she now wants a new prescription for the same medication.

Current Findings Gait is unsteady—sipping on water to speak clearly—untidy, with a strong body odour—thought processes and speech are slow—flat emotional state.

Multidisciplinary Diagnosis	Planning/Goals
Adverse medication reactions related to current medication regimen (12 medications/day)	Senedu will decrease her daily medication intake to five medications/day (selected by the physician) within 1 month.

THERAPEUTIC INTERVENTIONS

Interventions	Rationale	Team Member
1. Have Senedu put every medication, vitamin, or substance she takes into a brown paper bag and bring it to the clinic.	To assess each medication's name, dosage, use, indications, adverse effects	Psy, Nsg, MD
2. Review each medication with Senedu and her caregiver; explain the need for decreasing medications.	To treat current adverse effects and prevent adverse reactions	Nsg, Pharmacist
3. Explore Senedu's emotional reactions to giving up half of her medications.	Provides reassurance, acceptance of feelings, improves chances of adherence	All
4. Help Senedu develop a system for taking the remaining five medications each day.	A routine improves adherence and monitoring	Nsg, Pharmacist
5. Teach Senedu and her caregiver about the correct use and monitoring for each remaining medication. Provide written instructions and contact information of a health care provider for all substances.	Helps determine therapeutic effectiveness, monitor for adverse effects, adverse reactions, medication interactions	Nsg, Pharmacist, Soc Svc

Evaluation After 3 weeks, Senedu was alert with a steady gait and clear speech. She can identify each medication and its common adverse effects. She will be seeing her primary care provider in 1 week to review her medication.

Critical Thinking Questions
1. How important is a knowledge base for each drug (substance)?
2. Does Senedu need to be referred to home care services? Why or why not?

A complete patient care plan includes several other diagnoses and interventions.
Nsg, nursing staff; *MD,* physician; *Psy,* psychologist; *Soc Svc,* social services.

Mental Health Promotion and Prevention

Many problems of older persons can be prevented or minimized if they are discovered early. Health care providers must work together and grasp every opportunity to promote healthful practices in their older patients. They should assess patients for changes in social, emotional, behavioural, and physical functioning and intervene early. Care providers should not hesitate to help satisfy patients' needs, even though it may take some creative planning. Interventions such as improved diet and increased physical activity have proven to be beneficial. Newer interventions, such as using dolls and stuffed animals to provide comfort (doll therapy) and life review (reminiscence therapy), are proving effective with many older persons. Sample Patient Care Plan 16.1 focuses on an older person who is having trouble coping with her medication and OTC medication use.

All care providers play a major role in the mental health care of older individuals. Interventions often require the services of several specialists, such as nurses, physiotherapists, social workers, and occupational therapists. Sharing information and coordinating care promote quality in the lives of older persons. Health care providers also have the opportunity to make a significant difference in public policies regarding older persons, as well as in the lives of all persons they touch.

KEY POINTS

- Older adulthood, or maturity, is the period of life from 65 years of age until death.
- According to the theorist Erikson, older persons with a well-developed sense of personal integrity accept the worth and uniqueness of their own lifestyles.
- Although short-term memory and speed begin to decline in the 40s, mental capabilities such as judgement and wisdom continue to improve as one grows older.
- Physical problems can lead to changes in mental status.
- Older persons experience several physical and social losses.
- Problems with housing for older persons range from having too much house to having none at all.
- The availability of health care for the older population is an important factor in maintaining both physical and mental health.

- One of the greatest mental health challenges is coping with the loss of loved ones and friends.
- The misuse or abuse of drugs and alcohol is a complex issue for older persons who receive a great number of prescription medications to treat multiple and chronic health problems.
- Polypharmacy refers to the use of multiple medications inappropriately.

- Elder abuse is defined as any action on the part of a caregiver to take advantage of an older person, their emotional well-being, or property.
- Depression is one of the most common mental health disorders of late adulthood.
- Care for older persons cannot be effective without respect, courtesy, consideration, and the esteem due each individual who has reached this stage of life.

ADDITIONAL LEARNING RESOURCES

Go to your Evolve website (http://evolve.elsevier.com/Canada/Morrison-Valfre/) for additional online resources, including the online Study Guide for additional learning activities to help you master this chapter content.

CRITICAL THINKING QUESTIONS

1. An 80-year-old female patient arrives at the emergency department with her son and daughter-in-law, with whom she lives. She is found to have a broken arm. Her son and daughter-in-law seem very agitated with the patient. When questioned about how it happened, she drops her head and mumbles that she doesn't really know. What are the staff's legal obligations?

2. What are the main principles of the care for older persons?

REFERENCES

Abraham, M. K., & Cimino-Fiallos, N. (2019). Falls in the elderly: Causes, injuries, and management. *Medscape.* https://reference.medscape.com/slideshow/falls-in-the-elderly-6012395

Ahn, H., Bailey, C. S., Rivers, C. S., et al. (2015). Effect of older age on treatment decisions and outcomes among patients with traumatic spinal cord injury. *Canadian Medical Association Journal, 187*(12), 873–880. http://www.cmaj.ca/content/187/12/873

Burke, M. M., & Laramie, J. A. (2004). *Primary care of the older adult: A multidisciplinary approach* (2nd ed.). Mosby.

Can your patient name her drugs? *Nursing, 32*(8), (2002), 33–34 [Seminal Reference].

Centre for Addiction and Mental Health (CAMH). (2006). *Responding to older adults with substance use, mental health and gambling challenges a guide for workers and volunteers.* Author. https://doi.org/10.1503/cmaj/150085 [Seminal Reference].

Centre for Addiction and Mental Health (CAMH). (2020). *Medication use in older adults.* Author. https://www.camh.ca/en/health-info/guides-and-publications/medication-use-in-older-adults#:~:text=Although%20adults%20aged%2065%20and,one%20medication%20at%20a%20time

Conroy, S. (2017). Family violence in Canada: A statistical profile 2015. Section 5: Police-reported family violence against seniors. https://www150.statcan.gc.ca/n1/pub/85-002-x/2017001/article/14698/05-eng.htm

Doidge, N. (2015). Our amazingly plastic brains: Mental and physical exercise can keep the brain fit and help it recover capacities lost to disease and trauma. *Wall Street Journal* February 6.

Edelman, C. L., & Kudzma, E. (2018). *Health promotion throughout the life span* (9th ed.). Mosby.

Erdmann, A., & Schnepp, W. (2016). Conditions, components and outcomes of integrative validation therapy in a long-term care facility for people with dementia. A qualitative evaluation study. *Dementia, 15*(5), 1184–1202. https://doi.org/10.1177/1471301214556489. https://journals.sagepub.com/doi/abs/10.1177/1471301214556489?rfr_dat=cr_pub%3Dpubmed&url_ver=Z39.88-2003&rfr_id=ori%3Arid%3Acrossref.org&journalCode=dema

Giger, J. N., & Haddad, L. G. (2020). *Transcultural nursing: Assessment and intervention* (8th ed.). Mosby.

Government of Canada. (2016). Elder abuse: It's time to face the reality. https://www.canada.ca/en/employment-social-development/campaigns/elder-abuse/reality.html

Government of Canada. (2017). Provincial and territorial public drug benefit programs. https://www.canada.ca/en/health-canada/services/health-care-system/pharmaceuticals/access-insurance-coverage-prescription-medicines/provincial-territorial-public-drug-benefit-programs.html

Government of Canada. (2019a). *Canada's dietary guidelines. Section 1.* Foundation for healthy eating. https://food-guide.canada.ca/en/guidelines/section-1-foundation-for-healthy-eating/

Government of Canada. (2019b). *Cannabis legalization and regulation.* Department of Justice. https://www.justice.gc.ca/eng/cj-jp/cannabis/

Kramer, M. K. (2001). A trio to treasure: The elderly, the nurse, and music. *Geriatric Nursing, 22*(4), 191–195 [Seminal Reference].

Lee, E. E., Depp, C., Palmer, B. W., et al. (2018). High prevalence and adverse health effects of loneliness in community-dwelling adults across the lifespan: Role of wisdom as a protective factor. *International Psychogeriatrics, 31*(10), 1447–1462. https://doi.org/10.1017/S1041610218002120. https://www.cambridge.org/core/journals/international-psychogeriatrics/article/high-prevalence-and-adverse-health-effects-of-loneliness-in-communitydwelling-adults-across-the-lifespan-role-of-wisdom-as-a-protective-factor/FCD17944714DF3C110756436DC05BDE9

Roussotte, F. F., Jahanshad, N., Hibar, D. P., et al. (2015). Altered regional brain volumes in elderly carriers of a risk variant for drug abuse in the dopamine D2 receptor gene (DRD2). *Brain Imaging and Behavior*, *9*(2), 213–222. https://doi.org/10.1007/s11682-014-9298-8

Ruholl, L. (2003). Tips for teaching the elderly. *RN*, *66*(5), 48–52 [Seminal Reference].

Statistics Canada. (2018). Living arrangements of seniors. https://www12.statcan.gc.ca/census-recensement/2011/as-sa/98-312-x/98-312-x2011003_4-eng.cfm

Statistics Canada. (2019). Analytical products, 2016 census: Working seniors in Canada. https://www12.statcan.gc.ca/census-recensement/2016/as-sa/98-200-x/2016027/98-200-x2016027-eng.cfm

Stergiopoulos, V., & Herrmann, N. (2003). Old and homeless: A review and survey of older adults who use shelters in an urban setting. *Canadian Journal of Psychiatry*, *48*(6), 374–380. https://doi.org/10.1177/070674370304800603 [Seminal Reference].

Subramaniam, M. (2017). Responsible gambling among older adults: A qualitative exploration. *BMC Psychiatry*, *17*(1), 124. https://doi.org/10.1186/s12888-017-1282-6

Williams, P. A. (2019). *Basic geriatric nursing* (7th ed.). Mosby.

17

Cognitive Impairment, Alzheimer's Disease, and Dementia

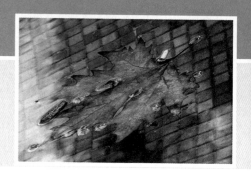

OBJECTIVES

Upon completion of this chapter, the student will be able to:
1. Describe two normal age-related changes in cognition.
2. Identify three main categories of confusion.
3. Explain why medication use can lead to confusion in older persons.
4. Describe at least three signs or symptoms of delirium.
5. Identify seven main symptoms of dementia.
6. Describe the signs and symptoms seen during the progression of Alzheimer's disease.
7. List three mental health care goals for patients with Alzheimer's disease.
8. Describe the gentle persuasive approach.
9. Describe communication techniques for communicating with a patient who has dementia.

OUTLINE

KEY TERMS

affective loss (ă-FĔC-tĭv lŏs) (p. 203)
Alzheimer's (AWLTZ-hī-mĕrz) disease (AD) (p. 202)
catastrophic (KĂT-ə-STRŎF-ĭk) reactions (p. 203)
conative (KŎN-ə-tĭv) loss (p. 203)
confusion (kŏn-FŪ-shən) (p. 197)
delirium (dĭ-LĬR-ē-ŭm) (p. 197)
delusions (p. 199)
dementia (dĭ-MĔN-shə) (p. 197)

functional assessment (p. 205)
gentle persuasive approach (GPA) (p. 201)
hallucinations (p. 199)
neurocognitive disorder (NCD) (p. 197)
sundown syndrome (SŬN-dŏwn SĬN-drōm) (p. 201)
vascular dementia (VaD) (VAS-kyuh-ler dĭ-MĔN-shə) (p. 202)

CONFUSION HAS MANY FACES

The words *cognition* and *cognitive* describe activities of the mind involved in thinking and thought processes. Cognition refers to intelligence, learning, judgement, reasoning, knowledge, understanding, and memory—all higher brain functions. A cognitive impairment is a disruption in higher brain functions that results in confusion. The patient's ways of knowing and understanding the world have changed. This chapter focuses on confusion, its causes, and its treatments.

Normal Changes in Cognition

It was once thought that mental aging was normal. Now we know that the brain, with good mental and physical exercise, can function well into advanced age. According to Greider and Neimark (2016), "some people simply don't experience any mental decline. Older people can continue to have extremely rich and healthy mental lives." The most common changes seen with aging are slower response times and changes in short-term memory. More time is needed to process, store, and retrieve information.

Several other factors influence how one ages mentally. Culture, education, general health, genetics, diet, physical and mental activity, and living conditions all have an influence on one's cognitive (intellectual) abilities. We all age individually, but one thing is certain: *confusion is not normal.* Although it most often occurs in older persons, individuals of any age can become confused. No matter what the age, *confusion demands investigation.*

The Three "D's" of Confusion

The word **confusion** is a very general term that is difficult to define. Commonly, it means mixed-up, bewildered, or uncertain. For health care providers, confusion is a symptom of an underlying problem that requires immediate attention. Confusion can be traced to physical, biochemical, social, or cultural sources. It can be acute, subacute, chronic, reversible, or irreversible. Sources of confusion are grouped into three broad categories. To help you remember the causes of confusion, use the three "D's": delirium, dementia, and depression (Toronto Region Best Practice in LTC Initiative, 2007; Table 17.1). See Figure 17.1 for characteristics of each group.

Delirium from injuries or conditions that cause a lack of oxygen (*hypoxia*) to the brain can lead to confusion. Exposure to certain chemicals, infections, toxic substances, or diseases can cause brain damage and confusion. Anything that interrupts or alters the blood supply or nerve pathways in the brain can result in acute or lasting confusion.

People can experience confusion caused by depression. When one's focus is inner sadness, outside stimuli can be misinterpreted or misunderstood. The individual becomes labelled "confused," and the depression is ignored. Chapter 21 offers a more thorough discussion of depression. Here, remember that confusion (especially in older persons) can be caused by depression and other mood disorders.

Dementia is a progressive loss of multiple abilities, including memory, language, and the ability to think and understand (judgement and abstract thought). It is a broad term that describes a group of symptoms relating to a severe loss of intellectual functions. Personality and behavioural changes may also be present. The losses are severe enough to interfere with daily living activities as well as social and work functioning. Unlike delirium, with dementia there is no change in one's level of consciousness.

In the *Diagnostic and Statistical Manual of Mental Disorders,* 5th edition (*DSM-5*), the word *dementia* is preserved only for continuity and easier adaptation of diagnostic criteria by clinical teams. The new term is **neurocognitive disorder** (NCD). NCD is a much broader term than dementia and includes neurocognitive decline from a wider etiology. NCD includes conditions related to loss of multiple cognitive abilities (dementia) or a few or even a single cognitive ability (complex attention, executive function, recognition of emotions, learning and memory, etc.). Delirium also belongs to the group of NCDs.

Other examples of NCD include Alzheimer's disease, frontotemporal lobar degeneration, Lewy body disease, vascular disease, traumatic brain injury, substance- or medication-induced disorders, HIV infection, Prion disease, Parkinson's disease, Huntington's disease, and another medical condition, multiple etiology, and unspecified. All of these have a different etiology, course, treatment, and prognosis.

To illustrate the main techniques and approaches used in caring for people with different neurocognitive diseases, we will focus here on delirium and the most prominent disease leading to the manifestation of dementia—Alzheimer's disease (AD).

Medications and the Older Population

Many medications and drugs cause confusion, especially in older people. Metabolism is slower in older persons. This means that medications are eliminated more slowly and can build up in the body to toxic levels if not closely monitored. People who take several medications are at risk for confusion resulting from medication interactions. Over-the-counter (OTC) medications, especially those with anticholinergic adverse effects, can cause confusion, disorientation, and memory loss.

Practitioners are becoming more careful with the prescribing of psychotropic medications. Most often, their use is appropriate and helps improve behaviours that pose a risk to self or others. However, these powerful medications can cause sedation and confusion, so patients must be carefully monitored for effectiveness and adverse effects. Confusion is often the first sign of a medication reaction.

! MEDICATION ALERT

MEDICATIONS THAT CAN CAUSE CONFUSION

Medications Used to Treat	Over-the-Counter Medications Used to Treat
Allergies	Cold and flu
Arthritis	Diarrhea
High blood pressure	Hay fever
Irritable bowel syndrome	Insomnia
Migraine headaches	Constipation
Pain	
Parkinson's disease	
Antipsychotics	
Sedatives	
Hypnotics	

PATIENTS WITH DELIRIUM

Delirium is a change of consciousness that occurs quickly, typically as a result of a medical emergency, altering brain functions. A few typical agents that can cause such an effect include different toxins from infections (urinary tract infection, lung infection, or skin infections), rapid changes in blood oxygenation (exacerbations of chronic obstructive

TABLE 17.1   Recognizing Delirium, Depression, and Dementia (3 D's)*

	Delirium	Depression	Dementia
Definition	• Delirium is a medical emergency that is characterized by an acute and fluctuating onset of confusion, disturbances in attention, disorganized thinking, and/or decline in level of consciousness. • Delirium cannot be accounted for by a pre-existing dementia; however, it can coexist with dementia.	• Depression is a term used when a cluster of depressive symptoms (as can be identified using the SIG-E-CAPS mnemonic depression screening criteria) is present on most days, for most of the time, for at least 2 weeks, and when symptoms are of such intensity that they are out of the ordinary for that individual. • Depression is a biologically based illness that affects a person's thoughts, feelings, behaviour, and even physical health.	• Dementia is a gradual and progressive decline in mental processing ability that affects short-term memory, communication, language, judgement, reasoning, and abstract thinking. • Dementia eventually affects long-term memory and the ability to perform familiar tasks. Sometimes there are changes in mood and behaviour.
Onset	• Sudden onset: hours to days	• Recent, unexplained changes in mood that persist for at least 2 weeks	• Gradual deterioration over months to years
Course	• Often reversible with treatment • Often fluctuates over 24-hour period and often worse at night	• Usually reversible with treatment • Often worse in the morning	• Slow, chronic progression, and irreversible
Thinking	• Fluctuations in alertness, cognition, perceptions, thinking	• Reduced memory, concentration, and thinking; low self-esteem	• Cognitive decline with impairments in memory, plus one or more of the following: aphasia, apraxia, agnosia, and/or impaired executive functioning
Sleep	• Disturbed but with no set pattern. Differs night to night	• Disturbed • Early morning awakening or hypersomnia	• May be disturbed with an individual pattern occurring most nights
Mood	• Fluctuations in emotions—outbursts, anger, crying, fearful	• Depressed mood • Diminished interest or pleasure • Changes in appetite (over- or undereating) • Possible suicidal ideation/plan; hopelessness	• Depressed mood, especially in early dementia • Prevalence of depression may increase in dementia; however, apathy is a more common symptom and may be confused with depression
Laboratory tests	Delirium workup includes the following tests: • Hgb, WBC, Na, K, Ca, O_2 sats, blood gases, urea, creatinine, liver function tests, chest X-ray, urinalysis and culture, alcohol/drug/toxicology screen	Depression workup includes the following tests: • TSH, B_{12}, folate, Ca, albumin, FBS, ferritin, ion, Hgb, K, ESR	Dementia workup includes the following tests: • CBC, TSH, blood glucose, electrolytes including Ca
Next steps	Notify: • Attending physician as soon as possible (consider delirium as a medical emergency; may require transfer to an emergency department)	Refer to: • Attending physician, and if suicidal risk, consider transfer to emergency department • Geriatric Mental Health Outreach Team • Psychogeriatric Resource Consultant (PRC)	Refer to: • Attending physician • Geriatric Mental Health Outreach Team • Psychogeriatric Resource Consultant (PRC)

*Individuals may have more than one D present at the same time, and symptoms may overlap.

B_{12}, vitamin B_{12}; *Ca,* calcium; *CBC,* complete blood count; *ESR,* erythrocyte sedimentation rate; *FBS,* fasting blood sugar; *Hgb,* hemoglobin; *K,* potassium; *Na,* sodium; O_2 *sats,* oxygen saturation; *SIG-E-CAPS,* Sleep, Interest, Guilt, Energy, Concentration, and Appetite, Psychomotor, and Suicidal ideation; *TSH,* thyroid-stimulating hormone; *WBC,* white blood cell count.

Excerpted and modified from Toronto Region Best Practice in LTC Initiative. (2007). *Recognizing delirium, depression and dementia (3D's).* https://connectability.ca/Garage/wp-content/uploads/2012/11/ThreeDcomparison-TPADD-CONFERENCE.pdf

Delirium
- Acute onset
- Causes: metabolic disorders, diseases, infections, fever, dehydration, pain, drug reactions, lack of oxygen to the brain
- Reversible if treated early

Dementia
- Slow onset
- Causes: cardiovascular disease, HIV, metabolic problems, Alzheimer's disease; more than 60 causes
- Usually not reversible

Depression
- Subacute onset
- Causes: loss, drugs, inner sadness, metabolic imbalances
- Usually reversible

Fig. 17.1 The three "D's" of confusion.

pulmonary disease [COPD]) or asthma, acute metabolic problems (from kidney and lever malfunctions to bad drug interactions and oncology), and many other potential causes. The signs and symptoms of delirium include "disorganized thinking, a decreased attention span, lowered or fluctuating level of consciousness, disturbances in the sleep-wake cycle, disorientation, and changes in psychomotor activity" (Henry, 2002). Individuals with delirium may have a psychosis. *Psychosis* is a symptom that may present itself as delusions with or without perceptual abnormalities (*hallucinations*). **Delusions** are false beliefs that are not a part of that person's cultural–social affiliation and resist change following presentation of evidence. **Hallucinations** are perceptional abnormalities (malfunctions) in a one or more of the five senses—the patient can see, hear, smell, test, and feel/touch things that are not based in reality. Patients with delirium who also experience perceptual abnormalities are often agitated. However, hypoactive behaviours, such as lethargy and reduced activity, are common but often overlooked behaviours.

The onset of delirium is rapid (acute), occurring in hours to days. *Delirium is reversible if treated early.* Once the underlying cause is found and treated, full recovery of mental functions occurs. It is important for health care providers to recognize the signs of delirium. Box 17.1 lists a method for assessing delirium.

Finding the Cause

Delirium is associated with various medical conditions, a variety of medications and their interactions, or other problems. Infections, fevers, and dehydration are common causes of delirium. Metabolic and endocrine conditions, such as diabetes, thyroid problems, and kidney or liver disease, may all result in delirium. Reactions to certain medications are common causes in older individuals. Delirium can also occur when people abruptly stop taking their medications. It can occur after surgery, especially in older persons. Pain, constipation, extremely high or low body temperature, alcohol use, a lack of oxygen to the brain, and malnutrition can all trigger delirium.

BOX 17.1   Assessing Delirium

Obtain information from a family member or someone who knows the patient and their usual behaviours.

Onset and Course
Questions to ask: Has there been an acute change in mental status? How long ago was the change first noticed? Do the behaviours fluctuate (come and go) during the day? Are behaviours worse at night?

A positive (yes) answer to any question may indicate delirium.

Attention
Questions to ask: Does the person have trouble paying attention? Can they keep track of what is being said? Are they easy to distract?

A positive (yes) answer to any question may indicate delirium.

Thinking
Questions to ask: Is thinking unorganized? Is there an illogical or unclear flow of ideas? Do they switch from subject to subject? Does their conversation ramble?

A positive (yes) answer to any question may indicate delirium.

Level of Consciousness
Questions to ask: Overall, how would you rate their level of alertness (consciousness) compared with usual levels? Are they alert? Vigilant? Hyperalert? Drowsy but arousable? Difficult to arouse?

Any answer other than "alert" may indicate delirium.

Data from Henry, M. (2002). Descending into delirium. *American Journal of Nursing, 102*(3), 57.

The causes of delirium, sometimes called *acute confusion,* are many. As Henry (2002) notes: "In order to identify delirium, clinicians must be familiar with the patient's baseline mental status and the characteristics of any changes." Delirium is a frightening experience that can last from hours to days.

CASE STUDY

Josef is an alert, outgoing 80-year-old man who lives with his cat in a senior citizens' complex. Despite several chronic conditions, he remains active and volunteers at the senior centre. His daughter visits weekly.

Today she was called by another volunteer at the senior centre and told that Josef had not been there for 3 days. Although she had visited only 2 days before and found her father "his usual cheery self," she rushed to her father's home. On her arrival, she finds that he does not know who she is. He tells her that he is afraid she has come to steal his late wife's jewellery. He is inattentive and drowsy. The daughter calls his physician and takes him to the emergency department.

The medical workup shows continuing confusion and a slight fever. Blood and urine tests indicate an infection. The physician diagnoses acute delirium related to a urinary tract infection. Orders are given for intravenous (IV) antibiotics and fluids. After a few days' hospitalization, Josef's confusion is completely gone, and he is ready to return home.

Treating Delirium

The treatment of delirium depends on its cause. The first priority is to *treat the source*. Antibiotics are given for infections. Older persons lose their sense of thirst, and delusions often subside quickly as water and minerals are replaced. If medications are the culprit, they are withdrawn (gradually in some cases) and the patient is monitored closely. At times, antipsychotic medication can be given briefly to deal with intense emotional suffering and aggression.

The second focus of care is supportive. Providing an environment that has low stimuli helps patients remain calm. Have patients wear their hearing aids and glasses. Encourage fluid intake to prevent dehydration. Use clocks and calendars to help orient patients. Allow patients to be involved with their care. Ambulate patients frequently if allowed, and balance rest with activity. Always protect the patient from injury.

Do not attempt to talk patients out of their delusions or convince them that they are false. Their reality is different at this time, but it is real to them. Use a low, calm voice, and maintain eye contact. Project a calm, unhurried manner. Validate patients' emotions (but not patients' beliefs): "How does that make you feel?," "That sounds scary," "That must be very difficult for you," "I am so sorry for what you are going through," "That must be very frustrating; how are you feeling?" Use simple orienting statements, such as "It is warm for June" or "Isn't it a nice evening?" Patients with delusions require close monitoring and supervision. As the cause of the confusion is corrected, patients will become more oriented and cooperative.

PATIENTS WITH DEMENTIA

Currently, approximately 564 000 Canadians live with a diagnosis of dementia (Alzheimer Society of Canada, 2019a).

Symptoms of Dementia

There are seven A's that represent the seven main symptoms of dementia. Different types of dementia have different

BOX 17.2 Challenging Behaviours of Patients With Dementia

Agitation and Aggression

Agitation: Repetitive motor, verbal, or vocal activity that is judged by an outside observer to be inappropriate relative to the needs

Aggression:
- Physically nonaggressive behaviours: general restlessness and repetitive mannerisms
- Verbally nonaggressive behaviours: constant requests for attention, interrupting
- Physically aggressive behaviours: kicking, biting, hitting
- Verbally aggressive behaviours: screaming, cursing, and temper outbursts

Catastrophic Reaction

Characterized by an excessive sudden emotional response, usually expressed as angry outbursts or physical aggression

Disinhibition

Impulsive and inappropriate behaviour due to poor insight and judgement: behaviours include euphoria, verbal aggression, sex disinhibition (talk/act), self-destructive behaviour, intrusiveness, impulsiveness, and motor agitation

Wandering

Wandering: tendency to move about in a seemingly aimless or disoriented fashion or in pursuit of an unobtainable goal
Repetitive checking of the whereabouts of caregiver
Trailing/stalking (extreme form of checking)
Pottering or rooting (walking around the house)
Repeated attempts to leave

Data from Krishnamoorthy, A., & Anderson, D. (2011). Managing challenging behaviour in older adults with dementia. *Progress in Neurology and Psychiatry, 15*(3), 23–26. https://onlinelibrary.wiley.com/doi/pdf/10.1002/pnp.199

etiologies, so not everyone who suffers from dementia will have all seven of these:
- Anosognosia: Loss of self-awareness. Patients may not know what they don't know, and may forget that they forget.
- Aphasia: Loss of language: speaking and comprehending (first frontal and second parietal lobe).
- Agnosia: Loss of recognition across all sensors: perception (sound, smell, test, vision), people, places, objects and what they are for.
- Apraxia: Loss of purposeful movement despite intact ability for physical activity; difficulty with initiating a task, inability to sequence steps of a task, lost sense of right/left, up/down, back/front, etc.
- Altered perceptions: Loss of reality test: hallucinations and illusions, loss of colour definition, depth.
- Attentional deficit: Loss of ability to maintain attention (easily distracted) and ability to shift attention (perseverative).
- Apathy: Loss of motivation; lack of concern; unable to initiate speech; unable to initiate activities without encouragement.

Dementia is responsible for some challenging behaviours (Box 17.2).

In the early stages, dementia is difficult to differentiate from age-associated memory impairment. Persons with age-associated memory impairment tend to learn and recall things more slowly. Yet, if given extra time, they are able to function. Individuals with dementia are increasingly unable to process new information. At the same time, they are losing the ability to retrieve and use the information accumulated through their lifetime.

Each person is unique, and no two people react the same way to dementia or follow the same course. A person's general health, intelligence, personality, and social situation all influence the behaviours seen in dementia. However, all people with dementia have progressive difficulties with memory, judgement, and abstract thinking.

Dementia has a slow, gradual onset. In the beginning, only small changes are noticeable. Individuals often attempt to hide their impairments. There is often an associated depression at this stage. The most common early symptom is a declining memory. For example, the patient may ask the same question repeatedly and then promptly forget the answer. Problems with abstract thinking follow. For example, an accountant becomes unable to balance his chequebook because he forgets what numbers are and how to use them. A homemaker can no longer plan meals or put together a shopping list. Problem-solving skills are lost. Things are misplaced and then forgotten. Familiar routines and tasks are no longer performed. Behaviours that demonstrate poor judgement become common. Communication problems and personality changes follow.

Sundown syndrome describes a group of behaviours characterized by confusion, agitation, and disruptive actions that occur in the late afternoon or evening. The cause is unknown, but sundowning is associated with dementia, loss of cognitive functions, and physical or social stressors. As visual cues and social interactions decrease with the onset of nighttime, individuals become more confused, irritable, and agitated. The signs and symptoms and interventions for patients with sundown syndrome are listed in Box 17.3.

When doing an assessment of older patients, remember to do so thoroughly and routinely. You must know the patient's baseline or usual behaviour. Family members and caregivers become a valuable resource for gathering information. The minor observations of one caregiver can make a difference. The label "dementia" should never be applied until after patients and their abilities have been thoroughly investigated.

The incidence of dementia increases with age, although a healthy diet with routine physical and mental exercises appears to slow the decline. Alzheimer's disease, a form of dementia, is often called "the long good-bye" because it slowly robs the individual of their memory, intellect, and personality.

Gentle Persuasive Approach

The **gentle persuasive approach (GPA)** reframes challenging behaviour associated with dementia to be interpreted as self-protective/defensive or responsive behaviour that occurs as a result of unmet needs; staff are encouraged to assess the meaning of the behaviour and work alongside the resident or

---

> **BOX 17.3 Caring for Patients With Sundown Syndrome**
>
> **Assess for:**
> Hunger, thirst, pain, the need to eliminate.
> Feelings of fear, insecurity.
> Isolation, little contact with other people.
> A recent move or change in routine.
>
> **Therapeutic (Nursing) Interventions:**
> Maintain comfort, toilet as necessary, keep dry.
> Control pain with nonmedication interventions (back rub, massage, touch, distraction).
> Reduce environmental stimulation during late afternoon and evening.
> Maintain daily routine.
> Provide environmental cues, turn on lights before dusk, provide a nightlight.
> Provide soothing music.
> Provide reassurance and companionship during evening hours.

> **BOX 17.4 Practical Interventions Using the Gentle Persuasive Approach (GPA)**
>
> *Validate:* You think your purse has been stolen? I understand why you are so upset.
> *Join:* You need to keep looking for your purse? Well, I am trying to find something too. Let's look together.
> *Distract:* Let's look for your purse over there, where people are having coffee.
> *Redirect:* This coffee smells good; do you want a cup?

---

patient. The ancient Greek physician Hippocrates (about 400 BCE) noted, "It is more important to know what sort of person has a disease than to know what sort of disease a person has." Keeping Hippocrates' advice in mind, here are some GPA strategies that health care providers and caregivers can use when caring for patients with dementia:

- Search for the meaning: Look for previous life experience, country of origin, interests and hobbies, family life, and significant others.
- Use unconditional positive regard, despite the patient's level of behaviour.
- Use nonverbal communication.
- Respect personal space.
- Use a reassurance position and a supportive stance.
- Take time to connect.
- Give brief, one-step directions.
- Use empathic listening.
- Practise validation.

Box 17.4 presents some practical GPA interventions.

Dementia Care

Recent research shows that we do not stop being a person when we lose our memory; we still have wishes and desires and still can enjoy things. Even "meaningless" exchanges of sound (which may seem incoherent) are helpful for maintaining

BOX 17.5   Possible Causes of Dementia

Remember: MEND A MIND

Metabolic disorders

Electrical disorders

Neoplastic disease (cancer)

Degenerative disease

Arterial disease

Mechanical disorders

Infectious disease

Nutritional disorders

Drug toxicity

CULTURAL CONSIDERATIONS

Alzheimer's Disease	Vascular Dementia
More common in North America and northern Europe	More common in China and Japan
Higher rates among Black people	
Higher rates in women	No gender differences
Rates increased for Japanese who immigrated to North America	Rates declined for Japanese who immigrated to North America

personhood. Those "meaningless" sounds become filled with some meaning for the person. Simple smiles between two people can be a powerful exchange. Social etiquette, table manners, and other types of etiquette remain a significant part of human life for a long time.

Encourage nonverbal (body language and paraverbal) communication with patients to help maintain their quality of life. Knowledge of patients' biography and history may help in understanding patients' behaviour and in making changes as needed to allow patients to cooperate with care. Patients' hobbies are also important to know, as they may preserve them. It is important to know what was significant for the person in their life; even if memory disappears, something meaningful remains inside. Religious practice or belief usually continues as well.

Causes of Dementia

NCD and its main presentation—dementia—can be primary, as with AD, or it may occur secondarily, as a result of disease. Cardiovascular disease, stroke, HIV/AIDS, and problems with circulation in the brain are also linked to dementia. For instance, normal pressure hydrocephalus occurs when there is a "gradual buildup of spinal fluid in the brain. The resulting swelling and pressure over time can damage brain tissue" (Rosen, 2014) and cause signs of dementia. In fact, there are more than 60 causes associated with dementia, including depression, metabolic problems, hormonal abnormalities, infections, brain traumas, and tumours. Pain; sensory deprivation; toxic alcohol and drug reactions; anemia; chemical intoxication; medication interactions; and nutritional deficiencies, such as those of vitamin B_{12}, folic acid, or niacin, can all result in dementia. Refer to Box 17.5 for an easy way to remember the causes of dementia.

The two most common types of dementia are **vascular dementia (VaD)** and AD. VaD occurs as a complication of cardiovascular disease causing extensive or very small cerebral vascular accidents when not enough blood is nourishing the brain to keep it functioning properly. The courses of VaD may be characterized by steep decline of function and long periods with no changes, whereas the course of AD usually has a gradual but constant decline. Memory impairment and executive dysfunction are well-known early features of AD, and persons with VaD tend to show a faster rate of cognitive decline.

ALZHEIMER'S DISEASE

Dementia of the Alzheimer's type presents special challenges. **Alzheimer's disease (AD)** is a progressive, degenerative disorder that affects brain cells and results in impaired *memory, thinking, and behaviour.* In 1907, Alois Alzheimer, a German psychiatrist, first described the unique characteristics of this condition. He related the case of a 51-year-old woman who had a severely impaired ability to encode information, compromised language functions, and delusions. When she died from this severe form of progressive dementia, an autopsy of her brain revealed that it was shrunken, contained abnormal tangles of nerve fibres, and was filled with clusters of degenerated nerve endings. Since this first description, the pathology of AD has been the subject of intense study and research.

Scientists divide AD into early onset and late onset. People younger than 65 who develop Alzheimer's have the early-onset form. Although this group is relatively small in number, it spans a wide age range. There are rare instances where people in their 30s have developed AD (Peterson, 2002).

According to a report form the Government of Canada (2017), "the onset of AD usually begins after age 60, and risk goes up with age. In Canada, 7.1% of all older people above 65 years of age suffer from some type of dementia, including AD. About two-thirds of Canadian seniors living with dementia are women." It is important to note, however, that AD is not a normal part of aging.

The cause of AD is unknown. Because people with AD can live more than 20 years after diagnosis, many older people living with AD need extensive care. Care providers need to be knowledgeable about the effects and treatment of AD and other dementias.

Symptoms and Course

The diagnosis of AD is not clear-cut. Therefore, a diagnosis is made by exploring and ruling out all other causes of dementia. A patient's confusion or dementia may be the result of a drug interaction or reaction. Other times, dementia occurs as the result of a medical condition. A careful and thorough history, physical examination, and mental status examinations are performed. The diagnosis of AD is made only after all the findings are considered. Today researchers are working

TABLE 17.2 Assessment of Alzheimer's Disease

Signs and Symptoms	Example
Memory loss	Especially short term; forgets and never remembers; trouble with associations
Difficulty performing familiar tasks	Forgets what order to put clothes on; prepares meal but then never serves it; leaves the car running
Problems with language	Forgets simple words; substitutes the wrong word; uses unusual words; hard to understand what is wanted because of word usage
Poor judgement	Inappropriate dress; buys unneeded items; forgets to watch child and leaves house for the day
Problems with abstract thinking	Stops paying bills; cannot balance chequebook; stops reading; has difficulty following a conversation
Misplaces things	Puts things in unusual places, such as a sandwich in the underwear drawer, milk in the oven, a watch in the freezer
Disoriented to time and place	Gets lost on one's own street; forgets where they are or how they got there
Loss of initiative	May become passive; sits in front of TV for hours; does not want to go places or see other people; loses interest in hobbies; sleeps more than usual
Changes in mood or behaviour	May have rapid mood swings; may show less emotion than usual
Changes in personality	May become anxious, angry, apathetic, depressed, fearful, irritable, suspicious; may become agitated in situations where memory problems are causing difficulties

intensively to develop a diagnostic test for AD. Promising results have been seen with a type of skin testing, brain imaging techniques, and genetic studies.

AD involves a gradual, progressive death of one's brain and its functions. The incidence increases as age advances. The signs and symptoms of AD are listed in Table 17.2. AD progresses slowly and involves a loss in every area of functioning. In normal aging, cognitive (intellectual) and psychomotor (physical) changes are to be expected. Reaction times slow, and lapses of memory commonly occur. Learning new skills requires more time and practice, but intelligence and understanding remain intact. People living with AD, however, lose their cognitive abilities and experience many intellectual losses.

Losses of Alzheimer's Disease

AD slowly robs an individual of their "personhood," and each decline is accompanied by a loss. Individuals living with AD become unable to make even the simplest decisions or choices. Following a conversation becomes impossible because speech becomes disjointed, simplified, and empty. The intellectual losses of AD are accompanied by the slow drain of one's personality (affective loss). Emotional control declines as the individual fades into childlike, antisocial, or emotionally labile behaviours. As the disease progresses and the ability to process information fades, people with AD become lost and absorbed in themselves. Some may even experience delusions, hallucinations, and feelings of paranoia.

Another loss for people with AD relates to the ability to make and carry out plans (conative loss) even for the simplest activities. The everyday tasks of living, such as dressing, grooming, and bathing, become overwhelming challenges. The harder they concentrate on the activity, the more difficult the activity becomes to perform. Stress, anger, and frustration increase fatigue levels because everything requires so much energy. Short-term memory fades, and everything seems to be happening for the first time.

Finally, there is the loss of the ability to withstand stress. People with AD become less and less able to cope with stress as the disease progresses. Minor anxieties cascade into full **catastrophic reactions,** in which the person becomes increasingly confused, agitated, and fearful. They may wander, become noisy, act compulsively, or behave violently. Because of the lowered stress threshold, it takes fewer and fewer stimuli to produce these overwhelming behavioural reactions. For this reason, care for patients with AD centres around providing a low-stimuli environment with as few stress-provoking situations as possible.

Stages of Alzheimer's Disease

The progression of AD is divided into four stages. Disease progression, however, is not orderly, because each individual is unique. Sometimes, symptoms seem to plateau for a time, but slow, progressive decline is the usual course.

The *early stage* begins with the loss of recent memory. An inability to learn, to process, and to retain information, followed by language problems, occurs. Judgement and abstract thinking decline. Individuals in the early stage forget where they put things and begin to have difficulty performing the activities of daily living. Many individuals react to their loss of memory and control with irritability, agitation, or hostility. Individuals are still social at this time, but family members begin to report strange behaviours and mood swings.

In the *intermediate stage,* patients cannot recall any recent events or process new information. Remote memory is affected but not totally lost. As the disease progresses, they usually develop aphasia (loss of language), apraxia (loss of ability to perform everyday actions, activities), and visual agnosia (loss of recognition of previously known or familiar people and objects). Individuals become increasingly forgetful and may require assistance with toileting, bathing, dressing, and eating. Behaviour becomes further disorganized. Wandering, agitation, and physical aggression often occur.

TABLE 17.3   Alzheimer's Disease In-Home Caregiver Skills and Responsibilities

Skills	Responsibilities
• *Good organization*—tracking medical, legal, financial records, medication schedules, physician appointments, and other caregivers' schedules • *Physical stamina*—coping with custodial duties, lifting, carrying the person; going without a regular eating and sleeping schedule yourself • *Emotional stamina*—coping with your own feelings, the feelings of the person with Alzheimer's disease (AD), feelings of other family members and friends; distancing yourself from the intense emotional responses of others • *Ability to cope with repetitive, distasteful tasks*—in early stages exercises to slow person's mental and speech decline; continual supervision is necessary; most work in the middle and late stages is focused on feeding, elimination, personal hygiene, and ensuring safety while person is still ambulatory • *The need to manage your life*—protecting your own health and well-being; making peace with death and dying; shifting focus to your own life and future	• *Early stage*—being alert to any changes; helping with memory and communication problems; being attentive to the person's needs; providing a stable, routine environment; financial and estate planning, if possible • *Middle stage*—adapting home for safety and convenience; making legal and financial decisions; managing medication schedules; managing hygiene, elimination, feeding, and exercise needs; coping with the changing personality and behaviours of the loved one • *Severe stage*—being attentive to needs that can no longer be expressed; arranging for long-term care; maintaining medication schedules; preparing for eventual death • *Final stage*—complete physical care required; saying good-bye in your own way; preparing for the future

Data from Larkin, M., *Alzheimer's outreach.* http://www.zarcrom.com/users/alzheimers

By now, individuals have lost all sense of time and place. However, they are still ambulatory and at high risk for falls and other accidents.

The *severe stage* of AD is characterized by an inability to do anything. Patients are usually incontinent, unable to walk, and entirely dependent on others for care. Memory, both recent and remote, is completely lost. An inability to swallow increases the risk for developing pneumonia and malnutrition. Many develop mutism (inability to speak) or communicate only in grunts.

In the *end stage*, patients slip into a coma, and death from pneumonia or other infection occurs.

After the Diagnosis

On hearing the diagnosis of AD, most patients and their loved ones experience shock and denial (the beginning of the grieving process). People with AD may live from 2 to 20 years after diagnosis. The average is about 8 years. Although they are in great emotional turmoil, family members must cope with the reality of the disease and begin planning for a challenging future.

Some day-care facilities are available to care for AD patients while family members or caregivers work or attend to other obligations. Most people with AD are cared for in their home by family members until placement in long-term care becomes necessary. Table 17.3 lists the skills and responsibilities of in-home care providers. There are many challenges in caring for a loved one living with AD.

In the early stages, responsibilities for care are to supervise the person and maintain their safety. As the disease progresses, assistance is required with dressing, bathing, and other activities of daily living. When the demands of care become too great or the individual's safety is threatened (e.g., by wandering, smoking, combative behaviour), most people

TABLE 17.4   Medication Treatment for Alzheimer's Disease

Generic Name	Brand Name Examples
donepezil	Aricept
rivastigmine	Exelon
galantamine	Reminyl ER
memantine	Ebixa
Anti-inflammatory medications (may slow the rate of decline)	Advil, Naprosyn

are admitted to long-term care facilities. Some arrive earlier if family support is unavailable; people with AD cannot be left alone.

Once the patient adjusts to the new surroundings, their quality of life often improves. Family members are frequently relieved because the tremendous responsibility of constantly providing every need of their loved one (often without recognition or thanks) is lifted from their shoulders and their loved one is in a safe environment.

Principles of Management

Treatments for AD are presently limited to providing physical and emotional support. Medication therapy showing promise involves medications that improve cognition, behaviour, and functioning (Table 17.4). Alternative therapies, such as ginkgo biloba, vitamin E, and coenzyme Q-10, are currently under investigation.

Researchers are aggressively investigating AD, and four potential therapies that may be useful include a nasal spray that seems to stop cognitive decline, a vaccine that stimulates the immune system to attack toxic proteins, intravenous infusions of human gamma globulin proteins that have halted

---

BOX 17.6 **A Functional Assessment**

Conduct and document initial and ongoing assessments of the following patient areas:

Daily functions: Eating and drinking, sleep patterns, personal hygiene, bathing, dressing, mobility, toileting and continence, ability to manage own medications, finances

Cognitive status: Mental status examination, memory, orientation, judgement, abstract thinking, intellectual functioning, state of consciousness

Medical conditions: Current medical problems, high blood pressure, diabetes, heart disease, etc.

Behavioural problems: Agitation, anger, fear of being alone, frustration, insensitivity to others, irritability, loss of inhibitions, jealousy, paranoia, suspicion

Psychological status: Personality changes, mood swings, flat emotional responses, psychotic symptoms, depression

Psychosocial status: An initial psychosocial history and ongoing assessments of communications, interactions with others, spiritual needs

---

BOX 17.7 **Interventions for Patients Living With Alzheimer's Disease**

1. Treat the person, not the condition.
2. Support the relationship between patient and caregiver.
3. Treat each person as an individual.
4. Establish and maintain communications.
5. Provide physical care, rest, and exercise.
6. Maintain a safe and supportive environment.
7. Maintain routine and consistency.
8. Manage difficult behaviours without reacting.

---

the progression of AD in a small number of patients, and genetic manipulation that boosts levels of nerve growth factors to restore healthy brain functioning (Martine & Duda, n.d.). New developments will undoubtedly change the face of AD. Until then, we must apply our current knowledge to providing the best possible care.

Institutional long-term care is necessary for the majority of individuals with AD. As a result, the therapeutic environment has become an important aspect of treatment. Some long-term care facilities have 1960s-style surroundings, and residents seem comforted by an environment with memories of younger times. Others employ music therapy and audio and video recordings of family members to calm agitated patients. Regardless of the environment, the daily management of people with AD is focused on providing the highest quality of life possible during the slow progression of the disease.

THERAPEUTIC INTERVENTIONS

Therapeutic care for patients with AD has three major goals:
1. To provide for patients' safety and well-being
2. To manage patients' behaviours therapeutically
3. To provide support for family, relatives, and caregivers

People living with AD are unable to care for themselves, even in the most basic ways. Bathing, grooming, eating, and physical activity for persons with AD all require interventions tailored to the individual. Older persons with AD have no sense of safety or idea of danger. When they wander, they may walk in the street, step out in front of moving vehicles, or sit on railroad tracks. Because of this absent sense, many facilities that care for AD patients have restricted or locked environments. Here patients are safe from the threats of both physical harm and overstimulation.

Several interventions help manage patient behaviours therapeutically. When behaving inappropriately, patients are gently redirected to less stressful activities. Music therapy, validation therapy, and exercise have all been used successfully to reduce stress and quell agitation.

Assessment

On admission to a long-term care facility or health care service, a patient undergoes a **functional assessment**—an analysis of each patient's abilities to perform the activities of daily living. Areas of assessment are listed in Box 17.6. How does the patient eat, bathe, move, and provide for their hygiene? What are the cognitive patterns, communication patterns, and sensory deficits? Are there any psychotic symptoms or signs of depression? What are the current medications and treatments? In short, what is the patient's physical, intellectual, psychosocial, and emotional level of function? This information helps to establish an important baseline for comparisons later as the patient deteriorates.

The assessment should also include the patient's support system and identify the primary caregiver and the patient's treatment and financial decision-making capacity. The family and caregivers are an important source of information. They should be included in the planning and care process whenever possible.

Nurses usually perform functional assessments. In many facilities, a dietitian, physiotherapist, occupational therapist, and an activity therapist also assess the patient. The multidisciplinary team then meets. Information from each specialty is shared and goals for care are developed.

Interventions for Patients Living With Alzheimer's Disease

Care for the individual with AD is based on gradually increasing services for both the patient and family or caregiver. The case management process allows for continual monitoring and modification of services as needed. Cultural beliefs are taken into account as care is planned. Specific interventions for each patient are developed on the basis of current abilities.

Care for the person with AD takes place in the home, a day-care centre, a long-term care facility, or an acute care facility. The main goal of care is to preserve as much function as possible by promoting good care provider–patient relationships within a safe and supportive environment. Treatment goals change as the patient's functional abilities decline. Box 17.7 lists several basic interventions for patients at all stages of this devastating disease.

Early Stage

Therapeutic interventions in the early stage focus on preserving mental abilities. Scientists have found that the neurotransmitter *acetylcholine* is greatly decreased in people with AD. Researchers then developed a class of medications, called *cholinesterase inhibitors,* that help prevent the breakdown of acetylcholine and thus preserve cognitive functions. Cholinesterase inhibitors are used only in the mild to moderate stages of Alzheimer's—generally 3 to 6 years after diagnosis (Alzheimer Society of Canada, 2019b; National Institute on Aging, 2018).

! MEDICATION ALERT

COMMON CHOLINESTERASE INHIBITORS

These are used during the early stages of Alzheimer's disease to improve cognition, memory, and disease-related behaviour.

Generic Name	Brand Name	Adverse Effects
Donepezil	Aricept	Generally mild; include nausea, vomiting, diarrhea, dizziness, headache, insomnia, high or low blood pressure, urinary problems, cough, rash, seizures
Rivastigmine	Exelon	Tremors, confusion, insomnia, depression, anxiety, headache, sleepiness, fatigue, dizziness, nausea, vomiting, anorexia, diarrhea, constipation, increased sweating, urinary tract infection, weight changes
Galantamine	Reminyl	Tremors, insomnia, depression, dizziness, headache, sleepiness, fatigue, anemia, slow heart rate, blood in urine, nausea, vomiting, anorexia, gas, diarrhea, urinary incontinence, weight decrease

---

Cognitive training, which focuses on preserving learning and memory, may be started. Frequent orientation to time, place, and person is needed. A calendar with large letters and a clock with large numbers are helpful.

Care providers need to monitor the patient's personal hygiene and daily activities and help them keep a daily routine. Be sure the environment is safe, and monitor for falls and other accidents.

Establish good communications in the early stages. Know the patient's personal history and link present behaviours to past events. *Do not react to inappropriate behaviours.* Work with the person to discover what the negative behaviours are attempting to communicate. Box 17.8 offers several specific techniques for communicating with individuals with AD.

BOX 17.8 Communication Techniques for Persons With Alzheimer's Disease

1. Always approach from the front—make no surprise appearances.
2. Speak in a normal tone of voice, and greet the person as you would anyone else.
3. Face the person as you talk.
4. Minimize hand movements.
5. Avoid a setting with a high level of sensory stimulation, such as a big room with many people, a high traffic area, or a noisy place.
6. Maintain eye contact, and smile. A frown will convey negative feelings.
7. Use simple familiar words and short, simple sentences.
8. Ask yes-or-no questions.
9. Allow plenty of time for a response.
10. Repeat important information.
11. Be respectful of personal space, and observe the patient's reaction as you move closer. Maintain a distance of 1 to 1.5 m initially.
12. If a person is a pacer, walk with them, in step, while you talk.
13. Use distraction if a situation looks like it may get out of hand, such as if the person is about to hit someone or is trying to leave the home or facility.
14. Use a low-pitched, slow speaking voice, which older persons hear best.
15. Ask only one question at a time. More than one question increases confusion.
16. Repeat key words if the person does not understand the first time.
17. Nod and smile only if what the person said is understood.

Data from Elder Care Online at www.ec-online.net

Maintaining a supportive environment is an important goal of care. Individuals who are cared for in the home need an environment that is simple, free of clutter and other safety hazards, and familiar. Orienting cues help individuals remember where they are and decrease agitation. Box 17.9 offers several interventions that help keep patients oriented to their environments.

A simple daily routine is soothing to people with AD. Daily activities, such as eating, toileting, bathing, and exercise, should follow a consistent schedule. Individuals with AD depend on their routines and structure. They do not adapt well to change, and the consistency of a stable environment helps keep stress levels more manageable.

Simple physical exercises and activities are included in the daily routine for as long as the patient is ambulatory. Exercise helps maintain balance, induce fatigue and restful sleep, prevent constipation, and reduce wandering. Sports, card games, musical activities, painting, and gardening can be enjoyed by individuals well into the moderate stage of AD.

Some therapies that have been helpful for patients with AD are listed in Table 17.5.

Middle and Late Stages

Physical care is increasingly necessary as behaviour gradually becomes more disorganized. Personal hygiene, eating, and

BOX 17.9   Orienting Environmental Cues

- Keep the environment simple and "user-friendly."
- Keep the environment safe: ramps for stairs, grab bars in bathroom, no throw rugs, etc.
- Put large signs that identify each room on the doors.
- Label each drawer with its contents. Use large letters and simple words. Tape the list to the drawer.
- Have clocks and calendars with large letters and numbers in several rooms.
- Colour-code hot and cold faucets red and blue, respectively. Adjust water heater to 48.8°C (120°F).
- Install a brightly coloured toilet seat (it will be easier to see).
- Keep rooms brightly lit with no glare.
- Use nightlights in hallways, bedrooms, and bathrooms.
- Cover doors with curtains or posters to discourage wandering.

TABLE 17.5   Therapeutic Interventions for Alzheimer's Disease

What Is It?	How Does It Work?
Validation therapy	Caregiver buys into patient's illusions and plays along (validates it) until opportunity to refocus behaviours is present, based on the premise that the patient's illusion cannot be changed, but it can be directed
Music therapy	Use of familiar tunes to induce relaxation, alter moods, improve social interactions, and change maladaptive behaviours
Life review	A systematic reflection on one's personal history in which one learns to evaluate, integrate, and accept life as it has been lived; increases quality of life and helps prevent despair and depression
Comfort touch	Skin-to-skin touch with the purpose of bringing comfort; results in improved well-being, self-esteem, and socialization
Doll therapy	Use of dolls and stuffed animals to provide tactile stimulation and comfort
Audio presence intervention	Playing of audio-recorded memories by family members to help decrease agitation

elimination become totally neglected without caregivers (see Sample Patient Care Plan 17.1). All sense of time and place is lost by the middle stage of AD. Behavioural disorganization occurs with behaviours such as agitation, hostility, physical aggression, uncooperativeness, and wandering. Individuals remain ambulatory throughout the middle stage, but they are at a much greater risk for falls and accidents as a result of their confusion.

Wandering is a serious and common problem with persons with AD. About 40% of people with dementia get lost outside their home at least once (Bowen, McKenzie, Steis, et al., 2011). Because of this, there is a growing use of Global Positioning System (GPS) to ensure dementia patients' location and safety.

By the time patients enter the third stage of AD, they are usually unable to walk, totally incontinent, and incapable of self-care. Memory is completely lost. Speech becomes limited to one or two words and is soon lost altogether. Patients become unable to swallow or eat, which leads to a high risk for malnutrition, pneumonia, and bedsores. Placement in a long-term care facility becomes necessary because full-time care and monitoring are now required. Eventually, the individual slips into a coma and dies.

Caregiver Support

Caring for an older person with dementia radically changes the lives of the primary caregiver, family members, and friends. Caring for a loved one with AD is probably the most difficult of all caregiving experiences. It has often been said that AD is worse on the caregivers who must stand by and watch the person they love fade into a vague, unconscious existence.

The majority of people with AD are cared for in the home by family, friends, and home care agencies. Tremendous physical and emotional burdens accompany the home care of a loved one with AD. "Caregivers are more likely to suffer from depression and other negative health issues" (Fowler, 2014). Caregivers must learn to find a balance between personal needs and providing care for their loved ones. Various sources of support help family members through this difficult journey.

Informal support groups consist of family members, friends, people at work, social groups, and faith communities. Members of these groups knew the individual with AD before the illness. Often, they are a great source of respite, strength, socialization, and support for the primary caregivers.

Formal support groups are offered by various home care agencies, elder care centres, and hospices. The local chapter of the Alzheimer Society of Canada (https://alzheimer.ca/en/Home) supports family members and provides information about dementia. It offers both emotional and educational support groups. Stress management groups are helpful in recognizing stress and developing successful coping strategies. Many long-term care facilities now offer *respite care*, where the loved one with AD is safely cared for while caregivers receive a much-needed break. As a care provider, never forget that those who care for the cognitively impaired need your attention as much as your patient does. The support from family, friends, and resource people makes a difference in the quality of life for those caring for loved ones with AD.

Caregiver Education

Studies have found that when caregivers are educated about care for their loved one, stress levels in the home decrease. Caregiver training prepares family members to provide appropriate care for their loved one. Topics such as environmental safety, personal care, coping with difficult behaviours, and care provider stress are addressed, and sources of support are explored.

AD and other dementias are serious conditions, but with continued research and good care we may someday be able to lessen the sad effects of these devastating conditions.

SAMPLE PATIENT CARE PLAN 17.1   Self-Care Deficit

Assessment

History Tess is a 70-year-old retired accountant who is being admitted with a diagnosis of Alzheimer's disease. She had been cared for in her daughter's home until she began to wander. Now the family fears for her safety.

Current Findings Functional assessment reveals an ambulatory woman who is unable to follow directions. She is oriented to person only and has self-care deficits in bathing, dressing, eating, and toileting.

Multidisciplinary Diagnosis

Self-care deficit related to cognitive impairment

Planning/Goals

Tess will dress correctly daily.
Tess will consume 50% or more of each meal by September 15.

THERAPEUTIC INTERVENTIONS

Intervention	Rationale	Team Member
1. Lay out clothes in order of dressing, underclothes first to sweater last.	Provides routine, easier to dress appropriately	Nsg
2. Assist as needed, and praise all efforts.	Positive feedback increases the likelihood that the desired behaviours will be repeated.	All
3. Determine her favorite foods.	She will eat the foods she likes.	Diet, Nsg
4. Evaluate speech and swallowing.	Determines level of impairment	ST
5. Assist Tess with eating.	Ensures nutrition is received	Nsg
6. Document intake, output, and amount of food consumed.	Monitors fluid and nutritional status	Diet, Nsg

Evaluation By the seventh day on the unit, Tess was dressing herself appropriately with cues from caregivers. She currently consumes more than 70% of her meals when she is fed.

Critical Thinking Questions

1. How does providing a daily routine benefit Tess?
2. What can be done to provide support for Tess's daughter?

A complete patient care plan includes several other diagnoses and interventions.
Nsg, nursing staff; *Diet,* dietitian; *ST,* speech therapist.

▎ KEY POINTS

- AD and other dementias are behavioural or mental health problems caused by a medical condition.
- The most significant losses in aging are slower response times and decreased short-term memory.
- The causes of confusion are delirium, dementia, and depression.
- Many medications and drugs cause confusion, especially in older persons because metabolism is slower, drugs are eliminated more slowly, and they can reach toxic levels quickly.
- The signs and symptoms of delirium include disorganized thinking, a decreased attention span, lowered or fluctuating level of consciousness, disturbances in the sleep–wake cycle, disorientation, and changes in psychomotor activity.
- The treatment of delirium depends on its cause. The first priority is to treat the source. The second focus of care is supportive.
- Dementia is a loss of multiple abilities, including short- and long-term memory, language, and the ability to understand. Persons with dementia are unable to process, retrieve, and use information. All have progressive difficulties with memory, judgement, and abstract thinking.

- AD is characterized by memory loss, difficulty performing familiar tasks, problems with language, poor judgement, problems with abstract thinking, misplacing things, disorientation to time and place, loss of initiative, changes in mood or behaviour, and changes in personality.
- Dementia can be primary, as with AD, or it may occur as a result of disease or other conditions, such as HIV (secondary).
- AD is characterized by memory loss, difficulty performing familiar tasks, problems with language, poor judgement, problems with abstract thinking, misplacing things, disorientation to time and place, loss of initiative, changes in mood or behaviour, and changes in personality.
- AD is accompanied by losses in every area of functioning.
- The progression of AD is divided into four stages—early, intermediate, late, and end stage.
- The gentle persuasive approach (GPA) is the model of care that is recommended for dementia patients who display potentially disruptive behaviours.
- Informal support groups consist of family members, friends, and people who knew the individual with AD before the illness. Formal support groups are offered by various home care agencies, elder care centres, hospices, and the Canadian Alzheimer Society.

ADDITIONAL LEARNING RESOURCES

Go to your Evolve website (http://evolve.elsevier.com/Canada/Morrison-Valfre/) for additional online resources, including the online Study Guide for additional learning activities to help you master this chapter content.

CRITICAL THINKING QUESTIONS

1. Using GPA principles, describe how you would care for a patient with dementia who requires his scheduled medication and blood pressure check when he is determined to find his way "out from that place to go to work."
2. An older female patient on the mental health unit who was admitted to treat her depression suddenly becomes upset because she can't remember where she is; she says, "I can't think straight." The staff has never witnessed this behaviour in the patient before, and this type of complaint is not documented in her nursing history. What is this patient most likely experiencing?
3. A 91-year-old female patient with dementia is being seen by the home health nurse. She no longer recognizes her husband or children. She also has forgotten how to eat and dress herself, and she wanders through the house both day and night. The nurse notes that the caregiver is noticeably tired, yet he is adamant that he wants his wife to be in her home. What should be the priority focus of the nurse's communication with the husband?

REFERENCES

Alzheimer Society of Canada. (2019a). *Dementia numbers in Canada.* https://alzheimer.ca/en/Home/About-dementia/What-is-dementia/Dementia-numbers

Alzheimer Society of Canada. (2019b). *Drugs approved for Alzheimer's disease.* https://alzheimer.ca/en/on/About-dementia/Treatment-options/Drugs-approved-for-Alzheimers-disease

American Psychiatric Association (APA). (2013). *Diagnostic and statistical manual of mental disorders* (5th ed.). American Psychiatric Publishing.

Bowen, M. E., McKenzie, B., Steis, M., et al. (2011). Prevalence of and antecedents to dementia-related missing incidents in the community. *Dementia and Geriatric Cognitive Disorders, 31*(6), 406–412. https://doi.org/10.1159/000329792

Fowler, C. (2014). Caring for the caregiver. *Nursing, 44*(5), 60.

Government of Canada. (2017). *Dementia in Canada, including Alzheimer's disease.* https://www.canada.ca/en/public-health/services/publications/diseases-conditions/dementia-highlights-canadian-chronic-disease-surveillance.html

Greider, K., & Neimark, J. (2016). *Making our minds last a lifetime.* https://www.psychologytoday.com/articles/200910/making-our-minds-last-lifetime

Henry, M. (2002). Descending into delirium. *American Journal of Nursing, 102*(3), 57.

Hippocrates. (about 400 BCE). *Brainy quote. Hippocrates quote.* https://www.brainyquote.com/quotes/hippocrates_132701

Martine, R., & Duda, J. (Eds.). (n.d.). *Parkinson's disease: Mind, mood & memory.* National Parkinson Foundation. http://www3.parkinson.org/site/DocServer/Mind_Mood_Memory.pdf?docID=191

National Institute on Aging. (2018). *Alzheimer's disease medication fact sheet.* https://order.nia.nih.gov/sites/default/files/2018-03/alzheimers-disease-medications-fact-sheet.pdf

Peterson, R. (2002). *Mayo clinic on Alzheimer's disease.* Mayo Health Clinic Information.

Rosen, M. D. (2014). Am I losing my mind? *AARP Bulletin, 55*(3), 18.

Toronto Region Best Practice in LTC Initiative. (2007). *Recognizing delirium, depression and dementia (3D's).* https://connectability.ca/wp-content/uploads/2012/11/ThreeDcomparison-TPADD-CONFERENCE.pdf

Patients With Psychological Challenges

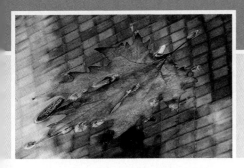

18

Managing Anxiety

OBJECTIVES

Upon completion of this chapter, the student will be able to:
1. Describe the continuum of responses to anxiety.
2. Identify three types of coping mechanisms used to decrease anxiety.
3. Compare the difference between normal anxiety and an anxiety disorder.
4. Discuss the difference between phobic and obsessive-compulsive behaviours.
5. Examine three features of post-traumatic stress disorder.
6. Explain the importance of monitoring medication use for patients with high levels of anxiety.
7. Examine three methods for recognizing and preventing anxiety.

OUTLINE

KEY TERMS

Anxiety is a feeling of uneasiness, uncertainty, and helplessness. It is a state of tension. Sometimes it is associated with feelings of dread or doom. Anxiety is the *normal emotional response* to a real or imagined threat or stressor. It is just as normal a response as joy, surprise, or pity.

Anxiety serves several purposes. It is a warning of impending danger. Mild anxiety can increase learning by helping with concentration and focus. Anxiety can also provide motivation. However, uncontrolled anxiety often leads to ineffective and maladaptive behaviours. Anxiety is a normal part of survival and growth. How individuals use and control anxiety is a measure of mental health and illness.

CONTINUUM OF ANXIETY RESPONSES

Reactions to anxiety occur along a continuum of behavioural responses (Stuart, 2013). *Adaptive responses* to anxiety result in positive outcomes. New learning and greater self-esteem result from coping successfully with anxiety. Positively focused anxiety helps us to adapt, learn, and grow from our experiences. *Maladaptive responses* to anxiety are ineffective attempts to cope. They do nothing to resolve the problem or eliminate uneasy feelings (Fig. 18.1).

Responses to anxiety occur on four levels, ranging from mild to panic (Table 18.1). During periods of anxiety, physical, intellectual, emotional, and behavioural responses help us cope. In periods of severe anxiety, the autonomic nervous system stimulates the fight-or-flight response, which triggers many physical changes. Use Table 18.1 as a basis for assessing the anxiety levels of patients. Decreasing anxiety is an important intervention in every health care situation.

Types of Anxiety

Anxiety occurs as the result of a perceived threat to one's self. The threat itself may be real or occur in response to what we think is happening. The actual object of anxiety often cannot be identified, but the feelings associated with the experience are all too real.

For the sake of discussion, anxiety is classified by types. **Signal anxiety** is a learned response to an anticipated event. The usually calm student who becomes nauseated during examinations illustrates signal anxiety. An anxiety state occurs when one's coping abilities become overwhelmed and emotional control is lost. Many emergencies, accidents, and traumas are associated with anxiety states. Last is an **anxiety trait**, which is a *learned* component of the personality. Persons with anxiety traits react with anxiety in relatively low

stress situations. The adolescent who always gives reasons for their behaviour, even when not requested, illustrates an example of a person with an anxiety trait.

Anxiety is similar to fear, but anxiety is usually less specific. Following are a few facts about anxiety (Newman, 2017):
Feeling anxious is normal, but it should not interfere with everyday life.
Excessive, persistent anxiety is an issue for many people.
There are a range of coping mechanisms and strategies to alleviate anxiety.
Sometimes, anxiety may be diagnosed as a particular anxiety disorder.

Types of Anxiety Responses

People often feel anxious when they face uncertainty. New situations, unfamiliar environments, or tasks for which we are not prepared are often associated with anxiety.

The physical symptoms of anxiety include muscle tension, fidgeting, headaches, and problems with sleep. Higher levels of anxiety trigger the fight-or-flight reaction and result in nausea, dizziness, sweating, increased heart rate, and elevated blood pressure.

Most individuals deal with anxiety by using a number of behaviours or **coping mechanisms** that help decrease discomfort. All coping methods reduce anxiety, but if used to extreme, serious mental and physical health challenges can result.

Coping Methods

Coping mechanisms in the *physical* realm include efforts to directly face and handle the problem. The woman who fights the thief who is attempting to snatch her purse, for example, is directly dealing with the source of her anxiety. Running away or removing oneself from the stressor is another physical way to reduce anxiety. Many individuals exercise to reduce anxiety. Physical exercises, such as running or other aerobics, can reduce the effects of the fight-or-flight response by lowering blood pressure and neurochemical levels. Stretching and yoga exercises release muscle tension and encourage relaxation.

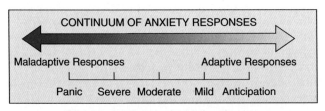

Fig. 18.1 Continuum of anxiety responses.

TABLE 18.1   Levels of Anxiety

Anxiety Level	Physical	Cognitive/Perceptual	Emotional/Behavioural
Mild	• Vital signs normal • Minimal muscle tension • Pupils normal, constricted	• Perceptual field is broad • Awareness of multiple environmental and internal stimuli • Thoughts may be random, but controlled	• Feelings of relative comfort and safety • Relaxed, calm appearance and voice • Performance is automatic; habitual behaviours occur
Moderate	• Vital signs normal or slightly elevated • Tension experienced may be uncomfortable or pleasurable (labelled as "tense" or "excited")	• Alert; perception narrowed, focused • Optimal state for problem-solving and learning • Attentive	• Feelings of readiness and challenge, energized • Engages in competitive activity and learns new skills • Voice, facial expression interested or concerned
Severe	• Fight-or-flight response • Autonomic nervous system excessively stimulated (vital signs increased, sweating increased, urinary urgency and frequency, diarrhea, dry mouth, appetite decreased, pupils dilated) • Muscles rigid, tense • Senses affected; hearing decreased, pain sensation decreased	• Perceptual field greatly narrowed • Problem-solving difficult • Selective attention (focuses on one detail) • Selective inattention (blocks out threatening stimuli) • Distortion of time (things seem faster or slower than actual) • Dissociative tendencies; vigilambulism (automatic behaviour)	• Feels threatened; startles with new stimuli; feels on "overload" • Activity may increase or decrease (may pace, run away, wring hands, moan, shake, stutter, become very disorganized or withdrawn, freeze in position/unable to move) • May seem and feel depressed • Demonstrates denial; may complain of aches or pains; may be agitated or irritable • Need for space increased • Eyes may dart around room, or gaze may be fixed • May close eyes to shut out environment
Panic	• The preceding symptoms escalate until sympathetic nervous system release occurs • Person may become pale, blood pressure decreases, hypotension • Muscle coordination poor • Pain, hearing sensations minimal	• Perception totally scattered or closed • Unable to take in stimuli • Problem-solving and logical thinking highly improbable • Perception of unreality about self, environment, or event • Dissociation may occur	• Feels helpless with total loss of control • May be angry, terrified; may become combative or totally withdrawn, cry, run • Completely disorganized • Behaviour is usually extremely active or inactive

Intellectual coping mechanisms are aimed at making the threat less meaningful by *changing* one's *perception.* If we do not define the event as threatening, then anxiety is not produced. A good example is the individual who sees everyone in the audience smiling when he is about to give a speech. The threat (audience disapproval) is reduced by the perception of smiling faces. Another coping mechanism in the intellectual realm is meditation, which helps clear and refocus one's mental energies.

Spiritual coping methods include faith, prayer, and ritual. Attending religious services or communing with nature can reduce anxiety. Many cultural rituals also help individuals cope.

Emotional responses include crying, communicating or sharing one's feelings of anxiety, and using ego defence mechanisms.

Defence Mechanisms

The psychological strategies that help to lessen anxious feelings are called (ego) **defence mechanisms**. These are normal psychological self-preserving behaviours. Their purpose is to reduce or avoid negative states such as conflict, frustration, anxiety, and stress. They are used when one feels threatened. Employing defence mechanisms helps to avoid negative emotional states, but usually individuals are not consciously aware of their use. No matter which mechanism is used, the goal is to reduce uncomfortable negative emotions. Table 18.2 lists several commonly used ego defence mechanisms.

Crisis

When one's ability to cope with anxiety is overwhelmed, a crisis results. One's defence mechanisms are no longer useful. No efforts to cope with the situation lessen one's anxiety. During a crisis, new coping behaviours must be developed to successfully resolve the source problem. Review Chapter 8 for a more thorough discussion of crisis and its therapeutic interventions.

TABLE 18.2	**Common Defence Mechanisms**	
Mechanism	**Definition**	**Example**
Compensation	Attempt to overcome feelings of inferiority or make up for deficiency	A girl who thinks she cannot sing studies to become an expert pianist.
Conversion	Channelling of unbearable anxieties into body signs and symptoms	A man's arm becomes paralyzed after impulses to strike another person.
Denial	Refusal to acknowledge conflict and thus escapes reality of situation	Persons living near a volcano disregard the dangers involved.
Displacement	Redirecting of energies to another person or object	A husband shouts at his wife, the wife then berates her child, who then scolds the dog.
Dissociation	Separation of emotions from situation; removal of painful anxieties from conscious awareness	A soldier casually describes the battle in which he lost his legs.
Fantasy	Distortion of unacceptable wishes, behaviours	A teenager doing poorly in school daydreams about owning a private jet.
Identification	Taking on of personal characteristics of admired person to conceal own feelings of inadequacy	Adolescents dress and behave like the members of a popular singing group.
Intellectualization	Focusing of attention on technical or logical aspects of threatening situation	A wife describes the details of nurses' unsuccessful attempts to prevent the death of her husband.
Isolation	The splitting-off of emotional components from a thought to cope unemotionally with topics that would normally be overwhelming	A medical student dissects a cadaver without being disturbed by thoughts of death
Projection	Placing of one's own unacceptable thoughts, wishes, emotions onto others	A sportsman, unable to accept that he has hostile feelings about his competitor, says, "He doesn't like me."
Rationalization	Use of a "good" (but not real) reason to explain behaviour to make unacceptable motivation more acceptable	A student justifies failing an examination by saying that there was too much material to cover.
Reaction formation	Development of conscious attitudes and behaviour patterns that are *opposite* to what one really would like to have (Stuart, 2013)	A young man with homosexual feelings, which he finds to be threatening, engages in excessive heterosexual activities.
Regression	Coping with present conflict, stress by returning to earlier, more secure stage of life	A 4-year-old boy whose parents are going through a divorce starts to suck his thumb and wet his pants.
Restitution	Giving back to resolve guilt feelings (paying up with interest)	A man argues with his wife and then buys her roses.
Sublimation	Unconscious channelling of unacceptable behaviours into different but constructive and more socially approved areas	A hostile young man who enjoys fighting becomes busy with extra activities, preventing from him from socializing and being exposed to the potential to be in a fighting situation.
Substitution	Suppressing anxiety by replacing or substituting inappropriate behaviour or/and a difficult-to-achieve goal with one that is more acceptable or/and easy to achieve	A person who cannot go to a medical school for lack of funds or sufficient merit may opt to go to the College for Occupational Therapists instead.
Suppression	Removal of conflict by removing anxiety from consciousness	A woman with a family history of breast cancer "forgets" her appointment for a mammogram.
Symbolization	Use of an unrelated object to represent hidden idea	A girl who feels insignificant draws a picture of her family in which she is the smallest character.
Undoing	Distractive or inappropriate behaviour or thought that is followed by acts to take away or reverse action and decrease guilt and anxiety	The most famous example for this defence mechanism is confession. A person attempts to diminish anxiety about their own distractive behaviour or thoughts by a secret admission.

Ineffective Coping

While anxiety is a normal part of everyday life, sometimes it is not dealt with in an effective manner. Ineffective coping expresses itself differently across different cultures (see Cultural Considerations box).

CULTURAL CONSIDERATIONS

Anxiety appears to occur in most cultures, if not every culture. Expressions of anxiety, however, differ greatly:
- Japanese people tend to somatize or handle anxiety by becoming physically ill.
- Mothers in the Dominican Republic cope with the anxiety of the "evil eye" by wearing red and saving the infant's umbilical cord.
- Greek men consider body hair a sign of manhood. Shaving their hair in preparation for a surgical procedure can result in great anxiety.
- When a Vietnamese individual has a panic attack outdoors, they are said to be trug gio (hit by the wind).

Anxiety is a protective state that motivates us to pursue goals and respond to threats. However, too little or too much anxiety can lead to ineffective coping behaviours and cause more problems. Too little anxiety can result in a lack of attention or focus in important situations. Too much anxiety can overwhelm and immobilize an individual and result in an inability to accomplish important tasks. When ego defence mechanisms become the primary means of dealing with anxiety, they replace problem-solving and other positive ways of coping. The use of ineffective coping behaviours can lead to too much anxiety and result in an anxiety disorder.

Self-Awareness and Anxiety

A basic characteristic of anxiety is that it is contagious. Like a cold or influenza virus, anxiety is easily transmitted to others. Patients have an uncanny ability to focus on the anxiety levels of their health care providers. Sometimes the patient becomes the therapeutic agent for an anxious care provider.

The therapeutic relationship is built on trust. Inherent in that trust is the care provider's responsibility to listen and communicate effectively. High levels of anxiety can impair our ability to interact therapeutically with the patient. For this reason, it is important for care providers to recognize and cope effectively with their own anxieties. Remember, we may not choose our anxieties, but we do choose how we deal with them. The following Case Study provides an example of how a health care provider's anxiety can affect the therapeutic relationship.

THEORIES RELATING TO ANXIETY

A number of theories have been developed since Sigmund Freud first listed anxiety as a defence mechanism. Today the causes of anxiety are still uncertain, but research indicates that a combination of biological, psychosocial, and environmental factors is involved. A few of the more well-known theories of anxiety are discussed here.

CASE STUDY

Cathy's appointment with her physician was for 10 a.m. By the time she had waited for more than 2 hours, Cathy was feeling frustrated. After a 2.5-hour wait, she was downright anxious. Just as she began to leave, her name was called, and she was ushered into a rather impersonal examination room where she changed into the paper gown and waited, shivering, for her physician.

After what seemed another hour, the door finally opened. Her physician, a woman of many words, began the interaction with "My gads, what a day! One thing goes wrong in the morning, and I spend the rest of the day chasing myself to catch up."

Noting her physician's tension and rapid speech, Cathy responded, "You certainly look tired. Sounds like you have been working too hard." Her physician countered with, "That's not the half of it," and then proceeded to share each of her day's frustrations.
- Who was the therapeutic individual in this situation?
- How did the physician's behaviour affect therapeutic interactions with this patient?
- How do you think the interaction affected Cathy's anxiety?

Biological Models

The biological group of theories attempts to find a biological or physical basis for anxiety. The work of Charles Darwin first posed the possibility of a link between emotions and the ability to adapt. Later, Hans Selye demonstrated a connection between the perception of stress and physical changes in the body with his fight-or-flight response. During the 1990s, "the decade of the brain," many advances in the understanding of emotions and mental illness were made. Today we are beginning to gain an understanding of the role that emotions play in health and illness as researchers unveil new information.

One of the most popular current theories of anxiety relates to the role of neurochemicals. Research into the role of these body chemicals, called *neurotransmitters,* has resulted in evidence that emotions may be linked to changes in brain biochemistry. Anxiety is thought to result from the dysfunction of two or more neurotransmitters. Some studies have demonstrated inappropriately activated norepinephrine and imbalances between this and other neurotransmitters. Further research is being done to investigate specific medications designed to alter neurotransmitter activity.

Other ongoing studies are investigating the role of the autonomic nervous system in the development of anxiety. Anxiety commonly occurs with other challenges. Many medical disorders, hormonal imbalances, problems with substance use, eating and sleeping disorders, headaches, and even fatigue are related to anxiety.

Psychodynamic Model

According to Freud, anxiety results from a conflict between two opposing forces within the personality—the ego and the id. Neurotic or maladaptive behaviours are the result of attempts to defend oneself against anxiety, just as adaptive behaviours do. Psychotherapists today have broadened the psychoanalytic theory to define anxiety as the result of a conflict between two opposing forces within an individual.

Interpersonal Model

With the interpersonal model, anxiety is explained in terms of interactions with others. Anxiety develops when early childhood interactions with significant others result in negative outcomes, such as disapproval. Over time, an individual's responses to anxiety form the basis for low self-esteem and poor self-concept.

Interpersonal theorists work with a broad definition of anxiety. Harry Stack Sullivan believed that children acquire the values of their parents because they are dependent on others for approval or disapproval. In adulthood, individuals cope with anxiety on the basis of their perceptions in addition to how they were taught to cope with conflict as children. Thus, from the perspective of this interpersonal model, early assessment of and intervention for children who are anxious are important.

Behavioural Model

The behavioural theories consider anxiety a learned response. Children who have experienced anxiety in one situation link those feelings to more general situations. Anxiety results when individuals encounter a signal that reminds them of earlier anxious times. Thus, individuals learn to react with anxiety by linking anxious experiences.

Other Models

Other theories explain anxiety as the result of a loss of life's meaning (*existential* theory). Environmental models tie anxiety to uncontrollable events or situations. Fires, floods, and other natural disasters, along with assaults and human-induced traumas, all serve as stressors for the individual.

Many health care providers have chosen to view anxiety from a *holistic* mode. Anxiety can be viewed as influencing every realm of human functioning. Physical reactions, such as the fight-or-flight reaction, result from anxiety. Strong emotional responses occur when one is anxious. Social areas of functioning can become impaired because of anxiety, and even one's spirituality comes into question during times of great or prolonged anxiety. By considering each area of functioning, care providers are better able to plan and implement effective therapeutic interventions for relieving anxiety.

ANXIETY THROUGHOUT THE LIFE CYCLE

Anxiety is a universal experience. It begins early in life, as soon as one becomes capable of realizing that something could go wrong. Responses to anxiety grow and evolve with the individual. Behavioural reactions to anxiety change as effective (anxiety-reducing) actions are added to current coping mechanisms. Responses or behaviours that are ineffective or serve no purpose are discarded. An understanding of how individuals at various developmental stages perceive and cope

with anxiety can help care providers plan and implement individualized care for all patients.

Anxiety in Childhood

Children learn to cope with anxiety by watching and imitating others. Most children are happy, active individuals with few anxieties. However, if their needs for nurturing are not met, high levels of anxiety can result. Children's needs for love and belonging are so great that later-life emotional difficulties are often related to unmet needs in childhood. Although children are not strangers to stress, some children appear to be more vulnerable than others (Hockenberry & Wilson, 2014). Recognizing signs of childhood stress and intervening early are important as doing so can prevent anxiety from becoming overwhelming and help teach children how to cope successfully.

Anxiety is experienced in relation to a child's *developmental level*. Infants feel a sense of discomfort if their needs are not immediately met. Toddlers become anxious when they perceive something larger or more ferocious than themselves that is capable of harming them. Their anxiety relates to power and lasts until the balance of power can be restored. Anxiety in preschool children revolves around the experience of separating from the security of parents. As children learn that separations are not permanent, anxieties lessen and coping abilities improve. School-age children learn to cope with the anxieties of becoming members of a group outside the family.

The development of certain habits early in childhood appears to help children relieve anxiety. Thumb sucking, nail biting, hair pulling, and rhythmic body movements are examples of behaviours that seem to soothe and lessen anxiety for young children. Excessive anxiety appears to develop when children resist their feelings of anxiety and focus them elsewhere. Problems associated with anxiety in childhood include compulsions, phobias, separation anxiety disorder, overanxious disorder, and avoidant disorders.

Separation anxiety disorder is diagnosed when children are unable to be without their parents for any length of time. By about 6 months of age, infants are able to recognize their parents' absence from the room and protest. They soon become very aware of their mother's activities. They learn to identify behaviours that indicate their mother is leaving the area. By 11 months, most children begin to protest before their mother leaves. During the next 4 years, children learn to tolerate varying degrees of separation from parents. By school age, most children separate from parents easily and their focus changes to coping with school life.

Children with separation anxiety disorder, however, experience severe anxiety that can develop into panic when separated from significant others. Physical complaints such as headaches, nausea, or vomiting are common when children anticipate separation. Nightmares occur frequently. Associated fears of death, animals, monsters, and harmful situations are seen in children with separation anxiety disorder.

Overanxious disorder appears during childhood with unrealistic levels of anxiety lasting longer than 6 months—a long time in the life of a child. These children worry about everything from past events to future expectations. Overanxious disorder often occurs in children whose parents focus on overachievement and downplay their children's actual accomplishments.

Children can also experience severe anxiety during times of great change in the family. Reactions to divorce, death, or separation often lead to situational anxiety or **avoidance behaviours** in which the child refuses to cope with the anxiety-producing situation by ignoring it.

Sadly, children are not immune to the effects of unresolved anxiety. Occurrences of post-traumatic stress disorder (PTSD), depression, and suicide are on the rise in children. Children with behavioural issues often have underlying anxieties. For children to grow and mature into effective, adaptable individuals, we must recognize and treat the signs of anxiety early.

Anxiety in Adolescence

Coping skills learned in childhood continue to be refined throughout adolescence. If teens have successfully handled anxieties in childhood, the distresses of becoming adults offer opportunities for personal growth and maturation. Adolescents who ineffectively cope with anxiety often express themselves inappropriately. Running away from home; becoming angry, defiant, aggressive, or manipulative; experimenting with drugs; and engaging in high-risk behaviours often occur. They frequently use denial to cope and resist attempts to explore the anxiety-producing perceptions that lead to understanding. When anxieties are extreme, adolescents may engage in self-mutilating behaviours or develop the behaviours of anorexia nervosa or bulimia (see Chapter 23).

Many initial symptoms of schizophrenia and other psychoses begin in adolescence. Signs of maladaptive behaviours, such as flights from reality, ritualistic behaviours, or withdrawal from others, may actually be symptoms of serious mental health challenges.

According to the Canadian Institute for Health Information (CIHI), 10% to 20% of Canadian children and youth may develop a mental disorder (CIHI, 2019). Health care providers who work with adolescents must assess adolescents' anxiety levels and offer early intervention and education before anxiety becomes the fuel for more serious mental health issues.

Anxiety in Adulthood

By young adulthood, coping behaviours are well established. Adults commonly encounter situations that provoke anxiety as they move through their worlds of work, family, and community. Some adults appear to lead a "charmed life," with few stresses and anxieties. Others seem to continually struggle, only to rebound from one misfortune after another. Like their younger counterparts, adults handle anxiety using earlier, established coping mechanisms.

Adults must cope with many anxiety-producing situations. Developmental tasks, such as establishing a career and family, present numerous stressors. The loss of income, spouse, or physical ability can lead to severe anxiety. Uncontrollable situations, such as fires, floods, earthquakes, or wars, often result in long-lasting anxiety. Unless resolved, it can evolve into post-traumatic stress syndrome. When adult anxieties are not successfully managed, a number of mental health challenges may result. Generalized or situational anxiety disorders are diagnosed when individuals become overwhelmed and nonfunctional because of their anxieties. Other maladaptive responses include panic disorders, phobias, behavioural addictions, obsessions, and compulsive activities.

Anxiety in Older Persons

Older persons tend to express anxieties in less overt ways than younger people do. Elders often deny their anxiety. They may *somatize* (physically express) their feelings (this is called **somatization**). Social desirability factors, such as looking good to others and projecting an image of self-reliance, commonly influence their expressions of anxiety.

Although few actual statistics are available, anxiety appears to be a common issue for many older persons. Elders face a combination of anxiety-producing life hazards. They must cope with an uncertain future as well as the problems of the present. Issues about loss of health, self-determination, and control can cause much anxiety in older individuals.

Many of today's older persons have experienced difficult times when work and food were scarce. Socially, they were taught that it is inappropriate to share one's fears and anxieties. Because older persons are less likely to share feelings directly, it can be more difficult to recognize the signs of anxiety in older patients.

Behaviours indicating the presence of anxiety include apathy; changes in eating, sleeping, and ability to concentrate; impatience; and fatigue. To promote an atmosphere that allows for expression of what is being experienced, state your observations of behaviours that indicate anxiety. One of the most effective methods for assessing anxiety in older persons is to simply ask the patient to explain or describe their anxious feelings. Older people usually appreciate the interest of concerned care providers.

ANXIETY DISORDERS

If anxiety is a normal human response, when does its expression become a disorder? An **anxiety disorder** exists when anxiety is expressed in ineffective or maladaptive ways and one's coping mechanisms (behaviours) do not successfully relieve the distress. People cope with anxiety using every area of functioning. In the physical realm, one deals directly with the source. Intellectual efforts involve analyzing the situation, problem-solving, or changing the meaning of the problem. Many individuals call on their spiritual resources in an effort to cope with anxiety-producing issues. When efforts in these areas fail, ego defence mechanisms are used in an attempt to reduce the emotional distress.

The diagnosis of an anxiety disorder is based on a description of the behaviours that express distress. The fifth edition of the *Diagnostic and Statistical Manual of Mental Disorders* (*DSM-5*) (American Psychiatric Association [APA], 2013) classifies anxiety disorders by the objects or situations that induce anxiety and the individual's perceptions of or reactions to them. Because these disorders are encountered in every culture, society, and health care setting, it is important to understand their nature.

Separation Anxiety Disorder

A person who becomes inappropriately fearful and anxious when separated from an important person or object may be diagnosed with separation anxiety. To meet the criteria for diagnosis, the anxiety must be long-standing with inappropriate or extreme reactions. These individuals fear that great harm may come to them when they and the attached figure are apart. Nightmares and physical symptoms, such as upset stomach, nausea, vomiting, and sleep disturbances, may occur.

Signs of separation anxiety are commonly seen following a loss or traumatic event. The individual becomes reluctant to leave the attachment figure and withdraws from social activities. Children may avoid school and social activities. Adults can be protective and dependent. They may dislike travel. Many have difficulty coping with changes, such as marriage or a new baby.

Selective Mutism

The hallmark of selective mutism is a repeated, consistent failure to speak when one is expected to do so and is able to speak in other situations. Children may speak to family members in the home but remain silent in front of all others, including relatives and close friends. Their lack of speech limits their ability to do well in school and in other situations. Sometimes an individual will "outgrow" selective mutism but still suffer from a social anxiety disorder.

Specific Phobia

A **phobia** is an internal fear reaction. Phobias involve specific situations or objects. They can stem from a fear of people, animals, objects, situations, or occurrences. For example, a *social phobia* is an unrealistic and persistent fear of any situation in which other people could be judging. Individuals with social phobias are constantly worried about looking foolish. They fear their hands will tremble if they try to write, their voice will quaver if they attempt to talk, or they will vomit if they start to eat. Some are especially anxious in the presence of authority figures or persons with high social contacts. Even eye contact (or the lack of it) from others can be misunderstood as scrutiny and rejection. When the anxieties associated with the social phobia are intense, a full-blown panic attack often results. Persons with severe social phobias often avoid contact with anyone outside their immediate family. Life for many socially phobic individuals can be a lonely and isolated existence.

Phobias differ from common fears. First, phobias are obsessive in nature. Individuals with phobias tend to dwell on their object of fear almost to the point of fascination.

Thinking may take the form of fantasies about the fear, such as the person with thanatophobia (fear of dying) rehearsing their funeral.

People with phobias handle their anxieties differently. Craighead and Nemeroff (2010) note, "A phobia typically produces so high a level of anxiety that it is immobilizing, preventing the person from acting in a way that could prove effective in alleviating the anxiety." The anxiety or fear that is normally protective immobilizes the individual with a phobia.

The characteristics of phobias vary with the culture. In some cultures, fears of hexes, spells, magical spirits, and unseen forces result in phobic reactions. Health care providers should remember cultural backgrounds when assessing patients for phobic responses to anxiety.

CRITICAL THINKING

A patient has reported an intense fear of "needles." Even a view of the needle can cause significant discomfort.

At this time, you are preparing the patient for surgery and have to install an IV line.

- How would you react to your patient's anxiety associated with the "needle"?
- Which therapeutic interventions would you choose as a care provider?

Social Anxiety Disorder

Social anxiety disorder is a severe form of anxiety that causes impairment in social, occupational, or other aspects of a person's functioning. The anxiety is related to a person's fear of a potential judgement by others during social exposure (meeting, gathering, or even been observed causally). The individual fears that they will show signs of anxiety that will be judged and that they will be rejected by others.

These can be shy individuals, speaking with an overly soft tone of voice, using inadequate eye contact, not being open in conversations, and employed in work that does not require social contact. Blushing can be their typical response to a social environment.

Panic Disorders

Panic disorders offer a challenge to health care providers because their signs and symptoms are difficult to distinguish from actual physical dysfunctions. People living with a panic disorder suffer from recurrent, *unanticipated* panic attacks. A **panic attack** is a brief period of intense fear or discomfort. At least one such attack would be followed by a persistent worry that it may happen again. That worry will lead to a significant change in a person's behaviour to avoid the situation associated with a panic attack or unfamiliar situations, even though each time it is unexpected. The person may reorganize their whole life to have somebody always available to help, and may restrict their own activity in order "to be safe." A panic attack is always accompanied by at least 4 of 13 physical and emotional reactions (Box 18.1). The duration of the actual attack

BOX 18.1   Panic Attack Criteria

A panic attack is a period of intense fear or discomfort in which *at least four* of the following symptoms develop abruptly and reach a peak within 10 minutes:

1. Palpitations, pounding heart, or accelerated heart rate
2. Sweating
3. Trembling or shaking
4. Feeling short of breath, smothering
5. Feeling of choking
6. Chest pain or discomfort
7. Nausea or abdominal distress
8. Feeling dizzy, unsteady, lightheaded, or faint
9. Chills or hot flushes
10. Paresthesias (numbness, tingling sensations)
11. Derealization (feelings of unreality) or depersonalization (being detached from oneself)
12. Fear of losing control or going crazy
13. Fear of dying

is short (usually 1–15 minutes), with a peak in anxiety after about 10 minutes.

Panic disorders are more common than once thought. Research has shown that many patients seen in primary care settings suffer from panic disorders. These disorders are often misdiagnosed or inadequately treated. Panic disorders are more common in women (70%), people who are separated or divorced, and people between ages 24 and 44. Typically, an individual with a panic attack presents with physical complaints that may indicate a life-threatening situation.

If agoraphobia is a part of panic attack, then this condition is given a separate diagnosis of agoraphobia.

Panic Attack Specifier

One single panic attack is not indicative of a separate mental disorder. Yet, panic attack can be a part of other mental disorders (e.g., depression, PTSD) or medical conditions (e.g., cardiac, gastrointestinal). A panic attack differs from severe anxiety by its very distinguishable severe symptoms (outlined in Box 18.1), abrupt nature, and brief duration. Panic attacks can be expected or unexpected. Expected panic attacks are easier to avoid because they have an identifiable trigger.

Agoraphobia

Agoraphobia is anxiety about possible situations in which a panic attack may occur. People with agoraphobia avoid people, places, or events from which escape would be difficult or embarrassing. Fear accompanies a sense of helplessness and embarrassment with the thought of a panic attack occurring. Typically, agoraphobia is associated with public situations, such as being in a crowd, standing in line, or travelling on a bus or plane. Standing on a bridge or being afraid to leave the house alone is also associated with agoraphobia. The presence of chronic stressors complicates the picture for treatment and improvement.

Treatment for panic disorders has three goals: educate patients about the nature of the disorder, block the panic attacks pharmacologically, and assist patients in developing more adaptive ways of coping with their anxieties. Cognitive therapy can help individuals identify their emotions and behaviours. Psychotherapy allows them to explore social or personal difficulties. Education and emotional support are important therapeutic measures for patients who experience panic disorders. Many have found meditation, biofeedback, aromatherapy, and other stress-reducing techniques helpful.

Generalized Anxiety Disorder (GAD)

A **generalized anxiety disorder** is diagnosed when an individual's anxiety is broad, long-lasting, and excessive. It is primarily a disturbance in the emotional area of functioning. Eventually it affects every other aspect of one's world. People with GAD are worried and anxious more often than not. They tend to *fret* about numerous things and find it difficult to control their worries. They are so anxious that they often cannot concentrate on a task long enough to complete it. Emotional responses are far out of proportion to the actual situation. Physical signs and symptoms usually accompany the anxiety. They can range from muscle tension to full fight-or-flight responses.

Children with GAD tend to worry about their school performance and social interactions, whereas adults with generalized anxiety concentrate on worrying about everyday events.

There are three main things separating GAD from non-pathological (natural) anxiety. GAD involves the following:

1. Worries cause a significant malfunction of daily life.
2. These worries are more pervasive, cause a serious distress, last much longer in time, and include a massive range of personal life circumstances (finances, career, family, social, etc.).
3. The worries are usually accompanied by physical symptoms (restlessness or feelings of being keyed up or on edge).

OBSESSIVE-COMPULSIVE AND RELATED DISORDERS

Obsessive-compulsive and related disorders include obsessive-compulsive disorder, body dysphoric disorder, hoarding disorder, trichotillomania (hair-pulling disorder), excoriation (skin-picking) disorder, substance-/medication-induced obsessive-compulsive and related disorder, obsessive-compulsive and related disorder due to another medical condition, other specified obsessive-compulsive and related disorder, and unspecified obsessive-compulsive and related disorder.

Obsessive-Compulsive Disorder (OCD)

An **obsession** is an irrational distressing, persistent *thought and/or image that causes excessive anxiety and discomfort*. A **compulsion** is recurring *behaviour that a person executes to diminish that anxiety and discomfort*. Compulsions are not just habits; they are specific behaviours that *must* be performed to reduce anxiety. All of us have repeated worries and routines that we recognize as not entirely sensible. However, persons with obsessive-compulsive disorder (OCD) are consumed by self-destructive, anxiety-reducing thoughts and actions.

To diagnose an individual with OCD, they must have obsessions, compulsions, or both that take up at least 1 hour per day or cause significant distress or impairment. For behaviours to be called obsessions and compulsions, they must meet the criteria listed in Box 18.2.

Obsessive-compulsive disorders were thought to be relatively rare, but recent studies have demonstrated that OCD occurs in many more individuals than previously thought. Symptoms of OCD can occur as early as 3 years of age, but usually they begin in adolescence. Men and women seem to be equally affected, though symptoms frequently appear an average of 5 years earlier in men. A high rate of OCD occurs in persons with other mental health challenges, especially depression and schizophrenia.

The most common obsessions relate to cleanliness, dirt, and germs; aggressive and sexual impulses; health concerns; safety concerns; and order and symmetry. Obsessions can take the form of thoughts, doubts, fears, images, or impulses. People with OCD use the ego defence mechanisms of repression to cope with distressing obsessions. They focus anxieties into compulsive actions (*displacement*) and engage in undoing behaviours to relieve stress. They know, intellectually, that their attempts to relieve anxiety are maladaptive, but they feel emotionally compelled to yield to their distressing obsessions. Many people with OCD are unable to maintain social relationships because their compulsions are too time-consuming or inappropriate.

Individuals with OCD may have different degrees of insight into their condition. The majority have good insight (e.g., the person believes that hands are clean without washing them seven times). Only less than 4% actually have delusional beliefs (e.g., believe that hands are clean only when they have been washed seven times). It is very common for individuals with OCD to avoid situations (people and places) that can trigger obsessions and compulsions.

People with OCD often have other dysfunctional beliefs that are unrelated to their obsession. They frequently have an inflated sense of responsibility and a tendency to overestimate threat. They are often perfectionists and cannot tolerate uncertainty.

Comorbidity is very high for people with OCD. Up to 30% of people with OCD (mostly males) have a lifetime tic disorder; 76% also have a diagnosis of anxiety disorder; 63% live with depression and bipolar disorder; and 23 to 32% of people with OCD have obsessive-compulsive personality disorder (discussed below).

Suicidal risk is high for individuals with OCD: 50% of them report having suicidal thoughts and 25% have made a suicidal attempt.

OCD is seen in families. Many studies are exploring possible genetic and hormonal causes. Treatment for OCD consists of a combination of medication and behavioural therapy. A number of antidepressants and selective serotonin reuptake

---

BOX 18.2 Obsessions and Compulsions Criteria

Obsessions

1. Recurrent and persistent thoughts, urges, or images that are intrusive or inappropriate, unwanted, and cause marked anxiety or distress.
2. The person is aware that those thoughts are irrational and attempts to ignore, suppress, or neutralize such thoughts with other thoughts or actions (compulsions).

Compulsions

1. Repetitive behaviours (e.g., hand washing, walking in a special way, checking locks) or mental acts (e.g., praying, counting, repeating words) that the person feels driven to perform in response to an obsession or according to rigid rules.
2. The behaviours or mental acts are aimed at reducing distress or preventing some dreaded event or situation from occurring; however, they are not realistically connected with what they are designed to neutralize or they are clearly excessive.

---

inhibitor (SSRI) antidepressant medications have been used successfully to treat OCD.

OCD and **obsessive-compulsive personality disorder (OCPD)** are two different diagnoses. The main difference is that with OCPD, the person deploys a set of actions to tightly control their environment and actually believes in the benefits of these actions. For example, a person with OCPD might keep everything tidy, clean, and extremely well organized; however, at the same time, this attitude may generate serious challenges in other aspects of the person's life, including in social interactions and work performance. These controlling actions are not as specific and repetitive as OCD compulsions and they will not meet the criteria for compulsion. Despite the challenges they face, a person who has OCPD will not look for help because they feel that nothing is wrong. On the other hand, a person with OCD usually has good insight and knows that their hands are clean, but obsessive thoughts about their hands being unclean generate a high level of anxiety. Performing the action of washing the hands (the compulsion) diminishes that anxiety. This person is usually aware of their compulsion and may look for help. OCPD is discussed in more detail in Chapter 30.

Body Dysmorphic Disorder

People with body dysmorphic disorder (BDD) become obsessed with a perceived defect or a flaw in their body. Features such as the nose, ears, hair, breasts, genitalia, or feet can be the objects of their fixation. They become preoccupied with their physical appearance and may avoid social situations. The flaw causes significant distress and interferes with the activities of daily life. People with BDD will frequently examine themselves in the mirror and believe their flaw makes them ugly. This repetitive examination causes significant distress or impairment in the person's functioning. Family relationships or other aspects of the person's life may suffer. They may seek unnecessary cosmetic surgery or other treatments. In many cases, depression, eating disorders, and suicidal behaviours are also seen.

The two main components of treatment are pharmacology and intense cognitive-behavioural therapy (a type of psychotherapy in which negative patterns of thought about the self and the world are challenged in order to alter unwanted behaviour patterns or treat mood disorders such as depression). Ongoing treatment with SSRIs not only helps to alleviate symptoms but also can prevent a relapse (Hollander & Hong, 2016).

Hoarding Disorder

Hoarding disorder is the persistent difficulty in parting with or discarding possessions, regardless of their value, because of the intense anxiety this act generates. Persons may hoard certain items, but to the person with hoarding disorder accumulating possessions becomes a way of life. Their environments become cluttered, dirty, and unusable. If one hoards animals, the home quickly becomes unsafe due to the accumulation of animal refuse.

People with hoarding disorder may understand their behaviour or show no insight by being completely convinced that no problem exists. Complications of hoarding disorder include unclean living conditions; inability to perform basic living tasks; increased risk of falls, fires, or injury; insect and rodent infestations; social isolation; and possible legal problems.

Treatment may be difficult if the patient does not recognize or admit to a problem. When individuals are cooperative, antidepressant medications and psychotherapy are prescribed. The goals of therapy are to help the individual understand the need to hoard and develop a plan for eliminating the clutter without undue anxiety.

Hair-Pulling Disorder (Trichotillomania)

We all pull on our hair at one time or another, but people with **trichotillomania** suffer from a disorder that involves repeated, persistent pulling of hair from the body despite efforts to stop. For some, the urge to pull out hair is mild and manageable, but others become overwhelmed and develop a compulsive focus, resulting in hair loss and significant distress.

The age at onset is usually in the early teens. Women are affected more than men, and the behaviour can be lifelong. Complications include problems with social functioning, skin and hair damage, bald spots, infections, and hairballs when individuals eat the pulled hair.

Treatment is focused on changing the self-destructive behaviours through cognitive and acceptance therapies. Antidepressant medications may be prescribed.

Excoriation Disorder (Skin Picking)

The key feature of **excoriation disorder** is repeated picking of the skin with fingers, needles, or other objects despite efforts to stop. The skin picking causes lesions, scabs, tissue damage, and infections. Individuals may spend hours a day involved in thinking about or engaging in picking. Many avoid social situations or going out in public. Feelings of boredom, anxiety, or tension are often relieved by picking. Pain does not usually accompany the skin-picking behaviours.

Treatment includes ruling out any physical causes or drug use. Antibiotics may be used to treat infections. Psychotherapy and support groups help to identify the anxieties involved and replace them with healthier, stress-reducing behaviours.

Substance-/Medication-Induced Obsessive-Compulsive and Related Disorder

To diagnose this condition the above-described symptoms of OCD and related disorders (skin picking, etc.) must be observed, in addition to clear evidence for substance intoxication or withdrawal or presence of a substance that can produce such symptoms.

Obsessive-Compulsive and Related Disorder Due to Another Medical Condition

To diagnose this condition the above-described symptoms of OCD and related disorders (skin picking, etc.) must be observed, in addition to clear evidence for presence of another medical condition (e.g., Sydenham's chorea).

Other Specified Obsessive-Compulsive and Related Disorder

For this diagnosis, the clinician chooses to communicate the specific reason why that presentation does not meet the criteria for any obsessive-compulsive and related disorder.

Unspecified Obsessive-Compulsive and Related Disorder

For this diagnosis, the clinician chooses not to communicate the specific reason for why that presentation does not meet the criteria for any obsessive-compulsive and related disorder.

TRAUMA- AND STRESSOR-RELATED DISORDER

People relate to traumatic events in different ways. Some cope and move on, and others become fearful and anxious. When exposure to an especially traumatic event occurs and an individual becomes so anxious that daily living activities are affected, a stress-related disorder is diagnosed. The exposure to a traumatic event is a clear diagnostic criterion for these disorders.

Reactive Attachment Disorder

Reactive attachment disorder is a disorder of early childhood or infancy that is characterized by inappropriate attachment behaviour in which a child almost never seeks out comfort, protection, and support from an attachment figure. The main feature is underdeveloped attachment between the child and caregiver.

The following criteria *must be present* for a diagnosis of reactive attachment disorder:
A. A consistent pattern of withdrawn behaviour toward the adult caregiver is demonstrated by the child not seeking

comfort when in distress, and the child shows no response when comfort provided.

B. A persistent social or emotional disturbance characterized by at least two of the following:
   1) Minimal social and emotional responsiveness to others
   2) Limited positive affect
   3) Episodes of unexplained irritability, sadness, or fearfulness, even during nonthreatening interactions with caregivers

C. The child has experienced severely insufficient care as evidenced by at least one of the following:
   1) Serious emotional neglect or deprivation (e.g., persistent lack of having basic emotional needs for comfort, stimulation, or affection met by caring adults)
   2) Frequent change of primary caregivers that prevented or severely limited opportunities to form attachments (e.g., frequent changes in foster care)
   3) Being reared in unusual settings that severely limited opportunities to form attachments (e.g., institutions with high child-to-caregiver ratios) (APA, 2013; Ellis & Saadabadi, 2020)

Disinhibited Social Engagement Disorder

The main feature of a child (9 months of age or older) with **disinhibited social engagement disorder** is a pattern of culturally inappropriate, overly familiar, behaviour with strangers. Diagnostic criteria (APA, 2013) include the following:

A. A pattern of behaviour when a child actively approaches and interacts with strangers, and exhibits at least two of the following:
   1) The absence of any reservation or shyness with unfamiliar adults
   2) Overfamiliarity (physical or verbal) which is outside of the child's cultural norms
   3) Absent checking back with an adult caregiver in unfamiliar settings or after exploring a new environment
   4) Willingness to go off with a strange adult without hesitation

B. The behaviours listed in criterion A are not limited to impulsivity (e.g., as a result of attention-deficit/hyperactivity disorder [ADHD]) but include social disinhibited behaviour.

C. The child has experienced insufficient care as evidenced by at least one of the following:
   1) Caregiver's emotional neglect (lack of comfort, stimulation, affection)
   2) Limited ability to form stable attachments as a result of frequent changes of primary caregiver (e.g., frequent changes in foster care)
   3) Being raised in an unusual setting that severely limits opportunities to form selective attachments (e.g., in an institution with a high child-to-caregiver ratio)

D. The care in criterion C is responsible for the behaviour in criterion A (e.g., disturbances identified in criterion A began after deficient care experienced in criterion C).

E. The child has a developmental age of at least 9 months of age.

Adolescents with this disorder experience more superficial peer relationships and more peer conflicts.

Post-Traumatic Stress Disorder (PTSD)

Post-traumatic stress disorder (PTSD) "usually occurs after the individual experiences or witnesses severe trauma that constitutes a threat to physical integrity or life" (Gore, Lucas, & Lubit, 2018). People who are involved in natural disasters, terrorist or other violent incidents, serious accidents, or sudden loss of loved ones have high rates of PTSD. Combat veterans, refugees, and victims of sexual assault can experience rates as high as 30%. Patients who have been treated for major physical traumas, and the nurses who provide their intensive care, also have higher rates of PTSD. Many times, individuals will self-medicate with both prescribed and illicit drugs and alcohol.

Individuals may become *emotionally numb,* extremely alert, and guarded. They can be easily startled. Eating and sleeping disturbances are common. Different environmental clues that remind the person of the traumatic event through one or more of the person's five senses can trigger **flashbacks**, which are vivid recollections of the event in which the individual relives the frightening experience. Flashbacks can last from a few seconds to hours. They can vary in severity, from a brief reminder of the trauma to dissociation (a loss of awareness of present surroundings). During a flashback, the experience is vividly real and life-threatening to the individual. Health care providers must remember this when caring for a patient who is experiencing a flashback. Interventions must ensure everyone's safety and reorient the patient to their present surroundings. Different techniques for such reality orientation are called *grounding.* There are also a variety of techniques that allow a person with PTSD to take control over the duration or even the scenario of the flashback so that it can be less distracting. Vivid recurrent dreams about the traumatic event are called *nightmares.* There are medications (like Prazosin) available that work to diminish nightmares.

Flashbacks, nightmares, and dissociation may severely compromise quality of life for the person who suffers from PTSD. Anxiety, depression, and nightmares can complicate the picture. Individuals may reduce their involvement with others as their responsiveness to life numbs. Frequently, people with severe PTSD isolate themselves from society. Suicide rates are higher among people living with PTSD. Children with PTSD may express themselves through disorganized or agitated behaviours. Long-term interventions include medication therapy, cognitive-behavioural and group therapy, anger management, and ongoing emotional support.

Acute Stress Disorder

An acute stress disorder is diagnosed when an individual repeatedly relives or reacts to the anxiety from a traumatic event. Distressing memories and dreams often occur. One may experience an altered sense of reality and engage in efforts to avoid anything associated with the traumatic event.

There is a persistent negative mood along with an inability to experience happiness or other positive feelings. Sleep disturbances, irritability, and problems with concentration are common.

Treatment focuses on reducing stress, ensuring a safe environment, promoting effective coping mechanisms, and providing emotional support.

Acute stress disorder and PTSD have a similar presentation. *The main difference between acute stress disorder and PTSD is that acute stress disorder lasts up to 1 month.*

Adjustment Disorder

An identifiable stressor (e.g., a new diagnosis, job, or relationship challenge) can generate emotional or behavioural symptoms up to 3 months from that event. This condition is called *adjustment disorder*. The symptoms cause social, occupational, or other impairments. After the stressor or its consequences end, it can take up to 6 months for the symptoms to disappear. The risk of suicide is high with this condition.

Other Specific Trauma- and Stressor-Related Disorder

Other specific trauma- and stressor-related disorder is diagnosed when a patient's clinical presentation does not meet the full criteria for any of the specific trauma- and stressor-related disorders and the clinician chooses to indicate the specific reason why criteria are not met.

Unspecified Trauma- and Stressor-Related Disorder

Unspecified trauma- and stressor-related disorder is diagnosed when a patient's clinical presentation does not meet the full criteria for any of the specific trauma- and stressor-related disorders but the clinician chooses not to specify the reason why criteria are not met.

THERAPEUTIC INTERVENTIONS

The most effective way to cope with anxiety is to *prevent* it. Learn to recognize the signs and symptoms of anxiety in yourself and others. Include an anxiety assessment for every patient. Be especially alert to the signs of anxiety in children. Talk with them about their concerns. Teaching children to cope appropriately with their anxieties can prevent or minimize a number of mental health challenges later in life. There are a few self-administered questionnaires and surveys that are used by clinicians for assessments. They also can be used as outcome measures following therapy. One that is popular in Canada and is used in many outpatient clinics is the Patient Health Questionnaire (PHQ-9) (see https://www2.gov.bc.ca/assets/gov/health/practitioner-pro/bc-guidelines/depression_patient_health_questionnaire.pdf). There are many others (e.g., Hamilton Anxiety Rating Scale, Yale-Brown Obsessive-Compulsive Scale [Y-BOCS], Obsessive Compulsive Inventory [OCI]), some of which may be self-administered, and some of which must be administered by experienced staff and are specific to a particular condition.

Therapeutic interventions for individuals with maladaptive responses to anxiety involve a combination of mental health therapies and medications. Psychotherapy helps patients to discover the basis for their anxiety. Three behavioural therapies that are successful in treating phobias and other anxiety-related problems are cognitive-behavioural therapy, systematic desensitization, and flooding.

Cognitive-behavioural therapy (CBT) helps patients intellectually understand the ineffective behaviours used to cope with anxiety and replace them with more successful behaviours. The core idea of CBT is that our feelings follow our thoughts and that even though we have no control over our feelings, we can exercise better control over our thoughts. The goal of therapy is for patients to "learn healthier ways of coping with stressful situations. They gain awareness and change how they think in critical situations, gradually confronting their anxiety and becoming less afraid" (Symonds & Janney, 2013). Changing the way of thinking brings about a change in feelings.

With **systematic desensitization (SD)**, patients learn to cope with one anxiety-provoking stimulus through gradual exposure until the stressor is no longer associated with anxiety. This step-by-step method progressively removes the anxiety from the distress-causing event and allows patients to develop more effective ways of perceiving their anxiety.

Flooding is just the opposite. This method for treating phobias rapidly exposes patients to the feared object or situation and keeps up the exposure until anxiety levels diminish. However, this method often creates severe psychological distress, and although it is more cost-effective than SD because of the short intervention time, this method remains ethically questionable because of the distress it causes patients.

Animal therapy is proving effective in reducing anxiety. Lavin (2011) notes that it is a "relatively new therapy [that] involves providing specially trained service dogs to assist veterans with combat-related PTSD." Therapy animals help anxious individuals, not just veterans, feel more secure and help decrease many of the physical responses to stress.

Anxiety is also treated with various medications, including benzodiazepines, antidepressants, antihistamines, beta-blockers, and the anxiolytic medication buspirone. Because each type of medication is associated with possibly severe adverse effects, nurses must monitor their patients' responses to medication therapy. The adverse effects of commonly used antianxiety agents, benzodiazepines, and suggested therapeutic interventions are listed in Table 18.3. Table 18.4 lists the adverse effects for various other medications used to treat anxiety.

> **! MEDICATION ALERT**
>
> CAUTION: Benzodiazepines and other anxiety-reducing medications can be dangerous when taken in combination with alcohol. Patients must be instructed about the possibility of sedation, decreased mental activity, and decreased coordination when alcohol is consumed while taking these medications.

TABLE 18.3 Adverse Effects of Benzodiazepines and Nursing Care

Adverse Effects*	Nursing (Therapeutic) Interventions
Central Nervous System Dizziness, drowsiness, sedation, headache, tremors, depression, insomnia, hallucinations	Ensure safety, prevent falls, assist with ambulation, and use side rails. Reassure patient that symptoms are common when first beginning the medication. Assess mental status routinely.
Gastrointestinal Dry mouth, anorexia, nausea, vomiting, constipation, diarrhea	Give medication with food or milk. Ensure frequent oral care. Offer hard candy, gum, sips of water frequently.
Cardiovascular Electrocardiogram changes, *orthostatic hypotension, tachycardia*	Monitor intake and output if anorexia, vomiting, or diarrhea occur. Assess blood pressure, pulse (lying and standing); if systolic pressure drops >20 mm Hg, hold medication, notify physician. Monitor complete blood count and other laboratory studies during long-term therapy.
Eyes, Ears, Nose, Throat *Blurred vision,* ringing in ears	Provide reassurance. Ensure safety.
Integument (Skin) Itching, rash, dermatitis	Encourage use of tepid baths without soap. Assess rash and report to the physician.
Emotional Feelings of detachment, irritability, increased hostility	Encourage social interactions. Assess for loss of control over emotions and aggression.
Long-Term Effects Increased medication tolerance, physical and psychological dependency, rebound anxiety and insomnia	Medication dose is tapered slowly after 4 months of treatment. Help patient identify the difference between symptoms of medication withdrawal and original feelings of anxiety.

*The most common side effects are in italics.

TABLE 18.4 Adverse Effects of Various Medications That Treat Anxiety

Medication	Adverse Effects
Antihistamines	Drowsiness, headache, thick bronchial secretions, nausea, diarrhea, constipation
Benzodiazepines	Groggy, sleepy feelings, uncoordinated movements, slurred speech, impaired thinking, metabolized slowly so may accumulate in the body and cause oversedation
Selective serotonin reuptake inhibitor (SSRI) antidepressants	Nervousness, dizziness, drowsiness, headaches, nausea, diarrhea, dry mouth, urinary retention, sexual dysfunction, low blood pressure when standing, high blood pressure, acute renal failure
Buspirone	Dizziness, headache, depression, nausea, upset stomach, constipation, diarrhea, insomnia, fast heart rate, blurred vision, nasal congestion, sweating, rash, weakness, chest congestion

After a complete nursing history and thorough physical examination, the most appropriate problem statements are selected. Information is then brought to the health care team, overall patient goals are established, and therapeutic interventions are chosen.

One of the first priorities of care is to protect the patient from injury to self and others. Establishing a trusting therapeutic relationship helps patients to explore their distresses and learn to link their behaviours to the sources of their anxiety. Problem-solving techniques can assist patients in developing more effective coping mechanisms. Relaxation techniques, such as meditation, and stress-reducing exercises can help patients counter their anxieties. Sample Patient Care Plan 18.1 provides an example of a care plan for anxiety responses.

Health care providers are in an excellent position to help patients cope effectively with the effects of stress and anxiety. Handling small, everyday distresses successfully is the key to preventing complicated mental health challenges that arise as maladaptive expressions of anxiety.

SAMPLE PATIENT CARE PLAN 18.1 Anxiety

Assessment

History Sebastian is a 44-year-old man who has lost his wife, his job, and his car within the past 3 months. Last night, after Sebastian and his buddies "had a few drinks," Sebastian became suspicious and accused his friends of trying to steal "what little I have left. I just know something awful is going to happen." Today Sebastian is seeking treatment for his upset stomach and inability to sleep.

Current Findings An untidy man who appears older than his stated age. There is an odour of alcohol. Vital signs are increased, with a pulse rate of 116 beats/min. He complains of shortness of breath, upset stomach, frequent urination, and lack of sleep. When questioned about the recent changes in his life, he replies, "It's no big deal. I'll get by."

Multidisciplinary Diagnosis	Planning/Goals
Anxiety related to loss of wife and job.	Sebastian will identify the causes of his anxiety and make two attempts to decrease the level of anxiety he is experiencing by October 10.

THERAPEUTIC INTERVENTIONS

Interventions	Rationale	Team Member
1. Establish trust with Sebastian.	Trust helps patient to explore new ways of coping.	All
2. Contract with him to refrain from hurting himself and others for the duration of therapy.	To ensure safety of Sebastian and others during expressions of anxiety.	Nsg
3. Use active listening to encourage Sebastian to link his anxiety with recent experiences.	Allows time to assess Sebastian's perspective; helps Sebastian to connect his emotions with his feelings of anxiety.	All
4. Assess Sebastian's statements of self-worth, and reinforce personal strengths that he has identified.	Helps determine Sebastian's perception of himself; energy flows where it is focused.	All
5. Help Sebastian identify areas of his life over which he has control.	Learning to direct one's energies decreases anxiety, promotes relaxation, and increases a sense of control.	All
6. Give positive feedback for attempts to reduce anxiety.	One small success builds on another when recognized.	All
7. Encourage Sebastian to continue established relationships.	Established relationships can be a source of comfort and support.	All
8. Help identify areas of strength and limitations in social interactions.	Positive reinforcement encourages appropriate actions; the first step in changing behaviours is identifying them.	Soc Svc, Nsg
9. Encourage Sebastian to undergo job skill and employment testing.	A source of income helps satisfy basic needs.	Soc Svc, OT
10. Monitor for therapeutic response, adverse effects of buspirone.	Medication has several adverse effects that can be disturbing for patient.	Nsg

Evaluation Sebastian attended four counselling sessions before he recognized that he was anxious. By the seventh session, he was able to reduce his anxiety about 15% of the time.

Critical Thinking Questions

1. What is the purpose of helping Sebastian link his feelings of anxiety to recent events?
2. How does identifying strengths help decrease anxiety?

A complete patient care plan includes several other diagnoses and interventions.
Nsg, nursing staff; *OT,* occupational therapist; *Soc Svc,* social services.

KEY POINTS

- Anxiety is a diffuse feeling of uneasiness, uncertainty, and helplessness; it is a normal emotional response to a threat or stressor.
- Adaptive responses to anxiety result in positive outcomes, new learning, and greater self-esteem.
- Maladaptive responses to anxiety are ineffective attempts to cope that do nothing to eliminate feelings of anxiety.
- To decrease stress, people use physical, intellectual, spiritual, and emotional coping mechanisms.
- An understanding of how individuals at various developmental stages perceive and cope with anxiety is important for health care providers.
- The specific causes of anxiety are still uncertain, but research indicates that a combination of physical, psychosocial, and environmental factors is involved.
- An anxiety disorder exists when one's coping mechanisms or behaviours do not relieve anxiety's distress.
- A generalized anxiety disorder (GAD) is diagnosed when anxiety is broad, long-lasting, and excessive.
- A panic attack is a brief period of intense fear or discomfort accompanied by physical and emotional reactions.
- A phobia is an unnatural fear of people, animals, objects, situations, or occurrences.
- An obsession is a distressing, recurring, persistent thought.
- A compulsion is a distressing recurring behaviour.
- People with body dysmorphic disorder (BDD) become obsessed with a flaw in their body.
- Hair pulling and skin picking are obsessive-compulsive disorders that may result in physical alterations.
- Hoarding disorder is the persistent difficulty in parting with or discarding possessions, regardless of value.
- Stressor and trauma disorders include traumatic stress reaction, acute stress disorder, adjustment disorder, and post-traumatic stress disorder (PTSD).
- One of the first priorities of care is to protect the patient from possible injury to self and others.
- Medications for treating anxiety include benzodiazepines, antihistamines, buspirone, beta-blockers, and selective serotonin reuptake inhibitor (SSRI) antidepressants.
- Establishing a trusting therapeutic relationship is a therapeutic intervention that helps patients explore their distresses and learn to connect behaviours with the sources of their anxiety.
- Problem-solving techniques assist patients in developing new, more effective coping mechanisms.
- Relaxation techniques help patients counter the anxieties currently being experienced.

ADDITIONAL LEARNING RESOURCES

Go to your Evolve website (http://evolve.elsevier.com/Canada/Morrison-Valfre/) for additional online resources, including the online Study Guide for additional learning activities to help you master this chapter content.

CRITICAL THINKING QUESTIONS

1. Consider the physical symptoms of a panic attack. How would you distinguish between panic attack and acute myocardial ischemia (MI)? What would be differences in intervention? What would be a commonality in intervention?
2. What are the main principles of cognitive-behavioural therapy?
3. What are the main symptoms of post-traumatic stress disorder and how might they interfere with a patient's daily life?
4. What treatment modality would be suitable for a patient with a phobia about using an elevator?

REFERENCES

American Psychiatric Association (APA). (2013). *Diagnostic and statistical manual of mental disorders* (5th ed.). Author.

Canadian Institute for Health Information (CIHI). (2019). Child and youth mental health in Canada—infographic. https://www.cihi.ca/en/child-and-youth-mental-health-in-canada-infographic

Craighead, W. E., & Nemeroff, C. B. (Eds.). (2010). *The Corsini encyclopedia of psychology and behavioral science* (4th ed.) Wiley.

Ellis, E. E., & Saadabadi, A. (2020). *Reactive attachment disorder.* StatPearls. https://www.ncbi.nlm.nih.gov/books/NBK537155/

Gore, A. T., Lucas, J. Z., & Lubit, R. H. (2018). Posttraumatic stress disorder, practice essentials. http://emedicine.medscape.com/article/288154-overview

Hockenberry, M., & Wilson, D. (2014). *Wong's nursing care of infants and children* (10th ed.). Mosby.

Hollander, E., & Hong, K. (2016). Relapse prevention and the need for ongoing pharmacological treatment in body dysmorphic disorder. *American Journal of Psychiatry, 173*(9), 857–859. https://doi-org.uhn.idm.oclc.org/10.1176/appi.ajp.2016.16050624

Lavin, J. (2011). Surviving posttraumatic stress disorder. *Nursing, 41*(9), 41–44.

Newman, T. (2017). *Causes and coping techniques for anxiety.* Medical News Today. https://www.medicalnewstoday.com/articles/7603.php

Stuart, G. W. (2013). *Principles and practice of psychiatric nursing* (10th ed.). Mosby.

Symonds, A., & Janney, R. (2013). Shining a light on hoarding disorder. *Nursing, 43*(10), 22–28. https://doi.org/10.1097/01.NURSE.0000434310.68016.18

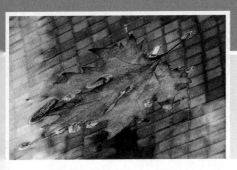

19

Illness and Hospitalization

OBJECTIVES

Upon completion of this chapter, the student will be able to:

1. Explain the difference between health and illness.
2. Outline the five stages of illness.
3. Identify how denial is used as a protective mechanism during illness.
4. Explain why hospitalization is considered a situational crisis.
5. Describe the three stages of the hospitalization experience.
6. Compare hospitalization for psychiatric issues with hospitalization for physical problems.
7. Discuss how emotional support of significant others affects the outcome of a patient's illness.
8. Identify three nonmedication methods for managing pain.
9. Examine the importance of discharge planning for hospitalized persons.

OUTLINE

KEY TERMS

body image (p. 229)
denial (p. 230)
discharge planning (p. 234)
health (p. 228)
hospitalization (p. 230)

illness (p. 228)
pain management (p. 234)
sick role (p. 229)
situational crisis (p. 230)

Do you remember the first time you visited a hospital? Perhaps you were a visitor or maybe a patient. Can you recall how you felt? First, the hospital appeared to be huge. Even small hospitals are confusing, with mazes of hallways and mysterious little rooms everywhere. The odours were different—extra clean, antiseptic smells, like no other odours. The workers there were all dressed in ceremonial garb and paraded through the hallway mazes with businesslike efficiency. Then there was the equipment—the machines and strange items that do one thing or another. It seemed that every piece came with a bell, whistle, or other annoying tone to periodically remind us of its presence. Generally, a health care facility can be a scary, intimidating place, not one in which most people would choose to spend time.

For those of us in the health care professions, however, the hospital (or long-term care facility or clinic) is a known environment, filled with the familiar. We often forget that the thought of "going to the hospital" brings immediate anxiety to the hearts of many. For these people, hospitalization can be an overwhelming and threatening experience. This chapter explores the mental health aspects of illness and the situational crisis of hospitalization. It describes the process of illness and its psychosocial adaptations, and it offers several therapeutic interventions for decreasing or eliminating the anxieties that can accompany the illness and hospitalization experiences. Most important, it reminds us of the discomforts shared by the individuals who must cope with and adapt to the inpatient environment—a world we health care providers take for granted.

It is important to note that this chapter discusses the impact that any illness and any hospitalization has on a person and their family. Whether a patient is admitted to a medical, surgical, psychiatric, oncology, orthopedic, cardiology, labour and delivery, or any other hospital department, some of their psychological challenges will be similar.

CASE STUDY

Mark is an 82-year-old retired printer living in a small retirement village with his wife, who has diabetes. He has enjoyed excellent health throughout his life. Other than periodic visits to his physician, he has had no contact with the medical community.

One evening, Mark noticed that he was bleeding when he urinated. After referral to a specialist, he was scheduled for a simple operative procedure to remove the extra tissue that was blocking the flow of urine and causing the bleeding. Mark and his wife were instructed to arrive at the hospital early on the next morning.

On admission, the nurse, noting Mark's age, assumed that he had some experience in a hospital—after all, he was more than 80 years old. Mark was quickly admitted and prepared for surgery.

The surgical procedure was completed without problems. Mark was taken to the recovery room in good condition with a Foley catheter to drain urine and an intravenous line in his right forearm. The first hour after the procedure was uneventful; however, the minute Mark regained consciousness, he insisted on going home. Nurses reassured him that he would be discharged as soon as the physician saw him. He nodded and then dozed off. Seeing him sleeping, they turned their attention to other patients.

Mark suddenly hopped off the gurney and detached himself from the intravenous line and Foley catheter. He was seen walking out the door to his car in his hospital gown and bleeding from the urethra. As a result of this mishap, Mark was chased down, "captured" against his will, and, following a conversation with his care team, he agreed to be hospitalized for 2 days to control the bleeding from the traumatic catheter removal. You can imagine what a challenging time that was for Mark and his wife, not to mention his health care providers.

Regrettably, not one health care provider had assessed this man's previous experiences relating to hospitalization or medical treatment. Mark was under the false assumption that once the task was completed, he was free to return home.

- What actions could have prevented this situation from occurring?
- How could the lessons from this study be applied to your practice?

THE NATURE OF ILLNESS

Health is a dynamic state of physical, mental, and social well-being. "Each person has a personal concept of health" (Potter, Perry, Stockert, et al., 2019) that is based on their values, lifestyle, and personality. Our state of health constantly changes as we respond and adapt to the challenges of life. This

constant change and adaptation process is called *homeostasis,* and it serves us well throughout our lives. When individuals become unable to adapt or to regain the balance of homeostasis, they become ill and must mobilize critical energies to return to a state of health.

Illness is a state of imbalance. It is an "abnormal process in which aspects of the social, physical, emotional, or intellectual condition and function of a person are diminished or impaired, compared with that person's previous condition" (*Mosby's dictionary,* 2013). For instance, when you are ill or sick, you feel poorly. The body is not working correctly, energy is sapped, and spirits are low. Activities performed yesterday without a thought now loom as obstacles. Getting dressed for work becomes such a challenge that you seriously wonder how you will make it through the day. You need some rest, but your will is reminding you of your commitments and obligations. Does this sound familiar?

Illness is the body's way of communicating its need for attention. The body will adjust to the demands placed on it until it is no longer capable of compensating. Illness also has strong psychosocial aspects. The example of the person with hallucinations who collapses from malnutrition because his visions told him he should not accept food reminds us of the complexity of the mind–body interaction.

CRITICAL THINKING

Remember the last time you were feeling ill but went to work or school anyway.
- How well did you perform that day?
- How sharp was your mental acuity?
- How did you cope with the physical, intellectual, and emotional demands of the day?

Stages of the Illness Experience

The experiences associated with illness and disability are very personal. Some individuals consider being ill a minor annoyance. Others analyze their sickness for hidden evidence of certain doom or destiny. The illness experience is roughly divided into five stages. Each stage is associated with certain perceptions, decisions, and behaviours (Table 19.1).

Because nurses and other health care providers support patients throughout their institutional stays, it is important to be familiar with the emotional and behavioural reactions during each phase of the illness experience, be it physical or mental in origin.

Stage 1: Symptoms

The illness experience begins when one becomes aware that something is not right. It may be a physical or emotional discomfort, but something is perceived as wrong. During this stage, there is an undesirable change. That change is analyzed and evaluated. A decision is made that the change indicates an illness. Actions are then taken to remedy the situation based on the decision and the accompanying emotional response.

TABLE 19.1	Stages of the Illness Experience	
Stage	**Decision**	**Behaviour**
Symptom experience	Aware that something is wrong	Symptom control, over-the-counter medicines, self-medicates
Assumes sick role	Gives up normal roles	Seeks support for sick role
Medical care contact	Seeks professional advice	Seeks sick-role approval from an authority, negotiates treatments and procedures
Dependent-patient role	Accepts health care treatment	Receives treatment, follows regimen
Recovery and rehabilitation	Gives up sick role	Resumes normal roles and responsibilities

Data from Potter, P. A., Perry, A. G., Stockert, P., et al. (2013). *Essentials for nursing practice* (8th ed.). Mosby.

Many factors, such as the nature of the symptoms, the knowledge of the individual, and the availability of treatment resources, enter into determining whether an illness exists. Emotional responses often govern behaviour during this stage. If symptoms are mild, one may self-medicate with various over-the-counter medications, visit a local cultural traditional healer, pray, meditate, or ignore the situation. For symptoms that are more serious, the individual may seek medical care or continue to deny that a problem exists. When an individual recognizes the presence of a health problem, they begin to move into the second stage.

Stage 2: The Sick Role

Once a person acknowledges the presence of an illness, they seek to confirm it by talking with other people. Family members, fellow workers, and friends are all consulted for their opinions. If the social group supports the presence of an illness, the individual either assumes the **sick role** actions and behaviours of a person who is ill or continues to deny the illness.

Assuming the sick role serves several purposes. First, the person is excused from everyday duties and responsibilities. Other people "take up the slack" by assuming the ill person's roles. Second, permission is given for the individual to rest and conserve energy for healing. Third, the social responsibilities of interacting with others are relieved during the illness. In short, permission is given for the individual to focus on restoring health. In the context of the recent pandemic, social responsibilities are also relieved so that the individual can go into quarantine to protect others from acquiring the illness.

Stage 3: Medical Care

If symptoms of the illness persist and home remedies fail, the person usually becomes motivated to seek medical intervention. Using knowledge and expertise, a health care provider can confirm the presence of an illness, provide treatment, and inform the individual about the causes, course, and future implications of the illness. At this time, the individual can either accept the provider's advice and the diagnosis and follow the plan of treatment or continue to deny the problem. Many people consult several different health care providers (shop around) in an attempt to receive a diagnosis more to their liking or until they finally accept the professionals' opinions.

Stage 4: Dependency

In the dependency stage, the ill individual accepts the attentions of other people. A dependent role is assumed in which one must rely on the kindness and energies of others. "Care, sympathy, and protection from the demands and stresses of life" (Potter et al., 2019) are provided by family, friends, health care providers, or a combination of these individuals. The individual is relieved of obligation, allowed to be passive and dependent, but expected to get well. The sick person may feel ambivalent: grateful for the help but resentful of the limitations imposed by the illness. People in this stage have a particular need to be informed and emotionally supported.

Stage 5: Recovery and Rehabilitation

Movement into the recovery and rehabilitation stage can occur suddenly (e.g., a response to medication therapy or the breaking of a fever) or more slowly (e.g., recovery from a stroke or mental disorder). If recovery is rapid and complete, the individual gradually gives up the sick role and resumes their normal obligations and duties. For those whose recoveries are prolonged, long-term care is usually necessary. Whenever possible, arrangements are made for people to recover in their homes. When this is not an option, the individual is usually transferred to another institution for further rehabilitation or care.

Not all people pass through every stage of the illness experience. Progression through the stages occurs at a very individual rate. However, care providers who understand the emotional aspects of the illness experience are better able to plan and implement effective patient care.

Effects of Illness

Illness is not an isolated event. It affects the activities of the individual as well as those who come in contact with the sick person. When illness occurs, it challenges the resources and changes the activities of all those involved. Short-term acute illnesses, such as the flu or a cold, have little effect on one's behaviour, but a serious health challenge (physical or mental) can lead to major emotional and behavioural changes for all involved. Individuals may react to illness with anxiety, anger, denial, shock, or withdrawal (Box 19.1).

An illness involving a change in physical appearance will have a strong impact on the individual's **body image** (one's concept of one's body). Threats to body image occur with surgery, extensive diagnostic procedures, and acute and chronic illness. One's self-concept also becomes threatened if the illness progresses beyond the expected time. Tension and conflict with other family members can further erode the ill person's confidence, and a depressed mood may begin to take hold.

Psychosocially, illness has an impact on all family members. Changes in routine can add more pressure to an already threatened family. Because the obligations and responsibilities of the ill individual cannot be met, family members often take on heavier workloads during times of illness. If the illness is prolonged, family members may experience situational stress, leading to an imbalance in family stability (Dames, Luctkar-Flude, & Tyerman, 2021) until new roles and habits are established.

Illness has many faces. Remember, when assessing the physical signs and symptoms of illness, we are touching only the tip of the iceberg. Underneath lie the emotions, reactions, and behaviours that arrive with the package called "illness."

Illness Behaviours

During each stage of the illness experience, people are faced with several emotional choices. Some emotions serve to protect us from further stresses or mobilize resources to be devoted to healing. Emotions can be destructive, however, if they block efforts toward resolving health problems. For example, the emotion of denial can be useful or paralyzing.

Denial is a psychological defence mechanism (see Table 18.2) used to ward off the painful feelings associated with problems. Denial can be helpful when it allows the time to collect and reorganize thoughts and plans, but it can be deadly when it clouds judgements and prevents individuals from taking the needed steps to restore themselves to health. Patients who are in denial require patience and understanding. They are struggling with the emotional aspects of illness

and attempting to restore themselves to a more comfortable state of functioning.

Fortunately, most people experience illness, recover to previous levels of functioning, and move on with their lives. They have taken part, actively or passively, in returning themselves to a state of homeostasis. Becoming ill and experiencing disability is not a comfortable experience. Health care providers, especially nurses, should remember that illness is the most important priority for the individual who is experiencing it.

THE HOSPITALIZATION EXPERIENCE

The great majority of illnesses are successfully treated in the home. However, some individuals require an inpatient setting for treatment. **Hospitalization** is the placing of an ill or injured person into an inpatient health care facility that provides continuous nursing care and an organized medical staff.

People have vastly different experiences relating to stays in a hospital. Attitudes are also affected by what one hears. The relative who drags out minor historical facts about the hospital experiences of every family member and the horror stories from tabloid news outlets can add to one's concerns about receiving care in a hospital.

People who are hospitalized experience several emotional threats to their well-being and progress through different stages throughout their hospital stays. During each stage, certain anxieties and emotional issues surface and challenge the patient's coping abilities. Care providers should be aware of these issues and include them in the patient's plan of care. Hospitalized individuals are faced with physical, emotional, and environmental challenges all at the same time. For most of us, being hospitalized is seen as a crisis, an event with which we are unable to cope.

Situational Crisis

People are generally hospitalized in one of two ways: either the admission is planned in advance, or it is an emergency that requires special health care resources. In the case of the planned admission, one has time to experience the anxieties and work with the complications that will occur as a result of the individual's absence. Although emotional reactions may be intense and the event is seen as a crisis, people who elect to be hospitalized have the luxury of time to prepare themselves and their loved ones, both physically and emotionally. For those individuals brought to the hospital through the emergency department, no time was allowed for preparation. Their lives have suddenly been disrupted. If the health problems require complicated or long-term treatment, major adjustments in lifestyles must be made quickly.

It is helpful to review the principles of crisis intervention discussed in Chapter 8 and apply them to the crisis of hospitalization. Remember, a **situational crisis** is one that relates to external or environmental problems. In the case of the patient who has been coping with an illness or dysfunction before admission, the precrisis behaviours consist of efforts to deal with the health issue. For the individual whose admission was an emergency, the precrisis behaviours were a healthy person's usual activities of daily living with no thought given to illness or injury.

The actual crisis in both cases, however, is about being removed from one's familiar home environment to be cared for by strangers in an impersonal, uncomfortable setting. All hospitalized patients have one thing in common—the feeling of being out of control and dependent on the mercy, knowledge, and expertise of unknown care providers. If care providers are sensitive to the fact that their patients are experiencing a crisis, therapeutic interventions will meet with greater success.

Stages of Hospitalization

The process of becoming a patient is peppered with challenges. Hospitalization becomes more anxiety provoking as the admission process transforms a person from an individual into a patient. The name band around the patient's wrist provides a means of identity; now care providers can identify the person by an armband. The demand for paperwork reduces a person to an account number and can sap what little energy they have. Next, with the donning of an institutional gown the sick person exchanges their role as a functioning adult for that of a patient (Fig. 19.1). The focus of treatment may be on the physical body, but care providers must be aware of the psychosocial aspects of every patient's health problems and hospitalization experiences.

Individuals who are experiencing hospitalization tend to progress through three stages. The first stage is the sense of being *overwhelmed*. The intensity of being separated from loved ones and left alone in an unfamiliar environment can leave many individuals exhausted. Energies needed to cope with the illness are diverted to surviving the admission process, separating from loved ones, and tolerating various diagnostic procedures. As a result, many patients withdraw into themselves and interact only when necessary. They must focus their attention inward in an effort to replace the energy that has been drained by the experiences of illness, crisis, and hospitalization.

During the second stage, *stabilization,* the hospitalized person gradually gains the strength to re-establish some personal identity. Individuals can become self-centred in this phase. The intellectual understanding that one is not the only person requiring care exists, but the emotional needs for reassurance and personal interest frequently must be asserted.

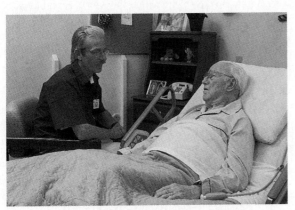

Fig. 19.1 Becoming a patient.

Adaptation marks the third stage. In this stage, the individual has regained enough of a personal identity to adapt. They often become interested in and willing to learn about health problems, coping techniques, or preventive measures. Energies are replenished. The body feels better and emotional responses are stable. Reorganization has taken place, and most people are again able to function effectively. For those persons who are transferred to another institution, the crisis begins again.

Common Reactions to Hospitalization

The rule of thumb for patients' reactions is "every person will react in their own way." The manner in which individuals respond to the stresses of hospitalization is determined by how they react to other threats or crises. The executive who controls a company commonly reacts by attempting to gain control over the hospital environment. The woman dominated by her spouse makes few decisions without the spouse's opinion, and the helpless individual often becomes more so in the hospital. It is important to remember that even though some of your patients' behaviours may be distasteful, they are coping to the best of their ability.

Hospitalization may also hold symbolic meaning. For some persons, hospitalization confirms the fear that this is no ordinary illness, that there may be something seriously amiss. For others, especially older people, the hospital is the place where one goes to die. It is also viewed as a place of respite where one is removed from the stresses of daily living. Attitudes and meanings concerning inpatient treatment for mental health challenges differ from those relating to institutional stays for physical problems.

Psychiatric Hospitalization

The experience of entering a psychiatric treatment facility differs from hospitalization for physical reasons in several ways. The individual and family must cope with the stigma of mental illness. Friends may be reluctant to discuss the illness or feel awkward about offering their support. Employers may question the individual's fitness for the job, and insurance companies may attempt to deny payment for treatment.

The ill person has received a diagnostic label that may follow them for years. Admission may be seen as a confirmation that one is truly "crazy," and the person may also have heard numerous stories about admission for psychiatric treatment.

If patients are alert and aware, they may fear other patients' behaviours. Odd or inappropriate behaviours can create anxiety and feelings of needing to protect oneself. Frequent contact and support from the health care staff during the admission and adjustment period can help patients cope with the anxieties of psychiatric hospitalization.

THERAPEUTIC INTERVENTIONS

Nurses and other care providers play a vital role in the care of sick persons within the hospital setting. Patients remember the people who provided their care. The care provider who went that extra mile for a personal favour, the therapist who made certain a patient's pet was fed, and the nurse who sat at the bedside when a patient was too anxious to sleep are remembered clearly. Unfortunately, the opposite is also true. Patients frequently remember the short temper, the cutting words, and the negative nonverbal messages more than the acts of kindness and concern. Psychosocial attention is just as important as good physical care. All health care providers need to be willing to meet both the physical and nonphysical needs of all patients. Problem statements that apply to the experience of illness and hospitalization should be considered with every patient admission.

Psychosocial Care

Good physical care is always the first place to start in meeting the emotional needs of ill persons. Therapeutic care communicates a willingness to focus attention on the patient, offers opportunities for interaction, and allows nurses to assess the patient's adaptation to the changes resulting from treatment. Good psychosocial care begins with an assessment of the patient's coping status. To perform a crisis assessment use the criteria listed in Table 19.2. This assessment helps you to identify problems *before* a crisis develops and plan preventive interventions.

Next, get to know your patients as individuals and real persons. Use active listening skills to encourage patients to discuss their anxieties and concerns. Clarify patients' perceptions of problems and their roles in treatment (Campbell & Anderson, 1999). *Listen* more than you talk. Most patients need to share their emotions about the illness experience. No matter what your personal opinions are, do not pass judgement on your patients' emotions and behaviours. Creating an accepting environment gives patients permission to share themselves and helps to build trust in the therapeutic relationship.

Assist patients in coping with the fight-or-flight response brought about by the illness or hospitalization. According to the theorist Richard Lazarus (2006), *stress* is defined by the individual's cognitive evaluation of the situation and the importance or significance they attach to it. Some individuals interpret the hospitalization experience as comforting and healing, whereas others may feel it is the first step toward dying. Teach and encourage patients to practise muscle relaxation techniques, imagery, and conscious sedation techniques to help ease their stress. If the patient practises a certain spiritual belief, notify the appropriate priest, minister, or spiritual practitioner. Also, be alert for any cultural practices that bring emotional support and comfort. The therapeutic (nursing) process applied to the hospitalized patient is illustrated in Box 19.2.

TABLE 19.2   Crisis Assessment

Assessment Steps	Description
Assess the patient's history of loss.	What types of losses (physical, psychological, social, or spiritual) has the patient experienced in the past? Who or what has helped the patient through crises in the past? Older and younger persons have more difficulty coping with crisis.
Assess what illness means to the patient.	What is the patient's understanding of the current situation? What has the patient been told about their condition, treatment, chances for recovery? How have the patient and family been affected?
Assess for other risk factors.	Assess the patient's level of support from supportive significant others and friends. How easily does the patient adapt to new situations? Assess for other crises. Other problems can exist in addition to the crisis. Older persons and children have more trouble cooperating and following therapeutic plans.

BOX 19.2   Therapeutic (Nursing) Process for Hospitalized Patients

Assessment
1. Perform a complete physical and psychosocial assessment, including previous hospitalizations. Have the patient describe each hospitalization and their reactions to and opinions of the experience.
2. Ask the patient to describe any particular concerns or fears about being hospitalized.
3. Ask if there is a special routine or ritual that is important to the patient.

Diagnosis
1. Diagnose general causes of the patient's symptoms.
2. Identify any risk the patient may face having these symptoms.

Planning
1. On the basis of the data obtained in the interview, develop a plan to decrease the patient's symptoms, concerns, and anxieties related to hospitalization.
2. Involve the patient and significant others in the planning process.

Implementation
1. Put a treatment plan into action. Convey respect and politeness when interacting with patients.
2. Maintain a pleasant environment. Pay attention to noise levels, lighting, and staff interactions.
3. Encourage the patient to cooperate and participate in their care.
4. Use therapeutic communications and offer emotional support. Listen to what the patient is saying.

Evaluation
1. Evaluate the patient's responses to the therapeutic interventions and treatment plan. Does the patient demonstrate a decrease in symptoms and level of anxiety? Have the patient's concerns been addressed?
2. Ask the patient to evaluate their hospital experience.

SAMPLE PATIENT CARE PLAN 19.1   Hospitalization

Assessment

History Paul is a 72-year-old man who has enjoyed excellent health until approximately 6 weeks ago, when he noticed a lump in the right abdominal area. Because of the possibility of extensive surgery, the physician would prefer to perform the biopsy at the hospital. Paul is being admitted the evening before surgery for preparation.

Current Findings A nervous, pale man, appearing his stated age. Appearance, speech, and motor activity are all within normal limits. Paul states he is "a little concerned" about the surgery. Although alert, oriented, and cooperative, he has difficulty following instructions.

Multidisciplinary Diagnosis

Anxiety related to situational crisis of illness, hospitalization, and outcome of surgery.

Planning/Goals

Paul will verbalize his concerns over his outcome and management of care by _____.

Paul will voice understanding and cooperate with his care by _____.

THERAPEUTIC INTERVENTIONS

Interventions	Rationale	Team Member
1. Address the patient by his preferred name.	Demonstrates respect and ensures that dignity will be maintained	All
2. Obtain a history of previous hospitalizations.	Helps plan care based on individual needs and experiences	Nsg
3. Actively listen to and accept Paul's feelings of anxiety and the threat it poses to his self-esteem.	Conveys respect, self-worth; assures him that his concerns will be addressed	All
4. Explain each procedure, and gain cooperation before beginning.	Helps decrease anxiety and fear of the unknown	All
5. Assist Paul in identifying and building on past successful coping mechanisms.	When added to newly learned ones, past successful coping mechanisms encourage Paul to use more effective skills	All
6. Help Paul identify new ways to cope with his anxiety.	Helps him manage anxiety	Psy
7. Inform Paul frequently of his status and progress made during hospitalization.	Knowledge of one's condition decreases anxieties associated with the lack of control during hospitalization	All

Evaluation By the morning of surgery, Paul was able to discuss his concerns with the nurse. Recovery from anesthesia was uneventful.

Critical Thinking Questions
1. How would the fact that Paul had never been hospitalized affect his anxiety?
2. How would the fact that Paul had never been hospitalized affect your planning of his care?

A complete patient care plan includes several other diagnoses and interventions.
Nsg, nursing staff; *Psy,* psychologist.

Support patients throughout each stage of the illness experience. Be alert to the behaviours associated with each stage of illness and hospitalization. Assist patients with the emotional discomforts of illness, whether physical or psychological. Sample Patient Care Plan 19.1 addresses some of these factors.

Supporting Significant Others

An individual's family is an important group in their life. Previously, the traditional family consisted of a mother, father, siblings, and relatives. Today, the family consists of whomever the patient calls family. Patients' families can have a significant impact on the outcome of their illness.

In many societies, the man is a symbol of strength and stability. When men from these societies are ill or hospitalized, their roles as providers change and they become receivers. Because they are unable to fulfill their roles, they can feel inadequate and humiliated. The role changes can leave family members bewildered and uncertain.

If the condition is serious or chronic, loved ones are also faced with the issues of long-term care placement or death. In addition, each family member is trying to cope with all the emotions associated with the illness of a loved one.

Care providers should be alert to how the family's interactions affect the patient. With a patient's consent, family members should be included and consulted for details about the patient's care. Following patient's consent, all family members should be kept informed about the patient's progress.

Also, remember that family members are people in crisis themselves. Gentle interventions provide some much-needed emotional support. When family members are satisfied that their loved one is receiving good care, the decrease in anxiety can help promote patients' recoveries.

Pain Management

An important component of any illness, hospitalization, or surgery relates to the concept of pain—that unpleasant sensation of nerve endings being unkindly stimulated. Pain is a subjective experience; it cannot be objectively seen, touched, or described. It cannot be shared. It helps us adapt to our environment by alerting us to an injury or other problem and reminds us that time is required to heal an injured body part.

People view pain individually based on their own experiences, attitudes, and anxieties. What one person considers unbearable, another identifies as mild or moderate pain. One's age, previous experiences with pain, coping styles, cultural background, and family support all influence how pain is perceived.

Pain is associated with many illnesses and hospital stays. Some people who are admitted to hospitals arrive with chronic pain. Others anticipate that hospitalization will be a painful experience. To manage patients' pain effectively, nurses must discover their patients' expectations of pain, what they think may happen to them, and how much they expect it will hurt. Many patients believe that if they complain, the physicians and nurses will be distracted from their real job—helping them to heal. Taking the time to learn about patients' viewpoints will help you plan and implement more effective pain relief measures.

An essential step in helping patients control their pain (**pain management**) is mutual goal setting. Because pain is a subjective experience, many tools have been developed to help patients assess their pain. One of the most helpful tools is the *body map*. Marking or drawing the location of the pain on a map of the body can significantly reduce miscommunications between care providers and patients (Dannemiller Inc., 2013).

There are many types of pain scales. Each has its advantages and disadvantages. For example, using a pain scale of 0 to 10, the patient is asked to pick a target, a "pain score." Remember, though, that people interpret pain differently. Pain for one person may not be pain for another. The more care providers know about patients' backgrounds in relation to pain, the more effectively they will be in relieving it.

It is important to assess a patient's pain frequently. If appropriate, try nonmedication remedies to decrease their discomfort before resorting to pain medications. Massage, visualization, distraction, and therapeutic touch are all helpful in relieving pain. Pain has an emotional component attached to it. If nurses and other care providers can decrease the anxiety associated with pain, the chances of a speedy recovery are much greater because energy that was once used to control pain can now be focused on healing.

Discharge Planning

To help patients cope with the hurdles of illness or dysfunction, early identification of and intervention for their challenges after hospitalization are essential. This process is called **discharge planning**. After the initial admission assessment, possible home care needs are identified. Then referrals are made to appropriate resources. For example, home care nursing is arranged for the patient who must recover from a fracture at home, or a social worker is notified if a patient needs psychiatric day care or housing. For patients who are living with others, discharge planning can help determine educational needs relating to the care of the recovering individual.

Leaving the facility affects the entire family group. New anxieties about the individual returning home must be addressed before release from the hospital. During the patient's hospitalization, make an effort to discuss home care requirements with the family. Note and correct any misleading or inaccurate information. Take time with family members to teach health care practices related to patient care. Most loved ones are more than willing to learn about good home care practices.

For people living alone, especially older persons, discharge planning is vital if individuals are to return to their home after leaving the health care institution. Basic needs are a high priority for persons living alone. When those needs are met, anxieties are diminished, and people can get on with the business of living. Discharge planning is an important component of every patient's care plan and a valuable tool for assessing and meeting patients' after-hospitalization needs.

Illness and hospitalization are stressful. Although thousands of people are treated in hospitals yearly, every admission can potentially be a crisis. Do not become so comfortable in your work environment that you cannot appreciate your patients' concerns and their situations.

KEY POINTS

- Health is a dynamic state of physical, mental, and social well-being based on a person's concept of health and their values, lifestyle, and personality.
- Illness is an abnormal process in which the social, physical, emotional, or intellectual functions of a person are diminished or impaired.
- The illness experience is roughly divided into five stages, with each stage associated with certain perceptions, decisions, and behaviours.
- During each stage of the illness experience, people are faced with several emotional choices and with reactions frequently involving feelings of denial, anger, frustration, shame, and helplessness.
- Denial is a psychological defence mechanism used to ward off the painful feelings associated with hospitalization.
- The situational crisis of inpatient treatment is about being removed from one's familiar home environment to be cared for by strangers in an impersonal, uncomfortable building.
- The stages of the hospitalization experience are being overwhelmed, stabilization, and adaptation.

- It is important for patients undergoing the psychiatric hospitalization experience to be emotionally supported because of the associated stigma and anxiety.
- Family interactions affect patients. With consent from the patient, family members should be included and consulted for details about the patient's care. They should be kept informed about the patient's progress.
- Health care providers must remember that psychosocial attention is just as important as good physical care.
- Pain is a subjective experience with physical and emotional components. Decreasing the anxiety associated with pain through the use of massage, visualization, distraction, and therapeutic touch increases the chances of a speedy recovery because the energy used to control the pain can be focused on healing.
- Discharge planning is the early identification of and intervention for possible challenges after hospitalization.
- Psychosocial care for hospitalized patients focuses on supporting patients and their families throughout the illness experience.

ADDITIONAL LEARNING RESOPURCES

Go to your Evolve website (http://evolve.elsevier.com/Canada/Morrison-Valfre/) for additional online resources, including the online Study Guide for additional learning activities to help you master this chapter content.

CRITICAL THINKING QUESTIONS

1. A single, 68-year-old patient just underwent urgent open-heart surgery. He is extubated now in a cardiac critical care unit, and has been told that he will be discharged home within a few days. He will have to gradually build up the strength to resume his usual activities, including basic home chores. His sister has arrived from out of town to care for him and help him with household chores. The patient is relieved to have the help but resents having to be cared for. Which stage of the illness experience is the patient exhibiting?

2. What is the psychological defence mechanism used to ward off the painful feelings associated with illness and hospitalization?

3. What, in large part, determines the manner in which patients respond to being hospitalized?

4. What is the stage of illness experienced when the person is relieved of obligation and is allowed to be passive but is expected to get well? What is the care provider's role in supporting the person in that stage?

5. What should care providers investigate to help a patient who is in pain?

REFERENCES

Campbell, D. B., & Anderson, B. J. (1999). Setting behavioral limits. *American Journal of Nursing, 99*(12), 40–42.

Dames, S., Luctkar-Flude, M., & Tyerman, J. (Eds.). (2021). *Edelman and Kudzma's Canadian Health promotion throughout the lifespan.* Elsevier.

Dannemiller Inc. (2013). A review of the evaluation of pain using a variety of pain scales. https://cme.dannemiller.com/articles/activity?id=318&f=1

Lazarus, R. S. (2006). Emotions and interpersonal relationships: Toward a person-centered conceptualization of emotions and coping. *Journal of Personality, 74*(1), 9–46.

Mosby's dictionary of medicine, nursing, & health professions (9th ed.) (2013). Mosby.

Potter, P. A., Perry, A. G., Stockert, P., et al. (2019). *Essentials for nursing practice* (9th ed.). Mosby.

20

Loss and Grief

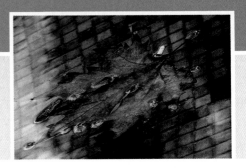

OBJECTIVES

Upon completion of this chapter, the student will be able to:
1. Describe two characteristics of loss.
2. Illustrate four behaviours associated with loss.
3. Describe the stages of the grieving process.
4. Explain the differences between anticipatory, healthy, and unresolved grief.
5. Compare the reactions of being diagnosed with a potentially fatal illness with those of having a terminal diagnosis.
6. Describe how cultural factors can influence attitudes about death, grief, and mourning.
7. Outline each stage of the dying process.
8. Explain the meaning of a "good death."
9. Describe the support given by nurses who provide hospice care for terminally ill persons.

OUTLINE

KEY TERMS

anticipatory (ăn-TĬS-ă-pă-TŎR-ē) grief (p. 239)
bereavement (bĭ-RĔV-mĕnt) (p. 238)
complicated grief (p. 239)
dying process (p. 241)
external (ĕks-TŬR-năl) losses (p. 237)
grief (p. 238)
grieving process (p. 238)

hospice (HŎS-pĭs) (p. 243)
internal losses (p. 237)
loss (p. 236)
magical thinking (p. 237)
mourning (MŎR-nĬng) (p. 238)
terminal (TĔR-mĬ-năl) illness (p. 240)
unresolved grief (p. 239)

Life is a series of situations, experiences, challenges, joys, and losses—a dynamic process that requires continual adaptation and adjustment. Life is filled with gains and losses on every level of functioning. Although change is interwoven throughout each life, reactions to change and the accompanying losses vary according to our sociocultural perceptions and personal experiences. We all tend to react to our world as we were taught. Culture influences attitudes about proper living, relationships with others, and what is considered important in life. It also has a strong influence on a society's attitudes and practices relating to loss, the expression of loss, and dying individuals.

This chapter explores reactions to loss. It offers several suggestions for assisting patients and their loved ones through the emotions of loss. It also encourages you to consider a patient-centered peaceful death as an appropriate therapeutic goal.

THE NATURE OF LOSS

The word loss has several meanings. It is a form of the verb which means "to become unable to find, to misplace; a failure to keep, win, or gain; or to have taken from one by accident, separation, or death." Add to this the attached emotional perceptions and one can see how loss becomes a very individual and personal experience.

Losses are an unavoidable part of life; everyone must cope with them. Emotional reactions and their resultant behaviours are learned from childhood observations and experiences. How individuals cope with problems, successes, and losses is influenced by the success or failure of their experiences, current attitudes, their genotype, and the situations they face. Thus people react and behave during times of loss in highly individual ways. Responses to loss can range from quiet withdrawal to angry rampages. What also matters is how the loss is perceived and valued by the person suffering the loss, as well as how it is supported by others.

Losses can be classified as external or internal losses. **External losses** include those outside the individual. They relate to objects, possessions, the environment, loved ones, and support. **Internal losses** are more personal and include losses that involve some part of oneself. An understanding of the characteristics of loss is important if care providers are to provide the psychosocial interventions that are so important in helping patients (and themselves) cope effectively with emotional times during loss.

Characteristics of Loss

In the health care professions, *loss* is defined as a state in which something valued that was formerly present is changed or gone. It can no longer be seen, felt, heard, known, or experienced. This broad statement requires some analysis.

First, loss is an actual or potential state. A loss can be real—an actual threat or a situation based in reality. For example, the family whose home burns in flames is experiencing an actual loss. Potential losses are defined by the individual experiencing them. The industrial worker who is facing a layoff is coping with the possibility of losing their means of providing for their family. A college student who loses confidence is faced with a less overt, but still important, potential loss. Losses can also be imagined—perceived as a loss. The case of a newlywed who loses her breast to cancer and imagines that her husband will reject her (even though that is not actually the case) illustrates an imagined loss resulting from an actual loss.

How a loss is defined depends on the value, importance, and significance of the item to the individual. Often the significance of a loss will be different for the patient and the care provider. For example, the young mother who has just experienced her fourth miscarriage may define her loss differently from the nurse who has never been pregnant. Thus it is important to remember to assess the *meaning* of loss for each patient.

The last portion of the definition, "can no longer be seen, felt, heard, known, or experienced," explains the state of loss. When the valued person, object, or concept is gone, something is changed. This change leads to certain emotional reactions and responses we call *grief*.

Losses may also be *temporary* or *permanent, expected,* or *unexpected.* They may occur suddenly or gradually. Illness, for example, results in the temporary loss of roles and obligations, but the loss of a limb is definitely a permanent loss. Expected losses arrive with many situations. To illustrate, a chronically ill 80-year-old does not expect to compete in the Senior Olympics because he knows he has gradually lost physical abilities. The individual diagnosed with a terminal illness is coping with an expected loss. Unexpected losses are just that. They are the unknown occurrences that arrive suddenly and without warning. The automobile accident, the diagnosis of human immunodeficiency virus (HIV), or the suicide of a cherished friend each illustrates unexpected losses.

Losses can also be *maturational,* in which an individual must give up something in order to gain a higher level of development. The 18-year-old who is moving into her own apartment loses the comfort and security of family to establish herself as an independent adult. The loss here is ideally offset by the gains in self-development and maturity.

Situational losses occur in response to external events. In a situational loss, the individual has no control over the event leading to the loss. The death of a loved one, a natural disaster, and the divorce of family members are typical situational losses.

Loss Behaviours Throughout the Life Cycle

Each of us reacts to loss based on our level of development, past experiences, and current support systems. To help patients cope with their losses, it is important to understand how people at various developmental stages react to loss.

Children's understanding and reactions to loss change as they mature. Newborns and infants feel the loss of their caregivers but show little emotional reaction to the loss as long as their basic needs are being met. Toddlers are concerned with themselves. Although they may repeat phrases such as "Daddy is gone," they have no grasp of the real meaning of loss. Because of their sense of time, preschoolers cannot understand a permanent loss such as death. Preschoolers use **magical thinking:** They believe that their thoughts can control events to explain their losses. This can result in a child carrying the burdens of shame, doubt, and guilt when their thinking is associated with the loss. To illustrate, Cesar, a 3-year-old, believes that if he were not such a bad boy, his mother would not have gone away. Younger children may react to the same loss more intensely than older children or adults because they have fewer coping mechanisms.

School-age children have some idea about cause and effect, but they still associate bad thoughts or misdeeds with losses. At this age, children experience great feelings of grief over the loss of a body part or function. They may feel overwhelming responsibility and guilt about an event, but they respond well to simple, logical explanations. Children around 6 or 7 years old often apply a broad definition to loss, especially death, by giving responsibility for the loss to the devil, God, or the bogeyman. By 9 or 10 years of age, most children have an adult concept of loss and death. They realize that some losses are permanent, whereas others are only temporary. Their attitudes, reactions, and responses to their losses are now firmly established.

Adolescents react to loss with adult thinking and childlike emotions. Although they can understand the concepts of loss and death, they are of the age group least likely to accept the situation. Adolescents grieve acutely over the loss of a body part or function and fear rejection from their peers. Death is particularly difficult to accept at this age because the developmental task of adolescence is to define who one is and to establish an identity. Threats of loss at this age may make a person stand out from the peer group, so many adolescents ignore the loss or deny their own mortality.

Adults facing loss are able to perceive events more abstractly than younger individuals. They can tell the difference between temporary and permanent losses. Most are able to accept their losses and grow from the experiences. As they continue to encounter and cope with various losses, most adults develop a "hardiness," a sense of self-confidence and understanding about life and death. This strength helps stave off the depression so common in older persons who have experienced significant losses. Hardy people are able to problem-solve. They are in control of their emotions, their lives, and their reactions to loss. By the time most individuals have reached old age, their emotional hardiness has carried them through many of life's losses.

THE NATURE OF GRIEF AND MOURNING

Although the terms *grief, mourning,* and *bereavement* are used interchangeably, each has a separate meaning. **Grief** is the set of *emotional reactions* that accompany a loss. **Mourning** is the *process* of working through or resolving one's grief, and **bereavement** is the *behavioural state* of thoughts, feelings, and activities that follow a loss. The period of grief and mourning after a loss can be intense and painful. It may last for a short period or remain as a deep emotional scar. Feelings of loss, grief, and mourning are deeply personal, and each of us has our own way of coping with these emotions. There is no right or wrong way to grieve.

The Grieving Process

To work through the emotional responses that come with loss, one must experience the **grieving process**—a method for resolving losses and healing. Grieving, mourning, and bereavement are normal, healthy responses to loss. Working through the grieving process allows people to "piece themselves back together," to reintegrate their lives, to find meaning in new relationships, and to re-establish a positive picture of themselves. It is a healing process that encourages individuals to continue on, even after the loss. The care provider's role during the grieving process is to provide emotional support and an atmosphere that helps patients accomplish the painful work of grieving (Meiner, 2014).

The grieving process was first studied by Sigmund Freud in the early 1900s. Since then, many theories have been developed to explain the work of grieving. Although various theories consider different aspects of grieving, all include stages that we experience while working through our grief.

Stages of the Grieving Process

The first step in the process of grieving is *denial.* It begins with a feeling of shock. One wants to reject the loss, to say "no," to refuse to give up the cherished object or person. Individuals may not even acknowledge that a loss has occurred. They behave as if nothing has happened or pretend that the loved object or person is still present. Denial at this stage provides an emotional buffer that allows people time to mobilize resources for the work ahead.

As the realization that the loss can no longer be ignored sets in, denial turns to *yearning.* The person may feel intense anger. During this stage, the reality of the loss begins to be realized and the griever becomes overwhelmed. Crying, self-blame, and anger are common, and some may even strike out at themselves or others. The griever "falls apart"—becomes disorganized, depressed, and unable to complete daily living activities. They may try to postpone coping with the loss by ignoring it. The person in this stage may feel that life is not worth living and consider or attempt suicide (Box 20.1). This is an extremely difficult time for people. They need the emotional support and caring of friends and family to remind them of all that still remains, even after loss and suffering.

As the impact of the loss is experienced in daily living, the third stage, *bargaining,* may occur for the grieving individual. This stage comes in a form of magical thinking, by asking, "What if?"; for example, "What if I never raise my voice again towards my wife? Would God cure her from cancer?"

With time, the *depression* stage settles over the grieving person. The work of mourning begins as the full impact of the loss is realized. Feelings of guilt and remorse are frequent as attempts are made to cope with the painful void left by the loss. The grieving individual may withdraw from social interactions, engage in unhealthy behaviours, or experience overwhelming loneliness. As time passes, however, most people become willing to share their memories and rely on the emotional support of others.

Acceptance and recovery begin when grieving individuals begin to focus their energies toward the living. The loss is a reality, but life continues, so they begin to reinvest their feelings in others and nurture their remaining relationships. Steps are taken to reorganize their lives by filling the void created by the loss. Eventually, a new self-awareness and inner strength evolve from the grieving experience. The good times start to outweigh the bad, and life slowly stabilizes.

The grieving process is dynamic; most individuals do not move through the process step by step. They may backslide or regress into earlier stages or make multiple adjustments at

---

BOX 20.1   Suicide Alert

Individuals who experience acute emotions of grief and loss often feel that life is not worth continuing. Any medications, over-the-counter medications, or other chemicals in the environment have the potential of being used for a suicide attempt. Grieving persons have ingested medications prescribed for the deceased with the purpose of committing suicide because their suffering is so great.

Sometimes grief is so intense that they will resort to slitting their wrists or using a weapon on themselves. Health care providers should be alert to the signs and symptoms of possible suicidal actions during the grieving process. See Chapter 27 for a more thorough discussion of suicide.

one time. The actual length of time required for the work of grieving varies considerably, depending on the severity of the loss and coping resources available. Some theorists state that the intense reactions of grief gradually decrease within 6 to 12 months, but active mourning may continue for 5 years or longer.

Recovering from an important loss is a slow process. Time is needed for people to mourn, to sort through their emotions, and then to cope with them. When the grieving process and its accompanying mourning behaviours are experienced successfully, people emerge with hope and a new sense of involvement with life. The loss has been recognized, accepted, and placed in memory. Although life may never be the same, a new appreciation and interest in current activities gradually replace the grief.

An individual who becomes aware of an impending loss, such as the loss of a body part or of a loved one through the diagnosis of a terminal condition, may experience **anticipatory grief**—the process of grieving before the actual event occurs. During divorce proceedings, for example, many persons grieve for the part of life that has been lost and what they know will be lost in the future. Anticipatory grieving allows individuals time to prepare for the loss.

Unresolved Grief

Mental health difficulties can result when the grieving process is prolonged or impairs functioning over time. **Unresolved grief**, also termed *dysfunctional grief* or *complicated bereavement,* describes unhealthy or ineffective grief reactions. People who experience unresolved grief are unable to shift their attention from their loss to the realities of everyday life. They become so preoccupied with the loss that they are unable to function effectively. Long-standing, unresolved grief can result in depression and complicated grief. Both are associated with distress about the loss, changes in eating or sleeping patterns, and changes in activity levels.

When the grieving person feels the loss so intensely that feelings of despair and worthlessness overwhelm everything in life, depression should be suspected. Every day is a grey fog with no light as one looks toward the future. Life becomes a burden, and each new day is faced with sadness and remorse. This attitude overshadows all else. The grieving individual experiences changes in eating, sleeping, and activity levels; angry or hostile moods; and an inability to concentrate or complete work tasks. There may be intense guilt, slowed body responses, and weight loss.

To complicate matters, individuals often become more and more socially isolated. They may react with hostility or anger when friends express concern. This type of grief may lead to suicidal ideation but responds well to treatment when it is recognized and interventions are begun early. A combination of psychotherapy and medication therapy has been shown to be effective. Emotional and social support are also important factors in patients' recovery.

Complicated grief is a persistent yearning for a deceased person that often occurs without signs of depression. Although the symptoms appear to be those of normal grieving, they are associated with impaired psychological functioning and disturbances of mood, sleep, and self-esteem. The grieving individual becomes preoccupied with the loss. There is a continuous yearning and longing for the lost loved one. Some may idealize and search for the lost person or object or relive past experiences. Some blame themselves for the death and wish to die so they can join the loved one. Because life in the present is not as desirable as past memories, the grieving person may become intolerant of others and socially isolated. The result is a loss of identity or purpose in life, feeling like a part of themselves died with the loved one.

Treatment for unresolved grief depends on the presence of depressive symptoms. A psychotherapeutic and psychopharmacological approach is used to treat depression. The grief can be eased by emotional support and having someone listen. Support groups and opportunities for social interactions add to the effectiveness of treatment in most cases.

CRITICAL THINKING

Your patient displays all the signs and symptoms of complicated grief. It is recommended that she attend a support group for widows, but she refuses. With gentle questioning, she confides that she has no money for transportation to the meetings and she will not ask for help.
- What therapeutic interventions would help this patient meet the goal of regularly attending the support group meetings?

The therapeutic interventions for grief involve listening, providing emotional support, and referral to appropriate resources. Nurses and direct caregivers are often the first to identify the signs and symptoms of unresolved grieving because of their focus on patients' activities of daily living. Therapeutic listening helps in understanding the needs of the grieving individual. It also offers an opportunity to provide emotional support and comfort. Sometimes when grieving individuals are encouraged to verbalize their feelings, the real healing begins. Health care providers are instrumental in referring their patients to the therapists, support groups, and educational opportunities that may help them work through the grieving process.

Caregivers' Grief

Care providers experience the same grief as others when faced with loss. Many nurses work with dying patients, some on a daily basis. Relationships are formed between care providers and patients that develop into understanding and rapport. The focus is on the patient, and the care provider acts therapeutically, but the bond between individuals grows with the relationship. When that relationship is lost, even if it was an expected loss, care providers grieve, and that is a necessary process for health. When the patient's loss of life was unexpected (e.g., they died by suicide), the staff may require a professional intensive intervention by a trusted clinician.

The care provider's role in offering support and comfort to grieving loved ones can become complicated if the provider's personal feelings of grief overshadow effectiveness. Care providers should share in the grief experience, but they need to remember that the primary goal is to provide support for the remaining loved ones. Many health care facilities offer support groups for nurses and other care providers who work with dying patients in an effort to assist them with their own grief experiences.

As a care provider, learn to appreciate the experiences of dying and grieving patients. Understand the steps of the grieving process. Identify how you cope with losses. Finally, do not forget to find a way to renew your energies. When we know and accept our own attitudes and feelings about loss and grieving, we are better able to provide the therapeutic interventions so needed by others.

THE DYING PROCESS

Dying is the last stage of growth and development. Like birth, it is an intensely personal process. Unlike birth, however, an individual is often aware and consciously takes part in the process. Death means different things to each of us. For some, it is a welcome relief from suffering. For others, it is the ultimate fear. The process of dying remains unchanged, but attitudes, beliefs, and behaviours surrounding death are as variable as the individuals who practise them.

CULTURAL CONSIDERATIONS

In Sri Lanka, a small island off the southeastern tip of India, quality of life is strongly preferable to quantity of life. Most of Sri Lanka's citizens are Buddhist (69%) and believe in reincarnation (the rebirth of a soul in a different body). They believe the suffering of this life will be relieved in the next incarnation, so there is no need for heroic lifesaving measures.

Dying persons in this culture are prepared for death by being helped to remember past good deeds of their lives and achieve a comfortable mental state. Because the body is no longer required after death, cremation is the preferred burial custom.

Death may occur suddenly or gradually. It may be expected or arrive as a total surprise. One may be fortunate enough to die in familiar surroundings, attended by loved ones and friends, or one may be forced to face the fate of dying alone and unloved. During earlier days in Canadian history, most families cared for their elders and ill members at home. Children witnessed the births of their siblings and the deaths of their grandparents. It was all accepted as part of living. Today, children know little about dying because older persons no longer live in the family home. More than two thirds of all deaths now occur in health care facilities, hospitals, and long-term care facilities (Touhy & Jett, 2015).

Age Differences and Dying

The impact of death is only as strong as one understands it. Before age 8, most children do not understand the permanency of death, but they do experience a sense of doom and danger associated with dying. By age 12, children are aware that death is irreversible, but they do not relate to their own deaths. Adolescents and young adults do not relate to death unless forced to. As people grow older, they begin to lose family and friends and must begin to face their own mortality.

Dying children need special care and communication. Children are remarkably observant and have an intuitive ability to understand the seriousness of their illness and its outcomes. However, their immediate concerns focus on how the illness affects their activities of daily living and limits their abilities. Children are also very aware of the family's reactions and may hesitate to discuss issues they think may be upsetting for the family. Whenever possible, parents should be encouraged to communicate with the dying child. Open discussions of the illness and its outcome help children cope with the feelings of isolation, anxiety, and guilt over causing distress in the family. Sharing feelings and insecurities helps to bond family members together and to give one another strength. Children who are able to share their emotions experience fewer behavioural problems, less depression, and higher self-esteem than those who suppress their feelings. They adapt to the difficulties of their disease and its treatment better than those who must cope with the isolation of dying emotionally alone. Siblings of the dying child also need extra attention during this time because feelings of jealousy, anger, and guilt are often present.

Parents and care providers should not hesitate to look for external assistance to help children work through the grieving process. For example, the Hospital for Sick Children (SickKids), in Toronto, has a free library of children's books specifically written to help children at different ages with different types of losses.

Terminal Illness

A **terminal illness** is a condition in which the outcome is death. The diagnosis of a terminal illness is perhaps one of the most difficult challenges an individual must face. The course of some diseases can be long, with periods of physical improvement and hope alternating with illness and suffering. Grieving occurs throughout the course of the illness.

How a person responds to and prepares for death depends on two factors: the meaning of death and the coping mechanisms used throughout life to deal with problems. If the individual is comfortable and satisfied with life, then death is usually accepted without fear; but if the person lived struggling and fighting, the experience of dying may be much the same. People tend to cope with dying in the same ways in which they coped with living.

The diagnosis of a fatal illness or condition is received with disbelief and shock—a true crisis. This is a time of great uncertainty because the patient and family are struggling to cope with the illness, its effects, and its final outcome. Crisis interventions can be very effective at this stage.

As the condition progresses, denial and hope allow the patient and family to slowly adjust to the reality of the situation. Hope is future oriented and helps individuals endure the suffering of the present because it offers the possibility that soon things will be better. Denial offers a way of coping with each little loss until the reality of the situation is finally accepted. During this time, the individual is encouraged to continue with daily activities until they are no longer able. In time, both the family and individual either accept the outcome and prepare for death or continue to deny the reality of the situation until it is no longer possible.

Receiving the diagnosis of a potentially fatal illness can bring forth a variety of reactions. Individuals who are young and feel healthy may refuse to accept that a problem exists. For others, the diagnosis of a potentially terminal condition acts as a wake-up call and a motivator to make major lifestyle changes. The following Case Study illustrates such a situation.

CASE STUDY

Brittany was just 35 years old when she received the diagnosis of severe coronary artery disease. She became short of breath one day while doing household chores and decided that she must be hanging on to the cold she had gotten from her 8-year-old a few weeks before. She decided to schedule an appointment with her family physician.

Dr. Singh had worked with Brittany's family for many years. He knew about her smoking, eating, and exercise habits. He had encouraged her to consider weight loss and had referred her to a smoking cessation program several times in the past few years, but to no avail. After a thorough physical examination and an electrocardiogram, Dr. Singh scheduled Brittany for a cardiac catheterization at the local hospital the following day. Brittany left the office in shock, stunned by the realization that she might actually not live long enough to see her children grow into adults. She knew in her heart that this was the warning call to take her life and health more seriously. She only hoped that she had the strength to make the changes she knew would be required if she wanted to live longer.

The results of Brittany's cardiac catheterization showed that three of her coronary arteries were seriously blocked and that the blood supply to her heart was inadequate. Her physician recommended surgery but firmly stated that this was only a temporary measure. Without major lifestyle changes, the threat to her health would reappear. At this point Brittany had to make some life-and-death decisions. As she saw it, she had two options: to continue with her easygoing, comfortable lifestyle and run the risk of dropping dead from a heart attack at an early age, or to change her diet, stop her unhealthy habits, begin to exercise, and learn to defuse her stress.

• What therapeutic interventions would help Brittany make a sound decision?

People often make the major changes necessary to prevent a condition from becoming fatal. Others value their present ways of living too much or feel that the work is not worth the extra time gained. The decisions about one's remaining time belong to and should be made by the individual. Care providers should accept and support patients' decisions about terminal illness. The goals of care are then structured to provide the best possible interventions within the realities of each situation.

Cultural Factors, Dying, and Mourning

Although death is a personal experience, it occurs within a cultural and social context. Cultural practices regarding dying, grief, and mourning have a strong influence on behaviours. To illustrate, many modern North Americans see death as the final loss in life. East Indian Hindus, however, believe that all creatures are in a process of spiritual evolution that extends through the boundaries of time and space. They view death as a passage from one existence to another (Giger & Haddad, 2020).

Culture also dictates many funeral, burial, and mourning practices. The length of time for mourning and public displays of grief are culturally determined. Special clothing is commonly worn during the grieving process to symbolize loss. To illustrate, traditional Chinese wear white as a sign of mourning, whereas black is the required colour for mourning among most individuals in North America and in many parts of Europe and Russia.

The beliefs, rituals, and practices of one's culture may be very important to one individual and barely matter to another member of that same culture. Thus care providers must be careful to assess and understand the meaning of each patient's cultural, religious, and social practices. Many variations exist in every group of people, no matter which culture they identify with. Do not assume how a patient feels about their cultural beliefs and practices. Find out what is important to them and, if at all possible, incorporate it into the patient's plan of care. Never take a person's cultural background for granted.

Stages of Dying

Unless death arrives suddenly, both individuals and loved ones progress through several psychological stages during dying. These stages or phases, called the **dying process**, allow people to cope with the overwhelming emotional reactions associated with dying and losing loved ones. Several theories about the process of dying have been developed, but the oldest and most well-known theory is Elisabeth Kübler-Ross's five stages of dying: denial, anger, bargaining, depression, and acceptance (Kübler-Ross, 1969). Later theorists simplified Kübler-Ross's five stages into three basic phases of resistance, working, and acceptance (Fig. 20.1).

During the *resistance* stage, the individual fights the issue through denial, avoidance, anger, and bargaining. The *working*, or review, stage broadens consciousness as one's life is reviewed. The resistance disappears, and the individual begins to deal with unfinished business. They reclaim a part of the self and become more in tune to the self of the present rather than that of the past.

In the last stage, called *acceptance*, the individual is comfortable and acknowledges death. They can discuss death with peace and calm. Increasingly greater amounts of time are spent focusing inward, moving one's energies away from outer reality. Some individuals have near-death experiences that they describe as a passage into another realm of consciousness or an intense personal journey when they were on the brink of death. Eventually, the dying person fades from this life, leaving only the body behind.

A broader perspective of the dying process is offered by Glaser and Strauss (1965). Their models of awareness of dying

Theorist   Stages

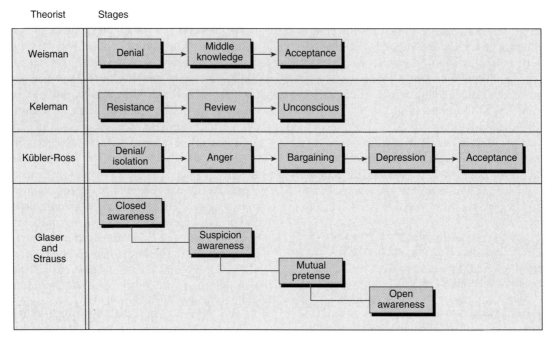

Fig. 20.1 Theories—stages of dying and grief. (Redrawn from Ebersole, P., & Hess, P. [2004]. *Toward healthy aging: Human needs and nursing response* [7th ed.]. Mosby.)

can be applied to family, friends, and those who care for the dying individual. They describe the closed awareness model as one in which medical personnel and family know that the condition is fatal but still "keep the secret" or withhold the information from the patient. Once the dying individual becomes suspicious of the truth, a battle for control of information ensues. This closed awareness model was commonly practised by health care providers in the past. Frequently, patients were not told of the seriousness of their illness because it was believed that the news was too upsetting. Most terminally ill persons know that they are dying. Many still experience death locked into a denial supported by care providers and loved ones.

The mutual pretense model is a "let's pretend" kind of awareness. Both caregivers and the dying individual are aware of the impending death, but nobody talks about it. Although no one really expects the patient to recover, it is easier to pretend that things will get better. Unfortunately, the true feelings of everyone remain hidden, unspoken, and unresolved.

In the open awareness model, the approaching death is openly acknowledged and accepted. The patient is resigned to dying and accepts each day as it can be lived. Family members, health care providers, and the dying have permission to discuss their fears, concerns, and experiences. The open awareness method of coping allows mutual support and comfort to be given and received. It also encourages loved ones to grieve with, rather than for, the dying individual.

THERAPEUTIC INTERVENTIONS

One of the most rewarding areas in health care is assisting an individual in experiencing a "good" death—one in which the dying and the living participate fully and completely. With

a good death, individuals control their own destiny. Patients decide when to stop aggressive treatments, refuse the one last surgical procedure, or end the discomfort of a painful therapy. Peace, serenity, and acceptance replace denial, fighting, and anger. Individuals value and cherish each day but look forward to the day when their suffering will end. They are not afraid of death—rather, it is the last step of the growth process, which draws a productive and fruitful life to a close.

Nurses and other health care providers bring their own attitudes, values, beliefs, and biases to the care of the dying. The way caregivers perceive "the act of dying, as painful, upsetting, indifferent, or a blessing, influences the treatment the dying patient will receive in the last days, whether in the hospital or nursing home" (Touhy & Jett, 2015). Thus it is important to explore your own attitudes about death; the quality of your patients' care depends on it.

Never limit your patients by placing labels on them. It is easy for nurses to focus on the dying person's biological or physical needs. It is nonthreatening to help relieve the physical symptoms associated with dying, but it is another thing to become involved in a meaningful therapeutic relationship that supports the dying individual. Box 20.2 lists problem statements (nursing diagnoses) that relate to dying patients.

Hospice Care

In the past, most dying individuals were cared for in the home by family and friends. As society gradually became more mobile, families separated from relatives when they moved to different locations. Dying at home was no longer an alternative for many people, so they were sent to hospitals and long-term care facilities. Health care providers assisted their patients through the dying process, providing comfort where they could, but realizing that there must be better ways to meet life's final challenge.

BOX 20.2   Problem Statements and Nursing Diagnoses Related to Dying

Physical Realm
Risk-prone health behaviour
Caregiver role strain
Ineffective coping
Knowledge deficit
Imbalanced nutrition
Insomnia
Social isolation
Risk for self-directed violence

Psychosocial Realm
Anxiety
Decisional conflict
Denial
Grieving, plus complicated grieving
Hopelessness
Knowledge deficient
Powerlessness
Self-esteem disturbance
Impaired social interactions

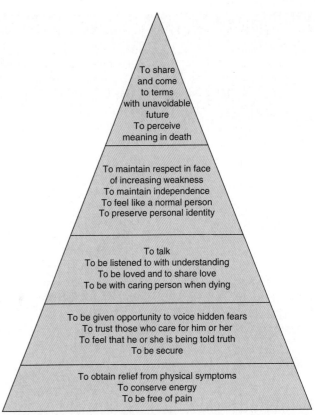

Fig. 20.2 Hierarchy of a dying person's needs. (Redrawn from Ebersole, P., & Hess, P. [2004]. *Toward healthy aging: Human needs and nursing response* [7th ed.]. Mosby.)

Finally, during the 1960s, a model for humane care of the dying was developed and tested at Saint Christopher's Hospice in London, England. Since then, the number of hospices has grown tremendously. In North America today, numerous patients receive hospice care. The term **hospice** symbolizes a philosophy of care for people with terminal illnesses or conditions and for their loved ones. The goal of hospice care is to make the remainder of an individual's life as meaningful and comfortable as humanly possible. Hospice care differs from institutional care in several ways. The focus of care reorients from curative to palliative (providing comfort). Hospice services are available 24 hours per day in institutional or home settings.

Hospice care helps the family retain control for the dying individual, and it allows individuals to experience death with the dignity they deserve. Hospice care helps redefine family relationships because care of the dying individual requires great energies of loved ones and friends. Many nurses and other care providers are choosing to specialize in hospice care because it is such a rewarding area of practice.

Meeting the Needs of Dying Patients

Dying patients have special needs during their final days (Fig. 20.2). One of the most urgent needs is to be free from pain and discomfort. This is usually accomplished by around-the-clock administration of pain-relieving medications. Addiction is not an issue in caring for the terminally ill population.

In 2016, the Parliament of Canada allowed eligible Canadian adults to request medical assistance in dying. Last reporting requirements came into effect November 2018, and now medical assistance in dying (MAiD) has become a part of our public health care system (Government of Canada, 2020).

Freedom from loneliness is not always so easily accomplished. Many dying individuals have already suffered numerous losses, both physical and emotional. The strange surroundings of an institution and unfamiliar care providers can add to a person's sense of isolation and loneliness. Dying patients need to know that someone who really cares for their welfare is there to help. Health care providers should assess for loneliness in patients and offer personal attention.

Individuals with terminal illnesses also need to preserve their self-esteem. The pride of a lifetime of work and struggle can be easily shattered by the thoughtless words or actions of a care provider. Respect is always an important factor in caring for patients, especially older persons. One of the most important principles to remember when working with terminally ill patients is that a dying person lives with the same needs as the rest of us. Life and its needs for love, friendship, and self-esteem continue even when an individual is in the process of dying.

As death approaches, many physical and emotional changes begin to take place (Tables 20.1 and 20.2). This is a time to provide comfort and solace and meet the physical needs of care, but most important, it is a time to support those who must say good-bye and those who are left behind.

Loss, Grief, and Mental Health

Loss is a part of living. The behaviours associated with grief and mourning help us heal after suffering a loss. For many people, death represents the ultimate loss. How effectively

TABLE 20.1   Signs and Symptoms Associated With Dying

Symptoms	Rationale	Interventions
Coolness, colour and temperature change in hands, arms, feet, and legs	Peripheral circulation diminishes to facilitate increased circulation to vital organs	Place socks on feet. Cover with a light cotton blanket.
Increased sleeping	Conservation of energy	Spend time with the patient; hold the patient's hand; speak normally to the patient even though there may be a lack of verbal response or consciousness.
Disorientation, confusion of time, place, or person	Metabolic changes	Identify yourself by name before speaking to patient; speak softly, clearly, and truthfully.
Incontinence of urine and feces	Increased muscle relaxation and decreased consciousness	Maintain vigilance, and change bedding as appropriate.
Congestion	Poor circulation of body fluids, immobilization, and inability to expectorate secretions causing gurgling, rattles, bubbling	Elevate the head, and gently turn the head to the side to drain secretions.
Restlessness	Metabolic changes and a decrease in oxygen to the brain	Calm the patient by speech and action. Reduce light; gently rub back, stroke arms, or read aloud; play soothing music. DO NOT USE RESTRAINTS.
Decreased intake of food and liquids	Body conservation of energy for function	Do not force the patient to eat or drink. Give ice chips, soft drinks, juice, and popsicles as appropriate. Apply moisturizing lubricant to dry lips. If the patient is a mouth breather, apply protective lubricant more frequently, as needed.
Decreased urine output	Decreased fluid intake and decreased circulation to kidneys	None
Altered breathing pattern	Metabolic and oxygen changes to respiratory centres	Elevate the head of bed; hold patient's hand, speak gently.

TABLE 20.2   Emotional and Spiritual Symptoms of Approaching Death

Symptoms	Rationale	Interventions
Withdrawal	Prepares the patient for release and detachment and letting go of relationships and surroundings	Continue communicating in a normal manner using a normal voice tone. Identify yourself by name: Hold the patient's hand; say what you want the person to hear from you.
Visionlike experiences (dead friends or family, religious vision)	Preparation for transition	Do not contradict or argue regarding whether this is or is not a real experience. If the patient is frightened, reassure them that they are not crazy but that these aberrations do occur.
Restlessness	Tension, fear, unfinished business	Listen to the patient express fears, sadness, and anger associated with dying. Give permission to go.
Decreased socialization	As energy diminishes, the patient withdraws and begins to make the transition	Express support; give permission to die.
Unusual communication: out-of-character statements, gestures, requests	Signals readiness to let go	Say what needs to be said to the dying patient; kiss, hug, or cry with them.

individuals cope with their losses has a large effect on their mental and emotional health. Sample Patient Care Plan 20.1 offers an example of a care plan for an individual who is coping with grief.

Many behaviours associated with the grieving process could be diagnosed as mental health disorders except for the fact that they are short-lived. Mental health issues arise only when a person is stuck or immobilized during a stage of the grief reaction for an extended period of time. Clinical diagnoses of depression apply only to those grieving individuals who are significantly impaired in their abilities to accomplish the activities of daily living. For persons who currently live with a

---

SAMPLE PATIENT CARE PLAN 20.1　Grieving

Assessment

History Cesar, 14 years old, lost his leg in an automobile accident 8 weeks ago. His attitude toward the loss of his leg was casual at first, but soon he became angry and withdrawn. Complaints of chronic fatigue, poor appetite, and an inability to concentrate have prompted his mother to seek further health care for him.

Current Findings An alert adolescent boy who complains that he is unable to sleep. Speech is slow with delayed responses. Left leg is amputated above the knee. Uses crutches for mobility.

Multidisciplinary Diagnosis

Complicated grieving related to loss of body part and physiological functioning

Planning/Goals

Cesar will attend each counselling session.
Cesar will identify his feelings of loss and anger by February 21.

THERAPEUTIC INTERVENTIONS

Intervention	Rationale	Team Member
1. Establish trust and open communication.	Adolescents must trust in the relationship before they commit themselves	All
2. Assure Cesar that his feelings are important, and give him permission to discuss them.	Shows interest and respect; helps maintain self-worth and dignity	All
3. Assist Cesar in acknowledging his feelings associated with losing his leg.	Helps Cesar to connect his anger with the loss and begin the work of grieving	All
4. Help Cesar and his family understand that anger is a normal response to loss.	Assures him that his emotions are a normal part of the grieving response	All
5. Assist Cesar in finding appropriate outlets for his anger rather than projecting it onto others.	Provides structure, gives a sense of control, helps him focus on more effective ways of emotional expression	Psy, Soc Svc
6. Encourage Cesar to make plans for the future and set goals.	Goals help change the focus from the past to the future	Psy, Nsg

Evaluation Cesar missed the first two appointments but has kept every appointment for the past month. Cesar is able to identify three reasons why he feels angry and frustrated. Cesar was unwilling to make any plans for the future at the time of evaluation.

Critical Thinking Questions

1. How would you help Cesar cope with his anger?
2. What interventions may help Cesar look toward the future?

A complete patient care plan includes several other diagnoses and interventions.
Nsg, nursing staff; *Psy*, psychologist; *Soc Svc*, social services.

---

mental health disorder, the stresses of loss and grief can overwhelm coping mechanisms and lead to further difficulties. For example, the 23-year-old with schizophrenia who has lived with her family all her life will likely experience great difficulty grieving the loss of her mother. Care providers must remember that people with existing mental health challenges require much emotional support during periods of loss or grieving.

How each human being copes with loss is unique and individual. Coping mechanisms may be effective and result in growth and healing. They may also be inadequate or dysfunctional, resulting in distress, depression, or other mental health issues. Health care providers need to assess their patients' abilities and resources to cope with their losses. By encouraging effective coping skills and providing physical and emotional support, health care providers become better able to help their patients (and themselves) successfully work through life's losses and grief.

KEY POINTS

- A loss can be actual, potential, or imagined; temporary or permanent; maturational or situational; expected or unexpected. Losses may occur suddenly or gradually.
- The significance of a loss is determined by the person experiencing it.
- Each person reacts to loss based on their level of development, past experiences, and current support systems.
- Grief is the set of emotional reactions accompanying loss.
- The steps of the grieving process are shock, disbelief, and denial; anger, bargaining, and reviewing; depression; and acceptance.
- Mourning is the process of working through or resolving one's grief.

- Bereavement is the emotional and behavioural state of thoughts, feelings, and activities that follow a loss.
- Anticipatory grief is the process of grieving before the actual event occurs.
- Dysfunctional (unresolved) grief can result in depression and complicated grief.
- The care provider's role in offering support and comfort to grieving loved ones can become complicated if the provider's personal grief overshadows effectiveness.
- To cope with your own feelings of grief, learn to appreciate the experiences of dying and grieving patients. Understand the steps of the grieving process. Discover how you cope with losses. Find a way to renew your energies.
- Dying is the last stage in the development of an individual.
- How an individual responds to and prepares for death depends on what death means and the coping mechanisms used throughout life.

- Terminally ill children who are able to share their feelings tend to experience fewer related emotional difficulties and adapt better than those who must cope with emotional isolation.
- One of the most rewarding experiences in health care is assisting an individual in experiencing a patient-centred, peaceful death, one in which the dying and the living participate fully and completely.
- The term *hospice* has come to mean a philosophy of care for people with terminal illnesses or conditions and for their loved ones.
- Dying patients have special needs during their final days, including freedom from pain and discomfort, freedom from loneliness, and preservation of self-esteem.
- One of the most important principles to remember is that a dying person lives with the same needs as the rest of us.

ADDITIONAL LEARNING RESOURCES

Go to your Evolve website (http://evolve.elsevier.com/Canada/Morrison-Valfre/) for additional online resources, including the online Study Guide for additional learning activities to help you master this chapter content.

CRITICAL THINKING QUESTIONS

1. What may be experienced by patients who have just survived a flood in which they lost their home, car, and all personal belongings?
2. What ideas may school-age children have about causes and events that they associate with loss?
3. What may determine the length of time for public displays of mourning, funeral, and grief?

4. What stage of grieving might the wife of a recently deceased patient experience when she states that she is going to return to work and rejoin her exercise class?
5. What would the best action for a care provider to support the dying patient who was overheard by her family speaking to her dead husband? The family has reported a concern that the patient is confused.

REFERENCES

Giger, J. N., & Haddad, L. G. (2020). *Transcultural nursing: Assessment and intervention* (8th ed.). Mosby.

Glaser, B., & Strauss, A. (1965). *Awareness of dying*. Aldine.

Government of Canada. (2020). Medical assistance in dying. https://www.canada.ca/en/health-canada/services/medical-assistance-dying.html

Kübler-Ross, E. (1969). *On death and dying*. Macmillan [Seminal Reference].

Meiner, S. E. (2014). *Gerontologic nursing* (5th ed.). Mosby.

Touhy, T. A., & Jett, K. F. (2015). *Ebersole & Hess' toward healthy aging: Human needs and nursing response* (9th ed.). Mosby.

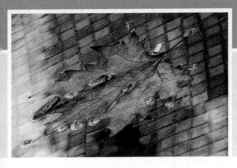

21

Depression and Other Mood Disorders

OBJECTIVES

Upon completion of this chapter, the student will be able to:

1. Describe the continuum of emotional responses.
2. Compare four theories relating to emotions and their disorders.
3. Explain how emotions affect individuals throughout the life cycle.
4. Compare the differences between a depressive episode and a depressive disorder.
5. List the diagnostic criteria for bipolar disorders.
6. Explain seasonal affective disorder.
7. Identify three medication classes used for the treatment of depression and other mood disorders.
8. Apply four nursing (therapeutic) interventions for patients with mood disorders.

OUTLINE

KEY TERMS

affect (p. 250)
affective disorders (p. 250)
bipolar disorder (p. 253)
cyclothymic (sī-klō-THĪ-mǐk) disorder (p. 254)
depression (dǐ-PRĚ-shǔn) (p. 250)
dysthymia (dǐs-THĪ-mē-a) (p. 252)
emotion (ē-MŌ-shǔn) (p. 248)
hypomanic (hǐ-pō-MĀ-nǐk) episode (p. 253)

major depressive episode (MDE) (p. 251)
manic episode (p. 250)
mood disorder (p. 250)
postpartum depression (p. 252)
religiosity (rǐ-LǏJ-ē-ĂHS-ǐt-ē) (p. 260)
seasonal affective disorder (SAD) (p. 252)
situational depression (p. 249)

The emotional realm affects all other areas of human functioning. Emotions can lead to physical changes, new intellectual perspectives, and altered social roles. An **emotion** is a feeling—a nonintellectual response. Emotions are *reactions* to various stimuli based on individual points of view. The following Critical Thinking box presents an example of how perceptions affect emotional reactions.

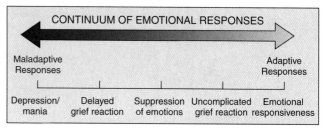

Fig. 21.1 Continuum of emotional responses.

CRITICAL THINKING

James and Justin, two neighbourhood teens, are working on building a model airplane in Justin's backyard. A piece of the model breaks, and they begin to argue about each other's clumsiness. The emotions grow, and soon scuffling, swearing, and fighting ensue. The commotion brings both fathers to the scene. Justin's father shakes his fist and shouts, "That's a boy! Punch him good. No son of mine is going to let someone get the best of him!" James's father, also seeing the scene, reacts with, "Boys! Stop fighting! There are better ways to solve your problems than beating each other up."
- How did each father's perception of the situation differ?
- What do you think caused the difference in their reactions?
- What do you think James and Justin learned from observing each father's response?

BOX 21.1   Possible Causes of Mood Disorders

- Genetic susceptibility
- Biochemical imbalances (neurotransmitters, hormones)
- Environmental and other stressors
- Childhood and adult experiences
- Social circumstances

CONTINUUM OF EMOTIONAL RESPONSES

The spectrum of human emotion ranges from elation to despair. Emotional responses can be growth promoting and adaptive, or they can lead to ineffective behaviours that could soon become maladaptive. Figure 21.1 illustrates the continuum of emotional responses. As individuals repeatedly react to behaviours, interactions, society, and the environment, they establish patterns of emotional responses that become moods.

Mood is described as a "prolonged emotional state that influences one's whole personality and life functioning" (Rollant, 1998). Mood may affect a person's outlook on life events, and vice versa. From this outlook, people interpret and react to the world around them. Some of the reactions are emotional, and the cycle continues. If a person experiences severe and prolonged stages of mood elevation or depression, or fluctuation of these stages without any correspondence to life's events, the person may suffer from a mood disorder.

THEORIES RELATING TO EMOTIONS AND THEIR DISORDERS

Mood disorders were once considered simple, correctable imbalances in behaviour. Current evidence suggests that a combination of physical, psychological, and environmental factors is involved in the development of mood disorders. Many theories about the cause of mood disorders have been offered throughout the years, but none fully explains the complexities of these conditions.

Biological Evidence

Much has been learned about the physical nature of mood disorders. The causes are complex. When sad moods deepen

and persist, the individual is unable to restore emotional equilibrium (balance) because of unusual stress or poor internal regulation. Box 21.1 lists the possible causes of mood disorders.

Defects in the immune system may be related to depression. Genetics may also be a factor in mood disorders. It has been shown that high rates of depression and bipolar illness are seen in individuals who have relatives with mood disorders.

Studies of the effects of neurochemical messengers (*neurotransmitters*) and hormones on behaviour have revealed that behaviours and body chemistries are interrelated. The monoamines norepinephrine and serotonin are major neurotransmitters that excite or inhibit the brain circuits involved in mood regulation. *Monoamines* are longer-acting neurotransmitters that actually modify the sensitivity of the neurons. When an imbalance in this complex system occurs, depression can result.

One of the ways the pituitary gland controls the secretions of hormones in the body is by balancing thyroid and adrenal hormones. This balance is often poorly regulated in those with mood disorders. Serotonin, estrogen, and progesterone imbalances may help explain the fact that women are more than twice as likely to develop depression. Investigators have also found that the biological rhythms of depressed persons differ from those of nondepressed persons. Depression is also related to physical illness. Many individuals who are being treated for a physical condition show signs of depression. As research efforts continue, new information about the biology of mood disorders will be uncovered.

Other Theories

Psychoanalytical theories state that mood disorders involve anger turned inward. *Behaviourists* view depression as a group of learned responses, whereas *social theorists* consider depression the result of faulty social interactions. A holistic viewpoint is usually used by health care providers because it considers all areas (realms) of human functioning and provides a framework from which to work with the whole person.

Many social factors have an influence on the development of mood disorders. Family relationships are important. Adults who were not nurtured as children are at a higher risk for depression. Losses, role changes, and physical illnesses all have an effect on the development of emotional difficulties. Poor social support, such as having few friends or no significant others, can heighten the loneliness of individuals. Repeated reactions to stress and crises wear down one's emotional resistance. Although the exact cause of depression and other mood disorders remains unclear, we do know that early recognition and treatment greatly improve the lives of people living with severe and prolonged emotional challenges.

EMOTIONS THROUGHOUT THE LIFE CYCLE

Emotional responses are a realm of human functioning. They develop and mature as the individual does. When we are young, emotions are often experienced but seldom controlled. Emotional control is slowly gained as we test and learn about the appropriateness of our emotionally expressive behaviours. By adulthood, most societies expect people to control their emotions and express them in appropriate ways. (See Box 15.2 for the characteristics of successful adults.)

Emotions in Childhood

When infants' basic needs are met, they feel a sense of contentment. Any delay in meeting those needs, however, is announced by verbal expressions of frustration or even anger. Toddlers struggle to cope with many newly experienced emotions, such as fear, helplessness, and anxiety. Many of these feelings are acted out because young children are often unable to express themselves verbally. School-age children learn to identify, express, and control their emotions. The emotional intensity of adolescence offers new challenges for learning emotional control.

Most depressive responses in children are tied to a specific event or situation. This type of depression is called *acute depression* or **situational depression** because it can be traced to a recognizable cause. Once the stressors are removed or decreased, the depression is expected to subside unless there are other factors creating stress. Situational depression occurs in all age groups.

Children who are depressed have a distinct way of thinking. Depression involves feelings of hopelessness, low self-esteem, and a tendency to take the blame for every negative event (Hockenberry & Wilson, 2014). They often respond with irritability, tearfulness, and sadness. Schoolwork and friendships suffer as increasing amounts of time are spent alone, especially watching television. Some children become clinging and dependent. Others engage in aggressive or disruptive behaviours. Many show changes in eating and sleeping behaviours. Fortunately, most acute episodes of childhood depression fade with family and social support.

A disruptive mood regulation disorder may be diagnosed in children who are persistently irritable and have frequent episodes of out-of-control, disruptive behaviours. These temper outbursts are usually in response to frustration. They occur both at home and school and may happen several times a week. Between outbursts, these children are chronically angry, irritable, and sullen.

During childhood, individuals begin to establish their self-esteem, coping mechanisms, and problem-solving abilities. If they have been successful in developing these skills, they are well prepared to handle the emotional distresses of later life. If self-esteem fails to grow or coping mechanisms and problem-solving abilities fail to develop, a mood disorder or other mental health issues may arise. The incidence of depression in childhood is increasing, thus health care providers should include an assessment of mood for all young patients.

Emotions in Adolescence

During the teen years, individuals struggle to identify, gain control over, and express emotions. The moods of adolescents commonly swing from feeling vulnerable and dependent to knowing that they are the smartest one in the family. Most adolescents establish their personal and social identities without significant psychological difficulties or emotional disorders. However, as stated earlier, a growing number of teens are showing evidence of depression.

Depression in adolescence is usually related to four factors: self-esteem, loneliness, family strengths, and parent–teen communication. While age and gender are lesser factors, adolescent girls and women with depression outnumber their male counterparts by two to one. Many individuals tend to react with a sense of helplessness and feelings of depression when self-esteem is low. They perceive the world as bleak and themselves as small and insignificant. Feelings of a poor self-image feed other negative emotions. A cycle of depression and low self-esteem is established. Grades drop as interest in school activities fades.

Loneliness is an aspect of depression in all age groups, but especially in adolescence. People need other people. As loneliness increases, so does depression. The emotionally isolated teen may be surrounded by others yet still feel emotionally alone.

Family relationships also have an influence on adolescent depression. Studies of mothers of depressed adolescents revealed that higher standards of achievement were expected, but the children were seldom rewarded. Often adolescents rebel against what they feel are impossible standards by withdrawing into depression.

Parent–adolescent communication patterns also have an influence on the teen's ability or willingness to discuss problems. Teens who can discuss their concerns with understanding parents have lower rates of depression.

The occurrence of depression and other mood disorders in adolescence reaches across gender and cultural lines. Teen depression must be recognized as serious. Depressions arising during adolescence tend to last, have a high rate of recurrence, and are associated with long-standing interpersonal problems. Teaching adolescents to cope effectively is essential if we are to protect the mental health of our greatest natural resource, our children.

Emotions in Adulthood

During adulthood, society expects people to practise emotional control. Unfortunately, some adults have difficulties with emotional control because of mood disorders or other issues: 5.2% of Canadians suffer from a mood disorder, and 4.7% from an anxiety disorder (Meng & D'Arcy, 2012). There are some common risk factors for mood and anxiety disorders, as well as some specific risk factors for specific mood disorders. The higher the number of risk factors, the higher the probability for disease (Box 21.2).

Adults must cope with a wide range of situations, events, developmental tasks, and responsibilities, as well as the emotional reactions that accompany each. Family interactions have a strong influence on adults. Many are also challenged with the problems of physical illness or dysfunction. Sometimes the practice of certain behaviours, such as medication use, dieting, or refusal to seek help for distressing symptoms, can result in the development of a mood disorder. Unfortunately, the public (and patients themselves) still stigmatizes people with mood disorders. These disorders are often seen as being caused by a lack of willpower or as a character flaw. Thus adults with depression or bipolar disorder must endure the additional burden of being stereotyped as "mentally ill." Being sensitive to this issue can assist health care providers in providing support for adults living with emotional difficulties.

Emotions in Older Persons

Depression is common in older people. The highest rates are found among older women, medically ill persons, and individuals who receive long-term care.

Depression is not a normal consequence of aging. Most older persons live full, active, and rewarding lives. When depression or another mood disturbance occurs *suddenly* in an older person, it is most likely linked to a physical cause. Depression can be treated, but a failure to recognize its symptoms prevents many elders from receiving therapy.

Older persons often express their feelings of depression in more subtle ways than younger persons do. Most do not complain or volunteer to share their feelings. Signals of depression in the older population include changes in daily routine, eating, sleeping, or activity patterns; decreased concentration, communications, and motivation; feelings of envy, failure, indecision, guilt, and hopelessness; loss of interest, self-confidence, and self-esteem; and worry or talk about death. Active listening, gentle questioning, and alert assessments can help nurses detect signs of depression in older persons.

Characteristics of Mood Disorders

Affect is the outward expression of one's emotions. Affects can be described as blunted (restricted), flat, inappropriate to the situation, and labile (rapidly changing) or euthymic (stable). A **mood disorder** is defined as a disturbance in the emotional dimension of human functioning. Mood disorders have also been called **affective disorders**. Problems with emotions occur when one is extremely happy or sad outside of any correlation with reality. We all experience emotional extremes, but when feelings interfere with effective living, they become maladaptive.

Difficulties with emotions range from manic episodes (mania) to depression. A **manic episode** refers to an emotional state in which a person has an elevated, expansive, and sometimes irritable mood accompanied by a loss of identity, increased activity, and grandiose thoughts and actions unsupported by reality. **Depression**, the opposite of mania, is characterized by feelings of sadness, disappointment, and despair. It is an illness that affects more than 10% of the adult population. Depression occurs in all ethnic groups, in all age groups, and at all socioeconomic levels. It affects twice as many women as men. Depression and other mood disorders are some of the most common mental health challenges occurring today.

DEPRESSIVE DISORDERS

Characteristics that are common to all depressive disorders are sadness and emptiness or irritability, accompanied by physical and cognitive challenges that severely impact an individual's ability to function. However, there are differences in the duration, timing, and etiology of these disorders.

Disruptive Mood Dysregulation Disorder

The main features of disruptive mood dysregulation disorder are onset before age 10; the disorder is chronic; severe outbursts and aggression (verbal, physical, or both) occur at least three times a week and in at least in two different settings (e.g., home and school); and irritable mood occurs every day and for most of the day (even without outbursts). The diagnosis applies to the age range of 7 to 18 years. This is the common

---

BOX 21.2   Common Risk Factors That Predispose Canadians for Mood or Anxiety Disorders

- Being young
- Having a low household income
- Being unmarried
- Experiencing a great deal of stress
- Having poor mental health
- Living with a medical condition

Unique Risk Factors

- Experiencing a major depressive episode and social phobia
- Experiencing panic disorder
- Having lower education (associated with panic and agoraphobia)
- Having poor physical health (associated with mania and agoraphobia)

Data from Meng, X., & D'Arcy, C. (2012). Common and unique risk factors and comorbidity for 12-month mood and anxiety disorders among Canadians. *Canadian Journal of Psychiatry, 57*(8), 479–487.

diagnosis for inpatient children and adolescents in mental health units. The majority of these patients are male.

Major Depressive Disorder

The main symptoms of depression are as follows, and must include one of the first two symptoms:

1. Feelings (that a person may report) or observation of sadness, emptiness, hopelessness (in children, this can be irritability)
2. Loss of interest or pleasure (reported by person or observed)
3. Significant weight loss, weight gain, or change in appetite almost every day
4. Insomnia or hypersomnia almost every day
5. Psychomotor agitation or retardation almost every day
6. Fatigue or loss of energy almost every day
7. Feeling of worthlessness or guilt almost every day
8. Decreased ability to think or concentrate, or indecisiveness, almost every day
9. Recurrent thoughts of death, recurrent suicidal ideation with or without a plan

When a combination of these symptoms (including one of the first two symptoms) presents for at least 2 weeks and causes significant distress and impairment, it is called a **major depressive episode (MDE)**. The diagnostic criteria depend on number of episodes (single versus recurrent), level of severity, presence of psychosis, and existence of remission (at least 2 months with no significant symptoms).

Depression is a "whole body" illness that involves emotional, physical, intellectual, and social challenges. It is a common and treatable mental disorder. Box 21.3 lists many of the behaviours associated with depression. A patient's nonverbal messages may be the only clues to the presence of this disabling disorder.

Major depressive disorder occurs twice as often in adolescent girls and adult women as it does in men. Symptoms may begin at any age, but the average age of symptom onset is

in the early 20s. The course of the disorder is variable. Some individuals experience depressive episodes that are separated by many years, whereas others suffer more frequent episodes as they grow older. Some people never have a remission, and some have many years between MDEs. People with a chronic pattern usually have an underlying personality disorder, anxiety disorder, or substance use disorder.

A substantial number of individuals who suffer first from MDE (even a few times) are later diagnosed as having a bipolar disorder. These individuals typically have an MDE diagnosed in adolescence with psychotic features and come from families with a history of bipolar disorder.

Suicidal risk exists at all times during an MDE. The major risk factors are the history of attempts, threats of suicide, or both.

Families that have one depressed family member are at an increased risk for other members also developing the disorder. Some families appear to be genetically vulnerable to depression.

Major Depressive Disorder With Specifiers

There are a few different specifiers that may characterize an MDE:

- **Anxious distress**: Individuals who suffer from MDE with this specifier have anxiety as a prominent part of their MDE. This feature is associated with a higher level for suicidal risk, longer duration of the depressive episode, and poor response to a treatment.
- **Mixed features**: Individuals who suffer from MDE with this specifier also have manic/hypomanic symptoms during their MDE. These patients are at a higher risk for developing bipolar I or bipolar II disorder.
- **Melancholic features**: The main characteristic of this specifier is full absence (not just reduction) of any pleasure during the MDE, even from the event most desirable

---

BOX 21.3 Behaviours Associated With Depression

Emotional	Physical	Intellectual	Behavioural
Anger	Abdominal pain	Ambivalence	Aggressiveness
Anhedonia	Anergia	Confusion	Agitation
Anxiety	Anorexia or overeating	Inability to concentrate	Alcoholism
Apathy	Backache	Indecisiveness	Altered activity level
Bitterness	Chest pain	Loss of interest and	Drug addiction
Dejection	Constipation	motivation	Intolerance
Denial of feelings	Dizziness	Pessimism	Irritability
Despondency	Fatigue	Self-blame	Lack of spontaneity
Guilt	Headache	Self-depreciation	Overdependency
Helplessness	Impotence	Self-destructive thoughts	Poor personal hygiene
Hopelessness	Indigestion or nausea	Uncertainty	Psychomotor retardation
Loneliness	Insomnia		Social isolation
Low self-esteem	Lassitude		Tearfulness
Sadness	Menstrual changes		Underachievement
Sense of personal	Sexual nonresponsiveness		Withdrawal
worthlessness	Sleep disturbances		
	Vomiting		
	Weight change		

Data from Stuart, G. W. (2013). *Principles and practice of psychiatric nursing* (10th ed.). Mosby.

for the individual. Patients who suffer from this specifier are more likely to be found in an inpatient setting than an outpatient setting. They are also more likely to have a psychotic feature (see below).

- *Atypical features*: The atypical characteristic of these patients with MDE is their mood capacity to react or even be cheerful as a reaction to a positive event. They may have an increased appetite and hypersomnia.
- *Psychotic features*: The main characteristic of this specifier is the presence of delusions, hallucinations, or both. These psychotic features can be *mood-congruent* (the content of delusions or hallucinations is consistent with patient's mood) or *mood-incongruent* (the content of delusions or hallucinations is not consistent with the patient's mood themes).
- *Catatonia features*: The main characteristic of this specifier is the presence of catatonia symptoms during most of the MDE.

The diagnosis of **postpartum depression** does not exist as a stand-alone diagnosis in the *Diagnostic and Statistical Manual of Mental Disorders*, fifth edition (*DSM-5*; American Psychiatric Association [APA], 2013). Instead, in recognition of the fact that 3 to 6% of women will experience the onset of an MDE before or after delivery (50% will develop it prior to delivery), the *DSM-5* offers a specification for this type of MDE as being "with peripartum onset" if the onset happens during the pregnancy or within 4 weeks after delivery (APA, 2013). When a woman has been diagnosed with *MDE with peripartum onset,* the risk of a similar diagnosis for the subsequent delivery is 30 to 50%. It is important for clinicians to remember that women may experience a mixed episode of MDE and obsessive-compulsive disorder (OCD) during the peripartum period, accompanied by intrusive thoughts of hurting themselves, their infants, or both. Thus, proper patient and family education regarding postpartum depression is important (Segre & Davis, 2013).

There is no unique diagnosis of **seasonal affective disorder (SAD)** in the *DSM-5*. However, the *DSM-5* recognizes the condition in which MDEs occur from fall to spring with a full recovery. When this has happened to an individual for the last 2 years, major depressive disorder "with seasonal pattern" specifier is diagnosed (APA, 2013). Usually, this MDE is characterized by notable energy, overeating and weight gain, and hypersomnia. SAD can vary in severity. Some individuals may have a subsyndromal S-SAD, also known as "winter blues." SAD occurs four times more often in women then in men. Those who live farthest from the equator in northern latitudes are most susceptible. For example, in Canada 15% of the population experiences winter blues and 2 to 6% experience SAD; in the United States, 1% of those who live in Florida and 9% who live in Alaska experience SAD; in the United Kingdom, 20% experience winter blues and 2% experience SAD (Melrose, 2015).

Persistent Depressive Disorder (Dysthymia)

Individuals diagnosed with persistent depressive disorder (**dysthymia**) have a depressed mood for most of the day,

for the majority of days and for at least 2 years (or 1 year for children and adolescents). The distress caused by persistent depressive disorder leads to impairment in a person's functions. Two of the following criteria must also exist for a diagnosis of this disorder:

1. Poor appetite or overeating
2. Insomnia or hypersomnia
3. Low energy or fatigue
4. Low self-esteem
5. Poor concentration or difficulty making decisions
6. Feeling of hopelessness

The symptoms of persistent depressive disorders resemble those of major depressive disorder, but they are not the same. Thus, if at any time a person's symptoms match those for major depressive disorder, then the person's diagnosis would be changed to major depressive disorder.

With dysthymia, because the feelings of depression have lasted so long, they become a part of everyday experiences for individuals who have them. Feelings of hopelessness become a part of daily life. Individuals with dysthymia have learned to see the world from a negative point of view and will often tell you that they have always been this way.

Dysthymic disorders can begin in childhood or as late as early adulthood. Because they develop slowly, dysthymic disorders are often difficult to recognize and diagnose. Persons with dysthymia can often carry out their daily living activities, but they are seldom able to enjoy them.

Premenstrual Dysphoric Disorder

Depressive, distressing emotions and behaviours linked to the menstrual cycle are the hallmark of premenstrual dysphoric disorder. Symptoms usually begin during the week before menses, reach the peak around the time of the onset of menses, rapidly improve during menses, and disappear within a week after menses.

Marked mood swings, sudden sadness, crying, irritability, anger, and feelings of tension all emerge. Physical symptoms, such as weight gain, breast tenderness, joint pain, and feelings of being "bloated," often add to the discomfort.

Substance-/Medication-Induced Depressive Disorder

Individuals who suffer from substance-/medication-induced depressive disorder have symptoms of a depressive disorder (e.g., major depressive disorder) and evidence linking those symptoms to the consumption of some sort of substance, toxin, or medication. The condition causes significant distress, impairment, or both.

Depressive Disorder Due to Another Medical Condition

Individuals who suffer from depressive disorder due to another medical condition experience a significantly depressed mood or low interest in the majority of normal life activities, persistently, for a long period of time. These symptoms are directly related to the known effect of some general medical condition (e.g., stroke, Parkinson's, or Huntington's diseases).

Other Specified Depressive Disorder

Individuals who have a diagnosis of other-specified depressive disorder suffer from symptoms of a depressive disorder that causes them significant distress but does not meet the full criteria for any of the other disorders, and the clinician chooses to communicate the specific reason.

Unspecified Depressive Disorder

Individuals who have a diagnosis of unspecified depressive disorder suffer from symptoms of a depressive disorder that causes them significant distress but does not meet the full criteria for any of the other disorders, and the clinician chooses not to communicate the specific reason.

BIPOLAR AND RELATED DISORDERS

The hallmark of a **bipolar disorder** is sudden and dramatic shifts in emotional extremes. From the perspective of symptomatology, family history, and genetics, this group of disorders is a connection between depressive disorders and schizophrenia spectrum and other psychotic disorders.

Bipolar I Disorder

The main diagnostic feature of bipolar I disorder is a manic episode. The occurrence of at least one manic episode must be identified to diagnose bipolar I disorder. A depressive or hypomanic episode may occur before or after the manic episode.

Manic Episode

A manic episode represents a persistently elevated or irritable mood with increased energy and goal-directed activity that causes a significant impairment in functions (or the need for hospitalization to ensure safety) for at least 1 week. During that period, at least three of the following symptoms must be present:

1. Inflated self-esteem or grandiosity
2. Diminished need to sleep
3. Much more talkative than usual (amount and speed of speech)
4. Objective (noted by an observer) flight of ideas or subjective (self-reported) experience of racing thoughts
5. Easily distracted by attention to unimportant or irrelevant stimuli
6. Significant increase in goal-directed activity (social, work, sexual, sport) or psychomotor agitation (non–goal-directed activity)
7. Uncharacteristic overinvolvement in high-risk activities (e.g., unrealistic business ventures, unrestrained buying sprees, sexual indiscretion) that have a high potential for painful consequences

The mood during a manic episode is often described as euphoric, excessively cheerful, or "feeling on top of the world." This often leads to poor judgement. In other cases, especially when the person's demands for unreasonable activity is denied, the mood may become extremely irritable. When the changes from euphoria to dysphoria and irritability happen rapidly over a short period of time, this is called *lability*.

Some individuals may shift mood rapidly not only from euphoria to irritability, but also from euphoria to depression. The depressive symptoms may last for hours or (rarely) days. This type of manic episode or hypomanic episode is labelled *with mixed features*.

Some individuals may have at least four mood changes during a period of 12 months that meet the criteria for a manic, hypomanic, or major depressive episode. This condition is labelled *with rapid cycling*. Females are more likely than males to experience mixed features and rapid cycling.

The difference between the lack of a need in sleep during a manic episode versus insomnia is that during insomnia the person has a need to sleep, wants to sleep, but cannot sleep. In contrast, it is common that during a manic episode the person does not perceive that they need sleep or that they are ill and need help.

Hypomanic Episode

The characteristics of a **hypomanic episode** are that *this episode does not cause marked impairment in functions*, but an external observer can note a significant change in functioning that is not characteristic of the individual. Those changes must happen throughout at least 4 consecutive days. During that period, the individual must experience an elevated level of mood or irritability, increased energy or activity, and at least three of the following symptoms:

1. Inflated self-esteem or grandiosity
2. Decreased need for sleep (e.g., feeling rested after only a few hours of sleep)
3. Much more talkative than usual (amount and speed of speech)
4. Objective (noted by an observer) flight of ideas or subjective (self-reported) experience of racing thoughts
5. Easily distracted by attention to unimportant or irrelevant stimuli
6. Significant increase in goal-directed activity (social, work, sexual, sport) or psychomotor agitation (non–goal-directed activity)
7. Uncharacteristic overinvolvement in high-risk activities (e.g., unrealistic business ventures, unrestrained buying sprees, sexual indiscretion) that have a high potential for painful consequences

Note that if psychosis is also identified during that episode, then, by definition, it becomes a manic episode.

Major Depressive Episode

An MDE is diagnosed when there is a combination of the following symptoms (for which one of the first two symptoms *must* be present) for at least 2 weeks and these symptoms cause significant distress and impairment to an individual:

1. Observed or reported feelings of sadness, emptiness, hopelessness (in children, this can seem more like irritability)
2. Loss of interest or pleasure (reported or observed)
3. Significant weight loss or weight gain, or change in appetite almost every day
4. Insomnia or hypersomnia almost every day
5. Psychomotor agitation or retardation almost every day

6. Fatigue or loss of energy almost every day
7. Feeling of worthlessness or guilt almost every day
8. Decreased ability to think or concentrate, or indecisiveness almost every day
9. Recurrent thoughts of death, recurrent suicidal ideation with or without a plan

Suicidal risk for individuals with bipolar disorder is at least 15 times higher than it is for the general population. Approximately 25% of all completed suicides are carried out by individuals who have bipolar disorder. A past history of a suicidal attempt and occurrence of depression symptoms during the past year are main risk factors.

CASE STUDY

Kevin felt extraordinarily good—full of confidence and vigour. He even convinced himself that this would be his lucky day. By the time he started dressing, he had already decided to "skip" work. He was going to the casino because he could do no wrong today. Too impatient to eat or finish dressing, he bolted from the house and jogged the 10 km to the casino.

By noon, Kevin had lost his pocket money and had consumed four scotch and sodas. He became angry with the cashier when she refused to cash a cheque without identification. "She should certainly know who I am. Why should I need identification? Everyone in town knows who I am! How dare they demand to see my ID!" Kevin shouted as he paced agitatedly.

After being forcibly removed from the casino, Kevin began a tour of every business in town. He demanded to see the owners and then offered them a contract to share a portion of his winnings if they financed his gambling now. By the time he visited the fourth gambling establishment, the police were waiting.

Kevin made his offer to both police officers and was promptly admitted to the local hospital for mental health care.
- What clues (signs or symptoms) in Kevin's behaviour indicate that he was in the manic phase of bipolar illness?

Psychotic symptoms that are usually seen in both the manic and the depressive phase are delusions, perceptual abnormalities (hallucinations), and different thought-form disturbances (ranging from the tangential form to word salad).

Bipolar II Disorder

Bipolar II disorder is a condition in which at least one hypomanic episode and at least one MDE have been identified. Because a hypomanic episode typically does not cause any significant impairment in the person's functioning, the person usually comes for help during the MDE of this disorder. Individuals and even their families see no pathology in the hypomanic episode. Thus, taking a proper medical history is necessary to identify a hypomanic episode and diagnose the condition as bipolar II disorder.

Individuals who have bipolar I disorder actually experience more hypomanic episodes than do individuals with

bipolar II disorder. However, those with bipolar II disorder experience a significantly higher number of MDEs, and this is what makes bipolar II disorder so debilitating.

Suicidal risk is *higher for people who have bipolar II disorder*. The rate of attempts is similar between bipolar II disorder and bipolar I disorder; however, the lethality rate is higher with bipolar II disorder.

Cyclothymic Disorder

Some individuals have periods with hypomanic symptoms that do not meet the criteria for a hypomanic episode and periods with depressive symptoms that do not meet the criteria for an MDE. If these symptoms present for the greater part of the preceding 2 years (1 year for children or adolescents), these individuals are diagnosed as having a **cyclothymic disorder**.

Cyclothymic disorder is usually diagnosed during adolescence. Individuals with this diagnosis have a 15 to 50% risk of developing a bipolar II disorder or bipolar I disorder.

Substance-/Medical-Induced Bipolar and Related Disorder

Individuals with substance-/medical-induced bipolar and related disorder suffer from severe and persistent mood disturbances that clinically resemble bipolar and related disorders, but there is evidence that the disturbances are the result of substance intoxication or withdrawal. Examples of substances that can cause this disorder are cocaine, alcohol, and amphetamines.

Bipolar and Related Disorder Due to Another Medical Condition

Individuals with bipolar and related disorder due to another medical condition suffer from severe and persistent mood disturbances that clinically resemble bipolar and related disorders, but there is evidence that these disturbances are the result of another medical condition (e.g., lupus erythematosus, stroke).

Other Specified Bipolar and Related Disorder

Individuals diagnosed with other specified bipolar and related disorder suffer from symptoms of bipolar and related disorders that cause them significant distress but do not meet the full criteria for any of the above disorders and a clinician chooses to communicate the specific reason.

Unspecified Bipolar and Related Disorder

Individuals with a diagnosis of unspecific bipolar and related disorder suffer from symptoms of bipolar and related disorders that cause them significant distress but do not meet the full criteria for any of the above disorders and a clinician chooses not to communicate the specific reason.

THERAPEUTIC INTERVENTIONS

Mood disorders present many treatment challenges. Perhaps the greatest challenge is that fewer than one half of the people with mood disorders receive any help for living with the disorder. Feelings of hopelessness and the stigma of having a mental illness prevent many people from seeking treatment. Others are misdiagnosed or treated for a medical illness because their symptoms are mainly physical.

Treatment and Therapy

The therapeutic plan for patients with mood disorders is divided into three phases. The *acute treatment phase* lasts 6 to 12 weeks. The goal during this phase is to reduce symptoms and inappropriate behaviours. Inpatient hospitalization may be required when patients are too impaired to continue with the activities of daily living or too suicidal to be left alone.

The goal of the *continuation phase* is to prevent relapses into distressing emotional states. This period usually lasts 4 to 9 months and treatment is given on an outpatient basis. Medications and psychotherapy are continued. Patients are educated about the nature of their conditions and their medications and are encouraged to try new coping behaviours.

The *maintenance treatment phase* concentrates on preventing recurrences in patients with prior episodes of depression or mania. Maintenance psychotherapy and medication treatment help prevent new episodes or recurrences (Table 21.1).

Current standard treatments for mood disorders include psychotherapy, pharmacological therapy, electroconvulsive therapy (ECT), transcranial direct current stimulation (tDCS), and repetitive transcranial magnetic stimulation (rTMS). Medication-free treatments for depression include exercise combined with group therapy, and the use of omega-3 fatty acids (UCLA Division of Geriatrics, 2015). Meditation and relaxation exercises have been shown to be helpful for alleviating depression.

During each phase of treatment, nurses and other health care providers play important roles because they are the ones who help teach, encourage, and guide patients toward living effectively with their disorders.

Psychotherapies

Various psychotherapies are effective in treating mild and moderate depression. Cognitive-behavioural therapy (CBT) is used to help patients identify and correct self-defeating thoughts and actions that keep self-esteem low. Interpersonal therapy assists patients with relationships and interactions, and psychodynamic therapy encourages the growth of personal insight. Support groups and organizations are also helpful for patients and families coping with mood disorders.

Electroconvulsive Therapy

Electroconvulsive therapy (ECT) involves the introduction of a controlled grand mal seizure by passing an electrical current through the brain while the patient is under general anaesthesia. ECT is used only in patients with severe, long-lasting depression after attempts to stabilize the depression with various medications and therapies have failed.

Each ECT treatment requires about 15 minutes, but the actual shock lasts for only a few seconds. Generally, 6 to 12 treatments are administered over a course of several weeks. Most individuals receive ECT two or three times per week.

ECT is not prescribed for patients who have had a recent myocardial infarction (heart attack) or who have heart disease, high or low blood pressure, stroke, heart failure, or increased intracranial pressure. The treatment slows heart rate and lowers blood pressure. This is followed by a reflex rise in heart rate and blood pressure. Each patient is evaluated for ECT on an individual basis, and the benefits must outweigh the risks before treatment is prescribed.

ECT is administered on an outpatient or inpatient basis. The preparation of the patient includes physical and emotional care, as well as education about the expected side effects of ECT. Consent forms need to be signed, and the patient is reminded that confusion and memory loss are common after treatment. Outpatient patients must be accompanied by a responsible adult to care for them following treatment.

Patients must eat nothing for at least 8 hours before treatment. Baseline vital signs are obtained. Cardiac, blood pressure, and oxygen monitoring begins. Sedatives and an anaesthetic drug are administered intravenously to alleviate pain, followed by short-acting muscle relaxants that help to prevent muscle and bone damage. The anaesthesiologist ensures proper lung ventilation during this short period of time.

Electroencephalogram (EEG) monitors and electrodes are positioned at certain points on the head by the physician. An airway is established, and an electrical shock, resulting in a controlled seizure of about 30 to 60 seconds, is delivered. The muscle relaxation drug often limits evidence of a seizure to only a flexing of the patient's great toes. Brain waves are monitored throughout the procedure and register the true duration of EEG impact on the brain. The patient sleeps for about 1 hour after the treatment.

Common side effects of ECT include headache, confusion on awakening from the treatment, and short-term amnesia, but the patient's mood improves rapidly. Many individuals can be managed on an outpatient basis with good postprocedure nursing management and appropriate patient teaching. The responsibilities of the nurse when working with patients undergoing ECT include initiating intravenous therapy, administering prescribed medications, and monitoring the patient's responses before, during, and after treatment.

TABLE 21.1	Phases of Treatment for Depression	
Phase	**Time Period**	**Goal of Treatment**
Acute treatment	6–12 wk	To reduce symptoms and inappropriate behaviours
Continuation	4–9 mo	To prevent relapses into distressing emotional states
Maintenance	Indefinite	To prevent recurrences

Transcranial Direct Current Stimulation

Transcranial direct current stimulation (tDCS) involves the use of a mild electrical current to stimulate the brain. Electrodes are placed on the patient's scalp and a weak current is delivered for 20 to 30 minutes per session. No anaesthesia or sedation is required. Sessions occur several times a week for several months. Although still in the experimental stage, studies have shown encouraging results with improvement in depressive symptoms, memory, and attention. According to Sabella (2014), "there is cautious optimism among researchers regarding its viability as a treatment for depression."

Repetitive Transcranial Magnetic Stimulation

Repetitive transcranial magnetic stimulation (rTMS) uses high-power short impulses to stimulate a particular area of the brain. Similar to tDCS, rTMS requires no anaesthesia. rTMS consists of around 40 minutes of treatment a few sessions per week for 4 to 6 weeks. The main difference between tDCS and rTMS is that tDCS uses a low-power current to tune brain function, whereas rTMS uses high power to activate the brain at each impulse. rTMS is approved for use in Canada and the United States to treat major depressive disorder; tDCS is still in the research phase and not yet approved for use.

Medication Therapies

Medications are a mainstay in the treatment of mood disorders. However, their use must be carefully assessed, monitored, and evaluated. These medications have many adverse effects and the potential for misuse. The most commonly used medications for treating mood disorders are antidepressants and mood-stabilizing medications known as *antimanics*. All of them work to increase neurotransmitter levels in the body and improve neuron capacity for neuroplasticity, which leads to improvement of depression.

Antidepressants

Antidepressants and mood-stabilizing medications are classified on the basis of their chemical composition. Each group alters a part of the brain's neurochemical balance. New medications for treating mood disorders are frequently being introduced. It is the responsibility of care providers to be familiar with each of their patients' medications.

Many antidepressants require 2 to 4 weeks' adherence before their effects are noted and the patient's well-being improves. For this reason, some patients believe that antidepressants are ineffective. They require education and reminders that these medications require time to take effect and encouragement to continue taking their medications. Box 21.4 lists examples of various antidepressant and mood-stabilizing medications.

Tricyclic antidepressants were once the first choice for the treatment of depression. The selective serotonin reuptake inhibitors (SSRIs) and related medications are now more often prescribed because of their low incidence of adverse effects. The last choices are the monoamine oxidase inhibitors (MAOIs) because of their severe and potentially fatal adverse effects. New antidepressants that are chemically unrelated to the other classes are routinely being marketed. Nurses who

---

BOX 21.4 Antidepressants and Mood-Stabilizing Medications

Tricyclic Antidepressants (TCAs)
amitriptyline (Elavil)
clomipramine (Anafranil)
desipramine (Norpramin)
imipramine (Tofranil)
maprotiline (Ludiomil)
nortriptyline (Aventyl)

Monoamine Oxidase Inhibitors (MAOIs)
isocarboxazid (Marplan)
tranylcypromine (Parnate)
phenelzine (Nardil)
selegiline (Eldepryl)

Selective Serotonin Reuptake Inhibitors (SSRIs)
citalopram (Celexa)
fluoxetine (Prozac)
paroxetine (Paxil)
escitalopram (Lexapro)
fluvoxamine (Luvox)
sertraline (Zoloft)

Serotonin-Norepinephrine Reuptake Inhibitors (SNRIs)
desvenlafaxine (Pristiq)
levomilnacipran (Fetzima)
duloxetine (Cymbalta)
venlafaxine (Effexor)

Serotonin Modulators and Stimulators (SMSs)
vilazodone (Viibryd)
vortioxetine (Trintellix)

Serotonin Antagonists and Reuptake Inhibitors (SARIs)
trazodone (Desyrel)

Norepinephrine Reuptake Inhibitors (NRIs)
reboxetine (Edronax)

Tetracyclic Antidepressants (TeCAs)
amoxapine (Asendin)
mirtazapine (Remeron)
maprotiline (Ludiomil)

Norepinephrine-Dopamine Reuptake Inhibitors (NDRIs)
bupropion (Wellbutrin, Zyban)

Mineral Mood-Stabilizing Medications
lithium carbonate (Carbolith)

Anticonvulsant Mood-Stabilizing Medications
carbamazepine (Tegretol)
lamotrigine (Lamictal)
oxcarbazepine (Trileptal)
valproic acid (Divalproex, Epival, Depaken)

Antipsychotic Mood-Stabilizing Medications
olanzapine (Zyprexa)
aripiprazole (Abilify)
ziprasidone (Zeldox)
quetiapine (Seroquel)
asenapine (Saphris)

---

administer these chemicals are responsible for maintaining current knowledge about their uses and effects.

Tricyclic antidepressants can produce severe central nervous system (CNS) depression when they interact with barbiturates, certain anticonvulsants, drugs, and alcohol. SSRIs act specifically to prevent the uptake of the neurochemical serotonin. They have fewer adverse effects than the tricyclics. Headache, nausea, nervousness, and insomnia are the most common adverse effects.

When MAOI antidepressants are combined with certain substances and foods containing the enzyme tyramine, the nervous system can become overexcited. This can lead to severely elevated blood pressure levels and hypertensive crisis. Refer back to Chapter 7 for a review of antidepressants, diet restrictions, and

TABLE 21.2 Adverse Effects of Antidepressants and Associated Nursing Care

Adverse Effects	Nursing Care
Tricyclic Antidepressants (TCAs)	
Fatigue, sedation, slow psychomotor reactions, poor concentration, tremors, ataxia	Give at bedtime; increase dose slowly; teach caution when using machinery; write instructions; document behaviours
Suicidal gestures	Institute suicide precautions; medication increases energy for suicide
Anticholinergic effects: dry mouth, decreased tearing, blurred vision (common)	Encourage frequent oral care, water, gum; use artificial tears; ensure that vision clears in 2 weeks; report eye pain immediately
Constipation, urinary hesitancy or retention, excessive sweating	Monitor food and fluid intake; promote high-fibre diet (more than 30 mg/day); encourage water intake of at least 2 500 mL/day; teach importance of adequate fluids, clothing, and sensible exercise; avoid hot showers, baths, dehydration; monitor urinary output, especially in older men
Selective Serotonin Reuptake Inhibitors (SSRIs)	
Dry mouth	Encourage fluids, good oral care
Nausea, diarrhea	Give medications with meals; maintain bland diet; encourage good hydration; administer lower dose
Drowsiness, dizziness, nervousness	Give at bedtime; keep active during day; institute safety precautions; instruct patient to avoid operating machinery
Sweating	Maintain good hygiene; wear cotton clothing; encourage fluids
Headaches	Teach relaxation techniques; administer mild analgesic for headache
Insomnia	Give medications early; encourage good sleep habits and relaxation
Serotonin-Norepinephrine Reuptake Inhibitors (SNRIs)	
Increased blood pressure	Monitor vital signs; report to physician if blood pressure stays high; may reduce dose
Weakness, sweating, sleepiness, dry mouth, nausea, vomiting, constipation, anorexia, blurred vision, anxiety, tremors	Refer to nursing care for other medication classes of antidepressants
Other Antidepressants	
Dizziness, drowsiness, anxiety, confusion, tremors, weakness, dry mouth, nausea, diarrhea, increased appetite, paralytic ileus, urinary retention	Ensure safety; monitor mental status, moods, affect, level of consciousness, increased symptoms; weigh weekly; monitor for weight gain; encourage fluids to 2 500 mL/day; monitor intake and output
Orthostatic hypotension, tachycardia, palpitations	Teach patient to rise slowly; monitor and report vital signs
Monoamine Oxidase Inhibitors (MAOIs)	
Increased CNS stimulation	Reassure patient; monitor for psychosis, seizures, hypoactivity
Postural hypotension	Teach patient to rise slowly; assure patient that symptoms will decrease
Muscle twitching	Vitamin B_6 (300 mg/day) is helpful
Fluid retention, urinary hesitancy	Monitor intake and output; administer thiazide diuretics as ordered
Insomnia	Give last dose as early as possible; encourage relaxation in evening
Food–medication interaction with tyramine (common amino acid)	Avoid tyramine-rich foods; avoid medications with epinephrine or stimulants

CNS, central nervous system.

education for patients receiving MAOIs. Profound CNS depression or severe anticholinergic effects can also occur.

Older male patients receiving antidepressants should be observed for urinary retention, which can develop quickly. Adverse effects such as blurred vision and dry mouth can cause problems with adherence because individuals stop taking their medications as a result of these bothersome effects. Atypical and other antidepressants can achieve the same effect using different mechanisms of action.

Antidepressants can exert their unwelcome adverse effects on both the central and peripheral nervous systems. Therapeutic interventions are thus often needed to help patients adjust to their medications. Table 21.2 lists common adverse effects of antidepressants and related care to minimize them.

Because antidepressants often may alter liver and kidney functions, hepatic and renal studies should be obtained monthly. Nurses should review all laboratory results for

TABLE 21.3   Adverse Effects of Lithium and Associated Nursing Care

Adverse Effects	Nursing Care
Abdominal discomfort, nausea, soft stools, diarrhea	Give lithium with food or milk; reassure that signs and symptoms are temporary and should subside
Edema, especially feet	Reassure that signs and symptoms are temporary; check with physician about salt restriction
Hair loss, hypothyroidism	Obtain thyroid function tests; reassure that condition is temporary; if continues, notify physician, who may discontinue medication
Muscle weakness, fatigue	Provide reassurance; give more frequent divided doses per physician prescription
Polyuria (can progress to diabetes insipidus)	Provide reassurance; increased output is expected; monitor intake and output; report if output greater than 3 000 mL/24 hr
Thirst	Encourage patient to quench thirst but maintain stable fluid intake
Tremors	Provide reassurance; eliminate caffeine; give slow-release form per physician prescription
Weight gain	Provide reassurance that weight gain is common; moderately restrict calories; advise patient against restricting fluids or salt

each patient. Often blood levels of certain medications are measured to determine the amount of medication still in the system. Toxic antidepressant levels can result if patients are not carefully monitored. Headaches, palpitations, changes in levels of consciousness, and stiffness in the neck should be reported to the physician immediately because these are signs of serious adverse effects.

Antidepressants and Suicide Precautions

Many patients who are depressed experience suicidal ideation and consider suicide to be a way to stop their suffering. However, often the low energy and poor cognitive functioning that results from depression are actually a barrier to carrying out a suicide plan. Medical interventions, as well as ECT, tend to improve functional and cognitive capacity faster than they improve mood. Care providers may see the following changes in their patients: better appetite, resumption of proper grooming, and even socialization. However, the patient's mood (and therefore suffering) may still remain as low as before. External improvement may simply mask the patient's internal suffering and hide it from staff's attention. At the same time, the patient's capacity to *carry out* a suicide plan has improved dramatically. Therefore, care providers should be aware that in terms of suicide risk, this is the most dangerous period of time during treatment for depression.

Antimanics

Lithium is a naturally occurring salt that helps stabilize and control mood. Because lithium does not bind to body proteins (like many other medications do), it does not need to be metabolized by the liver. Lithium is distributed throughout the body fluids, where it competes with sodium. It is excreted by the kidneys more rapidly than sodium. Therefore, an important interaction between the level of lithium in the blood and common table salt exists.

When patients who are taking lithium ingest large amounts of salt, lithium levels usually drop because of rapid kidney excretion of lithium. The opposite is also true. When patients decrease their salt intake or lose salt through

sweating, diarrhea, or altered kidney function, lithium levels in the blood are likely to increase. Because the range between therapeutic response and toxic effects is very narrow, patients must be instructed to avoid changing their diet or activity habits abruptly.

The narrow therapeutic index of lithium also requires close observation of patient responses. If blood levels of the medication are too low, manic behaviour returns. If levels are too high, an uncomfortable and possibly life-threatening toxicity may result.

While the mechanism by which lithium affects thyroid function is complex and not fully understood, with use over time, lithium is known to decrease secretion of thyroid hormone.

Most adverse effects of lithium are directly related to dosage and blood serum levels (Table 21.3). Polyuria (large urinary output) and polydipsia (increased thirst) are frequently seen in people beginning lithium therapy. Unwanted gastrointestinal tract reactions include a metallic taste, dry mouth, thirst, nausea, diarrhea, a bloated feeling, and weight gain. Sleepiness, light-headedness, drowsiness, and a mild hand tremor are common during the first weeks of therapy.

Because the signs and symptoms of lithium toxicity are the same as the adverse effects during the first weeks of therapy, all care providers should be aware of patients' responses to their lithium therapy. Most adverse effects disappear or decrease to a tolerable level by the sixth week of treatment. If they continue, care providers must be alert for the possibility of early lithium toxicity.

Blood tests for thyroid and kidney function, in addition to lithium levels, need to be routinely performed. Therapeutic blood levels of lithium range from 0.6 to 1.2 mmol/L. Toxic reactions occur when lithium levels in the blood are greater than 1.5 mmol/L. Lithium toxicity can be life-threatening, and no specific antidote exists. Because of this, one of the nurse's most important responsibilities is to frequently assess each patient's response during treatment and monitor for signs and symptoms of toxicity. See Table 21.4 and review Chapter 7 for more information about patient care and education. Study the procedure for a prelithium workup. Be alert to the special educational needs of patients who require lithium.

TABLE 21.4 Signs and Symptoms of Lithium Toxicity

Level of Toxicity	Signs and Symptoms
Mild Toxicity Blood serum fluid levels 1.5 mmol/L	Apathy, sluggishness, drowsiness, and lethargy; diminished concentration; mild incoordination, muscle weakness, muscle twitches, coarse hand tremors
Moderate Toxicity Blood serum levels 1.5–2.5 mmol/L	Nausea, vomiting, severe diarrhea; slurred speech, blurred vision, ringing in the ears; apathy, drowsiness, lethargy, moderate sluggishness; muscle weakness, irregular tremors, ataxia, frank muscle twitching, increased tonicity
Severe Toxicity Blood serum levels above 2.5 mmol/L	This is the life-threatening level. Nystagmus; irregular muscle tremors, fasciculations (twitches of single-muscle groups), hyperactive deep tendon reflexes; oliguria, decreased urine output, severe changes in level of consciousness, hallucinations; grand mal seizures, coma, death

Toxicity may set in rapidly unless the dose is reduced. Patients must be carefully monitored during the first weeks of lithium therapy. If little response is noted by the sixth week of treatment, the physician usually considers other mood-stabilizing medication therapies such as those listed in Box 21.4.

Nursing (Therapeutic) Process

Therapeutic care for patients with disturbances in mood focuses on the whole person. Patients are first assessed for the level of depression or mania. Next, a thorough history and physical examination are done to establish the database. Nursing diagnoses and therapeutic interventions are then chosen on the basis of the patient's most distressing symptoms (Box 21.5).

A holistic approach for patients with emotional challenges can be very effective. Therapeutic interventions for the *physical* realm focus on helping patients with personal hygiene, maintaining adequate nutrition, and encouraging physical activity. If patients are suicidal, special precautions and interventions are implemented.

In the *emotional* realm, care revolves around the therapeutic relationship. Acceptance and support are powerful tools in this area. Once trust is established, patients need encouragement and emotional support to cope with their problems.

Extreme emotional responses alter one's ability to think logically long enough to complete a task. In the *intellectual* realm of care, therefore, care providers should remember that these patients need extra patience. It is important to use gentle, nonjudgemental guidance when they are attempting to follow through on tasks. Give instructions slowly and clearly, and repeat them as needed. Do not become impatient. Remember, it is difficult to cope when one cannot think clearly.

Socially, most individuals with mood disorders are lonely and afraid of associating with others. Once medications have begun to stabilize the patient's moods, gentle encouragement to begin interacting with others is needed.

Manic patients commonly have delusions of **religiosity,** believing they have powers to communicate with God or

BOX 21.5 Nursing Diagnoses (Problem Statements) Related to Emotional Responses

Physical Realm
Ineffective coping
Risk for injury
Insomnia
Imbalanced nutrition
Self-care deficit—bathing/hygiene, dressing/grooming, feeding, toileting
Sexual dysfunction
Risk for self-directed violence

Psychosocial Realm
Anxiety
Impaired communication
Grieving and complicated grieving
Hopelessness
Risk for loneliness
Powerlessness
Disturbance in self-esteem
Social isolation
Disturbed thought processes

become a spirit. Therapeutic listening is a helpful intervention, but do not hesitate to contact a chaplain if the patient so requests.

Sample Patient Care Plan 21.1 offers a sample plan for patients with a mood disorder. Remember, each actual plan will be unique according to the needs of the individual patient.

Emotions, both positive and negative, add texture and meaning to the tapestry of our lives. While we may not yet understand the exact connections between mind and body, we do know that our emotions are determined in large part by the way we think, the way we perceive the world, and our self-talk. So powerful is an optimistic or pessimistic view that it determines not only our emotions but also the very condition of our physical and mental health. Thus, try to stay healthy by thinking positively. You and your patients will both benefit.

SAMPLE PATIENT CARE PLAN 21.1   Major Depressive Episode

Assessment

History Leanne is a 22-year-old woman with a diagnosis of major depressive episode after the loss of her infant son. Her childhood was uneventful, except for a domineering father. She reports no abuse during childhood but admits to being intimidated by her father's loud voice and gruff manner.

During her first year at university, she met and married Mark, a senior majoring in marketing. The first 10 months of the marriage went well, until Leanne discovered she was pregnant. The news of her pregnancy infuriated Mark, who insisted that she "do something." Leanne insisted on keeping the baby but was plagued by the guilt of adding an extra burden to Mark's load throughout the pregnancy. On May 10, she delivered a son.

Leanne's postpartum course was difficult. She was trying to care for her son, attend school, and appease her husband, who had become somewhat more interested in the baby. One morning she noticed that her son was too quiet. Attempts to revive him were unsuccessful, and the diagnosis of sudden infant death syndrome was made on autopsy. Three weeks later, Mark filed for divorce, stating that Leanne was not a "good mother."

Current Findings A dishevelled-appearing young woman with uncombed hair and wrinkled clothes. Speech is soft, almost inaudible. Does not maintain eye contact. Eyes red and swollen. Offers no information but when questioned admits to "being a complete loser" and "not worth the space I'm taking up." She describes her history as "filled with failures."

Multidisciplinary Diagnosis

Hopelessness related to loss of significant others as evidenced by an inability to perform activities of daily living

Planning/Goals

Leanne will use two effective coping methods to counteract her feelings of hopelessness by November 29.

Leanne will express three hopeful thoughts by December 15.

THERAPEUTIC INTERVENTIONS

Intervention	Rationale	Team Member
1. Assess risk for suicidal behaviours.	Suicide rates are high in depressed persons	Nsg, All
2. Establish a trustful and therapeutic relationship with Leanne to increase chances for her to ask for help before engaging in a suicide attempt.	Demonstrates caring and helps prevent suicidal gestures	Psy, Nsg
3. Assist with activities of daily living as needed.	Supports Leanne until she is able to care for herself	Nsg
4. Monitor fluid and food intake.	Depressed persons often do not eat or drink	Nsg, Diet
5. Use active listening to encourage her to identify and express feelings.	Gives her an opportunity to explore and vent her emotions realistically	All
6. Assess progress through the grief reaction and offer appropriate support.	Unresolved grief can cause depression; Leanne may not have grieved yet for the loss of her child	Psy, Nsg
7. Help her to focus on the positive aspects and support systems in her life.	When energies are positively focused, success is encouraged	All

Evaluation After 5 days on the unit, Leanne assumed self-care activities and appeared well groomed throughout the remainder of her stay. By December 1, Leanne was able to discuss her feelings with two staff members. On December 14, Leanne joined a support group for mothers who had lost children.

Critical Thinking Questions

1. What care provider behaviours can demonstrate to Leanne that she is not worthless?
2. How does the goal of "expressing hopeful thoughts" help Leanne cope with her current depression?

A complete patient care plan includes several other diagnoses and interventions.
Diet, dietitian; *Nsg*, nursing staff; *Psy*, psychologist.

KEY POINTS

- An emotion is a nonintellectual response in the affective realm of human functioning.
- A mood disorder is a disturbance in the emotional dimension of human functioning.
- Emotional responses grow and develop with the individual.
- Current evidence suggests that a combination of physical, psychological, and environmental factors is involved in the development of mood disorders.

- Depression is a "whole body" illness that involves emotional, physical, intellectual, social, and spiritual challenges.
- When depression is severe and lasts more than 2 weeks, it is called a major depressive episode.
- When major depressive episodes routinely repeat themselves (for more than 2 years), a depressive disorder is diagnosed.
- A dysthymic disorder is daily moderate depression that lasts longer than 2 years.

- Bipolar I disorder is characterized by episodes of depression alternating with episodes of mania.
- With bipolar II disorder, individuals experience major episodes of depression alternating with periods of hypomania.
- The therapeutic plan for patients with mood disorders is arranged into three phases: acute treatment phase, continuation phase, and maintenance phase.
- Various psychotherapies are effective in treating mild and moderate depression.

- The most commonly used medication classes for treating mood disorders are antidepressants and mood-stabilizing medications.
- Electroconvulsive therapy is used to relieve depression by inducing a controlled grand mal seizure by passing an electrical current through the brain.
- Transcranial direct current stimulation uses a mild electrical current to stimulate the brain.
- Therapeutic care for patients with disturbances in mood relates to each realm of functioning.

ADDITIONAL LEARNING RESOURCES

Go to your Evolve website (http://evolve.elsevier.com/Canada/Morrison-Valfre/) for additional online resources, including the online Study Guide for additional learning activities to help you master this chapter content.

CRITICAL THINKING QUESTIONS

1. What are the main differences in symptoms between bipolar I, bipolar II, or cyclothymic disorders?
2. What are the signs and symptoms of major depression?
3. Why is the risk for suicide increased upon initial improvement in a patient's condition, following their treatment for major depressive disorder with suicidal thoughts?

4. What are some challenges that patients who are taking lithium might experience?

REFERENCES

American Psychiatric Association (APA). (2013). *Diagnostic and statistical manual of mental disorders* (5th ed.). American Psychiatric Publishing.

Hockenberry, M., & Wilson, D. (2014). *Wong's nursing care of infants and children* (10th ed.). Mosby.

Melrose, S. (2015). NCBI. Seasonal affective disorder: An overview of assessment and treatment approaches. *Depression Research and Treatment, 2015,* 178564. https://doi.org/10.1155/2015/178564

Meng, X., & D'Arcy, C. (2012). Common and unique risk factors and comorbidity for 12-month mood and anxiety disorders among Canadians. *Canadian Journal of Psychiatry, 57*(8), 479–487. https://doi.org/10.1177/070674371205700806.

Rollant, P. D. (1998). *Mosby's review cards: Mental health nursing.* Mosby.

Sabella, D. (2014). Treating depression with transcranial direct current stimulation. *American Journal of Nursing, 114*(6), 66–70.

Segre, L. S., & Davis, W. N. (2013). Postpartum depression and perinatal mood disorders in the DSM. Postpartum Support International. https://www.postpartum.net/wp-content/uploads/2014/11/DSM-5-Summary-PSI.pdf

UCLA Division of Geriatrics. (2015). Drug free treatments for depression. *Healthy/Years, 12*(4), 4.

22

Physical Challenges, Psychological Sources

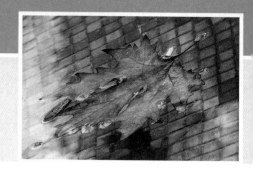

For centuries, humankind has questioned the interactions of mind and body and the roles that emotions play in health. In ancient China, around 2000 BCE, the emperor Huang Ti recorded his keen observations of the physical illnesses arising from emotional causes, in his book titled *Classic of Internal Medicine.* Hippocrates instructed people to care for the spirit as well as the body. Throughout the Middle Ages, magical and symbolic thinking kept body and mind inseparably linked. People whose behaviour or physical appearance differed were condemned as witches and workers of the devil.

Toward the end of the nineteenth century, scientific advances were made in biology, chemistry, and microbiology that shifted the focus of research to the cause and treatment of physical disease. By the time Freud's theories were introduced, the study of human beings had evolved into two distinct divisions: the biological (physical) and all other aspects of functioning (psychological).

In 1927, Dr. Julius Wagner-Jauregg was awarded the Nobel Prize in Medicine for his success with "pyrotherapy" in psychiatry (at that time, the terminology of "schizophrenia" was not yet being used). Dr. Wagner-Jauregg infected mentally ill patients who suffered from "general paresis of the insane" (GPI) with malaria; 15% of them died following that "treatment," but among the survivors were many with significant improvement in their symptoms (Lieberman, 2015). Their immune systems had gone through severe stress that allowed a dramatic recovery from schizophrenia for many of the patients. Today, we have enough evidence to connect at least some types of schizophrenia with malfunctions of the immune system.

Currently, researchers and practitioners alike know that no divisions between the mind and body exist; human beings are dynamic, complicated physical organisms that are affected by many nonphysical events. Each of us is a unique individual, a combination of genetics, culture, and experience. Each of us has psychological aspects to our being and our own way of coping with the stresses of life.

This chapter explores the connection between the physical and psychological aspects of people. It is an important chapter because patients with psychologically based physical symptoms are encountered in every practice setting. Health care providers who understand the role that emotions play in the development of health challenges are better able to assess patient needs and plan more effective care.

ROLE OF EMOTIONS IN HEALTH

Health is a concept embodying the whole person. It is a state of well-being in which the psychological realm is in balance with the physical realm. It is a state of **homeostasis**. All animals, including humans, must live with and adapt to stress. The antelope on the African savanna must deal with the stress of becoming some carnivore's lunch every day of its life. To do this, the antelope is equipped with a delicate internal mechanism of neurochemicals, all wired to the appropriate organs. When the animal is stressed, a response is activated and the antelope can run faster, jump higher, and endure the chase longer. In short, animals have evolved a stress response mechanism that protects them during times of threat or illness. It is called the fight-or-flight response, and it is an essential part of every animal's survival mechanisms.

ANXIETY AND STRESS

Human beings are also equipped with a **physiological stress response** mechanism. This biochemical fight-or-flight system is a biological survival tool designed to provide the energy to fight opponents or flee from the threat. The physical stress response served early humans effectively. However, as people became civilized and adopted rules for behaviour, fighting and running were replaced by more socially acceptable (but biochemically stifling) behaviours. Today the stressors of modern life are many, but outlets for the stress response are few.

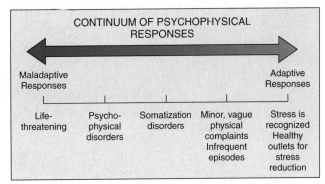

Fig. 22.1 Continuum of psychophysical responses.

In his book *Stress of Life*, Hans Selye "proposed that all humans show the same general bodily response to stress" (Craighead & Nemeroff, 2010). Selye studied the biochemical reactions of the stress response and their effects on various body systems; he called these reactions the **general adaptation syndrome** (Seyle, 1978). Today, it is known that stress activates primitive regions in the brain that also control eating, aggression, and immune responses. These responses to the stresses of modern life are biochemically identical to the responses that early humans experienced when fighting to stay alive. The problem today is that the fight-or-flight response occurs in non–life-threatening situations, stimulating the body for actions that never occur. The stress response mechanism can work overtime when people are routinely exposed to stressors.

When an individual perceives stress, tension, or anxiety, the body initiates a cascade of biochemicals (see Chapter 5, Fig. 5.2). The body's central command post, the hypothalamus, communicates to the pituitary gland, which in turn notifies the adrenal glands. The adrenal glands manufacture and release the body's four major stress hormones—dopamine, epinephrine, norepinephrine, and cortisol. Body functions are so responsive to these chemicals that even small changes in their levels can have a significant impact on one's state of health. Responses to stress exist along a continuum ranging from high-level adaptive responses to life-threatening disorders (Fig. 22.1).

Scientific investigations are discovering that the immune system is affected by stress levels. Several studies have demonstrated that significant immune function and blood pressure changes occur in people who display hostile or negative behaviours during periods of conflict. One study revealed that married couples who frequently argue had less effective immune systems. Other studies have demonstrated the importance of a positive attitude in physical healing.

Our psychological side has a strong influence on the ability to identify and successfully cope with stress. People who are able to recognize and defuse their stressors early on seldom experience the physical effects of stress. Others struggle with stressors and the body's response to them. For some individuals, stress affects body activities and functions, thus they develop physical challenges that arise from psychological sources. These challenges are called *somatic symptom disorders, psychosomatic illnesses,* **psychogenic** (i.e., nonorganic, functional) **disorders**, or *psychophysical disorders.*

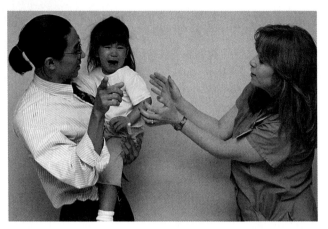

Fig. 22.2 The stress response is established early in childhood. (Courtesy T. C. Thompson Children's Hospital, Chattanooga, TN.)

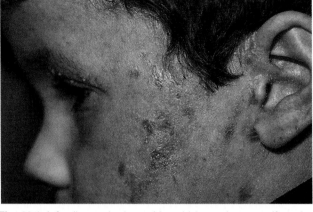

Fig. 22.3 Infantile atopic dermatitis, which can be a manifestation of stress. (Source: From Black, J. M., & Hawks, J. H. [2009]. *Medical surgical nursing: Clinical management for positive outcomes* [8th ed.]. Saunders.)

Childhood Sources

How an individual perceives and responds to stress is established in childhood (Fig. 22.2). The link between mind and body is made early in infancy. Infants require the routine attention of a consistent caregiver—someone who feeds, cuddles, and protects them. As children learn to cope with stresses, the brain becomes patterned. Biochemical reactions to stress alter the physical patterns of the brain and sensitize children to future stressors. This patterning sets up automatic chemical responses to stress. With each exposure to stress, the body responds with its biochemical program, even though the individual may not consciously feel stressed. Children who have experienced an unstable home environment, for example, may react to stress with exaggerated hormonal mechanisms as adults.

People experience stress according to their level of development. In infancy, mechanisms for coping with stress are limited. The only means of expression is through the body, so infants create physical signs and symptoms to help cope with their stresses. Conditions such as colic, atopic dermatitis, allergic reactions (Fig. 22.3), and obesity may all arise from the effects of stress.

Older children may express their stress by developing allergic skin reactions, asthma, gastrointestinal tract complaints, or joint aches and pains. Adolescents with anorexia or bulimia are coping with stress by gaining control over their bodies. Adults may express their stress through assorted physical symptoms or difficulties.

Families who emotionally support and encourage their children to effectively cope with their stresses tend to have fewer physical difficulties than do families filled with conflict and uncertainty, who often live with numerous physical challenges as well as psychological distress. Most psychosomatic issues and somatic symptom and related disorders (physical symptoms with emotional sources) start in childhood and become established during adolescence. By adulthood, individuals can be significantly impaired in their daily living activities because of their physical reactions to stress.

COMMON PSYCHOPHYSICAL CHALLENGES

The physical signs and symptoms of emotional distress are very real to the individual who is experiencing them. The discomfort of an upset stomach is the same, whether caused by too much pizza or a disturbing piece of news. The effects of emotionally caused illnesses are the same as those arising from physical sources.

When the body is under continual or repeated stress, it responds by overactivating its stress response mechanism, which can result in many physical signs and symptoms of an illness, disease, or disability. (Refer to the stress adaptation theory in Chapter 5.) In the past, these symptoms were often referred to as **psychosomatic illnesses**, meaning emotionally *(psycho)* related physical *(somatic)* disorders. Unfortunately, this term has come to mean an imaginary illness in popular vocabulary. The more recent term, **psychophysical disorders**, was coined to refer to stress-related physical symptoms. The physiological stress response affects many body systems (Box 22.1).

One of the systems that experiences much of the stress response is the gastrointestinal tract. Common stress-related symptoms include indigestion, vomiting, constipation, and diarrhea. Ulcerative colitis and gastric, peptic, and duodenal ulcers can also occur when the gastrointestinal tract is the focus of one's stress. The respiratory system can develop asthma, and the cardiac system can raise blood pressure when subjected to prolonged stress. Many mental health conditions, such as anxiety, are expressions of stress.

Theories of Psychophysical Disorders

Although we know that emotions play an important role in the development or prevention of illness, just how this connection works is uncertain. Several theories attempt to explain this relationship.

Biological theories include the stress response theory, which states that individuals are biochemically patterned to react to stress. During times of stress, the autonomic nervous system prepares the body for fight or flight. Because the threat is not

BOX 22.1   Physical Conditions Affected by Psychobiological Factors

Cardiovascular
Migraine headaches
Tension headaches
Hypertension (high blood pressure)
Angina (chest pain)

Musculoskeletal
Rheumatoid arthritis
Low back pain

Respiratory
Hyperventilation
Asthma

Gastrointestinal
Anorexia nervosa
Obesity
Peptic ulcer
Irritable bowel syndrome
Colitis

Skin
Neurodermatitis
Eczema
Psoriasis
Pruritus (itching)

Genitourinary
Impotence
Frigidity
Premenstrual syndrome

Endocrine System
Hyperthyroidism
Diabetes

From Stuart, G. W. (2013). *Principles and practice of psychiatric nursing* (10th ed.). Mosby.

external, no physical outlet for the biochemical response is usually possible. Consequently, nothing is done to relieve the conflict, and soon a cycle of biochemical stimulus–response is established. This pattern eventually results in physical disturbances within the body.

Carl Jung's *psychoanalytical theory* focuses on the symbolism attached to a symptom or illness. For example, the young executive who needs to vent his rage but feels that displays of anger are inappropriate may develop ulcerative colitis or high blood pressure as a way of coping with his anger.

Psychodynamic theories, such as Erich Fromm's theory, state that certain personality types are prone to developing certain illnesses. The hard-working, independent, overly ambitious executive is at high risk for the development of cardiac abnormalities because of his aggressive personality. The quiet, uncomplaining, overburdened clerk may suffer from ulcers, joint pain, or skin rashes.

Last is the *biological theory* of organic weakness, which states that every individual has one body system that is more

sensitive than other systems. When a person has underlying emotional challenges that affect functioning, the person may develop a physical illness as a means of coping with the unconscious issue.

Although these theories may appear unrelated, all of them have several concepts in common. First, unconscious emotional conflict that increases anxiety is the basis for many psychophysical difficulties. Second, the development of physical symptoms is the result of attempts to lower anxieties associated with conflict. Third, the illness is real to the person, regardless of whether organic changes exist. In some cases, physical changes can be life-threatening, so never treat a patient's complaints casually. Finally, the onset of the illness or condition is often related to a stressful event.

The physical signs and symptoms of an illness often relieve an individual's anxieties by masking inner emotional turmoil. This anxiety-reducing benefit is called **primary gain** because the symptoms reduce anxiety. There are other benefits, called **secondary gains**, to assuming the sick role. These include being relieved of responsibilities, receiving the special attention of others, and having dependency needs met. Most of the time, these gains tend to reinforce the pattern of psychophysical symptoms and encourage illness behaviours to continue.

SOMATIC SYMPTOM AND RELATED DISORDERS

The major common denominator for all patients with somatic symptom and related disorders is intense suffering and impairment resulting from somatic symptoms. Thus, the vast majority of these patient are found in medical/surgical departments and not mental health departments in the hospital. However, the main difference between these patients and patients who may suffer from similar somatic symptoms is that patients who have a **somatic symptom and related disorder** have an abnormal interpretation of and feelings about these somatic symptoms.

In the previous edition of the *Diagnostic and Statistical Manual of Mental Disorders (DSM-IV-R),* these disorders were called *somatoform disorders,* and there was an emphasis on the lack of medical explanations for these disorders. In the current edition, *DSM-5,* the focus is on the abnormal way in which patients perceive these somatic symptoms, rather than on the origin of those symptoms (American Psychiatric Association [APA], 2013). This is why the term *somatic symptom and related disorders* does not exclude the presence of a medical condition as being responsible for the somatic symptoms.

Most people formerly described as having hypochondriasis (which is also an old diagnosis from the *DSM-IV*) are now (based on the *DSM-5*) diagnosed as having a somatic symptom disorder, and the minority are diagnosed as having an illness anxiety disorder (APA, 2013).

Cultural Influences

Cultural differences are associated with certain illnesses, both physical and mental. Many somatic symptom disorders are

TABLE 22.1   Culturally Related Somatic Symptom Disorders

Cultural Group	Description
Japanese	*Gaman* means to internally suppress emotions, especially anger.
	Emotional distresses are expressed through physical signs or symptoms.
	Illness is a socially acceptable way of receiving care.
	Body functions are of concern, especially blood pressure.
	Headaches are related to depression.
Southeast Asian	Mental distress is not discussed but expressed via various physical ailments.
	Koro is fear of penis shrinking into abdomen, which results in death.
Latin American	*Mal ojo* (the evil eye) is associated with fever, headaches, diarrhea, restlessness, irritability, and weight loss.
East Indian (India)	*Dhat* syndrome consists of male reproductive signs and symptoms caused by fear and concern about losing semen.
Korean	The body is the property of the ancestors.
	Mental and emotional illnesses are expressed as physical (somatic) complaints.

culturally related, and their treatment depends on understanding the disorder within the patient's cultural context or framework (Table 22.1).

Health care providers who work with patients from different cultures must be aware of the meaning or importance that the illness holds for the person (Giger & Haddad, 2020). Many somatic illnesses are based in cultural or spiritual beliefs. Assessments and treatment plans must not threaten or challenge these beliefs if therapeutic interventions are to be effective. Culturally appropriate nursing interventions are based on knowledge of and respect for another's way of living (D'Avanzo, 2007). The effective health care provider does not hesitate to learn as much as possible about other cultures.

CULTURAL CONSIDERATIONS

Assessment of a patient's culture* should focus on the following:
- Biological variations
- Communications
- Cultural uniqueness
- Environmental control
- Social orientation
- Space
- Time

*See Figure 4.1 for a complete cultural assessment.

Somatic Symptom Disorder

A **somatic symptom disorder** is a condition in which a person's persistent symptoms suggest the presence of a medical illness for which no physical causes can be found (**somatization**) (APA, 2013). An individual can be diagnosed with somatic symptom disorder if for more than 6 months thoughts and/or feelings about a somatic concern impair major areas of their functions in at least one of the following abnormal ways:
1. Intense thoughts about the seriousness of the individual's condition
2. Intense anxiety/worry about this condition
3. Enormous and abnormal resources (time, finances, energy) assigned to this condition

It is important to stress here that for this diagnosis, it is not important whether or not the individual has any medical evidence for the somatic concern. What is really important is an authentic, excessive preoccupation with the concern and, as a result, impairment in daily life activities.

Typically, patient education about the seriousness of their symptom or symptoms does not help them, or it helps only for a very short time. An individual may assume that staff are not taking the symptoms seriously and thus lose trust in staff. This is why these patients may look for care from multiple care providers; all of these multiple treatments may only further aggravate their impairment. The disorder tends to affect females more than males.

⚠ MEDICATION ALERT

Nurses need to ask all patients if they are currently seeing any other health care providers, natural healers, or other practitioners.

Multiple medication use is common. Obtain a full medication/drug history from each patient, including the use of over-the-counter medications, home remedies, and herbs.

Illness Anxiety Disorder

Individuals who have an **illness anxiety disorder** have been preoccupied with worry/anxiety for at least 6 months about getting a serious illness. They may excessively seek medical attention and extra tests, or they may do the opposite and try to avoid medical checkups because of this intense worry that a serious illness will be discovered. Unlike with somatic symptom disorder, individuals who have an illness anxiety disorder may not suffer from any physical symptoms, or that suffering may be insignificant. The biggest function impairment with this disorder comes from the anxiety about getting a serious illness. An individual may change what illness they are afraid of contracting, but the anxiety remains constant.

As with somatic symptoms disorder, patient education and a real medical evaluation have no impact on the patient's beliefs and may only lead to a lack of trust in staff. Unlike somatic symptom disorder, the prevalence of illness anxiety disorder is similar for both males and females.

TABLE 22.2 Features of Somatic Symptom and Related Disorders

Disorder	Essential Features
Somatic symptom disorder	A history of intense focus (e.g., demands for excessive testing, soliciting multiple clinicians' opinions) on physical complaints, beginning before age 30 years, occurring over a period at least 6 months, and resulting in significant impairment in social or occupational functioning.
Illness anxiety disorder	Preoccupation with fears of acquiring a serious yet-undiagnosed disease, often without any somatic symptoms. The preoccupation persists despite appropriate medical evaluation and reassurance. It has existed for at least 6 months and causes clinically significant distress or impairment in functioning.
Conversion disorder	Symptoms or deficits affecting voluntary motor or sensory function. Psychological factors are often associated with the problem because the initiation or exacerbation of the symptom is preceded by conflicts or other stressors. The problem cannot be fully explained by a neurological or general medical condition and is not a culturally sanctioned behaviour or experience.
Factitious disorder	Somatic symptoms are unconsciously simulated on purpose to achieve some type of psychological (internal) gain (e.g., the caring from others when the sick role is assumed).
Malingering	Somatic symptoms are consciously simulated on purpose to achieve some type of tangible (external) gain (e.g., financial compensation, narcotic drugs, shelter, exemption from mandatory military service).

Conversion Disorder

The term *conversion* is derived from Freud's theory of conversion hysteria, which states that a psychosexual conflict is focused or converted into a physical disturbance. Today this is a relatively uncommon condition, called a **conversion disorder**. Individuals with a conversion disorder experience significant impairment in some aspect of their lives because of the breakdown in one or more of the voluntary or sensory body functions. At the same time, these individuals have no medical physiological mechanism explaining this breakdown (e.g., they experience blindness or paralysis or some other neurological symptom that cannot be explained by medical evaluation; laboratory and other diagnostic examinations show no specific abnormalities). In fact, it is the absence of diagnostic findings that helps to establish the diagnosis. It is important to note that these patients also do not fake these symptoms but really believe in them. (Individuals who intentionally fake symptoms will be discussed later under "Factitious Disorder" and "Malingering"; see also Table 22.2). Conversion disorder is also called *functional* or *psychogenic neurological symptom disorder.*

Conversion disorders appear more commonly in persons of lower socioeconomic status, those living in rural areas, and people with little health care knowledge. Approximately 1.2 to 11.5% of referrals to mental health clinics involve patients with conversion reactions (Psychology Wiki, 2020). When patients with conversion disorders are assessed, it is important to consider their social and cultural backgrounds.

Men and women differ in relation to conversion disorder: as many as 10 women for every 1 man are diagnosed as having conversion disorders. In men, conversion disorders are often associated with military service, industrial accidents, and antisocial personalities. The onset of problems is usually during late childhood through early adulthood, but almost always after 10 and before 35 years of age. There have been reports, however, of conversion reactions in persons in their 90s. Children usually present with gait problems or seizures.

In older individuals, the signs and symptoms usually appear as sensory or motor disturbances. Symptoms often appear suddenly, but they can also begin slowly and increase over time and typically last only a short time. In hospitalized patients, symptoms often disappear within 2 weeks. However, recurring episodes are common, and as many as 25% of patients have a return of symptoms within 1 year.

Conversion disorders are thought to be the result of an emotional (psychological) conflict. Situational factors, such as environmental stressors or interpersonal conflicts, can frequently trigger the appearance of conversion reactions.

Conversion signs and symptoms tend to be more in keeping with the individual's ideas of what the problems should be. For example, a "paralyzed" arm that is raised over the head by the care provider remains suspended for a moment, and then falls to the side rather than on its owner's head, or an extremity that is "paralyzed" moves automatically when the patient is not paying attention to it.

Conversion "seizures" vary in their activity. In short, the course of the signs and symptoms is not in keeping with physically based disease processes but rather with the patient's ideas about the seizures. Such seizures are *pseudo-seizures* or *psychogenic nonepileptic seizures (PNES)* and are very common. The main diagnostic differences from other seizures that can be immediately recognized by clinicians are that usually PNES patients have closed eyes and the ability to control their own body to avoid injury. With real grand mal seizures, the patient's eyes are open, and the patient typically cannot control their body. The treatment with short-term benzodiazepines can be helpful in both cases, as this group of medications has both antiepileptic and antianxiety effects.

An interesting feature of some individuals with conversion disorders is **la belle indifference**, which is a lack of concern or indifference about the signs or symptoms. Some individuals with conversion disorders appear totally indifferent to their symptoms, whereas others present their complaints in dramatic fashion. La belle indifference is not a diagnostic criterion for conversion disorder, however, because it may also be present with other disorders. Symptoms are more apparent during times of extreme psychological stress, such as with the loss of a loved one or change in fortune. People with conversion disorders are often very suggestible, and their symptoms can be modified or intensified by the reactions of others in their environments.

About 40 to 60% of people who suffer from somatic symptom and related disorders cannot find the words to describe the emotions they experience. This unique personality trait, called alexithymia, is not a part of the *DSM-5* diagnosis. The prevalence of alexithymia in the general population is 10%. Alexithymia includes difficulty identifying feelings, difficulty describing feelings to others, externally oriented thinking, and limited imaginative capacity. The Toronto Alexithymia Scale (TAS-20) is a self-report questionnaire used to assist in measurement of the degree of alexithymia that is present in a patient (Ricciardi, DeMartini, Fotopoulou, et al., 2015).

Treatment

Because the etiology of the conversion disorder includes the combination of unconscious and some pathophysiological processes, simple, abrupt patient education or awareness will not help. Treatment must include validation of the individual's real suffering, followed by sensitive and very gradual explanations about the connection between emotions and physical symptoms. The individual should be provided with examples of such connections (e.g., stress-related ulcers and hypertension, public speech and tachycardia, anxiety and leg restlessness). These conversations should be accompanied by gentle activation of the malfunctioning organs/sensors and reassurance. It is very important not to introduce any potential second gain from the condition, as that may aggravate symptoms.

Psychological Factors Affecting Other Medical Conditions

Individuals with the disorder called *psychological factors affecting other medical conditions* have some medical pathology (not psychiatric) leading to the presentation of medical symptoms. At the same time, these individuals have psychological factors that directly affect treatment, delay recovery, diminish medication adherence, create additional health risks, or in some way negatively impact the existing medical pathology to precipitate a worsening of the symptoms. These factors can include maladaptive behaviour, denial of treatment for an acute condition, or poor adherence to medication. The medical condition can be from any field of medicine (e.g., cardiology, oncology, gastrointestinal). The important diagnostic criterion is that a psychological factor creates an undeniable negative effect on the diagnosed medical pathological process.

Other Specified Somatic Symptom and Related Disorder

The diagnosis of other specified somatic symptom and related disorder is reserved for individuals with a clinical picture of somatic symptom and related disorder that causes a serious impairment of those individuals' functioning but does not fully meet the criteria for any of the previously mentioned diagnoses. In such cases, a clinician chooses to specify which criterion has not been met.

Unspecified Somatic Symptom and Related Disorder

A diagnosis of unspecified somatic symptom and related disorder is reserved for individuals with a clinical picture of somatic symptom and related disorder that causes a serious impairment of the individuals' functioning but does not fully meet the criteria for any of the previously mentioned diagnoses. In such cases, a clinician chooses to specify which criterion has not been met, usually due to very unusual circumstances and lack of information.

Factitious Disorder

In 1951, British endocrinologist and hematologist Dr. Richard Asher described the case of a patient who migrated from hospital to hospital seeking an admission and presenting fake symptoms and a fake personal medical history. Dr. Asher named this condition **Munchausen's syndrome**. In those days, parodied stories about the well-respected German army officer, Baron von Munchhausen, were very popular in England; in these stories, the original tales of this person's life were converted into funny and clearly unrealistic endeavours. They were written as if Baron von Munchhausen had made them up and believed in them himself.

Since the first publication of this case, many other providers have reported similar cases of patients faking their symptoms and personal history in order to be admitted to the hospital and, in some cases, even to undergo surgery. Today, these types of patients are diagnosed as having factitious disorder. (The term *Munchausen's syndrome* is now reserved for patients with factitious disorder who suffer from the most chronic and most severe physical symptoms.) Individuals with **factitious disorder** intentionally falsify the physical and/or mental symptoms or injuries that impair functioning in some aspect of their lives, but there are no identifiable rewards for claiming such impairment.

Despite the large number of cases and the cost of this disorder to the health care system, the etiology of this condition is still poorly understood. In the absence of any apparent benefits from faking an illness, some researchers suggest that patients may use their ill presentation as a defence mechanism against their own violent or sexual impulses. Some researchers think that undergoing painful surgeries, procedures, and tests can be a form of self-punishment for these patients. Other researchers believe that patients seek some emotional benefits from being in the "sick role," such as feeling protected, important, unconditionally accepted, and affiliated. Some researchers also think that the humiliating deception of physicians is an expression of Oedipal-based hostility toward authority figures.

Presenting complaints of factitious disorder include psychological signs and symptoms, self-inflicted illnesses or injuries, and exaggerated symptoms of actual physical problems. Examples include complaining of acute abdominal pain, producing abscesses by injecting saliva under the skin, ingesting medications to produce dramatic adverse effects, or pretending to have a seizure, with no actual history of epilepsy. The medical history of individuals with factitious disorder may be dramatic and colourful, but patients are vague and inconsistent when questioned about their condition. Often, they lie entertainingly about any aspect of their condition. Some may have extensive knowledge of hospital routines, diagnostic testing, and medical terminology. When the cause of the original symptoms is ruled out, individuals often develop new complaints and eagerly undergo invasive procedures. If they are confronted with evidence of their deceptive behaviours, they strongly deny it and discharge themselves from the institution or change health care providers.

Factitious disorder imposed on another, also called *by proxy,* is the deliberate production of signs and symptoms in another person. Situations most often involve a caregiver (mother, babysitter) who induces signs of illness in a child and then presents the child for medical care. The type and severity of signs and symptoms vary with the medical knowledge of the offender. Diagnosis is challenging because offenders commonly remove their victims as soon as the disorder is suspected.

OTHER CONDITIONS THAT MAY BE A FOCUS OF CLINICAL ATTENTION

The diagnostic group "other conditions that may be a focus of clinical attention" is a gathering of different conditions and problems that may affect other diagnoses, treatment, prognoses, symptoms, and patient care. They are not considered to be mental health disorders. If these conditions are diagnosed, it is important to keep them in the patient's record, to inform the interprofessional team and improve treatment outcomes. The diagnostic groups included in this category are as follows:

- Problems Related to Family Upbringing
- Other Problems Related to Primary Support Group
- Child Maltreatment and Neglect Problems
- Adult Maltreatment and Neglect Problems
- Educational Problems
- Occupational Problems
- Housing Problems
- Economic Problems
- Problems Related to Access to Medical and Other Health Care
- Nonadherence to Medical Treatment

There is one diagnosis from the very last category, "Nonadherence to Medical Treatment," called *malingering,* that we will discuss further here, as it is very similar to factitious disorder.

Malingering

The difference between a factitious disorder and malingering lies with the *intent* of the individual. As Spratt (2014) notes, "in factitious disorders, the simulated somatic complaints are done consciously but for unconscious reasons." The motivation to fake or to produce medical symptoms in **malingering** comes from *external conscious incentives.* In factitious disorder, it comes from internal and unconscious incentives.

The malingering individual consciously produces symptoms to meet a recognizable goal. The student who fakes a stomachache to be excused from school for the day is a common example of malingering. Producing symptoms to avoid military service, jury duty, or social obligations are examples. Frequently, patients will produce symptoms with the goal of receiving compensation, food, narcotic drugs, or shelter for the night. However, once the motive becomes apparent to others, the symptoms usually disappear because they no longer serve a purpose.

There is a combination of a few circumstances in which malingering should at least be suspected (Lebourgeois, 2007):

1. Medical examination in any legal context. An individual can be self-directed or referred by an authority, and their legal status and/or benefits depend on the results of this examination.
2. There is an obvious discrepancy between the individual's reported disabilities or level of distress and objective findings.
3. The health care team reports the individual's lack of effort or open lack of cooperation during diagnostic testing or treatment.
4. Diagnosis in the patient of an antisocial personality disorder.

IMPLICATIONS FOR CARE PROVIDERS

Caring for patients with somatic symptoms and related disorders is both challenging and rewarding. The first goal of care (in every case) is to rule out the presence of any physical disease or dysfunction. As physicians order and interpret diagnostic tests, nurses and other care providers observe and assess patients and their activities. Data are gathered and analyzed, physical dysfunctions are ruled out, and the health care team and nursing diagnoses are established.

The development of trust is an important goal in the treatment of patients with somatic symptoms and related disorders. Patients' suffering is very real to them, and health care providers must be aware of how their behaviours and attitudes affect the patients for whom they are providing care.

All care providers should attempt to understand the purposes served by patients' symptoms and work to encourage

BOX 22.2   Key Interventions for Patients With Somatic Symptom and Related Disorders

Convey an attitude of acceptance and understanding.

Meet all physical needs of the patient during acute feelings of illness.

Minimize secondary gains once the acute phase of the illness is resolved.

Use the patient's level of anxiety as a gauge to determine the amount and type of health teaching.

Acknowledge the patient as a responsible adult while indirectly addressing dependency needs.

Encourage the patient to talk about their feelings.

Assist the patient and family in enlarging their social network.

a trusting relationship. It is also important to encourage the expression of feelings and emotional states rather than physical complaints. Also, teach the importance of good nutritional, exercise, and sleep habits, using the patient's anxiety level as a guide for teaching. Meet physical needs when necessary, but encourage independence. Help patients fulfill their social needs, and encourage them to explore more adaptive ways of handling their stresses. Box 22.2 summarizes key interventions for patients with somatic symptom and related disorders. Sample Patient Care Plan 22.1 illustrates a patient plan of care. Finally, it is important to acknowledge patients as individuals and responsible adults who are capable of changing and developing more effective coping mechanisms.

SAMPLE PATIENT CARE PLAN 22.1   Psychophysical Responses

Assessment

History Jasmine is a 20-year-old university student. Last year during final examination week, she developed frequent bouts of nausea, followed by vomiting. Once final examinations were over, her symptoms subsided until about 3 days ago.

Current Findings A tense young woman, sitting stiffly in the chair and wringing her hands. On questioning, Jasmine reveals that she has "never had problems with her stomach." She believes that her nausea and vomiting are related to the "institutional food" she eats while on campus. She is here at the clinic to "get some of those nausea pills." Final examinations for her four classes are scheduled for next week. Jasmine states that school stresses "really have nothing to do with my stomach problems. It's the food that's the real problem here."

Multidisciplinary Diagnosis	Planning/Goals
Risk-prone health behaviour related to anxiety about school examinations	Jasmine will express her feelings verbally rather than through nausea and vomiting by July 2.

THERAPEUTIC INTERVENTIONS

Interventions	Rationale	Team Member
1. Assist Jasmine in identifying stressful situations by reviewing the events surrounding the development of nausea and vomiting.	Identifying events relating to internal conflicts helps reduce the anxiety that results in nausea and vomiting	Psy, Nsg
2. Help her see thoughts, feelings, and behaviours.	Helps Jasmine gain control over her expressions of emotion	All
3. Explore more effective ways of coping with her anxieties.	Preserves dignity and self-respect; encourages effective coping behaviours	Psy, All
4. Help her choose two new coping mechanisms for dealing with the stress of examinations.	Equips Jasmine with multiple ways to manage her anxieties and demonstrates the use of more effective behaviours	Psy, Nsg
5. Actively encourage Jasmine to test the new coping mechanisms and provide feedback.	Change requires time, emotional support, and positive reinforcement from others	All
6. Encourage physical activity and relaxation exercises.	Wellness requires a balance between physical and psychosocial needs.	Nsg
7. Assess eating and sleeping habits, and encourage her to follow a routine schedule.	A healthy, well-cared-for body functions more effectively during stress	Nsg

Evaluation During final examination week, Jasmine had two episodes of nausea but no vomiting. By the next final examination period, Jasmine had replaced nausea and vomiting with a 1-mile walk and 10 minutes of relaxation exercise during each examination day.

Critical Thinking Questions
1. How did Jasmine's coping behaviours affect her activities of daily living?
2. How would you assist her in developing more effective coping mechanisms?

A complete patient care plan includes several other diagnoses and interventions.
Nsg, nursing staff; *Psy,* psychologist.

KEY POINTS

- No real divisions between mind and body exist.
- The physical signs and symptoms of psychic (emotional) distress are very real to the individual who is suffering from them at the time.
- When the body is under stress, it activates its stress response mechanism, which protects the individual by preparing the body to fight or flee.
- When an individual perceives stress, the body initiates a cascade of biochemicals and releases the body's four major stress hormones—dopamine, epinephrine, norepinephrine, and cortisol.
- Common stress-related symptoms include indigestion, vomiting, constipation, diarrhea, asthma, high blood pressure, and mental health conditions.
- Theories about stress include the stress response, symbolism, personality, and organic weakness theories.
- Many somatic symptom disorders are culturally related and include *gaman* (Japanese), *koro* (South Asian), *mal ojo* (Latin American), and *dhat* (East Indian).
- *Somatization* is the term for feeling physical symptoms in the absence of disease or out of proportion to a given ailment.
- Patients with a conversion disorder present with problems related to sensory or motor function.
- The most important feature of factitious disorder is that symptoms are purposefully produced so that the individual can assume the sick role.
- The malingering individual purposely produces symptoms to meet a recognizable external goal.
- The goals of care for every patient with a somatic symptom disorder are to rule out the presence of any physical disease or dysfunction and to develop trust in the therapeutic relationship.

ADDITIONAL LEARNING RESOURCES

Go to your Evolve website (http://evolve.elsevier.com/Canada/Morrison-Valfre/) for additional online resources, including the online Study Guide for additional learning activities to help you master this chapter content.

CRITICAL THINKING QUESTIONS

1. What are the similarities and differences between factitious disorder and malingering?
2. How might anxiety affect physiological functions of the human body (e.g., heart rate, digestion, breathing)?
3. When does somatization become a mental health concern?
4. What are the main features that can help health care providers differentiate a somatic symptom disorder from a medical problem?
5. How might factitious disorder imposed on another present in an emergency department?

REFERENCES

American Psychiatric Association (APA). (2013). *Diagnostic and statistical manual of mental disorders* (5th ed.). American Psychiatric Publishing.

Craighead, W. E., & Nemeroff, C. B. (Eds.). (2010). *The Corsini encyclopedia of psychology and behavioral science* (4th ed.). Wiley.

D'Avanzo, C. (2007). *Mosby's pocket guide to cultural health assessment* (4th ed.). Mosby.

Giger, J. N., & Haddad, L. G. (2020). *Transcultural nursing: Assessment and intervention* (8th ed.). Mosby.

Lebourgeois, H. W., III. (2007). Malingering: Key points in assessment. *Psychiatric Times, 24*(5), 21, 27–29. https://www.psychiatrictimes.com/forensic-psychiatry/malingering-key-points-assessment

Lieberman, J. (2015). *From fever cure to coma therapy: Psychiatric treatments through time.* https://www.sciencefriday.com/articles/from-fever-cure-to-coma-therapy-psychiatric-treatments-through-time/

Psychology, Wiki. (2020). *Conversion disorder: Prevalence.* http://psychology.wikia.com/wiki/Conversion_disorder:_Prevalence

Ricciardi, L., Demartini, B., Fotopoulou, A., et al. (2015). Alexithymia in neurological disease: A review. *Psychiatry online. Journal of Neuropsychiatry and Clinical Neurosciences.* https://neuro.psychiatryonline.org/doi/10.1176/appi.neuropsych.14070169

Selye, H. (1978). *The stress of life.* McGraw-Hill (Original work published 1956).

Spratt, E. G. (2014). *Somatoform disorder: Factitious disorder and malingering.* http://emedicine.medscape.com/article/918628-overview

23

Eating and Sleeping Disorders

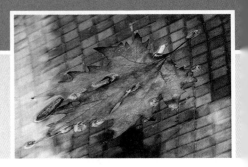

OBJECTIVES

Upon completion of this chapter, the student will be able to:
1. List three features of an eating disorder.
2. Describe three characteristics of a person with anorexia nervosa.
3. Define the complication of anorexia called refeeding syndrome.
4. Identify the criteria for the diagnosis of bulimia nervosa.
5. Forecast the prognosis (outcome) for a patient with an untreated eating disorder.
6. Explain why obesity can be considered an eating disorder.
7. Examine the main therapeutic goal for treating patients with eating disorders.
8. Develop four therapeutic interventions for patients with eating disorders.
9. Describe three functions of sleep.
10. Discuss the signs and symptoms of a patient experiencing insomnia.
11. Plan four therapeutic (nursing) interventions to assist patients with sleeping problems.

OUTLINE

KEY TERMS

anorexia (ĂN-ō-RĚK-sē-ă) **nervosa** (p. 274)
apnea (ap-NEE-uh) (p. 282)
binge eating disorder (p. 277)
body image (p. 273)
bulimia (bū-LĔM-ē-ă) **nervosa** (p. 276)
cataplexy (KĂT- ă-plĕk-sē) (p. 282)
compulsive overeating (p.278)
eating and feeding disorder (p. 273)
hypersomnia (p. 281)
hypersomnolence disorder (p. 281)
hypopnea (hahy-POP-nee-uh) (p. 282)
insomnia (ĭn-SŎM-nē-ă) (p. 281)
insomnia disorder (p. 281)
narcolepsy (NĂR-kō-lĕp-sē) (p. 282)

nocturnal sleep-related eating disorder (NSRED) (p. 283)
obesity (p. 277)
parasomnias (PĂR-ă-SŎM-nē-ăs) (p. 283)
pica (PĪ-kă) (p. 274)
polysomnogram (PŎL-ē-SŎM-nō-grăm) (p. 281)
purging (p. 276)
refeeding syndrome (p. 275)
restless legs syndrome (RLS) (p. 283)
rumination (ROO-mĭ-NĀ-shun) **disorder** (p. 274)
sleep-related hypoventilation (p. 282)
sleep terror (p. 283)
sleep–wake disorder (p. 281)
sleepwalking (p. 283)

FEEDING AND EATING DISORDERS

Every person has a **body image**—the collection of perceptions, thoughts, feelings, and behaviours that relate to one's body size and appearance. Body image is an important part of self-concept. *Positive body images* lead to behaviours that express confidence and self-assurance. *Negative body images* can contribute to shyness and social isolation. Anxiety, depression, anorexia nervosa, bulimia, obesity, and other mental health challenges are all interwoven with body image.

Eating disorders (EDs) are complex illnesses that people have always suffered from. The etiology of these illnesses is in the genetic predisposition of the brain structure and

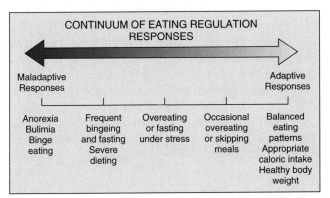

Fig. 23.1 Continuum of eating regulation responses. (From Stuart, G. W. [2013]. *Principles and practice of psychiatric nursing* [10th ed.]. Mosby.)

functionality. Changes in how society views body and dieting do not lead directly to eating disorders, but they can trigger the underlying predisposition to eating disorders and facilitate the occurrence of these illnesses. Many other theoretical models for what causes eating disorders point to increased levels of stress in modern society; they propose that people use food consumption as a maladaptive coping mechanism to deal with stress, which may ignite a predisposed eating pathology.

According to the National Initiative for Eating Disorders (NIED), EDs have the highest mortality rate of any mental health illnesses, estimated to be about 10 to 15% (Arcelus, Mitchel, Wales, et al., 2011; NIED, 2016). About one million Canadians meet the diagnostic criteria for some type of ED (NIED, 2016). As with everything in life, an occasional skipped meal or overindulgence is not a problem (Fig. 23.1), but when behaviours associated with eating interfere with an individual's quality of daily life, they become mental health disorders.

An **eating and feeding disorder** is an ongoing disturbance in behaviours, resulting in altered consumption or absorption of food that causes a significant impairment of a person's physical and psychological function (American Psychiatric Association [APA, 2013, p. 329]). Obesity, which is excessive body fat, is not a mental disorder. However, there are many mental health factors that can contribute to the development of obesity. Table 23.1 briefly defines the different types of eating and feeding disorders.

Although their etiology remains unknown, several theories and much research have attempted to explain the nature of eating disorders (Table 23.2).

TABLE 23.1 Types of Eating and Feeding Disorders

Disorder	Description
Anorexia nervosa	A disturbance in body perception resulting in an intense fear of gaining weight and a refusal to eat enough to maintain an adequate body weight. Prevalence is a 10:1 female-to-male ratio.
Avoidant/restrictive food disorder	Refusal to eat or apparent lack of interest in eating foods to the point where weight loss and nutritional deficiencies occur.
Binge eating disorder	Recurring episodes of eating large amounts of food in a short time with a sense of lack of control, followed by intense emotional distress. This is not associated with inappropriate compensatory behaviour, as in bulimia nervosa.
Bulimia nervosa	Recurrent ingestion of large amounts of food accompanied by a sense of lack of control, followed by efforts to compensate for overeating, such as purging, fasting, or exercise.
Other eating disorders	• Atypical anorexia—anorexia with a normal body weight • Limited bulimia nervosa—bulimia nervosa with less frequent episodes of bingeing and compensation • Limited binge eating—binge eating less than once a week and/or for fewer than 3 months • Purging disorder—recurrent purging to decrease weight • Night eating syndrome—recurrent eating of an excessive amount after awakening from sleep and following the evening meal
Orthorexia nervosa (a non-*DSM* diagnosis)	Fixation with eating "pure," "right," or "proper" foods leading to impaired function.
Pica	At least 1 month of persistent eating of nonfood substances, such as paper, hair, ash, clay, or chalk.
Rumination disorder	At least 1 month of repeated regurgitation of food back into the mouth after recent food intake. The food is rechewed, spit out, or reswallowed.

TABLE 23.2 Theories About Eating and Feeding Disorders

Theory	Description
Behavioural	Eating disorders are attempts to reduce anxiety; discomfort with body image creates more anxiety, feelings of guilt and disgust, and loss of self-protecting boundaries.
Cognitive	Eating disorders are the result of deficits in attention, concentration, and vigilance related to underlying anxiety and depression.
Developmental	The individual fails to develop an appropriate sense of self and body and has problems with autonomy and self-identity. The disorder is often brought about by a significant loss or crisis.
Sociocultural	Eating disorders are a response to a daily social emphasis on a stereotypical ideal of thinness. Social stereotypes serve as stressors that drive especially women and girls to harmful dieting behaviours. Anorexia nervosa is a way of mastering some control over the pressure on women to be successful in all areas of life.
Physical	The causes for eating disorders involve complex relationships among the body's neurotransmitters; there is evidence of altered serotonin function. Many of the same neuroendocrine findings are found in persons with depressive and bipolar disorders. Cortisol levels are altered in depression and eating disorders. Anorexia nervosa decreases levels of luteinizing hormone and follicle-stimulating hormone, which results in menstrual irregularities.

Pica

Individuals with **pica** eat non-nutritive substances (items not typically thought of as food) for at least 1 month, causing clinical concerns and attention. Eating the substance is not a part of cultural or social norms of their community. The typical substances are hair, soap, talcum powder, clay, or charcoal.

The prevalence of pica in the general population is unknown. The prevalence among individuals with intellectual disability is well documented, and the incidence increases with the severity of their disability.

Rumination Disorder

Rumination disorder, an uncommon condition most often seen in childhood, is defined as the regurgitation and rechewing of food. Partially digested food is brought up into the mouth and then either spit out or, more frequently, chewed and reswallowed. There are no signs of nausea, retching, or gastrointestinal disorder.

When rumination disorder affects infants, recovery may happen spontaneously. But if the course of the disorder continues, it may require medical intervention and nutritional supplementation, otherwise death from malnutrition can result. In older children and adults, malnutrition is less of a problem.

This disorder can occur continuously or appear at intervals. Psychosocial issues, such as lack of attention, neglect, or a stressful environment, may be risk factors. Other feeding disorders of childhood are discussed in Chapter 13. Refer back to Table 23.1 for a brief description of other, less common eating disorders.

Avoidant/Restrictive Food Intake Disorder

Individuals with avoidant/restrictive food intake disorder experience persistent challenges to achieving proper nutrition. These challenges manifest as a significant weight loss (or failure to achieve a proper weight), severe nutritional deficiency, dependence on enteral feeding (e.g., gastrointestinal feeding tube) or some oral nutritional additives, or serious involvement with psychosocial functioning (e.g., the person cannot eat with others or maintain relationships). Some individuals avoid food because of sense concerns or concerns about real or imagined consequences of eating.

Anorexia Nervosa

This is one of the most serious disorders among all mental health disorders. **Anorexia nervosa** is a condition in which an individual restricts energy intake to cause a significantly low weight because of their intense fear of becoming fat. Actually, the term *anorexia* (which in Greek means "want of appetite") is inaccurate because there is seldom an actual appetite loss associated with the disorder. The refusal to gain weight is part of a strategy to solve a deep psychological problem and maintain some form of control. Because of the secrecy and social stigma associated with the disorder, the exact number of persons with anorexia nervosa is unknown.

Anorexia nervosa was first identified in 1689 by English physician Richard Morton. In his work, he described an 18-year-old female patient "like a Skeleton, only clad with skin" (Wilkinson, 2018). Approximately 90 to 95% of people with anorexia nervosa are female, although men are not immune to the disorder.

Anorexia nervosa is a *life-threatening disorder*. The death rate associated with this disorder is far higher than for any other mental illness (Rikani, Choudhry, Choudhry, et al., 2013). Death usually results from dehydration, loss of critical muscle mass, electrolyte imbalances, or suicide. Often, patients are not seen by health care providers until the disorder has resulted in some other physical problem. The prevalence rate of anorexia in modern Western society is about 0.5%, which means that in Canada there are around 185 000 cases. The mortality rate is 10 to 15% (Arcelus et al., 2011; NIED, 2016), which means that between 18 500 and 27 750 people die from this disease across the country. It is very hard to determine the exact rate because often mental health causes are not listed on death certificates, for a variety of reasons. To put these numbers in perspective, however, by comparison, in 2017, about 5 000 Canadian females died from breast cancer (Canadian Cancer Society, 2020).

Anorexia nervosa is not often seen before puberty and rarely appears after 40 years of age. The average age of onset is about 17 years, but anorectic behaviours may be seen in 12-year-olds. People who are concerned with their appearance for professional or performance reasons, such as models, athletes, or flight attendants, are at a higher risk for developing anorexia nervosa. Early signs and symptoms of anorexia nervosa occur in children with depressive symptoms and obsessive behaviours. Anorexia primarily occurs in industrialized, Western societies but is seen with increasing frequency in other cultures (see Cultural Considerations box).

CULTURAL CONSIDERATIONS

The incidence of anorexia nervosa is rising in Asia. Studies of female Japanese students, dating back to 1982, have demonstrated that eating disorders are on the rise. According to Nakai, Nin, and Noma (2014), "on almost all measures, there were significant increases of a disordered attitude about fear of gaining weight, body perception disturbance and problem eating behaviours over time." Other countries that are adapting to Western influences are also seeing a rise in the incidence of eating disorders.

Certain *personality factors* appear to be associated with anorexia nervosa. The classic description of a person with anorexia nervosa is a tense, alert, hyperactive, rigid young woman who thinks, talks, and walks rapidly. She is ambitious and drives herself to perfection. She is sensitive, insecure, and serious, with a conscience that works overtime. Her neatness, self-will, and stubbornness can make her difficult to treat. She tends to have few friends, as she lacks warmth and friendliness toward others. As she struggles to gain a self-respecting identity, she engages in the pursuit of thinness. These behaviours eventually result in psychological and physiological disturbances.

The main issue is one of *control,* and the anorectic individual becomes constricted, conforming, and obsessed with the need to control body weight. Some teenagers have a fear of growing up and sexually maturing. With anorexia nervosa they can prevent the onset of adulthood by delaying menses and the development of secondary sexual characteristics.

Clinical Presentation

Weight concerns put adolescents at high risk for developing anorexia nervosa. Dieting, body dissatisfaction, current body weight below body weight ideals, and unusual eating patterns do not necessarily indicate an eating disorder. However, when the quest for thinness results in the refusal to maintain a normal body weight, anorexia is the result. To be diagnosed with anorexia nervosa, the individual must meet the three *DSM-5* criteria listed in Box 23.1.

The self-esteem of people with anorexia nervosa depends highly on body size and shape. Individuals often go to great lengths to monitor their body, such as weighing themselves three or four times each day, measuring body parts, and frequently looking in the mirror to check for areas of fat. The ability

---

BOX 23.1 Criteria for Diagnosis of Anorexia Nervosa

A. Restriction of energy intake relative to requirements, leading to significantly low body weight in the context of age, sex, developmental trajectory, and physical health.

B. Even though the individual is underweight, an intense fear of becoming fat exists and interferes with weight gain.

C. A distorted (inaccurate) significance is placed on body weight and shape (the person "feels fat" and perceives self as fat despite being underweight) or the ongoing lack of recognition of the seriousness of low body weight.

---

to lose weight is considered a sign of control and extraordinary self-discipline. Conversely, even the smallest gain in weight is seen as a threat and as a failure of self-control. Some individuals may actually acknowledge their extreme thinness, but they typically deny the seriousness of their condition. Refer to Figure 14.1 for signs and symptoms of a patient with anorexia nervosa.

Behaviourally, many anorectic persons have a preoccupation with food. They may save recipes or prepare elaborate meals and then cut their own food into small pieces and push it around the plate without eating. Some evidence suggests that anorexia nervosa may stem from a food phobia. Several family and twin studies suggest that a possible genetic link may increase the risk of developing anorexia. Obsessive behaviour with food often extends into other obsessive-compulsive activities, such as a preoccupation with studying, exercising, or cleaning. Often individuals with anorexia nervosa have poor sexual adjustment, with delayed sexual development or little interest in sex. They also may be unable to effectively cope with or solve problems. Their history frequently is positive for anxiety, depression, or substance abuse.

When severely anorectic individuals begin to resume eating after periods of starvation, the risk of developing **refeeding syndrome** increases. During prolonged starvation and lack of carbohydrate sources for energy, the body uses its own fat tissue and amino acids to survive. It no longer needs insulin because glucagon secretion is increased. The body shifts from a *catabolic* state (a state of breaking down tissues for nutrients) to an *anabolic* state (a state of rebuilding tissues and growth). This change in metabolism leads to secretion of many hormones that contribute to shifts in salts and fluids in the body. The body is so hungry for nutrients that in an effort to rebuild cells, it moves many salts from the blood to the growing cells. Low levels of salts such as potassium, phosphorus, and magnesium in the blood may lead to complications such as heart failure, abnormal heart rhythms (dysrhythmias), respiratory failure, muscle breakdown, and death (Eating Disorder Hope, 2018). For this reason, clinicians must be very careful during the refeeding process for anorexic patients.

Refeeding syndrome may happen on the fourth day of reinitiating nutrition. During refeeding, patients must be carefully and frequently monitored for physical and mental changes. Intense monitoring and resupply of electrolytes and vitamins are required.

People with anorexia nervosa need intervention, but they often deny the seriousness of their condition until extensive

TABLE 23.3 Key Features of Anorexia Nervosa and Bulimia Nervosa

Anorexia Nervosa	Bulimia Nervosa
Rare use of vomiting, diuretics, laxatives	Vomiting or diuretics, laxative abuse
More severe weight loss	Less weight loss
Slightly younger	Slightly older
More introverted	More extroverted, social
Hunger denied	Hunger experienced
Eating behaviour may be considered normal and source of esteem	Eating behaviour considered foreign and a source of distress
Sexually inactive	More sexually active
May be obsessive or compulsive	May have hysterical or borderline, as well as obsessive, behaviours
Death from starvation or suicide	Death from hypokalemia or suicide
Amenorrhea	Menses irregular or absent
Fewer behavioural abnormalities	Stealing, drug and alcohol abuse, self-mutilation, and other behavioural abnormalities

physical damage has taken place. All health care providers in every setting must be alert for the clues of anorexia nervosa because early intervention will often save a life that otherwise may literally waste away.

Bulimia Nervosa

Bulimia nervosa is a disorder of uncontrollable binge eating (intake of an amount of food that is larger than the amount required) followed by periods of food restriction (e.g., the use of inappropriate methods to prevent weight gain) at least once a week for 3 months. These food-restriction methods may include self-induced vomiting, fasting, excessive exercising, and misuse of laxatives or other medications. A bulimic person's self-evaluation is disproportionately influenced by body shape and weight.

Although anorexia nervosa may be a more dramatic disorder, bulimia nervosa occurs more commonly. The estimated incidence of bulimia nervosa varies with the population, method, and criteria used for study. An Ontario study of people aged 15 to 65 years, drawn from a community epidemiological survey, revealed a lifetime prevalence of bulimia nervosa of 0.13% for males and 1.46% for females (NIED, 2017).

Bulimia nervosa is most often found in young, white, middle-class and upper-class women. Men account for about one of nine cases. There is an increased frequency of anxiety, depression, and drug abuse among individuals with bulimia. Individuals suffering from bulimia nervosa often have other psychological challenges. About one third to one half also meet the diagnostic criteria for a personality disorder. Because it is difficult to detect, many individuals with bulimia nervosa go untreated. Like anorexia nervosa, bulimia nervosa appears to occur more frequently in modern industrialized countries.

Individuals with bulimia nervosa are usually ashamed of this illness and try to hide it. For some, the shame may lead to

the partial control of the condition (e.g., the person may not be able to stop binge eating when the phone rings or someone calls, but may stop when their spouse comes home).

The personality traits of persons with bulimia nervosa differ from those of persons with anorexia nervosa. The average individual with bulimia nervosa is a woman who is slightly older and more outgoing than her anorexic counterpart. She is socially and sexually active. She actually experiences hunger and feels distressed about her abnormal eating behaviours. Often her body weight is normal or even slightly above average. Other mental health challenges, such as substance abuse, self-mutilation, or hysteria, may be present at the same time. Refer to Figure 14.1 and Table 23.3 for a comparison of the key features of anorexia nervosa and bulimia nervosa.

When it comes to body image, people with bulimia nervosa typically view themselves as being either fat or thin. Being in the middle, or average, is generally not considered. Commonly, a woman with bulimia fears that she must follow a diet for the rest of her life if she gives up binge eating.

Perfectionism is an important trait in bulimic nervosa behaviours. Women with bulimia nervosa frequently have unrealistic expectations about themselves and how their lives should be. They become frustrated by their own inabilities to reach unrealistic goals. If they experience failure, they conclude that they were unable to reach the goal because they were weak, not trying hard enough, inadequate, or unlovable or had some other negative failing. In short, these individuals tend to think "I should have . . ." and are frequently not satisfied with their own efforts. Even when successful, they seldom can enjoy their accomplishments because they tell themselves that they should have done it better, sooner, or more efficiently. The desire to become the perfect person commonly leads to feelings of failure and uselessness. When life is based on the all-or-nothing principle, anything short of perfect is considered a failure. Perfection, in reality, is not attainable.

Clinical Presentation

The most essential feature of bulimia nervosa is recurring episodes of binge eating. Individuals are usually ashamed of their binges and often eat in secret. Episodes of binge eating may or may not be planned in advance. During the bingeing episodes, the individual feels out of control and often eats in a frenzied state.

Bingeing is followed by recurring inappropriate behaviours to prevent weight gain. The most popular method of purging is to induce vomiting (80 to 90%), which relieves the physical discomfort of a full stomach and the emotional fear of gaining weight. Sometimes the act of vomiting becomes a goal in itself. The person will binge to vomit or will vomit after eating only a small amount of food. Other methods of purging include the misuse of laxatives, diuretics, enemas, and syrup of ipecac. Some people use a combination of methods to purge, engage in strenuous exercise at inappropriate times, or follow semi-starvation diets after a bingeing episode.

In order for a diagnosis to be established, the eating binges must occur at least twice per week for at least 3 months (APA, 2013; see Box 23.2). Patterns of binge eating range from several episodes each day to a regular and persistent pattern of binge eating. Often episodes are triggered by a stressful event or experience.

BOX 23.2 Criteria for Diagnosis of Bulimia Nervosa

1. Recurring episodes of uncontrollable binge eating of an amount of food during a short period of time (e.g., a 2-hour period) that is significantly larger than most people would eat during a similar time period or in similar circumstances, and a sense of a lack of control over eating during that episode (e.g., the person feels unable to stop eating or control what or how much is eaten).
2. Binge eating is followed by recurring inappropriate compensatory behaviours to prevent weight gain (e.g., self-induced vomiting; misuse of laxatives, diuretics, or other medications; fasting; excessive exercise).
3. The eating binges and inappropriate compensatory behaviour both occur, on average, at least once per week for at least 3 months.
4. Excessive emphasis is placed on body shape and weight in determining self-esteem.
5. The disturbance does not occur exclusively during episodes of anorexia nervosa.

Bulimic individuals place excessive emphasis on body shape and weight in determining their self-esteem. They are dissatisfied with their imperfect bodies, have a fear of gaining weight, and often restrict their caloric intake or choose low-calorie foods between binge-eating episodes.

When purging behaviours are frequent, fluid and electrolyte abnormalities can result. The few persons who use syrup of ipecac are at risk for developing serious cardiac and skeletal muscle wasting. Bulimia nervosa is somewhat less lethal than anorexia; however, the underlying psychiatric concerns are often more severe than those seen with anorectic persons.

Many times, the signs and symptoms of anorexia nervosa and bulimia nervosa occur together in the same individual. Both disorders are complex and often interrelated with other mental and physical health issues.

Binge Eating Disorder

Binge eating disorder is defined as consuming (within a short period of time) an amount of food that is definitely larger than most individuals would eat in similar circumstances or during a similar time frame. During a binge, an individual often consumes large amounts of certain types of foods, usually carbohydrates. It is not unusual for the binger to eat as many as 5 000 calories in doughnuts, cakes, or other sweets in a single sitting. The binge lasts about 1 to 2 hours and then is followed by feelings of severe distress, guilt, and disgust. Unlike bulimia nervosa, however, binge eating disorder is not associated with the repeated use of this inappropriate behaviour to purge or to lose weight.

Obesity

The *Diagnostic and Statistical Manual of Mental Disorders,* fifth edition (*DSM-5*; APA, 2013) does not list obesity as a mental health disorder because it has not been established that obesity is consistently associated with mental health or behavioural challenges. However, obesity is linked to many physical and psychological difficulties that can cause distress for most overweight individuals. Like the person with bulimia, gambling addiction, or alcoholism, many overweight individuals lose control over their eating. They also live with the stigma that people with these diseases can actually control their behaviour and therefore deserve more judgement and less help. More than one in four adults in Canada are obese (Obesity Canada, 2019).

Obesity is defined as an excess of body weight. According to the Canadian Medical Association practice guidelines for obesity, primary care providers should recognize and treat obesity as a chronic disease, caused by abnormal or excess body fat accumulation (adiposity), which impairs health, with increased risk of premature morbidity and mortality (Wharton et al., 2020; Fig. 23.2).

Although body mass index (BMI) has its limitations, it remains a valuable tool for screening purposes and for population health indices. Canadian guidelines for adult body weight indicate six weight categories (Government of Canada, 2016). The calculation is based on BMI, which is calculated as weight in kilograms (kg) divided by height in metres squared (BMI = weight [kg]/ height [m²]). The six BMI categories are listed in Table 23.4.

There are several causes of obesity. In addition to overeating, other factors have been discovered that may help explain obesity. There is mounting evidence linking obesity to a strong genetic predisposition for the condition. The children of obese parents tend to be overweight themselves. Obese persons have larger fat cells in their bodies. Complicated neurochemical mechanisms that help to control appetite and eating behaviours may also be involved and are currently being studied. Finally, a lack of sufficient exercise contributes greatly to obesity. The Canadian Medical Association practice guidelines recommend obtaining a comprehensive history to identify the root causes of weight gain, as well as physical, mental, and psychosocial barriers. Physical examination, laboratory, diagnostic imaging, and other investigations should be carried out based on clinical judgement (Wharton et al., 2020).

Obesity is a progressive chronic condition, similar to diabetes or high blood pressure. Not knowing this and the genetic predisposition to obesity, many obese people blame themselves for what they perceive as a "lack of self-control," which may lead to a variety of psychological issues. For instance, overweight females commonly struggle with feelings of hopelessness and suicide, whereas males demonstrate more depressive moods. Studies of overweight adolescents revealed that obese teens often "had lower body satisfaction and decreased self-esteem" (Loth, Mond, Wall, et al., 2011). Thus health care providers need to maintain a nonjudgemental approach to a patient's weight.

In some cultures, by contrast, obesity is viewed as a positive trait (see Cultural Considerations box).

CULTURAL CONSIDERATIONS

The island nation of Nauru lies in the western Pacific Ocean south of the equator. Most Nauruans lead an inactive lifestyle because the island's phosphate mines are worked by immigrant miners. Almost all food and water are imported from Australia.

Eating processed foods is considered a sign of wealth in Nauru. Obesity is considered attractive, and overweight women are sought as wives. Nauru has the highest rate of diabetes in the world.

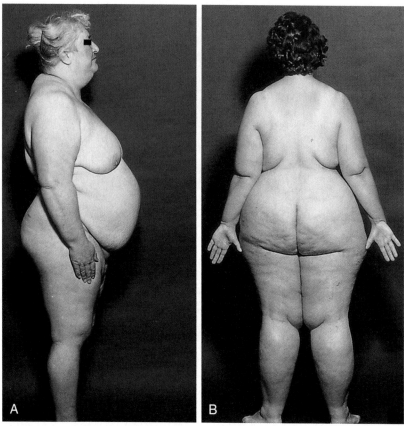

Fig. 23.2 Obesity. (From Seidel, H. M., Ball, J. W., Dains, J. E., et al. [2002]. *Mosby's guide to physical examination* [5th ed.]. Mosby.)

TABLE 23.4   Health Risk Classification According to Body Mass Index (BMI)

Classification	BMI Category (kg/m²)	Risk of Developing Health Problems
Underweight	<18.5	Increased
Normal Weight	18.5–24.9	Least
Overweight	25.0–29.9	Increased
Obese Class I	30.0–34.9	High
Obese Class II	35.0–39.9	Very high
Obese Class III	≥40.0	Extremely high

From Government of Canada. (2018). *Canadian guidelines for body weight classification in adults—quick reference tool for professionals.* https://www.canada.ca/en/health-canada/services/food-nutrition/ healthy-eating/healthy-weights/canadian-guidelines-body-weight-classification-adults/quick-reference-tool-professionals.html

Faulty eating behaviours appear to begin in childhood. Many overweight persons may once have relied on food to numb the discomforts of growing up. Throughout childhood, eating helped to relieve the emotional distresses of life. This pattern of lessening emotional pain by eating is called **compulsive overeating**. In time, food becomes like a drug, with a "fix" that temporarily lessens the psychological discomforts of an ever-growing desire for more food.

As the individual continues to find comfort in food, they grow physically more obese and less attractive to others and perhaps to themselves (according to Western cultural stigmas relating to obesity). This behaviour serves only to increase feelings of worthlessness, and the person again eats to relieve the pain. A vicious circle soon becomes established in which the individual replaces social relationships with the comforts of food.

Clinical Presentation

The first signs of obesity are often seen early in life. An estimate may be made by comparing the person's height and weight with a standardized chart. Children who are 20% over normal for their height and weight should undergo further evaluation. The evaluation should include a "height and weight history of the child, parents, and siblings, as well as eating habits, appetite, and hunger patterns, and physical activity" (Hockenberry & Wilson, 2014).

As overweight children grow and mature, they begin to sense society's disapproval of their obesity. Youngsters may begin to diet and exercise or react by continuing to find comfort in food. Dieting and other weight loss methods soon become a way of life for many overweight young people. Eating disorders may develop.

During adolescence, weight becomes an important part of a newly forming body image. Teens may rebel against parental nagging to lose weight or become unwilling to control their caloric intake. They may resort to unhealthy methods, such as prolonged fasting or purging, to gain some control

BOX 23.3 Nursing Diagnoses (Problem Statements) Related to Eating Disorders

Physical Realm

Altered activity tolerance
Failure to thrive
Imbalanced fluid and electrolytes
Imbalanced nutrition
Ineffective sexuality patterns
Nonadherence

Psychosocial Realms

At risk for self-directed violence
Disturbed body image
Disturbed thought processes
Ineffective coping
Denial
Risk-prone health behaviours
Self-esteem disturbances

over their weight. Often they will ignore their obesity and eat as though a problem does not exist.

The cycle of "I'm not attractive, so I'll eat because it makes me feel better" can become an ingrained way of coping in childhood. Many overweight individuals become even more obese as they grow older. Eventually, the many chronic health problems associated with obesity begin to appear. These problems can increase anxiety, causing the individual to seek the comfort that food has so frequently brought in the past. The cycle continues, and health care challenges may increase.

Guidelines for Intervention

The main therapeutic goal for all eating and feeding disorders is to establish behaviours that promote health for the individual. Although it sounds simple, this can be a lofty goal. People with eating disorders have learned to cope with their stresses by focusing on food in one way or another. Those with anorexia nervosa attempt to cope by controlling, and the highest form of control is the ability to determine one's body size. Individuals with bulimia learn to numb emotional pain by eating large amounts of food, then they suffer overwhelming guilt. Many persons who experience the discomforts of obesity have developed compulsive overeating habits to fill their need for love and belonging.

Treatments and Therapies

Treatment for eating disorders requires medical and mental health interventions. There are three immediate (short-term) treatment goals. The highest priority is to *stabilize existing medical problems*. The second goal is to *re-establish normal nutrition* and eating patterns. Last is to help the patient *resolve the psychological and emotional issues* that underlie their disordered eating behaviours.

Medical care is centred on nutritional management. Individuals with severe weight loss may require *parenteral nutrition* (PN) (also called *total parenteral nutrition* [TPN]). With PN/TPN, all necessary nutrients are administered through an intravenous (IV) line placed in a large blood vessel. For less severely malnourished patients, IV therapy or tube feedings may be ordered. However, the main focus is to encourage the patient to voluntarily consume food.

Patients are weighed daily, and supplemental vitamins are usually prescribed. Each patient is frequently monitored for signs of refeeding syndrome and closely observed for secret anorectic or bulimic behaviours. The long-term goals (for both underweight and overweight patients) focus on teaching patients about good nutrition and assisting them in developing appropriate eating habits.

The goals of mental health care focus on helping patients improve their self-esteem and develop more effective coping skills. Once patients are physically stable, they are encouraged to adopt proper eating habits. Behaviour modification techniques may help to reinforce healthful eating behaviours. Signs of depression are diagnosed and treated. Often family therapy is helpful. Individual or group therapy can help patients focus on the psychological conflicts that underlie their inappropriate eating behaviours.

Medication therapy can be quite effective, but only if it is combined with some form of psychotherapy (see Medication Alert). Amphetamines have been successfully used to treat obesity. However, their potential for addiction is high, so they are not frequently prescribed. Antidepressants or lithium has been used with success in the treatment of bulimia.

! MEDICATION ALERT

Administering antidepressants to patients who have anorexia nervosa before they regain weight may be hazardous if the individual has a history of cardiac problems or currently has a low serum potassium level. For this reason, the prescriber may order a trial dose of the antidepressant.

It is important to check the laboratory results of patients with eating disorders. Withhold the medication and notify the physician if the potassium level drops below normal limits.

Nurses and other health care providers play an important role in caring for individuals with altered eating patterns, in both hospital and community settings. The main goal is to assist patients in identifying and coping with the problems that led to inappropriate eating behaviours. Possible nursing diagnoses (problem statements) relating to eating disorders are listed in Box 23.3.

To accomplish the goals of care, rapport and trust with patients must first be established. Then patients are assisted in identifying how food is used to provide comfort and reduce anxiety. During the working phase of the therapeutic relationship, patients are helped to replace distorted body image ideas with thoughts and behaviours that build self-esteem. Problem-solving skills are taught, and patients are encouraged to identify the social support systems that promote healthful practices. Refer to Sample Patient Care Plan 23.1 for a care plan for patients with eating disorders.

Every individual with an eating disorder needs the understanding and compassion of health care providers. By nurturing and supporting more effective coping behaviours, providers may be able to help make the struggles of patients with eating disorders a little less difficult.

SAMPLE PATIENT CARE PLAN 23.1   Eating Disorder

Assessment

History Erica is a 15-year-old who is 9 kg (20 pounds) under her usual body weight. She has always been a "chubby child" who had no problems eating until the beginning of this school year. Three months ago, Erica told her mother to stop making "all those fattening foods" and began refusing most of her meals.

Current Findings A thin, tired-appearing adolescent girl who appears older than her stated age. Face is hollow, eyes are sunken, and skin is dry. Hair is fine and brittle. Skin is covered with lanugo (fine hair). Vital signs are low for age and size.

When questioned, Erica states that she "feels fine" and does not "know what all the fuss is about. Just because I choose to lose a few kilograms everybody gets upset. Sounds like this is their problem more than mine. I'm really still way too fat."

Multidisciplinary Diagnosis	Planning/Goals
Impaired nutrition: less than body requirements related to distorted self-image	Erica will voluntarily consume 2 000 calories/day by July 4. Erica will gain 0.5 kg of body weight per week.

THERAPEUTIC INTERVENTIONS

Intervention	Rationale	Team Member
1. Establish trust and gain Erica's cooperation.	Erica must first agree to work with the staff if other interventions are to achieve therapeutic results	All
2. Perform a complete nutritional assessment.	Establishes a baseline from which to judge progress	Diet, Nsg
3. Help Erica identify the consequences of her eating behaviours.	Helps her acknowledge the problem and its effects on her life	Psy, Nsg
4. Monitor physical status daily for signs of malnutrition.	To prevent further physical problems and decline	Nsg, MD
5. Explore other ways to achieve control over the parts of Erica's life that are causing distress.	When control is achieved in one area, it tends to spread to other areas; control builds self-image and confidence	All
6. Involve family members in therapy if possible.	Erica may benefit from supportive family members; offers an opportunity to assess family interactions	Psy, Nsg

Evaluation During the first week, Erica consumed an average of 1 000 calories per day, with much encouragement. By July 3, Erica was voluntarily consuming about 1 800 calories per day. Weight gain averaged 0.22 kg (0.5 pounds) per week.

Critical Thinking Questions
1. How do you think Erica's attitude influences her treatment?
2. Why do you think control is an important issue for Erica?

A complete patient care plan includes several other diagnoses and interventions.
Diet, dietitian; *MD*, physician; *Nsg*, nursing staff; *Psy*, psychologist.

SLEEP–WAKE DISORDERS

Sleeping patterns and routines change as we grow older. The 16 hours of nightly sleep required by infants dwindle to less than 8 hours by adulthood. The afternoon naps of childhood are soon replaced by the all-day demands of school and work. The ritual of the bedtime hour disappears altogether. For many people, by the time they have reach adulthood, their sleeping habits may have changed dramatically. Most young adults have few difficulties with sleeping. However, sleep disorders begin to occur more frequently as adults grow older. By older adulthood, it is unusual to have a full night of uninterrupted sleep.

Although no one knows exactly why we must sleep every night, researchers have found that sleep serves several purposes. During sleep, body functions and metabolic rate slow. The workload on the heart decreases. Muscles relax, and the body conserves energy during sleep. One theory states that sleep is important for the renewal and repair of body cells and tissues. Sleep also "appears to be a critical cycle of brain activity important for learning, memory, and behavioural adaptation" (Potter, Perry, Stockert, et al., 2019).

Dreaming is also important to good health. Dreaming helps us to gain insights, solve problems, work through emotional reactions, and prepare for the future. Many cultures place great meaning in dreams and use them to cope with the problems of everyday life.

Sleep occurs in cycles of about 24 hours, depending on each individual's personal body rhythms. There are two

CRITICAL THINKING

It has been said that dreams are the result of reflection or suggestion.
• What do you think is meant by this statement?
• Do you believe that dreams have meanings? Why or why not?

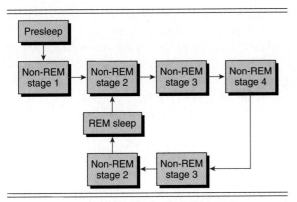

Fig. 23.3 Normal adult sleep cycle. *REM*, Rapid eye movement. (From Wold, G. [2012]. *Basic geriatric nursing* [5th ed.]. Mosby.)

phases to sleep: non–rapid eye movement (NREM) sleep and rapid eye movement (REM) sleep. NREM sleep is divided into four stages.

The average adult's sleep pattern begins with a presleep period, lasting about 10 to 30 minutes. During this time, a gradual drowsiness develops until the individual "drops off to sleep" or enters stage 1 of NREM sleep. As the sleeper moves through each stage of NREM, the quality of sleep becomes deeper. During stage 4, the sleeper is most difficult to arouse. After reaching stage 4, the sleep pattern reverses itself and the sleeper moves back through stage 3 into stage 2, in which REM sleep takes place. Figure 23.3 illustrates the normal adult sleep cycle and its stages. If the sleeper is interrupted or awakened at any time during the cycle, they must return to stage 1 and begin the process again. If the disturbances occur frequently enough, the individual will experience the signs and symptoms of sleep deprivation. Everyone has an occasional poor night's sleep. For people with sleeping disorders, however, this experience becomes an unwelcome and unwanted way of life.

A **sleep–wake disorder** is a condition or problem that repeatedly disrupts an individual's pattern of sleep. There are many different types of sleep–wake disorder. The core feature shared by all of them is daytime distress. Problems with sleep are common in modern societies where the pace of life is fast and demanding. Sleep disorders occur more frequently in older individuals, but all age groups are affected.

Children are especially vulnerable to sleep disorders because the "lack of restorative sleep can compromise the physical and emotional health of children and interfere with normal growth and development" (Gerber, 2014). Recommended nightly hours of sleep differ by age (Box 23.4). Children (and adults) who are well rested are easy to awaken in the morning and remain active and alert throughout the day.

The diagnosis of a sleep–wake disorder is based on a thorough history, physical examination, and the results of several tests. A **polysomnogram** monitors the patient's electrophysical responses during sleep. It includes measurements such as brain wave activity (electroencephalogram), muscle movement (electromyogram), and eye movements (electrooculogram). Many medical centers have specially

designed sleep laboratories in which patients can be monitored for the quantity, quality, and characteristics of their sleep.

Often sleep–wake disorders coexist with other medical and mental health disorders that directly influence the sleep–wake cycle. Thus, a careful patient examination is required to assess all aspects of the clinical presentation.

Insomnia Disorder

Insomnia disorder is a disorder of a severe impairment due to an inability to fall asleep (**insomnia**), maintain a sound sleep, and/or return to sleep after awakening early. To be diagnosed, an individual must experience this condition at least three times per week for a period of at least 3 months.

The diagnosis of insomnia disorder may coexist with other mental health and medical conditions (e.g., major depressive disorder, physical pain, chronic obstructive pulmonary disease [COPD]) that also lead to poor quality of sleep.

There are three classical manifestations of insomnia disorder: *initial insomnia* (difficulty initiating sleep), *middle insomnia* (awakening during the night), and *late insomnia* (early morning awakening without the ability to return to sleep). Insomnia is relatively rare in childhood and adolescence. Approximately 30 to 40% of adults have problems with insomnia, and the incidence increases with age. It occurs more often in women and usually begins in young adulthood or middle age with an initial period of poor sleep that progressively worsens over a period of months.

Hypersomnolence Disorder

Hypersomnolence disorder is an excessive sleepiness despite sleeping at night. Commonly called *hypersomnia*, the condition usually begins between 15 and 25 years of age, slowly progresses over a period of weeks or months, and then becomes chronic and stable. **Hypersomnia** is characterized by prolonged sleep episodes or frequent daytime sleeping that occurs daily for at least 3 months. Excessive sleepiness severe enough to cause significant impairment of daily living activities and that is not caused by any other physical or mental health disorder is also characteristic of hypersomnia.

In persons with hypersomnia, nighttime sleep may last from 8 to 12 hours, but it is often followed by difficulty awakening in the morning and excessive sleepiness during normal waking hours. During the day, these people may take long naps that last for more than 1 hour. After awakening, individuals do not feel refreshed or alert.

Hypersomnia can lead to significant distress in functioning. The long sleep and difficult morning awakenings make it nearly impossible to meet morning business or social obligations. Low levels of alertness result in decreased

BOX 23.4 Needs for Sleep
Adults need 7 to 9 hours a night
Ages 10 to 17 need 8.5 to 9.25 hours a night
Ages 5 to 10 need 10 to 11 hours a night

concentration, poor efficiency, and few memories of the day's events. Unplanned episodes of sleep can lead to embarrassing and even dangerous situations, such as falling asleep while driving. Daytime sleepiness can result in automatic behaviour in which tasks are carried out with little or no memory of having done them. Sadly, people with excessive sleepiness are often thought of as being lazy or indifferent.

Narcolepsy

Narcolepsy is an uncommon condition that disrupts the normal sleep–wake cycle. It is a chronic neurological condition in which an individual has repeated overwhelming attacks (lapses) of sleep or napping throughout most days at least three times per week for a period of at least 3 months. The severity of symptoms may change over time, but it is a chronic, lifelong condition once symptoms emerge (Psychology Today, 2017). This condition also comes with at least one of the three following symptoms:

1. **Cataplexy**, a sudden loss of muscle tone while a person is awake that leads to weakness and a loss of voluntary muscle that lasts for seconds to minutes at least a few times per month. It is often triggered by sudden, strong emotions such as laughter, fear, anger, stress, or excitement. In some patients (e.g., children), the onset of this disorder may happen without being triggered by any emotions, but just by grimacing or jaw-opening with tongue thrusting.
2. *Hypocretin deficiency* in the cerebrospinal fluid (CSF): Hypocretin is a neuropeptide that regulates arousal, wakefulness, and appetite; it is needed to help us stay awake. Individuals with narcolepsy experience an autoimmune loss of cells that produce hypocretin; 99% of these people carry the human leukocyte antigen HLA-DQB1*06:02 (vs. 12 to 38% in the general population). Human leukocyte antigens are responsible for immune system regulation.
3. *Short REM sleep latency* less than or equal to 15 minutes (as registered by nocturnal sleep polysomnography): Normal adult REM sleep latency is 50 to 150 minutes. *Sleep latency*, also known as *sleep-onset latency* (SOL), is the amount of time it takes for an individual to fall asleep when the light is switched off. *REM sleep latency* is the amount of time it takes for a sleeping individual to have a first episode of REM after sleep onset. Thus, REM sleep latency depends on SOL (Shrivastava, Jung, Saadat, et al., 2014).

Symptoms usually become apparent during adolescence, but a careful history often reveals a pattern of sleepiness dating back to preschool years. The onset of the disorder often follows a change in the person's sleep–wake schedule or a very stressful event.

The periods of sleepiness in narcolepsy are described as irresistible. Individuals fall asleep for about 10 to 20 minutes in any situation, whether it is appropriate to sleep or not. Episodes occur from two to six times per day. Some people with narcolepsy can "fight off" their sleep attacks, whereas others plan naps throughout the day to manage the condition.

At times, the sleepiness can be so severe and rapid that an individual may continue to carry out their activities in a semi-automatic way, without noticing the consequences. About 20 to 60% of individuals experience vivid hallucinations (Psychology Today, 2017) just before falling asleep or just after awakening. Vivid dreams and nightmares often happen as well. About 20 to 50% of patients experience sleep paralysis, during which they awake but cannot move or talk. However, many people in the general population may also experience this same paralysis when they are sleep-deprived (Monderer, Harris & Thorpy, 2014).

Narcolepsy is a long-term condition that requires careful and ongoing management.

Breathing-Related Sleep Disorders

Breathing-related sleep disorders are defined as sleep disruptions caused by abnormal ventilation during sleep. These disorder are discussed next.

Obstructive Sleep Apnea/Hypopnea

Obstructive sleep apnea/hypopnea is the most common breathing-related sleep disorder. During sleep, a partially obstructed upper airway causes periods of **apnea** (absence of airflow), **hypopnea** (reduction in airflow), or both that repeatedly awaken the individual. Sleeping patterns are characterized by periods of loud snoring, followed by periods of apnea lasting as long as 90 seconds. The apneic event ends when the individual gasps, moans, mumbles, or shakes with loud, air-gulping snores. Although the person may not fully awaken during these events, sleep is disrupted enough to result in excessive sleepiness during the day. People who are extremely overweight are at risk for this disorder. The term *Pickwickian syndrome* was coined to describe this disorder, based on an obese character in a Charles Dickens novel.

Central Sleep Apnea

Central sleep apnea is a condition characterized by periodic breathing, with periods of apnea and hypopnea. These periods may occur five or more times in an hour, leaving sleep fragmented with many wakenings during the night. It is thought that central sleep apneas are disorders of the respiratory system related to the control of ventilation.

Sleep-Related Hypoventilation

Sleep-related hypoventilation includes periods of decreased respirations resulting in elevated carbon dioxide levels in the blood. The individual is frequently awakened from sleep, and headaches or excessive sleepiness upon arising may be present due to low oxygen and high levels of the waste product, carbon dioxide. It is an uncommon disorder that is often associated with physical problems.

Circadian Rhythm Sleep–Wake Disorder

Circadian rhythm sleep–wake disorder is a persistent pattern of sleep disruption that results from a mismatch between personal body rhythms and environmental demands. This disorder is most often seen in persons who do shift work or must travel frequently.

Parasomnias

Parasomnias are sleep disorders that are characterized by abnormal behavioural or physical events during sleep. These conditions are a strong reminder that sleep and wakefulness are not mutually exclusive, and that much of our brain and body activity continues when we sleep.

Non–Rapid Eye Movement Sleep Arousal Disorders

Individuals who have NREM sleep arousal disorders suffer from serious distress and impairment due to recurrent and amnestic episodes of **sleepwalking** (rising from the bed while asleep and walking around with no ability to respond to others), **sleep terror** (terror or panic arousals from sleep without the ability to respond to others or to be comforted by others), or both. Usually, the individual does not awaken but continues to sleep. Sleep terror is often accompanied by the compulsion to escape and by intense autonomic signs of severe anxiety, such as increased heart rate, respiration, sweating, dilation of pupils, and tense muscle tone.

NREM sleep arousal disorders usually happen in childhood and diminish with age. Sleepwalking happens more often than sleep terror. From 10 to 30% of children have had at least one episode of sleepwalking, and 2 to 3% sleepwalk often (APA, 2015, p. 48).

Nightmare Disorder

Individuals with a diagnosis of nightmare disorder suffer from impairment caused by repeated extremely dysphoric and well-remembered, detailed dreams about their effort to survive a dramatic event. Upon awakening, they immediately become well oriented and alert, but their dysphoric feelings may continue, contributing to distress and lack of sleep (APA, 2015).

Nightmares can be diagnosed as an independent disorder or as comorbid with other medical conditions (e.g., coronary heart disease, cancer, pain) or other mental health disorders (e.g., post-traumatic stress disorder [PTSD], schizophrenia, anxiety) (APA, 2015, p, 56).

Rapid Eye Movement Sleep Behaviour Disorder

Individuals with this diagnosis suffer from impairment caused by repeated awakening during the REM phase of sleep, accompanied by vocalization, some complex motor behaviour (which may lead to injury), or both. These individuals are well oriented and alert upon awakening (APA, 2015).

Restless Legs Syndrome

Restless legs syndrome (RLS) is a sensorimotor, neurological sleep disorder that is characterized by an urge to move the legs in response to intolerable sensations (e.g., creeping, crawling, tingling, burning, itching). It is also called *Willis-Ekbom disease*. Individuals with the disorder suffer from significant distress and impairment due to this urge to move their legs. The urge increases during times of rest and is intensified in evenings or at night, and moving the legs actually relieves the urge (APA, 2015, p. 101). The distress comes from the poor quality of sleep (fragmentation and lack of sleep) that results from these disturbances.

Substance/Medication-Induced Sleep Disorder

Individuals with substance/medication-induced sleep disorder (APA, 2015, p. 102) suffer from significant distress and impairment due to serious disturbances in their sleep, and there is evidence that these disturbances are the result of the consumption of or withdrawal from substances or medications.

Other Sleep Disorders

An unusual sleep disorder is gaining clinical attention. **Nocturnal sleep-related eating disorder (NSRED)** involves binge eating during sleep. The person has impaired consciousness while preparing food and eating it, with little or no memory of these actions the next morning (APA, 2015, p. 48). During the sleep–eating episode, the individual quickly consumes a bizarre selection of high-calorie foods and nonfood items, such as cleaning products, animal food, or cigarettes. Diagnosis is difficult because of the patient's inability to remember or their embarrassment.

Other sleep disorders can be traced to specific causes. These include sleep disorders related to a general medical condition, a mental health condition, or the use of chemical substances. Sleep disorders can result from many physical problems. The presence of a neurological, cardiovascular, or respiratory disorder or an infection has a significant effect on sleep. Pain from musculoskeletal disease and anxiety related to coughing or difficult breathing can lead to prolonged periods of inadequate sleep.

Many mental health disorders are associated with sleep-related problems. Insomnia or hypersomnia is often seen in patients with major depressive, mood, anxiety, adjustment, somatoform, panic, and personality disorders. During flare-ups of schizophrenia, people have significant periods of insomnia.

Sleeping problems frequently occur during substance use (intoxication) or periods of withdrawal. Many prescription medications are associated with sleep disorders, including medications that treat hypertension, cardiac problems, inflammatory processes, neurological conditions, and respiratory diseases. Chemicals such as alcohol, cocaine, and various street drugs affect sleep. Even the medications prescribed to induce sleep (hypnotics and sedatives) can produce unwanted effects on the sleep cycle. Thus nurses and other care providers must be aware of how various medications and chemicals affect each patient's sleep.

Guidelines for Intervention

The first step in the treatment of sleep disorders is to teach prevention. Because many people do not regularly receive a good night's sleep, the need for good sleep hygiene habits is great. One of the best treatments for insomnia is to establish and maintain a regular sleeping routine by preparing both body and mind for the night's upcoming rest. Health care providers are in ideal positions to educate patients about the importance of receiving enough quality sleep. Box 23.5 offers several suggestions for developing effective sleep practices.

The main goal of care is to assist the patient in obtaining a restful night's sleep. Short-term goals focus on helping

BOX 23.5   Sleep Hygiene Strategies

Set a regular bedtime and wake-up time, 7 days per week.

Exercise daily; however, vigorous exercise too close to bedtime may make falling asleep difficult.

Schedule time to wind down and relax before bed.

Avoid worrying when trying to fall asleep.

Guard against nighttime interruptions. Earplugs may help with a noisy partner. Heavy window shades help to screen out light. Create a comfortable bed.

Maintain a cool temperature in the room. A warm bath or warm drink before bed often helps.

Excessive hunger or fullness may interfere with sleep. Avoid eating large meals before bed. If hungry, a light carbohydrate snack may be helpful.

Avoid caffeinated drinks, excessive fluid intake, stimulating drugs, and excessive alcohol in the evening and before bedtime.

Excessive daytime napping may make it difficult for some people to fall asleep at night.

Do not eat, read, work, or watch television in bed. The bed should be used only for sleep and sex.

Maintain a reasonable weight. Excessive weight may result in daytime fatigue and sleep apnea.

Get out of bed and engage in other activities if unable to fall asleep.

From Stuart, G. W. (2013). *Principles and practice of psychiatric nursing* (10th ed.). Mosby.

patients establish a regular and healthy sleep pattern. Nursing diagnoses or problem statements for sleep disorders include insomnia, high risk for injury, fatigue, disturbed thought processes, ineffective coping, ineffective breathing pattern, and deficient knowledge related to sleep hygiene practices.

Therapeutic interventions are aimed at promoting comfort, controlling physical disturbances, and maintaining a quiet, restful environment. Hypnotics (sleeping pills) may be administered as ordered but only after all other methods of inducing sleep have failed. Special care must be taken when administering hypnotics or sedatives to older persons because they react strongly to these classes of medications and adverse effects are common.

Research has demonstrated that morning bright-light therapy improves sleeping patterns by helping to re-establish natural biological rhythms. Other studies have revealed that the body has a naturally occurring sleep hormone, called *melatonin,* which helps to control our biological clocks. These findings may prove to be promising developments in the treatment of sleep disorders.

As a care provider you need to be aware of the importance of keeping the patient's environment dark during sleep and brightly lit during daylight hours. Read about new developments in the treatment of sleeping disorders, and apply them to yourself and your patients. We are learning more every day about the mysteries of sleep.

KEY POINTS

- Body image is the collection of perceptions, thoughts, feelings, and behaviours that relate to body size and appearance.
- An eating disorder is an ongoing disturbance in behaviours associated with the ingestion of food.
- The criteria for a diagnosis of an eating disorder are as follows: the problem interferes with a person's quality of daily life; the person does not maintain a normal body weight; there is a distorted significance placed on body weight and shape; and the person engages in inappropriate episodes of eating.
- One of the most serious eating disorders is anorexia nervosa, a condition in which an individual refuses to maintain a normal body weight because of an intense fear of becoming fat.
- Bulimia nervosa is a disorder of binge eating and the use of inappropriate methods to prevent weight gain.
- Binge eating disorder is the consuming (within a certain time) of an amount of food that is definitely larger than most individuals would eat in similar circumstances.
- Untreated eating disorders have a high mortality rate.
- Obesity is defined as an excess of body weight. Although not officially classified as an eating disorder, it presents health problems for a great number of people.
- The main therapeutic goals for treating all eating disorders are to establish eating behaviours that promote health and

- to assist patients in identifying and coping with the issues that led to their inappropriate eating behaviours.
- During sleep, body functions and metabolic rate slow. Muscles relax, and the body conserves energy. Renewal and repair of body cells and tissues occur. Sleep also appears to be a critical cycle of brain activity important for learning, memory, and behavioural adaptation.
- Dreaming allows us to gain insights, solve problems, work through emotional reactions, and prepare for the future.
- A sleep–wake disorder is a condition or challenge that repeatedly disrupts an individual's pattern of sleep.
- Dyssomnias are characterized by abnormalities in the amount, quality, or timing of sleep.
- Symptoms of insomnia include a preoccupation with the inability to sleep, which sets up a cycle in which one becomes negatively conditioned toward sleep.
- Sleep disorders characterized by abnormal behavioural or physical events during sleep are called *parasomnias.*
- Sleep disorders can also result from medical, psychological, or medication-induced conditions.
- Therapeutic interventions to promote sleep are to promote comfort, control physical disturbances, and maintain a quiet, restful environment.

ADDITIONAL LEARNING RESOURCES

Go to your Evolve website (http://evolve.elsevier.com/Canada/Morrison-Valfre/) for additional online resources, including the online Study Guide for additional learning activities to help you master this chapter content.

CRITICAL THINKING QUESTIONS

1. What are the major characteristics and risks of anorexia nervosa?
2. Which of the eating disorders are visible, and which ones are often difficult to detect?
3. How do you calculate a person's body mass index (BMI), and what are the six Canadian BMI categorizations?
4. The wife of an overweight patient who is being seen in the sleep clinic states that her husband snores terribly at night and that she has to shake him to get him to stop. The patient reports having a headache upon wakening and often falling asleep during the day when he sits for long periods. The patient also complains of poor concentration and irritability. What are potential reasons for the patient's daytime symptoms?

REFERENCES

American Psychiatric Association (APA). (2013). *Diagnostic and statistical manual of mental disorders* (5th ed.). American Psychiatric Publishing.

American Psychiatric Association (APA). (2015). *DSM-5 selections: Sleep-wake disorders.* American Psychiatric Publishing.

Arcelus, J., Mitchell, A. J., Wales, J., et al. (2011). Mortality rates in patients with anorexia nervosa and other eating disorders: A meta-analysis of 36 studies. *Archives of General Psychiatry, 68*(7), 724–731. https://doi.org/10.1001/archgenpsychiatry.2011.74

Canadian Cancer Society. (2020). *Breast cancer statistics.* http://www.cancer.ca/en/cancer-information/cancer-type/breast/statistics/?region=on

Eating Disorder Hope. (2018). *Refeeding patients with anorexia nervosa: What does research show?* https://www.eatingdisorderhope.com/information/anorexia/refeeding-patients-with-anorexia-nervosa-what-does-research-show

Gerber, L. (2014). Sleep deprivation in children: A growing public health concern. *Nursing, 44*(4), 50–54. https://doi.org/10.1097/01.NURSE.0000441881.87748.90

Government of Canada. (2016). *Canadian guidelines for body weight classification in adults—quick reference tool for professionals.* https://www.canada.ca/en/health-canada/services/food-nutrition/healthy-eating/healthy-weights/canadian-guidelines-body-weight-classification-adults/quick-reference-tool-professionals.html

Hockenberry, M., & Wilson, D. (2014). *Wong's nursing care of infants and children* (10th ed.). Mosby.

Loth, K. A., Mond, J., Wall, M., et al. (2011). Weight status and emotional well-being: Longitudinal findings from Project EAT. *Journal of Pediatric Psychology, 36*(2), 216–225. https://doi.org/10.1093/jpepsy/jsq026

Monderer, R., Harris, S., & Thorpy, M. (2014). Neurologic aspects of sleep medicine. In M. J. Aminoff, & S. A. Josephson (Eds.), *Aminoff's neurology and general medicine* (5th ed.) (pp. 1033–1065). Academic Press. https://doi.org/10.1016/C2012-0-03031-1

Nakai, Y., Nin, K., & Noma, S. (2014). Eating disorder symptoms among Japanese female students in 1982, 1992, and 2002. *Psychiatry Research, 219*(1), 151–156. https://doi.org/10.1016/j.psychres.2014.05.018

National Initiative for Eating Disorders (NIED). (2016). *About eating disorders in Canada.* https://nied.ca/about-eating-disorders-in-canada/

National Initiative for Eating Disorders (NIED). (2017). *Canadian research on eating disorders.* https://nied.ca/research-on-ed/

Obesity Canada. (2019). *Report card on access to obesity treatment for adults in Canada.* 2019 https://obesitycanada.ca/resources/reportcard/

Potter, P. A., Perry, A. G., Stockert, P., et al. (2019). *Essentials for nursing practice* (9th ed.). Mosby.

Psychology Today. (2017). *Narcolepsy.* https://www.psychologytoday.com/ca/conditions/narcolepsy

Rikani, A. A., Choudhry, Z., Choudhry, A. M., et al. (2013). A critique of the literature on etiology of eating disorders. *Annals of Neurosciences, 20*(4), 157–161. https://doi.org/10.5214/ans.0972.7531.200409

Shrivastava, D., Jung, S., Saadat, M., et al. (2014). How to interpret the results of a sleep study. *Journal of Community Hospital Internal Medicine Perspectives, 4*(5), 24983. https://doi.org/10.3402/jchimp.v4.24983

Wharton, S., Lau, D.C.W., Vallis, M., et al. (2020). Obesity in adults: a clinical practice guideline. *Canadian Medical Association Journal, 192*(31), E875–E891. https://doi.org/10.1503/cmaj.191707

Wilkinson, G. (2018). Richard Morton and anorexia nervosa—Psychiatry in history. *British Journal of Psychiatry, 213*(4). 626–626. https://doi.org/10.1192/bjp.2018.161

24

Dissociative Disorders

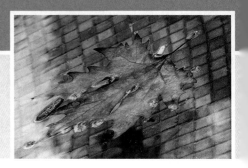

OBJECTIVES

Upon completion of this chapter, the student will be able to:

1. Understand the meaning and components of the term *self-concept*.
2. Describe the continuum of self-concept responses.
3. Compare the development of self-concept throughout the life cycle.
4. Classify the main characteristics of dissociative disorders.
5. Describe three types of dissociative disorders.
6. Explain the outstanding feature of a dissociative identity (multiple personality) disorder.
7. State the main goal of treatment for patients with dissociative disorders.
8. Plan three nursing diagnoses (problem statements) for patients with dissociative disorders.
9. Develop a care plan for a patient who has been diagnosed with a dissociative disorder.

OUTLINE

KEY TERMS

amnesia (ăm-NĒ-zhă) (p. 289)
depersonalization (p. 289)
derealization (p. 289)
dissociation (dĬ-SŌ-sē-Ā-shun) (p. 288)
dissociative (dĬ-SŌ-sē-ă-tĭv) **disorder** (p. 288)
dissociative identity disorder (DID) (p. 291)
dissociative trance disorder (p. 291)
fugue (fyūg) (p. 289)
identity diffusion (p. 288)

identity disturbance due to prolonged and intense
  coercive persuasion (p. 291)
personality fusing (p. 288)
personal identity (p. 287)
personality map (p. 287)
role performances (p. 287)
self-concept (p. 286)
self-esteem (p. 287)
self-ideal (p. 287)
trance (p. 291)

Human beings differ from animals in a significant way: they have a concept of *self*. As children grow, they learn to identify and define themselves as individuals. They develop a picture (a point of view) of who they are. Then they use that picture as a framework for perceiving, experiencing, and evaluating the world. This point of view becomes one's self-concept.

Self-concept is defined as all the attitudes, notions, beliefs, and convictions that make up a person's self-know-ledge. According to Stuart (2013), "it includes the individual's perceptions of personal characteristics and abilities, inter-actions with other people and the environment, values, asso-ciated experiences and objects, and goals and ideals."

The development of self-concept is influenced by many factors. The culture into which an individual is born and the society in which one lives have a strong influence on self-con-cept. The attitudes and beliefs of parents, siblings, and other significant people influence how an individual defines them-selves. The experiences of life also shape and influence one's picture of the self.

Self-concept is the frame of reference through which people view the world. It is the sum of several components: body image (the attitudes and feelings one has for one's body), **self-esteem** (an individual's judgement of their own worth), **self-ideal** (personal standards of how one should behave), **personal identity** (composite of behavioural traits and characteristics by which one is recognized as an individual), and **role performances** (socially expected behavioural patterns). All of these parts of an individual fuse and blend over time into the unique characteristics called self-concept.

CONTINUUM OF SELF-CONCEPT RESPONSES

People behave in a manner based in large part on their self-concepts. The range of behavioural responses relating to self-concept can be seen as occurring on a continuum. At the adaptive end, a healthy self-concept leads one toward self-actualization. Low self-concept results in maladaptive behavioural responses as individuals struggle to define who they are (Fig. 24.1).

The Healthy Personality

Persons with healthy personalities are able to effectively perceive and function within their world (Fortinash & Holoday-Worret, 2011). They have achieved a sense of peace and harmony within themselves that allows them to successfully cope with life's anxieties, traumas, and crises. A realistic self-ideal and a clear personal identity help to provide a sense of purpose and direction in life. High self-esteem and confidence levels provide the strength to handle anxieties and learn from life's highs and lows. Socially, such individuals are satisfied with the roles they play in society. They have the ability to intimately relate to others and share themselves without fear. In short, individuals with healthy personalities are able to struggle with life's challenges while feeling good about living.

CRITICAL THINKING

Using the five components of a healthy personality described in the text, assess yourself.
- How do your results compare with the description of a person with a healthy personality?

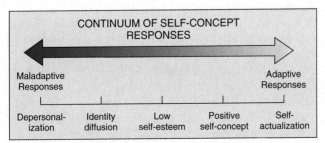

Fig. 24.1 Continuum of self-concept responses.

SELF-CONCEPT THROUGHOUT THE LIFE CYCLE

Self-concept develops over time, shaped by the influences within one's environment. The theorist Erik Erikson, in describing his eight stages of human development, stated that a psychosocial crisis or core task must be resolved for further personality development. As each task is completed, one's self-concept is affected. Mastery of core tasks builds self-confidence, worth, and esteem (Hockenberry & Wilson, 2014). If, however, one is unable to cope with a core task, ineffective or maladaptive behaviours result. This process, according to Erikson, continues throughout life.

Self-Concept in Childhood

Infants do not view themselves as separate from the rest of the world. Only after a period of time do they begin to distinguish themselves as different from their mothers. Infants learn to *trust* others when their needs are consistently met. After a series of social experiences, they develop stable relationships and learn to feel good about themselves. Rejection by significant others at this time has a strong negative effect on an individual's self-concept.

Toddlers' tasks are to explore the limits of their abilities, and these tasks include assessing the effects of their behaviours on others. Toddlers become independent by exploring their environments and testing their capabilities. They develop autonomy and a sense of self by experimenting with a variety of behaviours. Actions that get results are effective, even if inappropriate, and they are added to the general knowledge of the child. Behaviours that are not rewarded or do not get results are discarded. In this way, children learn about "right and wrong" and then use this information as a framework for their self-ideal. When parental reactions are routine and consistent, children develop a stable sense of who they are and a stable self-concept. When the reactions of significant others change or differ, children can become confused and have trouble establishing a positive identity and healthy self-concept.

School-age children become aware of different perspectives on life. They learn about social norms, peer pressures, and moral issues. Skill building and broadening social relationships keep them occupied with self-evaluations. Self-concept continues to develop as school-age children assess their skills and interactions with others and form mental pictures of themselves. If the picture is positive, the move into adolescence is generally graceful, but if self-concept is low or threatened, adolescence can be filled with anxiety and turmoil.

Self-Concept in Adolescence

By the early teen years, the comfortable self-concept of childhood is challenged. As adolescents mature, they begin to develop a more complex picture of themselves. Self-concept becomes more individual and based on one's special characteristics rather than on similarities shared by others. Thinking becomes more abstract, and much self-reflection is needed to digest all the physical, emotional, and social changes that are taking place at these times.

During adolescence, self-concept is influenced by many things. *Relationships* with family and peers play an important role in helping to define teens' confidence levels. The development of a *sexual identity* and the adjustment to a new adult body image must be included in the new concept of self. The struggle is to *define oneself* by combining previous roles and new emotions into a reasonably consistent and pleasing sense of self. Without the love, nurturing, and guidance of concerned adults, many teens do not finish the task of developing a comfortable self-concept. They become ill prepared to assume the many responsibilities of adult life because efforts to find themselves continue.

Self-Concept in Adulthood

Adults with strong, positive self-concepts can freely explore their environments because they have a background of success and effectiveness. Positive experiences further enhance self-concept, and the cycle of learning, succeeding, and growth repeats itself. Refer back to Box 15.2 to review the characteristics of a successful adult.

If one's self-concept is low or negative, individuals develop views of themselves as inadequate or unable. They can become easily threatened, which in turn increases anxiety levels. High anxiety forces them to become preoccupied with defending themselves. Soon this cycle becomes a way of life. Individuals find themselves caught in the trap of looking only at the negative or "down" side of life. The cycle of few successes and negative reinforcement becomes established, which reinforces a poor self-concept. Most adults, however, function somewhere between these two extremes.

Self-Concept in Older Adulthood

Self-concept is established in childhood, developed in adolescence, strengthened in adulthood, and refined in older adulthood. In later life, many occurrences and situations can threaten a positive self-concept. **Ageism,** the stereotyping of older persons as feeble, dependent, and nonproductive, contributes to older persons' self-concepts. Threats to the stability of one's lifestyle, such as changes in occupation, social standing, or environment, often lead to changes in self-concept. Health care providers can enhance older patients' feelings of self-worth through active listening and demonstration of concern.

DISSOCIATIVE DISORDERS

Dissociation is an attempt to cope with deep-seated emotional anxiety or distress. **Identity diffusion** is the failure to bring various childhood identifications into an effective adult personality. Individuals with identity diffusion are not sure who they really are because they have been unable to build a "picture" of themselves. They drift through life, unable to set a course or steer around obstacles. Identity diffusion is one criterion for developing borderline personality disorder.

Although people with identity diffusion feel emptiness and anxiety, they often exploit others. Feelings of empathy are often lacking. This leads to problems with intimacy and a lack of caring. Because the self-ideal is confused, moral codes or standards of behaviour are often missing (Keltner & Steele, 2014). Frequently, they are so desperate to define themselves that they attempt to bind their self-concepts to another. This type of identity diffusion is called **personality fusing.** When behaviours interfere with an individual's ability to function, a mental health challenge exists. The mental health issues that relate to anxiety and self-concept are called *dissociative disorders.*

Characteristics

Dissociation is a discontinuation of the connection between consciousness, identity, emotions, memories, perceptions, and even motor control and behaviour (American Psychiatric Association [APA], 2018). It is a complex neuropsychological process that ranges from normal, everyday experiences to those that disrupt daily living. Dissociation is a common, natural experience. Examples of normal dissociations are daydreaming or becoming so absorbed in an activity that one loses a sense of time and surroundings. Dissociation is also used as a coping mechanism to protect us from trauma. The victim of a mugging or severe accident is often unable to remember events surrounding the incident. Individuals who were abused in childhood may have only a few small, unrelated memories.

Children dissociate more easily than do adults. Faced with overwhelming abuse or trauma, children often psychologically flee their distresses by blocking emotionally damaging information from awareness. Dissociation, when routinely used as a defence in childhood, can later grow into a dissociative disorder. Thus, dissociative disorders are often found following an experience of trauma. Many of the symptoms create confusion and embarrassment and, as a result, the desire to hide them.

A **dissociative disorder** is a disturbance in the normally interacting functions of consciousness: identity, memory, emotion, perception, behaviour, and sense of self (APA, 2018). The most anxiety-producing aspects of the self are walled off or split from the remainder of the personality in an attempt to cope with severe anxiety or emotional trauma.

Although dissociative disorders were once considered rare, new evidence reveals that they are becoming more common, especially in those who were neglected or abused in childhood. Dissociative disorders are diagnosed more frequently in women.

In countries such as Japan, England, and France, the incidence of diagnosed dissociative disorders is low. In other cultures, dissociative trances are a part of religious or spiritual practices. Devout people enter into altered states or trances in which they interact with spirits or beings. Thus care providers who work with patients from different cultural backgrounds need to be alert to the customs and practices of their patients' culture. Several culturally defined mental health disorders involving dissociative states are described in Table 24.1.

TABLE 24.1 Cultural Aspects: Culturally Defined Mental Health Disorders With Dissociative States

Disorder	Culture(s)	Description
Amok	Malaysia, Laos, Philippines, Polynesia, Puerto Rico, Navajo	Period of brooding followed by outbursts of aggressive, violent behaviour; found only in males
Ataque de nervios	Latin American	Uncontrollable shouting, crying, fainting, and suicidal gestures after stressful event
Falling out	Southern United States, Caribbean groups	Sudden collapse; eyes are open, but individual is unable to see; hears and understands but feels powerless to move
Latah	Japan (imu), Philippines (mali-mali), Thailand	Excessive reactions to sudden fright; trancelike behaviour with command obedience, echolalia
Pibloktoq	Arctic and subarctic Inuit	Extreme excitement and irrational behaviour, followed by seizures and coma lasting up to 12 hr
Qigong psychotic reaction	Chinese	Acute episode of psychotic behaviours after folk practice of qigong, the exercise of vital energy
Shin-byung	Korean	Anxiety and somatic complaints that progress to dissociation and possession by ancestral spirits
Spell	Some people of African descent, some Europeans, Americans from the southern United States	Trance in which communication with deceased relatives or spirits takes place
Zar	Egypt, Ethiopia, Iran, Sudan	Spirit possession that interferes with daily activities; may develop long-term relationship with spirit and withdraw from reality

Dissociative disorders arise from two sources. If the problem lies with memory or consciousness, then amnesia or **fugue** (inability to remember important personal events or travels) results. If the disturbance is with one's identity, parts of the self assume separate personalities (also called *alters*), and a dissociative identity disorder (formerly known as *multiple personality disorder*) is diagnosed (APA, 2018). Post-traumatic stress disorder (PTSD), although considered an anxiety disorder, is actually a recall of past traumatic events alternating with detachment or dissociation. Traumatic experiences are the basis of all dissociative disorders. Behaviours are the result of repeated splitting of traumatic memories. Just as the body walls off the infection of an abscess, the mind walls off the extreme distresses of trauma and anxiety. Three types of dissociative disorders are classified by the *Diagnostic and Statistical Manual of Mental Disorders*, fifth edition (*DSM-5*; APA, 2013). They are depersonalization/derealization disorder, dissociative amnesia, and dissociative identity disorder.

Depersonalization/Derealization Disorder

During an episode of depersonalization, one feels detached or unconnected to the self. The individual may feel like a robot, working on automatic. There may be a sensation of being an outside observer and of not being involved. **Depersonalization** is a response to severe anxiety associated with a blocking of awareness and a fading of reality. One is unable to tell the difference between internal and external stimuli because the self-concept becomes disorganized. It is a sense of being outside oneself, a detachment from the body, as

if watching a movie. The body takes on an unreal quality. The person may feel absent or like they are an external observer.

Derealization (also called *depersonalization*) involves a detachment and feelings of unreality in relation to one's surroundings. People may feel as if they are outside their bodies and watching events happening to them (APA, 2013).

Depersonalization and derealization serve as defence mechanisms. However, they do nothing to relieve the cause of the distress, so they soon become maladaptive behaviours. In cases in which they become mental health issues, individuals attempt to "escape" distress and anxiety by losing their identities. Table 24.2 lists the physical, emotional, intellectual, and behavioural characteristics of this behavioural pattern.

Depersonalization is commonly associated with other mental health disorders, including acute stress disorder, panic disorder, obsessive-compulsive disorder, and schizophrenia. These disorders can suddenly develop after a life-threatening event or develop slowly after years of distress.

Dissociative Amnesia and Dissociative Amnesia With Fugue

Amnesia is a loss of memory. Dissociative amnesia is characterized by an inability to remember personal information that cannot be explained by ordinary forgetfulness. It is an attempt to avoid extreme stress by blocking memories from consciousness. Individuals with dissociative amnesia usually have gaps in their ability to recall certain events (localized amnesia) during their childhood. Most of these memory lapses relate to extremely stressful events. For example, a rape victim often has no memory of the attack but still experiences

TABLE 24.2 Behaviours Associated With Depersonalization/Derealization

Areas of Functioning	Description
Affective (emotional)	Feels identity is lost Lacks sense of inner togetherness Unable to feel pleasure or pride Feelings of detachment, fear, insecurity, shame, unreality
Behavioural (social)	Affect blunted; emotionally unresponsive and passive; not lively or spontaneous Communications odd or difficult to follow Loss of drive, decision-making abilities, impulse control Social isolation and withdrawal
Cognitive (intellectual)	Confusion; distorted thinking and memory Impaired judgement; disoriented to time
Perceptual (physical)	Dreamlike experiences of world Difficulty telling self from others Disturbed body image and sexuality May experience auditory and visual hallucinations

Modified from Stuart, G. W. (2013). *Principles and practice of psychiatric nursing* (10th ed.). Mosby.

the emotional numbness and depression associated with the trauma. Sights, sounds, odours, and images can trigger emotional distresses long after the event has occurred. Actual memories are too painful to consider, so they stay submerged, walled off, but still capable of inflicting pain.

Individuals with *generalized amnesia* suffer a complete loss of their own history. Personal identity is temporarily lost, along with previous skills and knowledge.

Dissociative amnesia may be associated with the rare, but dramatic, *amnesic fugue*. Some episodes may resolve rapidly, and some may take years. The word *fugue* means an escape from reality. The main characteristic of dissociative fugue is sudden onset, which can be followed by making an unexpected trip to a place some distance from one's original location and the person having no memory of how they got there or of their return. A fugue occurs in response to an overwhelmingly stressful or traumatic event. It is an extreme expression of the fight-or-flight mechanism, engaged to protect the individual.

Persons with dissociative fugue may travel a distance ranging from only a few miles away from home to another continent away. Individuals behave quite normally during periods of travel but are confused about their personal identity, which is what frequently brings them to the attention of authorities. Some individuals during that time assume entirely new identities (or alters), complete with a

new occupation and new significant others. Unlike in dissociative identity disorder, these alters are not stable and will disappear when the episode is resolved. The following Case Study describes an interesting case of fugue.

These patients require high levels of emotional support. Patient safety becomes a primary therapeutic goal because suicide attempts are common. Although memory may be gone, the emotional distress remains. Patients' connections with other human beings are sometimes the only link on the road back to stable mental health.

CASE STUDY

Amy was only 3 years old when she was first abused by her father. By the age of 4, she was hiding whenever she heard his footsteps coming down the hall. At 6 years old, Amy slipped out the window to escape. On those occasions when he could not be avoided, Amy played a game in her mind in which she would fly away to a land where everyone was kind and carried out no evil. She would wish and dream and hope during those times, ignoring the pain and distress of being repeatedly molested.

By the time Amy was 13, she had run away from home. Luckily, she found a youth shelter early in her wanderings, where staff members were understanding and had a genuine interest in seeing Amy survive her adolescence. She stayed at the shelter for about 7 months, learning the skills needed for adulthood. Soon Amy became very efficient in coordinating and supervising the daily household events.

Because of her newly learned organizational abilities, Amy was offered a job as a teacher's assistant at the local elementary school. There she remained for many years. By the time she was 30 years old, Amy had buried the memories of her abuse and forgotten the pain of her childhood. She was married and looking forward to a bright future.

Amy's father became seriously ill the following year. He was alone and in need of care. After no communications with Amy for more than 20 years, he wrote to ask if he could come and live with Amy and her family.

The letter arrived, and Amy stared, horrified, at the return address. The rest is a blank.

Six months later, she remembered nothing more: not the trip to San Francisco, not the bus ride to Colorado, not even her new fiancé. Today she can hardly remember who she really is.

- What do you think happened after Amy read the return address on the letter?
- If Amy were admitted to your unit, what interventions would you include in the care plan?

During an actual fugue, few personality changes are noticeable. Individuals may be more friendly and outgoing, but their behaviours remain appropriate. After the return to the prefugue state, individuals may experience aggressive impulses, conflict, depression, guilt, and suicidal wishes. There may be loss of memory of the events that occurred during the time of the fugue. Recovery is usually rapid, but some amnesia may remain. Psychosocial care and emotional support are important elements in recovery.

Dissociative Identity Disorder

When stress or trauma is repeated and severe, the personality attempts to protect itself. Abused children use dissociation to escape and defend themselves from the anxiety, trauma, and helplessness of reality. Major studies have confirmed that dissociative identity disorders are the result of severe physical, sexual, or emotional abuse.

A **dissociative identity disorder (DID)** is defined as the presence of two or more distinct identities or personalities that repeatedly take control of the individual's behaviour. DID develops as a defence against prolonged and inescapable trauma. The diagnosis of DID, which was formerly called *multiple personality disorder,* occurs more often. Some mental health professionals think that this is a result of better diagnostic tools, whereas others think that DID is overdiagnosed or view it as a culturally related syndrome.

The essential features of DID are associated with the presence of other personalities, or alters, in one individual. Individuals with DID often have a personal history full of time losses, unexplained possessions or changes in relationships, out-of-body experiences, and the awareness of other parts of the self. There may be feelings that emotions and behaviours are "not mine." Patterns of speech and actions, over which one has no control, may emerge. A history of abuse or trauma is not always identified because emotions are deeply buried.

When different alters do emerge, each has its own way of thinking about and relating to the world. Each alter is unique and often represents the individual at different developmental stages. The identities may be helpful, controlling, seductive, or destructive, but each serves a specific *protective* purpose. They may differ in age, gender, knowledge, state of health, speech, and behaviours. The primary alter (called the *host*) may or may not be aware of the presence of the other alters. Usually the transition from one alter to the other is sudden and related to stress. Sometimes the identities cooperate with each other, but more often they attempt to take control and refuse to share knowledge with the others. Hostility or open conflict can result among the more powerful alters.

Individuals with dissociative issues, especially DID, often have symptoms of PTSD (nightmares, flashbacks, extreme startle responses). Other mental or physical health challenges are frequently present, especially with some of the identities found in DID. The main goal of treatment is to help the patient integrate or combine all personalities into one functional individual, capable of coping with life's stresses in a healthy manner.

The controversy about this diagnosis among health care providers still leads to misdiagnosis or delays with a proper diagnosis. It is not unusual for patients to be treated for psychotic symptoms before they have been properly diagnosed with DID. The main reason for the controversy is the relatively rare prevalence of DID and, as a result, poor preparation of clinicians to diagnose this disorder.

Trance

Trance is defined as a state resembling sleep, in which consciousness remains but voluntary movement is lost. Some minor stereotypical behaviour may be present (e.g., finger or upper body movement). In many cultures, trances are expressions of spiritual or religious beliefs. Cultural trances are entered into voluntarily and cause no distress or harm to the individuals. Channellers, psychics, spirit guides, shamans, and the like rarely suffer from mental impairments while in a trance. Cultural influences also affect the type of trance, the associated sensory disturbances, and the behaviours exhibited during the trance. Culturally normative trances involve signs, symptoms, and behaviours that are expected by other members of the culture. During these trances, individuals do not lose their identities. Possession trances involve the appearance of one or more distinct identities that direct the individual to perform sometimes complex behaviours and activities, such as culturally appropriate conversations, gestures, or facial expressions. Amnesia after either type of trance state (with or without the loss of identity) is not uncommon, but it occurs more frequently with possession trances.

It is important to note that as long as these trance presentations do not cause a significant distress or impairment, these are normal and often culturally appropriate behaviours.

Other Specified Dissociative Disorders

There are a few presentations in which patients experience significant distress and impairment but do not meet the full criteria for the three main dissociative disorders. This diagnosis is used in cases when a clinician chooses to specify why exactly the presentation does not match any of the dissociative disorder diagnoses.

For example, a **dissociative trance disorder** exists when trances cause clinically significant distress or impairment. This presentation is characterized by full or partial loss of sense of surroundings and a lack of response to environmental stimuli. It is not a part of the dissociative disorders described earlier and is distinct from an acceptable, healthy trance involved in cultural or religious practice. If trances cause a great deal of anxiety and distress in an individual, the person can likely benefit from psychotherapeutic interventions.

Another example is an **identity disturbance due to prolonged and intense coercive persuasion**. This distress condition of identity alteration may happen following an experience of intense coercive persuasion, such as brainwashing while under fear and/or torture in captivity by a totalitarian regime, sect, or terrorist organization.

Table 24.3 lists the basic characteristics of each dissociative disorder.

THERAPEUTIC INTERVENTIONS

Treatment for dissociative disorders involves long-term therapy in an outpatient setting. Hospitalization is required in only three situations:

1. When anger, aggression, or violence is directed toward self or others and presents a danger

TABLE 24.3   Dissociative Disorders

Disorder	Characteristics
Depersonalization/Derealization disorder	• Loss of connection to self and reality • Unable to tell difference between internal and external stimuli • World is a dream • Associated with other mental disorders
Dissociative amnesia	• Loss of memory of personal information; gaps in memory • Blocks extremely stressful events from consciousness • Symptoms cause significant functional impairment
Dissociative amnesia with dissociative fugue	• Rare • Sudden travel with inability to recall the past • Occurs as a response to overwhelming stressor • Behaves normally during travel but confused about own identity • May assume new autobiographical identification
Dissociative identity disorder	• Presence of two or more distinct personalities who control the host • Gaps in recalling everyday events • Symptoms cause a significant impairment in function • Related to extreme childhood trauma • Host may or may not be aware of other personalities (alters) • Alters can be in conflict with each other • Often associated with post-traumatic stress disorder
Other specified dissociative disorder	• *Trance*—Functional impairment caused by trances, a state in which consciousness remains but voluntary motor activity is lost • *Mixed dissociative symptoms*—Mild dissociations or alteration of identity • *Identity disturbance due to prolonged and intense coercive persuasion*—The person may question their identity following indoctrination while captive, recruitment by sect or terror organization, or after torture • *Acute dissociative reactions to stressful events*—Acute conditions (ranging in duration from a few hours to a month) characterized by constriction of consciousness, depersonalization, derealization, short amnesia, brief stupor, and perceptual disturbances

2. When individuals are unable to function because of memory loss, rapid switching between identities, flashbacks, or overwhelming emotions
3. When medications need to be evaluated or adjusted

The stages of treatment for dissociative disorders relate to assessment, stabilization, and reworking past traumas. The most effective results are seen when patients are able to work with stable, established, and experienced multidisciplinary treatment teams.

Treatments and Therapies

Therapy for patients with dissociative disorders begins with assessment and stabilization. Because the work of coping with deeply seated trauma is difficult and emotionally demanding, an environment in which patients can safely examine their conflicts must first be established. A careful *assessment* includes the patient's history, symptoms, support systems, medical status, relationships, and challenges, and the presence of substance abuse and sleeping or eating disorders. Family history should include both the family of origin and the current family situation. Video-recording the alters (other personalities) often results in more diagnostic information.

In addition to trauma-focused therapy, DID patients need to receive special DID treatment. This treatment must include direct engagement with all of their alters to repair identity fragmentation and minimize dissociative amnesia (Brand, Loewenstein, & Spiegel, 2014). Staff can help a patient with DID establish a **personality map,** which is a full description of all alters (their full identity, triggers for appearance, views, and attitudes). Skillful staff can engage with a patient to achieve a good awareness about all alters and build trust, respect, and a consensus or, at least, a set of ground rules for behaviour among all alters. The goal is to bring peace, improve the quality of life for the patient, and achieve successful social functioning.

During the *stabilization* phase, the diagnosis is established as the patient gradually reveals the complexities of their nature. After each treatment team member assesses the patient, a plan for stabilization is jointly developed. Therapies are carefully chosen and may include individual psychotherapy, group therapy, family therapy, psychoeducation, and various expressive therapies, such as art, poetry, and dance. Contracts to ensure safety during therapy are established. During this time, patients and care providers develop trust in each other and build patient support networks. Although this part of treatment may last for more than 1 year, it is an essential step for the work to come.

Once the patient is stabilized, the next phase of treatment begins. This involves revisiting and *reworking* past traumas.

Once there is an awareness of other personalities and their purposes, the painful material is slowly and gently analyzed. Each identity is treated equally, with respect, and is encouraged to communicate with the others. Feelings of shame, guilt, anger, and grief are encountered as each traumatic event is relived. With time, patience, and hard work, the patient can eventually begin to integrate or combine the personalities into a unique individual who is able to effectively cope with life's stressors. This is the main treatment goal for patients with dissociative disorders.

Pharmacological Therapy

No specific medication exists at this time to treat amnesia, fugues, or other dissociative behaviours. Treatment is often based on symptoms. If high anxiety is apparent, antianxiety agents may be prescribed. When depression is intense, an antidepressant may be ordered. If hallucinations or delusions are commonly present, an antipsychotic medication may be administered. All medications are prescribed for only short periods to encourage the use of inner coping skills. Each medication prescribed must be monitored for adverse effects and unwanted reactions, so care providers must be vigilant in watching for these effects.

Nursing (Therapeutic) Process

As with all other mental health patients, assessments are routinely performed. Patients with dissociative disorders can present different pictures to various staff members to manipulate and divide their care providers. They may offer one side of themselves during one moment, and then, in the next moment, a personality that wants to pick a fight emerges. Assessments should describe the patient's behaviours, communications, anxiety, depression, social functioning, and the presence of amnesia (Shives, 2011). A much clearer picture is given with descriptions than with psychiatric "buzz words" or jargon.

Nursing diagnoses (problem statements) for patients with dissociative disorders are related to self-concept responses and depend on the identified issues of each patient. The expected outcome for each diagnosis is a patient who is able to obtain their maximum level of effective functioning and self-actualization. Problem statements or nursing diagnoses include disturbed personal identity, disturbed body image, low self-esteem, and ineffective role performance.

After patients have established trust with the staff, interventions are directed at helping them examine their situations and related feelings within an environment of safety and support. This process assists the growth of personal insight, which is the first step toward making behavioural changes. A problem-solving approach helps patients to gradually expand self-awareness, explore and evaluate the self, and eventually plan for actions that result in behaviour changes. Patients need to be emotionally supported and encouraged to actively take part in therapy.

Some patients with dissociative disorders engage in self-destructive behaviours. They may cut, bite, or repeatedly hit themselves or pull out their hair. Self-destructive behaviour is of great concern, and several interventions have been devised to assist patients in achieving control over these behaviours.

First, patients must be routinely assessed for self-destructive thoughts. The easiest way to find out whether such thoughts are occurring is to ask the patient. Contracts and agreements between the patient and staff help the staff and patient to develop trust in the therapeutic relationship and environment. During the admission process, ways of dealing with destructive behaviours should be discussed with the patient. If necessary, one-to-one support is provided until the patient can achieve self-control. If the patient is willing, a daily journal of thoughts and feelings is kept. This practice has been found to be a helpful self-control activity. In addition, care providers should be limited to a few personnel to provide a stable therapeutic environment (see Sample Patient Care Plan 24.1).

The care and treatment of individuals with dissociative issues are complex, time-consuming, and challenging. Individuals diagnosed with dissociative disorders are suffering from one of the worst human fears—not knowing oneself and being out of control of oneself. Although behaviours may be odd, unusual, or dramatic, each serves a purpose and communicates something about the person. Health care providers are challenged with the twin tasks of accepting and understanding the messages sent by dissociated individuals. Treatment of patients with backgrounds of trauma is often frustrating. At the same time, providing such treatment can be an extremely rewarding experience.

SAMPLE PATIENT CARE PLAN 24.1 **Maladaptive Self-Concept**

Assessment

History Inna is a 35-year-old wife and mother of three children, aged 15, 10, and 7 years old. Although she experienced severe sexual and physical abuse as a child, she has managed to complete community college, marry, and raise her family. She is being admitted to the clinic's mental health services for "several episodes of losing myself" that she has experienced in the past 5 months.

Current Findings A well-groomed woman who is distressed because she was unable to remember to pick up her daughter's dress at the cleaners yesterday. Because of this, her daughter refused to attend the school dance and threatened to run away. Lately Inna has felt like an "outside observer of my own life," "like a robot on automatic." During these episodes she is aware of reality but feels as though everything is mechanical. She feels that she may be "going insane" because the "spells" are becoming more and more frequent since her daughter has begun dating.

Continued

SAMPLE PATIENT CARE PLAN 24.1   Maladaptive Self-Concept —cont'd

Multidisciplinary Diagnosis	Planning/Goals
Disturbed personal identity related to increased anxiety and past history of abuse	Inna will decrease the number of depersonalization episodes to fewer than one per week by May 20. Inna will be able to recognize her anxiety and take steps to decrease it before it progresses to a depersonalization episode.

THERAPEUTIC INTERVENTIONS

Interventions	Rationale	Team Member
1. Establish therapeutic relationship; confirm her identity; support adaptive behaviours, identify strengths.	Provides a way of offering emotional support; builds trust; supports current adaptive behaviours	All
2. Assist Inna in describing thoughts and feelings.	Identification is the first step toward focused change	All
3. Identify stresses that bring about her "spells."	Known stressors can be handled more effectively	Psy, Nsg
4. Help to clarify faulty beliefs about self.	Builds confidence; helps focus energies in positive direction	All
5. Encourage Inna to make a plan for decreasing her anxiety during times her daughter is on a date; role-play mother-daughter roles.	Recalling and using successful strategies help to decrease anxiety levels, thus preventing depersonalization episodes	Psy, Nsg
6. Reinforce strengths, assets, and problem-solving abilities; encourage Inna to focus on her "positives."	Helps to improve coping abilities and ease the pain of feeling powerless	All

Evaluation Inna was able to decrease her episodes of depersonalization to less than one per week by May 29.

Critical Thinking Questions
1. In what ways will long-term therapy benefit Inna?
2. How would care providers go about helping Inna identify stressors in her daily life?

A complete patient care plan includes several other diagnoses and interventions.
Nsg, nursing staff; *Psy,* psychologist.

█ KEY POINTS

- Self-concept is defined as all the attitudes, notions, beliefs, and convictions that make up an individual's self-knowledge. It develops over time, shaped by one's developmental level and environmental influences.
- The continuum of self-concept responses ranges from a low self-concept, which results in maladaptive behavioural responses, to a healthy self-concept, which leads one toward self-actualization.
- Self-concept develops over time and is shaped by the influences within one's environment.
- Infants learn to trust others when their needs are consistently met.
- Toddlers develop autonomy by exploring their environments and testing their capabilities.
- School-age children assess their skills and interactions with others and form mental pictures of themselves.
- The adolescent's struggle is to define oneself by combining previous roles and new emotions into a consistent sense of self.
- Adults with strong, positive self-concepts can freely explore their environments. Those with low self-concepts tend to view themselves as inadequate or unable.

- Many occurrences and situations can threaten a positive self-concept of older persons.
- Low self-esteem is a common component of many mental health challenges.
- Identity diffusion is the failure to bring various childhood identifications into an effective adult personality.
- Dissociation is an interruption of a person's fundamental aspects of waking consciousness.
- Dissociative amnesia is characterized by an inability to remember personal information that cannot be explained by ordinary forgetfulness.
- Dissociative amnesia may be associated with a fugue, which is sudden, unexpected travel with an inability to recall the past.
- A trance is a state resembling sleep in which consciousness remains but voluntary movement is lost.
- A dissociative identity disorder (DID) is defined as the presence of two or more identities or personalities that repeatedly take control of the individual's behaviour.
- Treatment for dissociative disorders involves long-term psychodynamic/cognitive therapy.

- Treatment for DID consists of trauma-focused therapy, as well as special DID treatment that includes direct engagement with all of the individual's alters to repair identity fragmentation and minimize dissociative amnesia.

- There are no specific psychotherapeutic medications for the treatment of dissociative disorders.
- Therapeutic interventions for patients with dissociative disorders focus on safety, trust, communication, and problem-solving.

ADDITIONAL LEARNING RESOURCES

Go to your Evolve website (http://evolve.elsevier.com/Canada/Morrison-Valfre/) for additional online resources, including the online Study Guide for additional learning activities to help you master this chapter content.

CRITICAL THINKING QUESTIONS

1. A male patient was involved in an automobile accident several years ago in which his best friend was killed. He recalls nothing about the accident or the 1 to 2 months before and after the accident. The patient's son recently obtained his driver's license, and the patient is experiencing extreme emotional distress every time his son drives. When a care plan is developed for this patient, who suffers from dissociative amnesia, what would be the priority intervention?

2. What staff intervention would be appropriate for a DID patient whose multiple different alters are arguing among themselves and causing a significant impairment?

3. During the assessment before admission to a mental health facility, the patient states that he was found to have driven his car to another province but has no recollection of travelling there. What condition can lead to this behaviour?

REFERENCES

American Psychiatric Association (APA). (2013). *Diagnostic and statistical manual of mental disorders* (5th ed.). American Psychiatric Publishing.

American Psychiatric Association (APA). (2018). *What are dissociative disorders?* https://www.psychiatry.org/patients-families/dissociative-disorders/what-are-dissociative-disorders

Brand, B. L., Loewenstein, R. J., & Spiegel, D. (2014). Dispelling myths about dissociative identity disorder treatment: An empirically based approach. *Psychiatry, 77*(2), 169–189. https://doi.org/10.1521/psyc.2014.77.2.169

Fortinash, K. M., & Holoday-Worret, P. A. (2011). *Psychiatric mental health nursing* (5th ed.). Mosby.

Hockenberry, M., & Wilson, D. (2014). *Wong's nursing care of infants and children* (10th ed.). Mosby.

Keltner, N. L., & Steele, D. (2014). *Psychiatric nursing* (7th ed.). Mosby.

Shives, L. R. (2011). *Basic concepts in psychiatric–mental health nursing* (8th ed.). Lippincott.

Stuart, G. W. (2013). *Principles and practice of psychiatric nursing* (10th ed.). Mosby.

Patients With Psychosocial Challenges

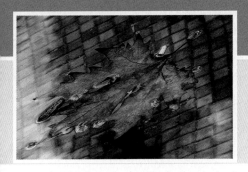

25

Anger and Aggression

OBJECTIVES

Upon completion of this chapter, the student will be able to:

1. Explain the differences between anger, aggression, and assertiveness.
2. Describe how anger is expressed by children, adolescents, young adults, and older persons.
3. Examine the impacts of anger and aggression on society.
4. Compare three theories that attempt to explain the causes of aggression.
5. Describe each of the five stages of the assault cycle.
6. Explain the main characteristics for three mental health disorders that relate to anger or aggression.
7. Outline the process for assessing patients who are angry or aggressive.
8. Develop four therapeutic interventions for patients who are experiencing anger or acting aggressively.
9. Consider six techniques for recognizing and coping with your own anger.

OUTLINE

KEY TERMS

acting out (p. 298)
aggression (ă-GRĔSH-ăn) (p. 298)
anger (p. 297)
antisocial personality disorder (p. 303)
assault (p. 299)
assertiveness (ă-SŬR-tĭv-nĕs) (p. 299)
battery (p. 299)
conduct disorder (p. 303)
impulse control (p. 299)

intermittent explosive (ĭn-tĕr-MĬT-ĕnt ĕk-SPLŌ-sĭv) disorder (IED) (p. 303)
kleptomania (p. 303)
oppositional defiant disorder (ODD) (p. 302)
passive aggression (p. 298)
pyromania (p. 303)
trauma-informed care (p. 306)
violence (p. 299)

Anger is a normal emotional response to a perceived threat, frustration, or distressing event. It commonly occurs in reaction to feeling threatened or losing control. Anger is felt, experienced, suffered, and expressed in many ways. In a crisis situation, anger is often one of the first coping behaviours employed.

Anger can be directed outward through overtly aggressive or violent behaviours, or it may be expressed through passive-aggressive behaviours. Anger can also be focused onto oneself. Some individuals turn their anger inward and become suicidal or depressed. Some live bouncing between aggression and helplessness, whereas others channel their anger in a way that produces physical symptoms. Figure 25.1 illustrates the continuum of anger responses.

Anxiety and loss of control are associated with anger. Anger can include feelings of hopelessness, powerlessness, and regret. It can arise intentionally as one "stews" about an event or situation, or it can result from unplanned circumstances. People tend to label anger as justified or unjustified according to their personal values. Anger can be rational and planned, or it can arrive in a blind fury of irrational rage.

Anger serves several purposes. It can be used as a *coping mechanism* to meet needs. According to Maslow's hierarchy (ladder) of human needs, when basic needs are threatened, a person may react with anger. The patient who feels powerless at the news of their prolonged recovery may react by insulting others, or the child who flies into temper tantrums may be attempting to meet basic needs.

People can be motivated or encouraged to act by anger. Consider the university student who, as a child, felt the anxiety and helplessness of watching her mother being abused. Now she studies to become a lawyer and champion of abused people. In this case, the use of anger motivated positive actions.

Table 25.1 lists many expressions of anger. Many of the listed emotions and actions are appropriate expressions of anger. However, when anger provides the motivation for inappropriate behaviours or violence, it becomes defined as a problem.

Aggression is a forceful attitude or action that is expressed physically, symbolically, or verbally. **Passive aggression** involves indirect expressions of anger through subtle, evasive, or manipulative behaviours. **Acting out** is the use of inappropriate, detrimental, or destructive behaviours to express current or past emotions.

Aggressive behaviours often are the result of angry feelings that are converted into action and expressed. Socially approved aggression is a basic element of many sports, such as hockey, football, and soccer (Stuart, 2013). Aggressive behaviour is socially approved for certain groups, such as journalists hot on the trail of some developing story. However, aggressive behaviours become inappropriate

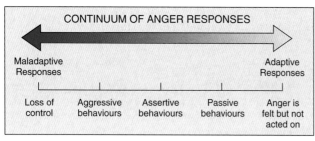

Fig. 25.1 Continuum of anger responses.

TABLE 25.1 Expressions of Anger

TURNED OUTWARD		TURNED INWARD	
Overt Anger	**Passive Aggression**	**Subjective**	**Objective**
Verbalization of anger	Impatience	Feeling upset	Crying
Irritation	Frustration	Tension	Self-destructive
Pacing with agitation	Tense facial expressions	Unhappiness	behaviour
Swearing	Pessimism	Feeling hurt	Self-mutilation
Hostility	Resentment	Disappointment	Substance abuse
Contempt	Jealousy	Guilt	Suicide
Clenched fists	Bitterness	Feelings of inferiority	
Insulting remarks	Complaining	Low self-esteem	
Intimidation	Deceptive sweetness	Sense of failure	
Bragging about violent acts	Unreasonableness	Humiliation	
Provoking behaviours	Intolerance	Somatic symptoms	
Sadistic acts	Resistance	Feeling harassed	
Maliciousness	Stubbornness	Envy	
Verbal abuse	Intentional forgetting	Feeling violated	
Temper tantrums	Noncompliance	Feeling alienated	
Violation of others' rights	Procrastination	Feeling demoralized	
Screaming	Antagonism	Feeling depressed	
Deviance	Belittling remarks	Resignation	
Rage	Sarcasm	Powerlessness	
Argumentativeness	Fault finding	Helplessness	
Overt defiance	Manipulation	Hopelessness	
Threats: words or weapons	Power struggles	Desperation	
Damage to property	Unfair teasing	Apathy	
Assault	Sabotage of others		
Rape	Domination		
Homicide			

From Keltner, N. L., & Steele, D. (2014). *Psychiatric nursing* (7th ed.). Mosby.

BOX 25.1   **Terms Relating to Anger**

BOX 25.1   Terms Relating to Anger

Expressions of anger depend on **impulse control**, the ability to express one's emotions in appropriate or effective ways.

Acting out is the use of inappropriate or destructive behaviours to express emotions.

Passive aggression involves indirect expressions of anger through subtle, evasive, or manipulative behaviours.

Violence is behaviour that threatens or harms other people or their property. A violent act is actions of force that result in abuse or harm.

Assault is a legal term that describes any behaviour that presents an immediate threat to another person.

Battery is the unlawful use of force on a person without their consent.

TABLE 25.2   Gender Violence Throughout the Life Cycle

Phase	Type of Violence Present
Prebirth	Sex-selective abortion (China, India, Republic of Korea); battering during pregnancy (emotional and physical effects on woman; effects on birth outcome); forced pregnancy (e.g., mass rape during war)
Infancy	Female infanticide; emotional and physical abuse; differential access to food and medical care for female infants
Girlhood	Child marriage; genital mutilation; sexual abuse by family members and strangers; differential access to food and medical care; child prostitution
Adolescence	Dating and courtship violence (acid throwing in Bangladesh, date rape in North America); economically coerced sex (African secondary school girls with "sugar daddies" to afford school fees); sexual abuse in the workplace; rape; sexual harassment; forced prostitution; sex trafficking of women
Reproductive age	Abuse of women by male partners; marital rape; dowry abuse and murders; partner homicide; psychological abuse; sexual abuse in the workplace; sexual harassment; rape; abuse of women with disabilities
Older person	Abuse of widows; elder abuse (in the United States, the only country in which data are available, elder abuse affects mostly women)

when they affect other people or their possessions. Several terms describe the characteristics of anger (Box 25.1). The legal concepts of assault and battery were established to define inappropriate aggression and to protect people from those who act on their emotions in ways that are threatening to others.

The terms *aggression* and *violence* are often used interchangeably, but they are different: *aggression* is generally defined as angry feelings or behaviour, whereas **violence** is the use of physical force with intent to injure a person, animal, or property. There are two forms of violence: *physical* (e.g., pushing, kicking, biting, grabbing) and *nonphysical* (e.g., verbal or nonverbal threat, verbal abuse). In Canada, most health organizations must ensure a violence-free environment for all employees and have violence-prevention policies in place to facilitate this. Violence is discussed in greater detail in Chapter 26.

Finally, the term **assertiveness** defines the quality for which we strive. Assertiveness is the ability to directly express one's feelings or needs in a way that respects the rights of other people yet retains one's dignity.

ANGER AND AGGRESSION IN SOCIETY

Anger and its expressions have a strong impact on a society. The histories of many cultures are peppered with accounts of uprisings and wars. Children were commonly sacrificed to keep the gods from becoming angry. Cultural expressions of anger differ, and care providers need the ability to recognize the signs of anger in the cultural groups with whom they work.

Gender Aggression

Violence against women has been tolerated since the beginning of history. Ancient and well-accepted beliefs that men were superior led to values that supported the abuse of women. Beatings and floggings of women were accepted practices throughout ancient Greek and Roman societies. By the fourteenth century, it was legal in France for a man to

beat his wife as long as he did not maim or kill her. In 1427, a nobleman encouraged his fellow Italians to treat their wives with as much concern and consideration as they did their livestock and fowl.

Today in Canada, an individual can legally press charges against their spouse or partner for abuse, regardless of gender. However, violence against women and children continues to occur throughout the world far too often.

Gender aggression and abuse are still practised everywhere. Many aggressive acts against women are centred on the concepts of virginity and fidelity. To illustrate, young women in some parts of Africa and the Middle East are still forced to undergo circumcision and other mutilating genital surgeries. Women of all ages can suffer from the effects of gender violence (Table 25.2).

Aggression Throughout the Life Cycle

Expressions of anger begin in infancy and end with death. Infants express unmet needs through diffuse rage reactions with "loud, uncontrollable crying and screaming, profuse perspiration, difficulty in breathing (sometimes turning blue), and flailing of arms and legs" (Keltner & Steele, 2014).

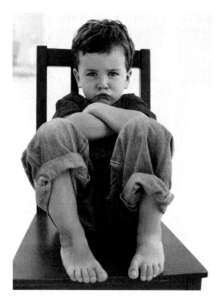

Fig. 25.2 Preschoolers generally direct their aggression toward peers. Time-outs are a disciplinary measure used to remove the child from an activity and allow the child to calm down and consider what was wrong in their actions. (Copyright Jupiter Images.)

Toddlers learn to use words to express their feelings. They often engage in temper tantrums (Fig. 25.2) in which they learn to focus their aggression on the person or thing they believe is responsible for their anger (Potter, Perry, Stockert, et al., 2019). Toddlers observe the behaviours of others in their environment and pattern their own actions after them. If toddlers observe shouting, fighting, or other forms of aggression, they understand that aggressive behaviours are acceptable. In some families, a show of aggression is encouraged in children as a way of teaching them to "stand up for their rights." Television and other forms of electronic media are other sources of witnessing aggression. Many studies of the effects of television (media) violence on children and teenagers have found that children may become "immune" or numb to the horror of violence, begin to accept violence as a way to solve problems, imitate the violence they observe on television, and identify with certain characters, victims, or victimizers. The greater the diet of violence in daily life, the more likely children are to engage in aggressive behaviours.

During preschool years, children often direct their anger toward others, especially peers or younger children. Children in the early school-age years assault or hit each other frequently. By preadolescence, most children stop hitting and learn to channel their aggression into physical activities, such as competitive sports or physical conditioning. Slander, gossip, and practical jokes provide other outlets for aggressive feelings during the school years. However, bullying has become a serious problem in schools today. At least one in three adolescent students in Canada has reported being bullied by peers (Canadian Institute for Health Research [CIHR], 2012).

In adolescence, fighting is organized, controlled, and purposeful. The peer group becomes the greatest source of influence on the teen. Peer groups can be focused on activities that promote cooperation, fair play, and respect. Examples include various after-school groups, such as the Boys and Girls Clubs, sports, and community volunteering. However, if the activities of the peer group are illegal or disruptive to others, then the adolescent peer group is known as a *gang.*

Generally, as an individual's age increases, so does their emotional control. According to Keltner and Steele (2014), "between 22 and 45 [years of age], most expressions of aggression and fighting occur within the family." After 45 years of age, few people engage in physical aggression. Sensory and cognitive (intellectual) impairments, such as dementia or Alzheimer's disease, may result in aggressive or hostile behaviours.

Scope of the Problem Today

Today, aggression and violence are worldwide concerns. Wife beating is still common in many countries. In Papua New Guinea, almost 67% of wives suffer from abuse.

Violent crime rates are very different in different countries. For example, in the United States, the rape rate is 16 times higher and the homicide rate 3 times higher than rates for these crimes in Canada (NationMaster, 2019).

Statistics are impressive, but they cannot tell the stories of how aggression and violence have changed the lives of so many individuals. It is our task, as health care providers, and human beings, to help others focus their aggression into more effective (and less violent) ways of coping with challenges they face in today's complex world.

THEORIES OF ANGER AND AGGRESSION

Theories about human aggression and violence attempt to explain why certain persons behave the way they do. Many theories about the nature of aggression have been devised, but most fall into one of three basic models: biological, psychosocial, and sociocultural theories.

Biological Theories

Models that see the cause of aggression and violence as physical or chemical differences are called *biological* or *individual theories.* Currently, research is focusing on the areas of the brain that influence emotional control and aggressive behaviours. The roles of certain neurotransmitters are being investigated as possible factors in the development of violence. Biological theories explain aggressive behaviour as a psychopathology—a disorder in the biological or physical makeup of a person.

Charles Darwin favoured his animal model, which stated that aggression strengthened human beings through natural selection. Sigmund Freud believed that the greater the death wish, the greater the need for aggressive behaviour. Other biological theories explain aggression as an innate (instinctual) drive. One thing, however, is certain: Physical sources of aggressive behaviours do exist.

Psychosocial Theories

The models based on psychosocial theories focus on an individual's interactions with the social environments. Violence arises from interpersonal frustrations. Psychosocial theories of aggression state that aggressive behaviours are learned responses.

Sociocultural Theories

In the sociocultural theories, aggression is explained from a social and cultural group viewpoint. Cultural theories state that aggressive or violent acts are a product of cultural values, beliefs, norms, and rituals. Many cultures have rules that endorse the use of violence.

The *functional model* states that aggression and violence fill certain functions in a society, serving as catalysts or motivators for action. Aggressive behaviours are often used to achieve fame, fortune, and power. Athletes, for example, must be aggressive if they are to excel.

Conflict theories assume that aggression is a natural part of all human interactions. They state that individuals, groups, and societies seek to further their own causes. This results in disagreements, conflicts, and aggressive actions. Because conflict is a natural part of human associations, that aggression will never be eliminated. It can only be controlled.

The premise of the *resource theory* is that aggression is a fundamental part of society. Therefore, the person who has the most resources can muster the greatest force or power. With this model, aggression is the result of having many resources and the power that goes with them.

The last theory of aggression is the *general systems model*. Here the feedback loop is used to demonstrate how aggression and violence perpetuate (feed on) themselves. Violence is viewed as a product of a system that must be stabilized and managed.

Many factors contribute to aggressive behaviours. Attitudes about work, education, the media, and religion all influence the development of anger, hostility, and aggression. Population challenges, such as overcrowding, can feed aggressive behaviours. Available community resources, or the lack of them, also play important roles in the occurrence of violent or criminal acts. Many attempts have been made to explain the nature of aggression and violence. No matter what the cause, however, society must learn to recognize and cope with the aggressive behaviours of some of its members that result in others' suffering.

THE CYCLE OF ASSAULT

Assaults are aggressive behaviours that violate others' person or properties. Behaviours that are considered assaultive include causing physical pain; certain criminal acts, such as rape, murder, suicide, robbery, theft, assault, and battery; passive-aggressive actions; and many forms of emotional abuse.

Studies have demonstrated that assault and violence occur in a predictable pattern of emotional responses. Each response pattern is called a *stage*. There are five stages in the assault cycle: trigger, escalation, crisis, recovery, and depression. Figure 25.3 illustrates the cycle of assault. This section

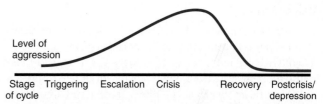

Fig. 25.3 The assault cycle. (From Keltner, N. L., Bostrom, C. E., & McGuinness, T. [2011]. *Psychiatric nursing* [6th ed.]. Mosby.)

TABLE 25.3	Levels of Intervention With Anger
Level	**Goal**
Level 1—Prevent violence	Use active listening skills. Remain calm, speak respectfully, listen carefully. Establish and maintain a trusting therapeutic relationship.
Level 2—Protect	Protect the patient, yourself, and others from potential harm. Suggest a "time-out" in a quieter place. Keep patient talking.
Level 3—Control violence	Patient is out of control. Protect patient and others through seclusion, restraints, and intramuscular medication.

describes each stage. Please refer to Chapter 8 to review the guidelines for crisis interventions.

Trigger Stage

During the trigger stage, a stress-producing event occurs, leading to stress responses, such as anger, fear, or anxiety. Coping mechanisms—behaviours to deal with the situation—are used in an attempt to achieve control. Individuals may withdraw, become irritable, and start complaining. For most people, these coping behaviours are appropriate reactions to stress. For persons who are assaultive, however, their coping behaviours can become automatic and are focused outward. Their ability to problem-solve or choose more effective options decreases as aggressive responses increase. Level 1 interventions for angry or aggressive patients are successful if begun early in this stage. Refer to Table 25.3 for a description of these interventions.

Escalation Stage

The escalation stage is the building stage during which each behavioural response moves a step closer to total loss of control. Repeated attempts to use aggressive behaviours to gain control become ineffective. This results in increasing frustration and greater anger. Intense emotions further flame the fires of aggression. Behaviours include rapid pacing, fist pounding, and complaining loudly. The person may swear, scream, and become irrational. Intervention is crucial at this stage if violence is to be prevented. Level 2 interventions are necessary here (see Table 25.3).

Crisis Stage

During the crisis stage, the potential for danger is increased. This is a period of emotional or physical blowout when actual assaultive behaviours occur. The ability to reason is lost, and many individuals act out, physically harm other people and animals, or destroy property. Others become verbally abusive or scream and shout. People in this stage are unable to listen to reason, follow directions, or engage in mental exercises. They are so controlled by their anger that they cannot respond to most outside stimuli. The best interventions at this stage are to protect the individual and others in the environment from physical harm (level 3 interventions). External control by care providers is needed.

Recovery Stage

The recovery stage is the cooling-down period that follows an emotional explosion. The individual slowly calms down and returns to normal behavioural responses and actions. Interventions during this stage include assessing for injuries or trauma and providing a safe, quiet environment in which the person can recover.

Depression Stage

The last stage of the assault cycle involves a period of guilt and attempts to reconcile (make up) with others. Aggressors are aware of the assault and genuinely feel bad about it. They may cry, apologize frequently, or provide loving care for the victim. They may spend large amounts of money on gifts or other offerings seeking forgiveness. With the passage of time, the assaultive event is slowly placed in the past. Life returns to normal—that is, until the next trigger that generates assault occurs, and the cycle repeats itself over and over again.

DISRUPTIVE, IMPULSE-CONTROL, AND CONDUCT DISORDERS

The majority of violence in modern Western society is not related to mental illness. The media often depicts mental health patients as being violent and unpredictable, which contributes to stigma. However, anger and aggression can be symptoms of many mental health disorders. Aggressive behaviours are commonly encountered in patients with disorders related to substance abuse, mood, anxiety, and depression. Some potential for violence exists in individuals with schizophrenia and other psychotic disorders. At the same time, the *failure to assess and treat schizophrenia patients on time leads to their risk for violence* (Pompili & Fiorillo, 2015). Patients with eating, sleeping, or somatoform disorders seldom behave aggressively toward others, but they are at great risk for suicide because they focus their anger and aggression inward.

All mental health disorders in some way lead to difficulties with emotion and behaviour regulation. In this chapter, we will discuss disorders in which these emotional and behaviour challenges violate other people's rights for safety and security.

> **BOX 25.2   Examples of Impulse-Control Disorders**
>
> Intermittent explosive disorder: Acting on aggressive impulses that result in assaultive or destructive behaviours
> Kleptomania: The impulse to steal objects when they are not needed for personal use or survival
> Pathological gambling: Maladaptive betting, wagering, or gambling
> Pyromania: Pattern of starting fires for pleasure or gratification
> Trichotillomania: Pulling out one's hair that results in noticeable hair loss

---

Impulse-control disorders are named for the impulse that is related to the specific manifestations of maladaptive behaviour. Box 25.2 lists five types of impulse-control disorders. Although all types involve some form of aggression, the impulse-control problems encountered by health care workers most often relate to patients with intermittent explosive disorder.

Oppositional Defiant Disorder

Oppositional defiant disorder (ODD) is a childhood disorder that is characterized by negative, defiant, disobedient, and often hostile behaviour toward adults and authority figures, primarily. Individuals who are diagnosed with ODD have persistently demonstrated four or more of following signs over a period of at least 6 months (Grohol, 2020):

1. Frequently lose temper
2. Frequently easily irritated or annoyed
3. Frequently become angry or resentful
4. Frequently argumentative with authority figures
5. Frequently refuse to cooperate with rules and requests
6. Frequently doing things to deliberately irritate or annoy other people
7. Frequently blaming others for their own mistakes or misbehaviour

It is very typical for these people to show these symptoms only with their own family members (e.g., in a home setting). Therefore, the disorder has three severity levels: mild severity—symptoms are confined only to one setting (e.g., at home, at school, at work, with peers); moderate severity—some symptoms are present in at least two settings; and severe—some symptoms are present in three or more settings (American Psychiatric Association [APA], 2013).

It is normal for people who have ODD *not* to see themselves as being generally angry or irritable. They always have explanations for how other people have made them feel and behave this way. Sometimes, when parents are truly hostile toward their child, it is difficult to differentiate between the impact of the disorder and the impact of the environment.

ODD usually begins during the preschool age. Many children will grow out of it and will have no disorder when they are older. Others will go on to develop conduct disorder, and anxiety, or major depressive disorder.

Intermittent Explosive Disorder

Intermittent explosive disorder (IED) is an impulse-control disorder characterized by sudden episodes of unwarranted anger, resulting in serious assaults, property destruction, or frequent verbal aggression in the form of temper tantrums or tirades (APA, 2013; Psychology Today, 2019a). Individuals who have been diagnosed with this disorder demonstrate a failure to control aggressive impulses, leading to frequent (at least twice a week) verbal or physical aggression toward people, animals, or property, without actual physical damage, during a period of at least 3 months, or at least three occurrences of physical aggression within 12 months, each time leading to destruction of property and/or damage to people or animals (APA, 2013). These outbursts are never planned and have no purpose. They are disproportionate to a potential provocation of anger and cause significant impairment in these individuals' function (occupational, social, legal, and financial). For example, an individual who has this disorder may strike the teller at the bank for making him wait in line too long, whereas most people would sigh and continue to wait quietly for their turn.

Outbursts typically have no prodrome period, come as an impulse reaction to some minor irritation from somebody (physically) close to the person, and last no more than 30 minutes. The disorder is more common in late childhood or adolescence and may continue for many years. IED has a very strong genetic predisposition.

Conduct Disorder

A **conduct disorder** refers to any of a group of antisocial emotional and behavioural problems in children and adolescents. Children with conduct disorders frequently behave in extremely troubling, socially unacceptable, and often illegal ways, though they feel justified in their actions and show little to no empathy for their victims (Psychology Today, 2017a). Individuals with this disorder have a pattern of violating the basic rights of others, social rules, and norms. To diagnose this disorder, an individual must demonstrate at least 3 of the 15 following criteria, grouped into four domains, for 12 months, and at least 1 in the past 6 months:

Aggression to People and Animals:
1. Pattern of bullying, threatening, or intimidation
2. Pattern of initiating physical fights
3. Pattern of use of a weapon
4. Physical cruelty to people
5. Physical cruelty to animals
6. Engaged in robbery involving a confrontation with a victim
7. Forcing someone to perform a sexual act

Destruction of Property:
8. Setting a fire to purposely cause damage
9. Destroying another's property using another method

Deceitfulness or Theft:
10. Burglary of a house, building, or car
11. Conning others in order to obtain goods or avoid obligations

12. Engaged in stealing without the confrontation or breaking-in (e.g., shoplifting)

Serious Violation of Rules:
13. Pattern of staying away from home during nights despite parents' prohibition, starting before age 13
14. Running away from home overnight at least twice, or at least once for a lengthy period of time
15. Pattern of being a truant from school starting before age 13

The diagnosis of conduct disorder for a minority of individuals may have a specifier of "with limited prosocial emotions," which is added if an individual exhibits at least two of the following symptoms over a period of at least 12 months:
- *Lack of remorse or guilt* (does not feel bad for hurting others, even when caught)
- *Callous—lack of empathy* (no concern for other people's feelings)
- *Unconcerned about performance* (at school or work, even when expectations are very clear)
- *Shallow or deficient affect* (no feelings about others; if some feelings are present, these are only to manipulate others and are not real) (APA, 2013)

Males who have a conduct disorder are prone to fight, steal, and commit vandalism. Females who have a conduct disorder are more prone to lie, be truants, run away, abuse substances, and engage in prostitution.

Antisocial Personality Disorder

Antisocial personality disorder describes a pattern of behaviour in which individuals consistently disregard and violate the rights of others around them. See Chapter 30 for a full description of this disorder.

Pyromania

Pyromania is a rare, pathological disorder that is characterized by intentional and repeated fire setting. People with pyromania are deeply fascinated by fire and related paraphernalia. They may experience feelings of satisfaction or a release of built-up inner tension or anxiety once a fire is set or when witnessing the result of a fire (Psychology Today, 2017b).

Kleptomania

Kleptomania is a condition in which an individual experiences a consistent impulse to steal items not needed for use or monetary value. They fail to resist this urge and feel immediate gratification and relief following the theft. The objects are stolen despite typically being of little value to the individual and are often given away or discarded after being taken.

Although someone with this disorder will generally avoid stealing when immediate arrest is likely, the individual usually does not plan out the thefts. People with kleptomania commonly feel depressed or guilty about the thefts after they occur (Psychology Today, 2019b).

About 0.3 to 0.6% of people are estimated to experience this condition, and it is more common among females than males (female-to-male ratio is 3:1) (APA, 2013).

GUIDELINES FOR INTERVENTION

It is important to keep in mind that diagnoses are only labels. As a health care provider, you are working with individuals—real people with real problems. Therapeutic interventions should always focus on the person, rather than on the diagnosis.

Assessing Anger and Aggression

The first step in controlling aggressive behaviours is to assess the patient's potential for engaging in inappropriate or violent behaviours. Approach the patient slowly and calmly. Use therapeutic listening techniques. Stay an arm's length away, and monitor the patient for signs of losing control. Obtain a mental status assessment, and if the patient is being admitted to a hospital or clinic, do this as soon as possible after admission. Use therapeutic communication skills to help patients feel at ease. Work to establish trust, and let patients know that they are respected, even when angry.

Mental Status Assessment

Basic mental status examinations (see Chapter 9) can be performed by any astute observer. During the mental status assessment, observe the patient's *general appearance* and note the state of dress, cleanliness, and use of cosmetics or jewellery. Be sure to observe the patient's activity and behaviours. Many times, the clues to violence are being communicated nonverbally. Health care providers need to be alert to detect such messages. What about the patient's *attitude*? Are interactions friendly and cooperative, or resistive and hostile? Listen for the quality, rate, and amount of verbal communications in the patient's speech. Pay particular attention to the individual's *mood, affect (emotional expressions), perceptions,* and *thoughts*. Have the patient describe their mood at the time. Listen to the patient's conversation for form and content. Does the person speak logically, with a flow of ideas that are easily followed? What is the issue according to the patient? Is the patient's *judgement* or *insight* clear and easy to follow, or does it follow a twisted path of fuzzy explanations for past inappropriate behaviours? Is the patient's reliability intact (do they give accurate information)?

Psychosocial Assessment

The next assessment to perform is a psychosocial assessment. Find out which internal or external *stressors* are present in the patient's life. Which *coping skills* are being used to adapt to the stressors? Encourage the patient to talk about important *relationships* and how they are affecting the situation. Do not forget the *cultural, spiritual,* and *occupational areas* of the patient's life. Is the patient a member of a specific cultural group, organized religion, or occupation? Is there a *value and belief system* that the individual feels is valuable, desirable, or worth following?

Observe the patient's reactions and behaviours during the interview. Their *reactions, behaviours,* and *attitudes* during this time offer many clues concerning the potential for aggression or violent behaviours. Remember, the key to effective

intervention begins with assessments. Assess patients often, and report new behaviours. Share your findings with other members of the health care team. Troubleshooting is always an easier task than controlling a full-blown violent reaction. Possible nursing diagnoses (problem statements) for aggressive behaviours are listed in Box 25.3.

Therapeutic Interventions

Therapeutic interventions for patients with anger and aggression focus on two basic areas: the patient and the care provider. Interventions for aggressive or potentially aggressive patient behaviours occur on three levels (see Table 25.3).

Level 1 interventions focus on the *prevention* of violence. The goal of level 1 interventions, one type of intervention for aggression, is to establish and maintain a trusting therapeutic relationship with clear and honest communications. This is accomplished using a number of simple communication strategies.

First, call the patient and any family members by name. No one likes to be an anonymous face in the crowd. Then, explain what is happening, the reason for any delays, and why testing is needed. Most important, listen actively, with your whole body, not just your ears. Communicate your concern nonverbally while listening. Maintain good eye contact (if culturally appropriate) while leaning forward slightly to communicate your interest. Give the patient time to respond. Concentrate on the message the person is trying to communicate to you. Paraphrase the problem to make sure that you have a good understanding of the patient's point of view. Finally, help identify the emotions associated with the problem and explore appropriate options. Refer to Box 25.4 for an effective communication strategy to use.

Level 1 interventions should be practised routinely as *preventive* measures. They are also appropriate for patients who are in the "trigger stage" of the assault cycle. If the patient is yelling and verbalizing anger, keep them talking. Being angry is tiring, and individuals will often wear themselves out. The majority of patients with difficult behaviour are motivated by fear. Often just the caring concern of someone who is willing to really listen is enough to prevent anger from turning into aggression or violence.

Level 2 interventions focus on *protecting* the patient and others from potential harm. These interventions are used when level 1 interventions are ineffective and signs of trouble are beginning to brew (see Case Study). Learn to recognize the verbal and physical signs of impending violence.

CASE STUDY

Randy, a hot-tempered 24-year-old man well known to the clinic staff, visits the clinic for weekly dressing changes for his right eye. Today he arrives seething with anger because his girlfriend just broke off their relationship.

"That _____! Just because we had a little fight, she can't stand to be with me now. You women are all alike. I could punch you out right now and feel just fine," he snarls through clenched teeth as he glares into your eyes.

"You sound pretty upset. Tell me about it," you calmly reply. As Randy tells you about his relationship with his ex-girlfriend, you can see him becoming angrier by the moment. He begins to pound his fists on the table and stomp around the room. You signal for other staff members who are keeping an eye on the situation to be prepared to help, but so far, Randy is acting out by ranting and raving. No damage is being done, and no person is in danger of harm.

After a few moments you reply, "Randy, I understand your anger, but stomping around is not appropriate. Let's take a couple of minutes to cool off, then maybe together we can think of some way to help you deal with this problem." Because you remained calm, quiet, and prepared, Randy responds to your request and takes a few minutes to regain his composure.

• How do you think Randy would have reacted if he had been approached by three staff members during his ranting?

Interventions during level 2 include measures to maintain a safe environment. It is important to take charge with a calm, but firm, attitude. Allow patients to act out, as long as they limit their behaviours to verbal assaults and harmless physical movements. Assure patients that they have a right to express angry feelings but not to impose them on others. Gently, but firmly, set limits on the patient's behaviours by suggesting that the patient take a time-out, a cooling-off period. If it appears that the time-out is not effective, offer prn (as-needed) medication. Only after all other measures have been tried are level 3 interventions implemented. As Stuart (2013) notes, "Nonviolent physical control and restraint should be used only as a last resort."

The last level of therapeutic measures (*level 3 interventions*) is reserved for those *patients who are out of control* (crisis stage of the assault cycle). Out-of-control patients fight, bite, kick, scratch, spit, and throw things. They are verbally abusive or physically aggressive. Without intervention, both patients and care providers are at an increased risk for

BOX 25.4   Communicating With Angry Patients

First, take a deep breath. Become calm, and introduce yourself to the patient. Speak slowly, and do the following:

1. *Listen actively.* Use active listening skills to communicate interest in helping the patient. Allow the patient to define the problem that is causing the anger or aggression.
2. *Identify emotions.* Try to understand what is causing the problem and why the patient is reacting with anger. Ask yourself what the patient may be feeling and ask, "How do you feel about that?" This gives the patient the chance to identify and discuss their emotions or problems. Do not tell the patient what you think they feel.
3. *Explore options.* Help the patient to regain some sense of control by brainstorming possible solutions to their problems. You may not be able to solve the problems, but you can assist the patient in finding their own solutions.
4. *Offer positive comments.* Increase the patient's self-esteem by finding something they do well and complimenting them. Many patients and their loved ones feel helpless, and the reassuring words of a concerned care provider can provide great comfort.
5. *Keep a 1.5-metre distance from the patient.* An arcing 45-degree angle of approach is safer and less threatening. Be aware of your physical environment (unobstructed access to exit, means to call for help). Keep your hands open and spread your fingers.
6. As soon as the patient raises any verbal or nonverbal threat, stop solo intervention, *retreat from the scene*, and, if needed, continue only as a team intervention.
7. *Be aware of your own automatic reaction toward threats and verbal violence,* including the use of offensive language about your own ethnicity, gender, orientation, or social status. Practise your capacity to depersonalize a patient's behaviour. Speak up about your own emotions with trusted colleagues or your supervisor to get their emotional support. This can diminish unwelcome automatic (unconscious) reactions and enable you to stay professional, thereby achieving better outcomes. This also contributes to your own emotional well-being.
8. *Utilize proper restraint techniques and equipment only as a last resort* to ensure everyone's safety and security.

injury. Few patients reach this stage if level 1 and 2 interventions are effective. However, for those who are engaging in violent behaviours, three interventions are available: seclusion, restraints, and medication.

A point to remember here is that using restraints and seclusion as interventions for the control of assaultive behaviours must be planned ahead. Both strategies involve federal and provincial/territorial laws, institutional policies, and special procedures. Study the procedures for applying restraints and placing patients in seclusion. This information is also available in any nursing fundamentals text. Remember to monitor the condition of the restrained patient at least every 15 minutes and use other, less drastic measures as soon as the patient has regained behavioural control.

Trauma-Informed Care

An important point to remember is that many mentally ill patients were themselves the victims of abuse at some point during their lives. Thus, it is necessary to use a trauma-informed care (TIC) approach when treating patients. **Trauma-informed care** refers to care focused on the patient's past experiences of violence or trauma and the role it currently plays in their lives. When a history of trauma is present, health care staff must be aware of this and avoid approaches or situations that may retraumatize or aggravate trauma symptoms in patients. Health care providers should assume that everyone has experienced trauma or abuse in their lives and should use this approach in any care modality as a general precaution. TIC is not a technique for treating or healing the trauma, but a general approach to take the fact of the trauma into the care consideration so that there can be improvement in the patient's health outcomes. Following are five main principles of TIC (Purkey, Patel, & Phillips, 2018):

1. *Awareness and validation*—Validate the patient's traumatic experience. This does not necessarily require validation of all small details of the trauma, but is an acknowledgement of the ongoing effect of the trauma on the patient's life and coping strategies. Validating patient experience opens the door to acknowledging the patient's coping strategies as having been adaptive at the time but being maladaptive now, when the threat of the trauma no longer exists. It is important to acknowledge the shame and guilt that often emerge when a patient shares a traumatic experience. Helping the patient understand the connection between the trauma experience and their current functioning can be very therapeutic.

2. *Safety and trustworthiness*—Make the patient feel emotionally safe. Consistency of the therapeutic relationship (primary nursing care, consistent physician care) and the predictability of the care procedures (clear departmental rules and procedures, predictable appointment schedule) are the first fundamental components for feeling safe. This is a stability component of a therapeutic relationship. The second fundamental component comprises all the other factors that contribute to safety: physical (absence of physical violence), financial, housing stability, and food security, among others.

3. *Choice, control, and collaboration*—Involve the patient in care. The typical reaction of a trauma survivor is submissiveness to authority. Care providers must make an effort to override that submissiveness by presenting all treatment choices to the patient (including the choice not to engage in care). A true collaborative approach with the patient may take significantly more time to develop, but it will result in a significantly better health outcome for the patient.

4. *Strengths-based and skills-building care*—Focus on the patient's strengths and resilience. This may require a change not only in the patient's but also the care provider's attitude to seeing the patient not as being weak and a victim but as someone who is strong and resilient, despite the trauma. The care provider must avoid becoming embedded in a health-system paternalistic approach.

The trauma experience is disempowering for the patient. Thus, the care provider's approach must be empowering, rewarding the patient for any demonstration of positive strengths and skills.

5. *Cultural, historical, and identity issues*—Incorporate processes that are sensitive to the patient's culture, ethnicity, and personal and social identity. Many patients experience a trauma related to their identity, such as marginalization based on their culture, sexual orientation, gender identity, ethnicity, religion, or disability. A care provider must demonstrate sensitivity to this potential systemic trauma of group marginalization.

Using a TIC approach is especially important during any coercive part of a patient's care. The Sample Patient Care Plan 25.1 offers suggestions for addressing aggressive behaviour.

Once the assaultive event has subsided and the patient is willing to discuss the problem, begin to enlist their help to modify the inappropriate behaviours. Table 25.4 offers an example of a patient education plan for controlling impulsive, aggressive behaviours.

Interventions for care providers focus on learning to effectively control their own feelings of anger. Even the most therapeutic care provider experiences anger. Learning to cope with personal feelings of anger and aggression allows care providers to be more successful in working with the angry emotions of others (see Critical Thinking box).

CRITICAL THINKING

There are several techniques for managing your own anger:

1. *Vent your feelings.* Yell, scream, shout, but do it in a safe place.
2. *Change your focus.* Distract yourself for a moment—listen to the radio, take a walk. Move your energies from the anger to another topic. Playing with a pet is a great tranquilizer. Even counting to 10 can be very effective.
3. *Use your anger constructively.* Take the energy that is used to be angry and do something else with it. Clean the house. Organize the junk drawer. Exercise. Meditate.
4. *Discuss* your anger with those involved. Talking it out (after you are calm) lets people know what is on your mind and how you feel. Discussion also offers opportunities for personal learning and developing more therapeutic behaviours.
5. *Forgive* those with whom you are angry. If harsh words were exchanged, apologize. Apologies are free; they are not a sign of weakness, and they communicate a willingness to cooperate in the future. Forgiveness is an underused therapeutic tool.
6. *Relax.* Take slow, deep breaths, and tell your body to relax and become calm. Remember the effects of our stress neurochemicals. Emotional responses have a strong influence on the physical body. Smile; it requires the use of fewer muscles and promotes positive reactions in yourself and others.

Practise your ability to cope with feelings and reactions at home and at work. As you enhance your skills, you will find yourself becoming more effective when working with the emotional responses of others.

SAMPLE PATIENT CARE PLAN 25.1 Risk for Violence

Assessment

History Bruce, a 15-year-old boy, has been sent to the mental health unit for psychiatric evaluation by the local police. Since age 13 he has been arrested several times for vandalism, drug possession, and menacing. His parents are cooperative but "feel helpless." His older sister is living away from home because she refuses "to be exposed to his violent behaviours."

Current Findings An unkempt, sullen adolescent boy with tattoos on each knuckle of the right hand. Head is shaved in a pattern. Smoking cigarettes despite the "no smoking" sign posted on the wall.

Multidisciplinary Diagnosis	Planning/Goals
Risk for other-directed violence	Bruce will demonstrate absence of aggressive or hostile threats or behaviours by October 10.

THERAPEUTIC INTERVENTIONS

Interventions	Rationale	Team Member
1. Approach Bruce with respect; avoid judging.	Adolescents need acceptance from adults as much as they need direction	All
2. Orient to unit routine and policies; give clear, specific rules and the consequences for breaking them.	Assists Bruce until he is able to gain internal control over his aggressive behaviours	Nsg
3. Assess for warning signs of increasing anger.	Behavioural changes often indicate an aggressive reaction; good assessment skills prevent injury to patient and others	All
4. Assess past acts of aggression, and determine the potential seriousness of present actions.	Knowledge of previous patterns of violence helps assess Bruce's tolerance for current stresses	All
5. Demonstrate acceptance of the painful feelings underlying Bruce's behaviours.	Helps to encourage Bruce's self-worth even though his behaviours are unacceptable	All
6. Use open-ended questions; avoid asking "why."	"Why" questions call for an explanation or defensive reaction; open-ended questions help explore feelings, thoughts, and reactions	All
7. Contract with Bruce for "no violence" while on unit.	Protects others from injury; encourages him to be responsible for his own actions	
8. Teach stress management and problem-solving techniques.	Redirects energy created by anxiety and anger into healthier responses	Psy, Nsg

Evaluation By September 15, Bruce no longer required daily time-out sessions. By October 2, Bruce was able to identify one source of his anger.

Critical Thinking Questions

1. What purpose does active listening serve when working with angry patients?
2. What care provider behaviours demonstrate respect for a sullen teen such as Bruce?

A complete patient care plan includes several other diagnoses and interventions.
Nsg, nursing staff; *Psy,* psychologist.

TABLE 25.4 Patient Education Plan: Modifying Impulsive Behaviour

Content	Instructional Activities	Evaluation
Describe characteristics and consequences of impulsive behaviour.	Select a situation in which impulsive behaviour occurred. Ask the patient to describe what happened. Provide the patient with paper and a pen. Instruct the patient to keep a diary of impulsive actions, including a description of events before and after the incident.	The patient will identify and describe an impulsive incident. The patient will maintain a diary of impulsive behaviours. The patient will explore the causes and consequences of impulsive behaviour.
Describe behaviours characteristic of interpersonal anxiety.	Discuss the diary with the patient.	The patient will connect feelings of interpersonal anxiety with impulsive behaviour.
Relate anxiety to impulsive behaviour.	Assist the patient to identify interpersonal anxiety related to impulsive behaviour.	

Continued

TABLE 25.4	**Patient Education Plan: Modifying Impulsive Behaviour—cont'd**	
Content	**Instructional Activities**	**Evaluation**
Explain stress reduction techniques.	Describe the stress response. Demonstrate relaxation exercises. Assist the patient in returning the demonstration.	The patient will perform relaxation exercises when signs of anxiety appear.
Identify alternative responses to anxiety-producing situations.	Using situations from the diary and knowledge of relaxation exercises, assist the patient to list possible alternative responses.	The patient will identify at least two alternative responses to each anxiety-producing situation.
Practise using alternative responses to anxiety-producing situations.	Role-play each of the identified alternative behaviours. Discuss the feelings associated with impulsive behaviour and the alternatives.	The patient will describe the relationship between behaviour and feelings. The patient will select and perform anxiety-reducing behaviours.

From Keltner, N. L., & Steele, D. (2014). *Psychiatric nursing* (7th ed.). Mosby.

KEY POINTS

- Anger is a normal emotional response to a perceived threat, frustration, or distressing event.
- Anger serves as a coping mechanism, a motivator, or an opportunity for learning.
- Aggression or hostile behaviours are angry feelings and impulses that are converted into action.
- Aggressive behaviours become inappropriate when they affect other people or their possessions.
- Assertiveness is the ability to directly express one's feelings or needs in a way that respects the rights of other people and retains the individual's dignity.
- Gender violence, which is the abuse of members of one gender by members of another, is seen in many cultural and social settings.
- The expression of anger occurs throughout the life cycle.
- Aggression and violence continue to be worldwide concerns.
- Theories about the nature of aggression fall into one of three basic models: biological, psychosocial, and sociocultural.
- Assaults are aggressive behaviours that violate others' person or properties.
- Assault and violence occur in a predictable pattern of emotional responses called the *assault cycle.*

- Stages of the assault cycle are the trigger stage, the escalation stage, the crisis stage, the recovery stage, and the depression stage.
- The *DSM-5* lists three categories of disorders relating to aggressive behaviours: conduct disorders, impulse-control disorders, and oppositional defiant disorder.
- The primary reason that a patient with a major mental illness may be violent is the lack of on-time diagnosis and inadequate treatment.
- The first step in controlling aggression is to assess the patient's potential for engaging in inappropriate behaviours.
- Interventions for aggressive or potentially aggressive behaviours are divided into three levels: preventing violence, protecting the patient and others, and secluding or restraining the out-of-control patient.
- There is no solo intervention with aggressive or threatening patients.
- Always use a trauma-informed care approach as a standard precaution when treating patients with a mental illness.
- Learning to cope with your own feelings of anger or aggression enables you to be more successful in working with the emotions of others.

ADDITIONAL LEARNING RESOURCES

Go to your Evolve website (http://evolve.elsevier.com/Canada/Morrison-Valfre/) for additional online resources, including the online Study Guide for additional learning activities to help you master this chapter content.

CRITICAL THINKING QUESTIONS

1. What are some common ways in which a patient may exhibit violence? How may it come across?
2. When can verbal violence be tolerated and when should it not be tolerated? What are examples of appropriate staff actions in different settings in response to verbal violence?
3. A patient is verbally violent toward a staff member in a one-to-one intervention. He is using offensive language about the staff member's ethnicity and then suddenly threatens him by saying, "I will kill you!" What should the threatened staff member do?
4. Together with your staff, you must restrain a 28-year-old female patient to the bed because she is behaving in a violent manner toward others around her. How would you apply the principles of trauma-informed care in this scenario?

REFERENCES

American Psychiatric Association (APA). (2013). *Diagnostic and statistical manual of mental disorders* (5th ed.). American Psychiatric Publishing (DSM-5).

Canadian Institute for Health Research (CIHR). (2012). *Canadian bullying statistics*. http://www.cihr-irsc.gc.ca/e/45838.html

Grohol, J. M. (2020). *Oppositional defiant disorder symptoms. PsychCentral, July 8.* https://psychcentral.com/disorders/oppositional-defiant-disorder-symptoms/

Keltner, N. L., & Steele, D. (2014). *Psychiatric nursing* (7th ed.). Mosby.

NationMaster.com. (2019). *Crime stats: Compare key data on Canada & United States.* https://www.nationmaster.com/country-info/compare/Canada/United-States/Crime

Pompili, M., & Fiorillo, A. (2015). Aggression and impulsivity in schizophrenia. *Psychiatric Times, 32*(7). https://www.psychiatrictimes.com/schizophrenia/aggression-and-impulsivity-schizophrenia

Potter, P. A., Perry, A. G., Stockert, P., et al. (2019). *Essentials for nursing practice* (9th ed.). Mosby.

Psychology Today. (2017a). *Conduct disorder.* https://www.psychologytoday.com/ca/conditions/conduct-disorder

Psychology Today. (2017b). *Pyromania.* https://www.psychologytoday.com/ca/conditions/pyromania

Psychology Today. (2019a). *Intermittent explosive disorder.* https://www.psychologytoday.com/ca/conditions/intermittent-explosive-disorder

Psychology Today. (2019b). *Kleptomania.* https://www.psychologytoday.com/ca/conditions/kleptomania

Purkey, E., Patel, R., & Phillips, S. P. (2018). Trauma-informed care: Better care for everyone. *Canadian Family Physician, 64*(3), 170–172.

Stuart, G. W. (2013). *Principles and practice of psychiatric nursing* (10th ed.). Mosby.

26

Outward-Focused Emotions: Violence

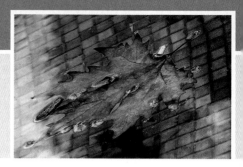

Aggressive, violent, and exploitive behaviours occur throughout the animal kingdom. Many animals battle violently for the right to mate and pass on their genes. Starlings exploit other birds by laying their single egg in another's nest. Animal aggression can serve to procure food, to mate, or to establish dominance. Animals' use of violence is predictable and useful; they seldom risk injuring themselves just to be violent.

Aggressive characteristics are also present in human beings, but they are expressed differently.

Human beings engage in aggressive or violent behaviours for a variety of reasons, similar to other mammals. This has been a *Homo sapiens* behaviour for all five million years of the species' existence. It was only about 50 000 years ago when *Homo sapiens* developed the unique capability of abstract thinking (the ability to think about something that does not exist in reality). This capacity allowed *Homo sapiens* to build new tools and new social structures; leave Africa for other continents; extinguish all other *Homo* species; and lead the worst outbreak of species die-off since the loss of the dinosaurs, 65 million years ago (Center for Biological Diversity, n.d.). The motives for killing are no longer always tangible. They include new motives for interspecies killing (the killing of *Homo sapiens* by *Homo sapiens*) and can involve concepts that do not exist in nature (e.g., morals, ethnicity, nationality, country, religion, money). It is important to underscore here, essentially, that our abilities for abstract thinking and creating material goods and social structures have caused tensions among our own species (*Homo sapiens*), as well as violence toward other species. All of this activity occurred during the last 50 000 years, which is a very short time in our evolution. We are not genetically predisposed to be as violent as we have been these last 50 000 years. Before this period, we were relatively peaceful animals with tangible reasons for interspecies violence (fighting for mating, for status inside a small group, and for hunting area). It appears that we are now witnessing a time when this ability for abstract thinking has started to lead us back to a more peaceful, nonviolent existence, with fewer wars than ever and less violence than that among our ancient ancestors.

In order to discuss violence, one must be familiar with its related terms, which change as social norms change. These terms were created and shaped by something that *Homo sapiens* made up—society. Society is an invented and constantly changing entity (sometimes the changes are very slow and sometimes very fast) due to multiple internal conflicts.

Likewise, the definitions of different terminology and norms change. For example, 100 years ago corporal punishment in Western schools was a norm that would not have met the definition of violence, but it does today. For most of our history, we have lived in separate societies, which has contributed to the great variety of norms. Technological progress has increased our mobility and communication, creating one global society. This sense of a global society has also led to changes in social terms, norms, and definitions, including those of violence.

The World Health Organization (WHO; the official representative of our global society) gives the following definition of **violence**: "The intentional use of physical force or power, threatened or actual, against oneself, another person, or against a group or community, that either results in or has a high likelihood of resulting in injury, death, psychological harm, maldevelopment or deprivation" (WHO, 2002).

Agitation is another common term used to describe some behaviour in neuropsychiatric disorders. Although this term is frequently used to describe the manifestation of many disorders, there is a surprising lack of consensus in the medical community regarding what "agitation" actually means. A group of international researchers formed an Agitation Definition Work Group (ADWG) to reach consensus on this term and, in 2015, after analyzing 928 respondents, they arrived at the following definition of **agitation**: "1) occurring in patients with a cognitive impairment or dementia syndrome; 2) exhibiting behaviour

consistent with emotional distress; 3) manifesting excessive motor activity, verbal aggression, or physical aggression; and 4) evidencing behaviours that cause excess disability and are not solely attributable to another disorder (psychiatric, medical, or substance-related)" (Cummings, Mintzer, Brodaty, et al., 2015). However, given the lack of final consensus among clinicians on what "agitation" means, it is important to avoid using this term in clinical descriptions. Instead, clinicians are encouraged to provide an exact description of a patient's presentation.

Another term used in the context of violence is **abuse**, the intentional misuse of someone or something that results in harm, injury, or trauma. Abuse can take place in the form of active harm or passive neglect.

Neglect is harm to another's health or welfare through a failure to provide for basic needs or by placing the individual's health or welfare at unreasonable risk. Neglect often occurs among the more vulnerable members of society, such as children and elders.

Exploitation refers to the use of an individual for selfish purposes, profit, or gain. Children who must labour with no time for study or play are examples of exploited individuals. Each of these terms describes some type of physical or psychological activity that is socially unacceptable.

The purpose of this chapter is twofold: (1) to help you understand the many ways in which violence is present in society, and (2) to provide you with the tools to effectively assess, intervene in, reduce, and prevent aggressive incidents.

SOCIAL FACTORS AND VIOLENCE

No one is certain exactly why violence occurs. We do know, however, that violent acts and their consequences are decreasing. According to the University of Oxford–based organization, Our World in Data, there is a correlation between the increased level of literacy, freedom, and democracy in the world and decreased levels of human-to-human violence, including during wars (Our World in Data, 2015). Essentially, despite our perception that there is a high level of violence in the world (e.g., when we hear about it through media), statistics actually show that *we live in the most peaceful time of Homo sapiens' history*. It is important to learn and understand as much as possible about the social sources leading to both increasing and decreasing violence in society.

The WHO estimated in 2002 that, globally, 815 000 people died from suicide and, in that same year, 310 000 people died as a result of direct conflict with other humans, mostly in very poor parts of the world (WHO, 2002). In Canada, death from homicide is an extremely rare event. In Canada, there are four times more deaths resulting from motor vehicle accidents and seven times more deaths resulting from suicide than there are deaths from homicide (Cotter, 2014).

Several cultural and social factors affect the type, rate, and approval or disapproval of violence carried out. Canada, as a multicultural country, has people from many cultures, many with subcultures. This makes Canadian society rich, vibrant, dynamic, tolerant, peaceful, and prosperous. In some

CULTURAL CONSIDERATIONS

In some poverty-stricken countries, children as young as age 4 years are forced to work in mining, rug mills, and other manufacturing businesses. They labour long hours in miserable working conditions and receive little pay. If a child does not work fast enough or does not have the courage to complain, they are physically punished. Children who are too outspoken about the poor working conditions have been known to "disappear."

Aggressive and violent acts are found in every group in society, and it appears that poverty plays a role in the development of aggressive behaviours. In many societies, productive and financially rewarding work is expected of most adults, especially men. A lack of fulfilling work often leads to poverty, frustration, and, in many cases, violence.

BOX 26.1   Characteristics of a Person With Machismo

Has an attitude of male pride
Engages in thrill-seeking behaviours
Employs competition as his guiding principle
Is egocentric (self-centred)
Is unable to express emotions openly, except anger and rage
Dislikes being gentle or vulnerable
Values sexual virility
Displays sexist attitudes
Treats women as objects or commodities
Sees women as objects of conquest
Insists on being dominant toward girls and women
Holds to unwritten law that infidelity by a woman must be avenged
Unable to cooperate with women
Agrees to sexual use and abuse of women
Glorifies war and violence, supports the use of military force
Enjoys contact sports
Uses aggression to physically solve problems

subcultures, however, the use of aggressive behaviour through beliefs and rituals is acceptable. And in some cultures, violent acts, such as suicide bombings, are considered heroic.

Theories of Violence

Several theories have attempted to explain the nature of violence. The *psychiatric/mental illness model* views violence as a mental illness. Both victim and abuser are considered mentally disturbed. Recent evidence, however, has found that the incidence of mental illness is no greater in batterers or their victims than in the rest of the population (Paddock, 2012).

Social learning theory states that aggressive and violent behaviours are learned through role-modelling others in the environment. Aggression is believed to be a learned behaviour based on the values, attitudes, and actions of role models within the individual's environment.

Sociological theories credit environmental and social factors as causes for violence. Environmental factors, such as overcrowding, lack of adequate housing, and poor hygiene, can increase the incidence of aggression. The social factors of unemployment, poverty, crime, substance or drug abuse, and isolation are believed to be related to violent acts.

Anthropological theories, which are based in the study of humans' social history, explain violence and aggression as being the result of cultural patterns, social organizations, or sexual differences. Some cultures encourage the use of aggressive behaviours, and their citizens learn to interact and cope aggressively. In other cultures, equality and harmony are stressed. Male and female roles are less defined in cooperative cultures than they are in cultures with hierarchies or degrees of power.

Finally, *feminist theories* use the concept of "machismo" (among others) to explain the occurrence of violence against women.

Machismo is defined as compulsive masculinity. Feminist theories state that males are socialized throughout childhood to behave more aggressively and violently. By the time boys have reached adolescence, they are preoccupied with physical strength, athletic prowess, and attempts to demonstrate daring, violent, or aggressive behaviours. Men who have a high degree of machismo demonstrate certain social,

behavioural, and sexual attitudes. Machismo is a strong influence on male behaviour in many countries. These theories do not imply that every man with a high level of machismo abuses other people. They do, however, remind us that the potential for abuse lies within the machismo belief system (Box 26.1).

Psychologists who study cyberspace and its effects on users are concerned that technology will change the way people think about themselves and their role in society. There is a temptation for young people to succumb to the temptation to leave "real life" behind for the more controllable realms accessed on the computer. As more people become members of the computer network society and interact on social media platforms, the number of "real" face-to-face relationships decreases. In these times of public isolation and anxiety over so many social forces, people are turning increasingly to the Internet's chat rooms or other information highways in search of social interaction and supportive relationships.

Social connectedness is more than just an obligation or a desire—it fills the basic human need to belong. Social relationships are important elements in preventing aggression and violence as the lack of supportive relationships has been linked to many negative consequences, including aggressive acts, mental illness, crime, and suicide. Supportive relationships also offer coping strategies to those suffering from challenging mental health. "Talk therapy" can help individuals reframe their current situation, when all they see in a moment of vulnerability is negativity and doom and gloom (Mental Health Foundation, 2020).

ABUSE, NEGLECT, AND EXPLOITATION WITHIN THE FAMILY

For far too long, physical abuse and emotional abuse within the family have remained unspoken issues. Traditionally, victims suffered in silence, unable to seek help for fear of being revealed as less than a real person. Today, communities are working to provide care and counselling for abused and exploited people. Family violence comes in several forms.

Domestic Violence

In Western society, the idea that "a man's home is his castle" has been inviolate. This principle has historically meant that the home is a private place. "What goes on inside one's home is nobody else's business" still remains a popular attitude today, even if activities endanger family members.

Domestic violence is defined as abuse and battering within a family. **Battering** is a term that describes repeated physical abuse of someone, usually a woman, child, or older person. Victims of violent or abusive acts often suffer from post-traumatic stress disorder (discussed later in this chapter).

In Canada, 26% of all violence is domestic or family violence. Experts believe that family violence is often underestimated and that only one in five people reports family violence to the police. Stigma and fear are the biggest obstacles to reporting domestic violence. Intimate partner violence against women is reported by 79% of police. Indigenous women are more likely than non-Indigenous women to experience spousal violence. Women who self-identify as lesbian or bisexual report significantly higher rates of violence by a partner than do heterosexual women. Girls are four to five times more likely than boys to be victims of child sexual abuse by a family member (Public Health Agency of Canada, 2018).

A functional family unit is described by what it does (its processes) to achieve its goals. These processes include clear and supportive communication among all family members, conflict resolution, the setting of goals, and the use of resources inside and outside the family (Potter, Perry, Stockert, et al., 2019). A dysfunctional family is described by its inability or unwillingness to fulfill its basic functions. Box 26.2 lists several characteristics of a dysfunctional family. Not all dysfunctional families have an element of abuse, but the inability of a family to meet the needs of its members greatly increases the potential for aggressive or violent behaviours. (For example, a father who has recently lost a minimum-wage job is too afraid to tell his wife and two children and instead spends his last paycheque to buy liquor. He then slaps his wife when she finds out that he has spent it on liquor instead of food and confronts him about this.)

The family is considered a social unit that is entitled to privacy and freedom from intrusion. Unfortunately, this doctrine has allowed untold numbers of women and children (and, occasionally, men) to suffer at the hands of their "loved ones." Violence within the family occurs in several ways. Common forms include physical, emotional, or sexual abuse and neglect of partners, children, and older members.

> ### BOX 26.2 Characteristics of Dysfunctional Families
>
> Family members are self-centred.
> Authority is inconsistent or lacking; parents feel they cannot control children.
> Roles are not clearly defined; it is unclear who is the parent, who is the child.
> Family members are unable to meet their own or others' needs, but each expects their own needs to be met.
> Individualism is not encouraged; autonomy and trust are lacking.
> No common goals are identified; the focus is on the present.
> The family appears chaotic, disorganized; no one is really aware of what is happening in the family.
> Communications tend to be cold and indifferent; family members feel pain and desperation; humour, caring, empathy, and intimacy are generally absent; few clear communications exist.
> Conflict is viewed as negative and is expressed through power struggles and sexual aggression.
> The family may confuse violence with caring.
> Family boundaries are rigid; family members feel threatened when outsiders try to enter the group; members are socially isolated; parents often married young and have few parenting skills.
> Family violence is often present.

> ### CASE STUDY
>
> At first, there were small arguments, but soon they grew out of proportion, and he was screaming. He began by "correcting" her; then it was directions about how to do it "the right way." When she forgot or refused, he tormented her by repeatedly reminding her of how stupid and worthless she was—how nobody would have her but him. He was relentless in his destruction of her self-esteem and confidence, but he never hit her.
> - Do his behaviours meet the criteria for abuse? Explain your answer.

Intimate Partner Abuse

No human enters a relationship with the intent of becoming a battered partner, but partner abuse is still considered an accepted part of marriage in many groups. Even in societies in which domestic violence is condemned, individuals have their own attitudes, personal agendas, and faults that may cause conflict within the family. The notion that "all is fair in love and war" promotes the idea that marriage is a private relationship and that the legal system should stay out of the picture—even when the picture includes assault, abuse, or injury.

While there is no "typical" abused partner, the victims of violence do have some characteristics in common. Perhaps the most common trait is a trusting nature. Many people were raised to be nonaggressive and traditional. They were brought up to believe that the partner who plays the role of the protector and the breadwinner of the household should have some exclusive right to commit violence. These people, in turn, often feel that submission is the way to "please your master." The problem is that most abusive partners cannot be pleased.

CRITICAL THINKING

Characteristics of Victims
Feel captive in the system (family, group, community)
Blame self for problems leading to abuse
Have low self-esteem; view self as unworthy
Feel helpless and powerless to change situation
Are financially, emotionally, or physically dependent on abuser
Are depressed, unable to see a future without abuse
- How many persons do you know who demonstrate these characteristics?
- What interventions would you choose for a patient who feels like a victim?

When abuse occurs, guilt, anger, and terror can shatter a person's self-esteem. The person suffers in silence, knowing that the consequences will be severe if they seek help. Once a person is repeatedly abused they becomes battered, and a vicious cycle of violence is soon established. Table 26.1 describes the cycle of domestic violence.

Abuser (batterer) behaviours have several characteristics. The profile of a typical abuser includes poor emotional control, a superior attitude toward women, a history of substance abuse, high levels of jealousy and insecurity, and the use of threats, punishment, and physical violence to control another's behaviour. This profile may easily be the picture of a patient, a patient's partner, a parent, a mate, neighbour, friend, or loved one. Early recognition of the characteristics of potential violence allows for interventions that are more effective. Box 26.3 lists several early signs of a potential abuser.

Abuse During Pregnancy

Pregnancy should be a time of great joy and anticipation, but for some women, pregnancy only increases their chances of being abused. While it is difficult to believe that fathers would intentionally harm the mother of their children, trauma is the leading cause of maternal death during pregnancy. Statistics on prenatal violence are difficult to gather. Studies in public prenatal clinics reveal that more than 15% of patients are physically abused during pregnancy, and about 60% of the women questioned had suffered two or more assaults, indicating that episodes of abuse were recurrent. The frequency and severity of abuse, as well as the potential for homicide, are significantly increased for White women.

The effects of abuse during pregnancy can be devastating. Because the mother is afraid to seek help, she often delays her entry into the health care system, thus denying both herself and her developing child the benefit of adequate prenatal care. Abused women of all ethnicities are twice as likely to postpone beginning prenatal care until the third trimester of pregnancy, too late to prevent or treat many complications. In addition, the frequency of low-birth-weight infants and preterm deliveries is almost doubled among women who have a history of abuse during pregnancy (Hockenberry & Wilson, 2014).

Child Abuse

Unfortunately, the most vulnerable individuals in society, our children, are often the most abused. Child abuse occurs in many cultures and in many different ways.

CULTURAL CONSIDERATIONS

The following is a popular saying in the red-light district of Bangkok, where children are often forced into prostitution:
"At 10 you are a woman.
At 20 you are an old woman.
And at 30 you are dead."

Misuse of children occurs through abuse, neglect, and sexual exploitation. Physical, sexual, emotional/psychological abuse, and neglect are the major categories of child abuse (Tracy, 2019). Child **pornography** involves writings, pictures, or other messages pertaining to children that are intended to sexually arouse. Child **prostitution** is the selling of sexual favours by children. Child sexual abuse exists all over the world (e.g., see related discussion about human trafficking later in this chapter). In Brazil alone it has been estimated that between 250 000 and 500 000 children are involved in the sex trade. The numbers are even greater in Asia, with more than half a million child prostitutes in Thailand. Most of them are girls under age 16 years, but in Sri Lanka many child prostitutes are boys who cater to older men.

Many children are sold into prostitution with the belief that they will not be infected with human immunodeficiency virus (HIV) or other sexually transmitted infections. Sadly, however, this is not the case. The Children's Rights Protection Center in Thailand claims that the AIDS rate among Thai child prostitutes is now greater than 50%.

Children are also bought, sold, and exploited as objects of trade. They are purchased cheaply in one country and sold for a handsome profit in another. Young girls from the Philippines are imported to Japan for prostitution in a business that makes more than one million dollars per day. Many Roma children are forced into begging, often bringing in hundreds of dollars each day while under the complete control of their abusers.

In some societies, female infants are considered undesirable. Girls commonly receive less food, attention, or education than their brothers. For example, according to the World Bank, the death rate for young girls in India outnumbers the death rate for young boys by more than 300 000 deaths per year. The majority of orphans in China are girls. After reviewing these facts, it is easy to understand why child abuse and neglect are important issues of our time.

TABLE 26.1 Example of a Cycle of Domestic Violence

Abuser	Victim
Tension Building	
He has excessively high expectations of her.	She is nurturing and compliant and tries to please him.
He blames her for anything that goes wrong.	She denies the seriousness of their problems.
He does not try to control his behaviours.	She feels she can control his behaviours.
He is aware of his inappropriate behaviours but does not admit it.	She tries to alter his behaviour to stay safe. She tries to prevent his anger.
Verbal abuse and minor physical abuse increase.	She blames external factors: alcohol, work.
Afraid she will leave, he gets more possessive to keep her captive.	She takes minor abuse but does not feel she deserves it. She gets scared and tries to hide (withdrawal).
He gets frantic and more controlling.	She may call for help as the tension becomes unbearable.
He misinterprets her withdrawal as rejection.	
Serious Battering Incident	
The trigger event is an internal or external event or substance.	In cases of long-term battering, she may provoke it just to get it over with.
The battering usually occurs in private.	She may call for help if she is afraid of being killed.
He will threaten more harm if she tries to get help (police, medical).	Her initial reactions are shock, disbelief, and denial.
He tries to justify his behaviours but does not understand what happens.	Fearing more abuse if police come, she may plead for them not to arrest him.
He minimizes the severity of the abuse.	She is anxious, ashamed, humiliated, sleepless, fatigued, and depressed.
His stress is relieved.	She may not seek help for injuries for a day or more and lies about the cause of injuries.
Honeymoon	
He is loving, charming, begging for forgiveness, making promises.	She sees his loving behaviours as the real person and tries to make up.
He truly believes he will never abuse again.	She wants to believe it will never happen again.
He feels that he taught her a lesson and she will not "act up."	She feels that if she stays, he will get help; the thought of leaving makes her feel guilty.
He preys on her guilt to keep her trapped.	She believes in the permanency of the relationship and gets trapped.

Spanking was, and in several countries still is, a main form of discipline for children. Unfortunately, spanking and other forms of physical punishment teach children that power and violence are approved coping mechanisms. Today the countries of Sweden, Finland, Norway, Austria, and Switzerland, in an effort to curb the growing rates of child abuse, prohibit all forms of physical punishment in schools and homes. Most other industrialized countries, except parts of Australia and Canada, and the United States and South Africa have banned physical punishment in schools.

The mistreatment of children can take several forms. **Physical abuse** is inflicted injury to a child, ranging from minor bruises and lacerations to severe trauma and death. **Sexual abuse** is the intentional engaging of children in sexual

BOX 26.3   Early Signs of an Abusive Personality

1. A push for a quick involvement
2. Jealously controlling
3. Unrealistic expectations
4. Isolates partner from family and friends
5. Blames others for own problems and mistakes
6. Makes others responsible for the person's feelings
7. Hypersensitive, easily insulted
8. Cruel to animals and children
9. "Playful" use of force during sex
10. Verbal abuse
11. Enforces rigid sex roles
12. Sudden mood swings
13. History of past battering
14. Threatens violence

acts. Sexual abuse can take the form of rape, incest, fondling, intercourse, or other forms of sexual contact. **Emotional abuse** involves rejection, criticism, terrorizing, and isolation. Although the scars of this type of abuse are seldom seen objectively, they result in deep and penetrating wounds for many individuals.

Neglect is the failure to provide the necessities of life. *Physical neglect* is the failure to provide a child's basic needs, such as food, clothing, shelter, and a safe environment. *Emotional neglect* is characterized by a lack of parent–child attachment. *Medical care neglect* is the refusal to seek treatment when it is needed. Delays in treatment are common among abused children. A rare form of child abuse, called *factitious disorder by proxy* (see also Chapter 22), occurs when caretakers simulate or create the signs and symptoms of illness in the child with the goal of receiving attention from health care providers for the caretakers' own psychological needs. Malingering by proxy is the same, but with some tangible goal for the individual (e.g., money, drugs, housing, etc.).

Abuse or neglect occurs during every stage of childhood. In infancy, shaken baby syndrome should be suspected in every infant with unexplained or vague injuries. **Shaken baby syndrome** is defined as vigorous shaking of an infant that leads to whiplash-induced bleeding within the brain with no external signs of head trauma. This syndrome is difficult to diagnose because of the lack of physical evidence and the parents' refusal to discuss the situation.

Every health care provider must be alert for the possibility of a "shaken baby" whenever there is a history of unexplained lethargy, fussiness, or irritability in an infant. Seizures or swelling in the head demands immediate investigation. Because the incidence of shaken baby syndrome is increasing, efforts must be made to educate parents and community members about the importance of handling the youngest members of our society with gentleness and care.

Children are victimized more often than adults. Types of violent behaviours associated with abused children include *pandemic aggression,* in which the majority of children are assaulted; *acute aggression,* in which children are abused,

neglected, or exploited; and *extraordinary aggression,* which usually results in death.

Everyone who interacts with children should be aware of signs of abuse. When a child has bruises or welts that fit a particular pattern, such as a belt buckle or a hand, teeth marks, or burns from a cigar or cigarette, physical abuse should be suspected. Children who have been sexually abused usually have general, nonspecific complaints, such as abdominal pain, bed-wetting, sleep disturbances, and phobias. However, the abuse usually goes undetected until the child discloses it.

A growing problem seen in today's schools is **bullying**, the intentional tormenting of others. This type of violence begins in childhood and can extend into adulthood. The definition of bullying is complex and not final, but includes actions within a relationship between a dominant and a less dominant person or group, where:

- An imbalance of power (real or perceived) is manifested through aggressive actions, physical or psychological (including verbal or social);
- Negative interactions occur that are direct (face-to-face) or indirect (gossip, exclusion); or
- Negative actions are taken with an intention to harm. These can include some or all of the following:
  - Physical actions (punching, kicking, biting);
  - Verbal actions (threats, name-calling, insults, ethno-culturally based or sexual comments); and
  - Social exclusion (spreading rumours, ignoring, gossiping, excluding).

The negative actions are repeated. Either the intensity or the duration of the actions establishes the bully's dominance over the victim.

Canada ranks in the middle of 35 countries that have been studied for levels of bullying. Between 10 and 20% of students have reported bullying in school. Boys report a slightly higher rate than do girls (Public Safety Canada, 2018a).

The victims of bullying are chosen because they are perceived as different in some way. They may be big or small for their age, overweight or underweight; belong to a different ethnic group or religion; live with a disability; or be sensitive, anxious, or insecure. Signs of being bullied begin with a change in behaviour. The individual becomes withdrawn, preoccupied, and anxious, leading to depressed moods and recurring somatic symptoms. Headaches and stomach aches, especially in the morning before school, are common. The child does not want to ride the bus or interact with other children. Torn or missing clothing and big after-school appetites are also clues. Some people who are bullied become reactive and lash out, often in a destructive or hurtful manner.

Bullies need to feel powerful, so they select their targets from those who can be easily intimidated. Often they blame the victims for the abuse. If repeated frequently enough, the victims accept that blame and begin to hold themselves responsible for the abuse.

Bullying behaviours can be physical, verbal, or via the Internet. They can involve harassment or exclusion from activities. Box 26.4 lists examples of bullying behaviours.

BOX 26.4   Examples of Bullying Behaviours

Physical Bullying
Choking, hitting, kicking, punching, pushing, tripping

Verbal Bullying
Hate talk, mocking, starting rumors, taunting, intimidating, teasing, threatening

Exclusion From Activities
Encouraging others to stay away from the targeted person, physically barring attendance

Social Media Bullying (Cyberbullying)
Using electronic media to deride others through hate talk, mocking, starting rumours, taunting, intimidating, teasing, threatening, and encouraging others to do the same

Motives for bullying are unclear, but research suggests that bullies have a strong need to be in control. They are quick to anger and find it easy to use aggressive behaviours when their self-image is threatened. Bullying has its roots in childhood and, unless adults intervene early and effectively, it can escalate to more seriously violent behaviours.

Adolescents who are involved in bullying experience poor psychosocial and emotional adjustment. They commonly have difficulty making friends, and they suffer increased loneliness. Victim reactions range from anxiety and avoidance to extreme fear and physical symptoms of illness. Often students may approach other staff members employed by the school, such as principals, teachers, educational assistants, volunteers, or parent volunteers, with headaches, an upset stomach, and other problems, hoping that someone will recognize their distress. Sleeping difficulties can also indicate that bullying is occurring. The best way to stop bullying is for responsible adults to recognize it when it occurs and to intervene early.

Adolescent Abuse

The incidence of abuse in adolescence is greater than once thought. Abuse of adolescents is often the most overlooked type of family violence. For this reason, abused teens are less likely to receive needed services and counselling.

Adolescence is a time of emotional development. But not all teens have severe mood swings, periods of depression, or suicidal thoughts, which can be signs of possible abuse. Too often, these signs go unnoticed by adults. At other times, they are recognized as natural outcomes of adolescent misbehaviour. "They had it coming" is still a widely held attitude when it comes to abusing adolescents.

Abused adolescents often have significant health risks. Emotional disorders often result from a history of insecurity and self-survival. The incidences of eating disorders, substance abuse, delinquent behaviours, post-traumatic stress disorder (PTSD), and suicide attempts are increased in adolescents who are abused (Loveisrespect.org, 2017). Premature sexual activity is common. All too often it leads to unwanted pregnancies, sexually transmitted infections, and AIDS. Worse yet, adolescent abuse can result in fatal accidents, murder, and suicide, the three leading causes of death for all adolescents. One in four violent crimes is committed by adolescents.

Girls are more likely to be abused than boys. Women who were abused in childhood are more likely to be abused as adults. Boys are more likely to suffer abuse outside the home by peers and others. Individuals who commit acts of violence as adolescents are often the same people in the nation's criminal justice system as adults. Sadly, studies have shown that many adults who were physically disciplined as children approve of the use of physical force for controlling another person's behaviour.

Adolescents who are maltreated are abused by parents, siblings, and persons outside the family. The most common form of violence within the home occurs between siblings. Violence between brothers and sisters is so common that it is often considered to be "normal" behaviour because parents take it for granted that "kids will be kids" and tend to ignore it. Yet this type of violence can have long-lasting effects.

Children learn to exploit and victimize each other during the early school years. By the teen years, the use of violence can become interwoven with daily activities. Peer pressure is great during adolescence. Those who are perceived as different suffer the consequences at the hands of their own peers. Of all age groups, adolescents often receive the most severe abuse, the kind that results in serious disability or death.

CASE STUDY

Sam is a quiet, thoughtful, and charming young man whose intelligence shines through his sarcastic and tough demeanour. At 17 years old, he is well developed and equipped to cope on the streets of Toronto. Sam is also the leader of a street gang and does not hesitate to use violence.

Sam comes from a family with two older brothers and a younger sister. In his early years, it was common to see his mother and father arguing and hitting each other. By the time Sam was 6 years old, his older brother had shot a neighbour and was "doing time." Throughout his childhood, Sam frequently vented his frustrations on his younger sister by hitting, pinching, and spitting on her.

At 8 years old, Sam was initiated into his brother's gang. By age 10, his intelligence and creativity had earned him the nickname "the brain." By 14 years old, he was destined for leadership. Today, at 17 years old, Sam sits in a hospital bed with three bullet holes in his body. His bruised and pregnant girlfriend sits at his side. As soon as he can walk again, he plans to "make a little visit and even the score" with the guys he believes are responsible for his attack.

- Can you see any learned patterns of behaviour in this family?
- What do you think could have been done to prevent this situation from occurring?

Often, however, the signs of family mistreatment are vague. A history of abuse is frequently found in teens who are runaways, homeless, or incarcerated (in jail or prison). The problems of teen violence and abuse can be prevented if health care providers are willing to invest in strategies directed at the level of a particular teenager's interest (similar between patient and health care provider), in an effort to form a therapeutic alliance.

Elder Abuse

The potential for older persons' maltreatment or neglect increases as the number of people grow older. The aggregate (physical, sexual, psychological, and financial abuse) prevalence for elder abuse in Canada in 2015 was 7.5%, representing 695 248 older Canadians (National Initiative for the Care of the Elderly [NICE], 2015).

Especially vulnerable older persons include those with chronic or disabling illnesses, aged individuals, and those who are poor or have few resources. The typical victim of elder abuse is an older woman who is living with a relative and is physically or mentally impaired. She has a history of unexplained bruises or injuries, burns in unusual places, sexually transmitted infection, or poor personal hygiene. She may experience extreme mood swings, be depressed, be fearful, and be extremely concerned about the cost of health care. Many times the families of abused older people "health care shop," miss appointments, and change health care providers frequently.

Family members are the most frequent abusers of older persons. The demands placed on caregivers often influence the development of abuse. Violence can erupt when caregivers feel stressed, pressured, or frustrated. In addition, many people who abuse their elders are coping with current substance-related or mental health challenges themselves.

Neglect and exploitation are also common among the older population. Neglect can take the form of not providing food, health care, or aids such as dentures, glasses, or hearing aids. Older persons who are unable to walk can suffer from long periods of isolation or abandonment. Neglect also includes deliberate efforts to cause emotional distress, such as threatening harm or withholding important information.

Exploitation of older individuals is often financial in nature. They are a favourite target for cons or extortionists. Many times, older persons are forced to sign over their properties, their pensions, or other assets. Older persons may be denied the right to vote or make their own decisions. On some occasions they are placed in a long-term care center without their consent.

Today, many jurisdictions have passed laws that require reporting of abusive incidents. Each health care provider can go a long way toward preventing elder abuse by recognizing the signs and symptoms of abuse. As a care provider, you need to become familiar with the laws governing mandatory reporting of abuse, and work to prevent violence in all settings. It is every person's responsibility to protect the aging members of society.

Sexual Abuse

A particularly devastating form of abuse is sexual abuse, the unwanted sexual attentions of another. When sexual activities or intercourse occurs between members of the same family (other than the parents), it is called **incest**. Sexual violence

has strong and lasting consequences for the victims. Children who are sexually abused suffer from a wide spectrum of mental health disorders, ranging from chronic headaches to depression, PTSD, and severe personality disorders. The effects of abuse are long-lasting and frequently follow the victim into adulthood.

Sexually abused adults are most often women. Most sexual assaults are made by women's partners. Date-rape drugs such as gamma-hydroxybutyrate (GHB) and Rohypnol are just a few of the central nervous system (CNS) depressants that can easily be placed in a drink because they are flavourless; they cause increased sensuality and sexual feelings and ultimately place the unsuspecting person who has ingested them in a happy, euphoric mood (Health Link BC, 2018). The most violent form of sexual assault, rape, occurs more frequently in relationships associated with other forms of physical aggression. Episodes of battering often include sexual and physical attacks—a deadly combination for many maltreated women.

Sexual abuse of older persons, especially women, occurs all too frequently. Because sexual mistreatment of older individuals is still a taboo subject, it often goes unrecognized by health care providers. Clues to the presence of sexual abuse in the older population include complaints of pain, itching, or soreness in the genital area; bruises or other evidence of injury around the genital area or elsewhere on the body; difficulty walking, sitting, or moving; the presence of unexplained venereal disease or genital infections; and stained, torn, or bloody underclothing.

Health care providers, especially nurses, should routinely assess all patients for a history of abuse or victimization and report any suspicious signs or behaviours to supervisors and required authorities. Regulated health care providers (RN, RPNs, social workers, respiratory therapists, occupational therapists) all have a duty to report it. An individual's well-being and dignity are worth the effort.

ABUSE, NEGLECT, AND EXPLOITATION WITHIN THE COMMUNITY

Violence Against Health Care Workers

The WHO has determined that between 8 and 38% of health care workers suffer from physical violence, much of which comes from patients and visitors; many more are threatened or exposed to verbal aggression (WHO, 2019). The workers who are affected most are nurses and those workers involved in direct patient care.

Strategies and recommendations for addressing abuse of health care workers include better management of violent patients and high-risk visitors. Interventions for emergency settings focus on ensuring the physical security of health care facilities. However, more research is needed to evaluate the effectiveness of these programs, especially in low-resources settings (WHO, 2019).

Violence, Trauma, and Crime

People are violent in many ways, in both legal and illegal ways. Today's society is confronted with a steady diet of violent behaviours. Although most **homicides** (taking the life of another person) are committed by family members or friends, a surprising number of them occur at the hands of complete strangers. Robbery has become common in most communities, and an unsettling trend of murder in the workplace is rising. Car theft and drive-by crimes are increasing. Children are being kidnapped with greater frequency, and the incidence of violent crimes by and against children and adolescents continues to soar.

Acts of violence are becoming commonly accepted in society. Radio, television, and the Internet flood people with examples of violence. Our children are immersed in tales of aggressive actions from the time they are first exposed to cartoons. Studies by television's cable network group have revealed that more than half of the programs on television are violent or aggressive in nature (American Academy of Child & Adolescent Psychiatry, 2014). In most programs, victims are harmed and the aggressor is seldom caught or punished. This steady diet has resulted in children who are more willing to solve their problems with the use of violence than with critical thinking or problem-solving.

Acts of violence seen on television pale in comparison with those that occur in real life (Fig. 26.1). Daily news sources announce a litany of the day's violent activities. Some people listen, shake their heads, and then continue with their own lives; others take action to address injustices they see playing out, highlighting tensions in society. To resolve these tensions, society will have to change itself, establishing new standards and norms of behaviour to achieve a new balance.

Violence breeds physical and emotional pain for its victims. The basic needs of trust and autonomy (control) are threatened when one is involved with violence. Victims react with anger, fear, denial, and shame. The well-meaning comments of friends and loved ones may even imply fault. Many victims of violence harbour feelings of unworthiness and contamination. Relationships with family and friends may become disturbed, or enhanced through support and care, as victims attempt to put the pieces of their lives back together.

Crime is a natural vehicle for violence. Many crimes are committed on impulse, whereas others are well planned. Crime may or may not involve physical aggression and violence, but the effect of being victimized by crime leaves deep emotional scars on most individuals.

Group Abuse

Throughout history, people have chosen certain groups of people to define as being different. Individuals within these groups may be kind and gentle, but association with the group stigmatizes them as "one of those people." This label somehow justifies the aggressive and violent reactions of persons who view the group members with hostility. Excellent examples of this twisted line of thinking can be found throughout history and in the "ethnic cleansing" that has occurred in many countries.

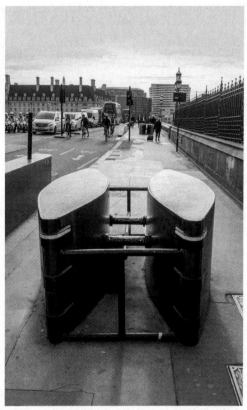

Fig. 26.1 Violence against a society: a protective barrier at the entrance to Westminster bridge in London, England. These protective barriers were installed as a result of the March 2017 terrorist attack, in which a driver drove a car along the sidewalk, knocking down pedestrians, before killing a policeman in the grounds of Parliament. (iStockphoto/Raylipscombe.)

Another form of group abuse is human trafficking, more commonly known as *slavery*. Sex trafficking and labour trafficking are the most common forms of this slavery. Victims may be so frightened that they refuse to talk to the authorities that can help them. We must all work to identify and put a stop to this billion-dollar industry. Although the extent of human trafficking in Canada is difficult to determine because of its undercover nature (Public Safety Canada, 2020), the following statistics from 2012 can provide some context:

- There were 25 convictions (41 victims) under human trafficking specific offences in the *Criminal Code* enacted in 2005.
- Approximately 56 cases were before the courts, involving at least 85 accused and 136 victims.
- At least 26 of these victims were under the age of 18 at the time of the alleged offence.

Over 90% of these cases involved domestic human trafficking; the remaining cases (less than 10%) involved people being brought into Canada from another country (Public Safety Canada, 2018b).

Aggression against certain groups also exists in more subtle ways. Admission to many schools and academic

TABLE 26.2   Stages of Recovery From Violence

Stage of Recovery	Time Frame	Emotions, Behaviours
Impact: disorganization	Minutes to days	Initial reactions: crying, confusion, denial, disbelief, fear, hysteria, helplessness, shock; may have physical responses, eating or sleeping disturbances; may be calm with others and then react in private
Recoil: struggle to adapt	Weeks to months	Slowly becomes aware of effect of event on their life; immediate danger is past, but emotional stress remains; may plan for revenge; tries to resume daily routines; needs to discuss details of violent event; may become dependent; needs much emotional support
Reorganization: reconstruction	Months to years	Emotions fade, but event is not forgotten; reviews event with "Why me?" questions; justifies own actions, then gains sense of control over life; grieves over losses; may experience lingering emotions, nightmares; realizes that life will always be different as result of violence; eventually integrates memories and learns to live with reasonable sense of safety and security; may develop mental health challenges if reorganization is not successful

Data from Keltner, N. L., & Steele, D. (2013). Psychiatric nursing (7th ed.). Mosby.

institutions often depends on belonging to the "right group." Job requirements may be structured to attract only a certain kind of applicant, and running for a political office can be done only if one "fits in." These forms of aggression against members of certain groups are all quiet, subtle, and usually unspoken, but they nevertheless influence the lives of many good people.

MENTAL HEALTH DISORDERS RELATING TO VIOLENCE

Crisis is a part of every violent act. One's usual coping skills are ineffective when dealing with the effects of a violent act. To recover from an act of violence, new coping behaviours must be found and then applied. The victims of violence suffer through a number of emotional and behavioural experiences that can take months or even years to resolve. Putting one's life back together after a violent act involves many changes that take place over time (Table 26.2). The process of recovery from violence is influenced by the severity of the trauma, the resources of the victim, and the help and treatment received immediately following the traumatic event.

Aggressive and violent behaviours are a part of numerous mental health disorders.

Post-Traumatic Stress Disorder

A full discussion of PTSD can be found in Chapter 18.

Rape-Trauma Syndrome

Rape-trauma syndrome is a related nursing diagnosis to PTSD that encompasses the essentials of care for the victims of this violent experience. Rape-trauma syndrome is not an actual *DSM-5* diagnosis, but rather a group of emotional, physical, and behavioural reactions to rape.

Rape is an act of sexual violence by one person against another. Although rape may involve sexual behaviours, it is an act of power that aims to cause pain at the most intimate level of one's being. Forced sexual attentions are a violation of one's person, whether they occur at the hands of a stranger or a loved one.

While a woman may be raped at any age, the ages of 15 to 24 years are associated with the highest risk. Rape is an underreported crime, with estimates of one in three women being raped at some time during her life. Although not as common, the incidence of men being raped by other men is rising, but it is rarely reported (Keltner & Steele, 2014).

Many victims of rape realize that they have lived through the experience but wish they had died. Body injuries may be minor or severe. Some individuals may have been tortured or injured during or shortly after the rape episode. A threat on the life of the victim or to return and commit the act again may have been made.

Survivors of sexual assaults feel severely violated. Feelings of anger, frustration, loss of control, fear, shame, and guilt haunt the victims of these violent acts. After the rape, most individuals feel the need to retreat to a safe place, clean themselves thoroughly, and remove all reminders of the event. Doing this, however, destroys most of the evidence that is useful in apprehending the offender.

Recovery from being the victim of a rape follows the same steps as the stages of recovery from other violent acts (see Table 26.2). Immediately after the incident, the individual tends to become disorganized, then attempts to adjust are made, and finally the experience is integrated into her life. The greater the force or brutality, the greater the psychological harm and recovery time. Many individuals do not report the assaults to the police. They carry their burden alone and suffer a silent rape-trauma syndrome.

Some nurses receive special training to become forensic nurses or sexual assault nurse examiners (SANEs). Often, though, nurses may be the first health care providers with whom a rape victim interacts. Strong support, gentle understanding, and nonjudgemental acceptance have a powerful influence on how well the victim copes with and successfully recovers from this violent assault. Because rape is a reportable crime, evidence must be gathered, with the victim's permission. Nurses should make sure to follow the same protocol every time they care for a patient who has been raped. Evidence that has been gathered carefully and good documentation are important tools if the case is taken to court.

THERAPEUTIC INTERVENTIONS

When working with victims of violence, there are two major goals. The first and longest-reaching goal is to prevent violence from occurring. The second goal revolves around early recognition and treatment of violated individuals.

Working with abused or victimized patients on a regular basis requires special education and training. Some health care providers become rape counsellors or advocates for abused and exploited patients. However, every care provider can apply special measures to care for the individuals who have the misfortune to become victims of violence.

Special Assessments

Whenever a suspected victim of violence enters the health care system, whether through the emergency department or clinic, special attention is required. The first priority of care is to ensure the patient's safety, but the preservation of evidence also is extremely important.

Forensic evidence is information that is gathered for legal purposes. It is the evidence that helps find and convict perpetrators of violent acts. When violence is suspected, the care provider's most effective tools are accurate observations, precise documentation, and notification of the appropriate authorities. By law, health care providers are required to report these incidents to the police. Although the law does not require victims of rape to report it, all evidence is important and must be gathered carefully.

When assessing a patient who has been a victim of violence, one must first obtain their consent. Then document the size, shape, colour, and pattern of any wounds, bruises, scars, or other marks. The skin records evidence well. Human bite marks leave a history. Look for them on the ears, nose, nipples, armpits, back, and genitals. Rings, belt buckles, and other items leave telltale marks behind when they are used as weapons. Other physical signs that may indicate violence or abuse include odd marks on the skin, hyperactive reflexes, and poor eye contact. Child abuse or neglect is not always

easy to spot. Table 26.3 lists numerous signs and symptoms of child abuse and neglect.

Care providers, especially nurses, must know how to assess suspicious injuries and describe their findings objectively. Figure 26.2 offers an example of an abuse assessment documentation form. One must document objective evidence as accurately as possible. Use quotation marks and the patient's own words. Do not guess or draw conclusions about the cause of any injury. If the patient is a rape victim, all specimens should be labelled and saved for analysis. It is wiser to err on the side of gathering too much information rather than not enough.

Ensuring use of the principles of trauma-informed care (TIC) can assist in optimal recovery outcomes and effective coping strategies for patients. The principles of TIC are discussed in detail in Chapter 25.

Treating Victims of Violence

Remember that the first priority of care for every victim of violence is to ensure their safety and security. Once a patient feels safe, other therapeutic interventions are more easily implemented.

Do not leave the patient alone. Many victims believe that their abusers may attempt to hurt them again, even when they are seeking help. Explain all procedures simply, and ensure cooperation before proceeding. Show respect. Allow the patient to maintain as much control as possible.

The care plan is developed on the basis of the individual patient, the type of abuse, and the resources available. Nursing diagnoses (problem statements) are chosen according to identified problems. Refer to Box 26.5 for a list of possible diagnoses and problem statements.

It is important to remember that each diagnosis or mental or physical health challenge has many interventions, and the selection depends on each patient's particular circumstances. However, all patients who have been abused, exploited, or neglected have certain care needs in common (see Sample Patient Care Plan 26.1).

Aggressive and violent actions are often seen in patients who are diagnosed with a mental illness. Treatment consists of assessing risk factors, developing interventions to reduce aggressive reactions, and helping patients learn more effective coping skills. Patients are often prescribed medications to help control aggressive and violent behaviours (Table 26.4).

Preventing Violence in Your Life

Given the statistics, it is likely that each of us will be exposed to some sort of violence at some time during our lives. As members of the health care profession, the odds of being involved in some type of violence are increasing. Health care providers are less immune to acts of violence than they were in the past. It is important to remain aware that violence can erupt in any patient situation.

TABLE 26.3   Signs and Symptoms of Child Abuse and Neglect

Category	Child's Appearance	Child's Behaviour	Caretaker's Behaviour
Physical abuse	**Bruises and welts:** on face, lips, or mouth; in various stages of healing; on large areas of torso, back, buttocks, or thighs; in unusual patterns, clustered, or reflective of instrument used to inflict them; on several different surface areas **Burns:** cigar or cigarette burns; glovelike or socklike burns or doughnut-shaped burns on buttocks or genitals indicating immersion in hot liquid; rope burns on arms, legs, neck, or torso; patterned burns that show shape of item (iron, grill, etc.) used **Fractures:** skull, jaw, or nasal fractures; spiral fractures of arms or legs; fractures in various states of healing; multiple fractures; any fracture in child under 2 yr **Lacerations and abrasions:** to mouth, lip, gums, or eye; genitals **Human bite marks**	Wary of physical contact with adults Apprehensive when other children cry Demonstrates extremes in behaviour (e.g., aggressiveness or withdrawal) Seems frightened of parents Reports injury by parents	Has history of abuse as child Uses harsh discipline Offers illogical, unconvincing, contradictory, or no explanation of child's injury Seems unconcerned about child Significantly misperceives child (e.g., sees child as bad, evil, a monster) Psychotic or psychopathic Misuses alcohol or other drugs Attempts to conceal child's injury or protect identity of person responsible
Neglect	Consistently dirty, unwashed, hungry, or inappropriately dressed Without supervision for extended time or when engaged in dangerous activities Constantly tired or listless Has unattended physical issues or lacks routine medical care Is exploited, overworked, or kept from attending school Has been abandoned	Engages in delinquent acts (e.g., vandalism, drinking, prostitution, drug use) Begs or steals food Rarely attends school	Misuses alcohol or other drugs Maintains chaotic home life Shows evidence of apathy or futility Mentally ill or of diminished intelligence Has long-term chronic illnesses Has history of neglect as child
Sexual abuse	Has torn, stained, or bloody underclothing Is experiencing pain or itching in genital area Has bruises or bleeding in external genitals, vagina, or anal regions Has venereal disease Has swollen or red cervix, vulva, or perineum Has semen on mouth or genitals or on clothing Is pregnant	Appears withdrawn or engages in fantasy or infantile behaviour Has poor peer relationships	Extremely protective or jealous of child Encourages child to engage in prostitution or sexual acts in presence of caretaker
Emotional maltreatment	Emotional maltreatment, often less overt than other forms of child abuse and neglect; indicated by behaviours of child and caretaker	Unwilling to participate in physical activities Engages in delinquent acts or runs away States they have been sexually assaulted Appears overly compliant, passive, undemanding Extremely aggressive, demanding, or full of rage Shows overly adaptive behaviours, either inappropriately adult (e.g., parents other children) or inappropriately infantile (e.g., rocks constantly, sucks thumb, is enuretic) Lags in physical, emotional, and intellectual development Attempts suicide	Has been sexually abused as child Experiencing marital difficulties Misuses alcohol or other drugs Frequently absent from home Blames or belittles child Cold and rejecting Withholds love Treats siblings unequally Seems unconcerned about child's problem

ABUSE ASSESSMENT SCREEN

1) Have you ever been emotionally or physically abused by your partner or someone important to you?

    Yes ☐   No ☐

    If yes by whom? _____

    Total number of times _____

2) Within the last year, have you been hit, slapped, kicked, or otherwise physically hurt by someone?

    Yes ☐   No ☐

    If yes by whom? _____

    Total number of times _____

3) Since you've been pregnant, have you been hit, slapped, kicked, or otherwise physically hurt by someone?

    Yes ☐   No ☐

    If yes by whom? _____

    Total number of times _____

4) Within the last year, has anyone forced you to have sexual activities?

    Yes ☐   No ☐

    If yes by whom? _____

    Total number of times _____

5) Are you afraid of your partner or anyone you listed above?

    Yes ☐   No ☐

MARK THE AREA OF INJURY ON A BODY MAP AND SCORE EACH INCIDENT ACCORDING TO THE FOLLOWING SCALE:

If any of the descriptions for the higher number apply, use the higher number.

1 = Threats of abuse including use of a weapon

2 = Slapping, pushing; no injuries and/or lasting pain

3 = Punching, kicking, bruises, cuts, and/or continuing pain

4 = Beating up, severe contusions, burns, broken bones

5 = Head injury, internal injury, permanent injury

6 = Use of weapon; wound from weapon

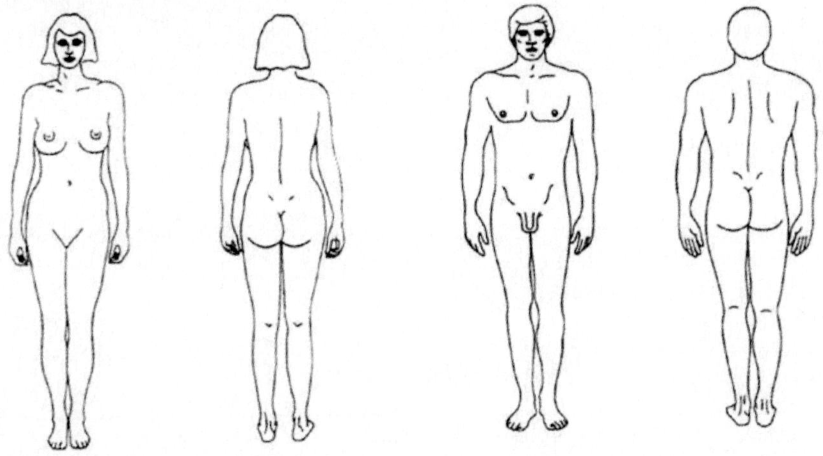

● ● ● ● Family Violence Prevention Fund

Fig. 26.2 Futures Without Violence abuse assessment screen. (Copyright © 2011, Futures Without Violence. All rights reserved.)

SAMPLE PATIENT CARE PLAN 26.1   Rape-Trauma Syndrome

Assessment

History Salima is a 19-year-old community college student who lives at home. Three weeks ago she met Ben, a road maintenance worker who was visiting a mutual friend. After a short visit, Salima said she was going to the gym for her workout. Ben offered to drive her because he was going in the same direction. Salima accepted, saying that she had to stop at her house first to change clothes.

On arrival, Salima left the car and walked into the house. She was surprised to see Ben following her and asked him to wait in the car. Later that day, Salima's mother found her beaten and tied to her bed.

Current Findings A stuporous young woman, lying in the fetal position. Numerous bruises and abrasions are noted on the face, both wrists, legs, and feet. Mother is at the bedside.

Multidisciplinary Diagnosis

Rape-trauma syndrome related to recent sexual attack and injury

Planning/Goals

Salima will be free of medical or physical complications of rape trauma.

Salima will establish a therapeutic alliance with the primary nurse by October 21.

THERAPEUTIC INTERVENTIONS

Intervention	Rationale	Team Member
1. Allow Salima's mother to remain with her at all times.	Mother has historically provided safety and security for Salima	Nsg
2. Assist with physical assessment and gathering of specimens after consent is obtained.	To assess the extent of her physical injuries, psychological trauma; to gather forensic evidence	Nsg
3. Let Salima know that she will not be blamed for the rape incident.	Violated persons often feel they will be held responsible for encouraging the assault.	Nsg, Psy
4. Convey an accepting, caring, nonjudgemental attitude regardless of the circumstances.	Helps to establish therapeutic communications and builds trust	All
5. Encourage Salima to acknowledge the pain and anger of the rape experience.	Releasing painful emotions lessens their intensity and power	Psy, Nsg
6. Explain the importance of seeking support and counselling for Salima and her family.	Provides emotional support during the process of returning to "normal"	Psy, Nsg
7. Encourage Salima to report the incident to the police.	May help to prevent other occurrences; may help to bring the perpetrator to justice	Psy, Nsg
8. Make referrals to a rape crisis centre, family counsellors (with permission).	Long-term emotional support will help Salima and her family effectively adapt	Soc Svc

Evaluation Salima tested negative for sexually transmitted infections 3 weeks after the incident. After 2 weeks of emotional support and encouragement, Salima attended her first crisis support group.

Critical Thinking Questions

1. What can be done to promote feelings of safety in Salima?
2. Why is long-term counselling important with rape-trauma victims?

A complete patient care plan includes several other diagnoses and interventions.
Nsg, Nursing staff; *Psy*, psychologist; *Soc Svc*, social services.

When interacting with patients, watch for signs of growing anxiety, frustration, or agitation, and then intervene quickly to prevent situations from escalating. Trust your own judgement or gut-level feelings, and seek assistance from other care providers when needed.

Prevent yourself from becoming victimized by patients or their family members, by enforcing your professional boundaries (see discussion of helping boundaries, in Chapter 11) and working within your legal and ethical parameters. The goal of providing emotional and mental health care is to assist patients in successfully coping with their difficulties. Remembering who "owns" the problem allows care providers to remain therapeutic without becoming victimized.

BOX 26.5 Problem Statements (Nursing Diagnoses) Related to Violence

Physical Realm
Risk-prone behaviour, risk-prone health
Risk for violence, self or other directed
Nonadherence
Rape-trauma syndrome

Psychosocial Realm
Anxiety
Ineffective coping
Denial
Impaired family processes
Fear
Hopelessness
Powerlessness
Self-esteem disturbance
Impaired social interaction

TABLE 26.4 Medications Used to Manage Aggression

Medication Class	Example	Care Implications
Atypical antipsychotics	clozapine, risperidone, olanzapine	Sedation
Typical antipsychotic	loxapine, haloperidol, zuclopenthixol	Sedation, drop in blood pressure
Beta-adrenergic blockers	propranolol	Drop in heart rate
Antianxiety agents	buspirone, lorazepam, benzodiazepines	Sedation
Anticonvulsants	valproic acid	Sedation

Work to prevent violence in your own life. Contact the sponsors of violent programs on television; write companies and protest. Support legislative actions that are designed to reduce violence. Volunteer at shelters, crisis hot lines, or support groups. Educate those who will listen about the effects of violence on children. Volunteer to teach a program on problem-solving at local preschools.

Learn to recognize aggression and violence in your personal thoughts, attitudes, and responses. Become aware of how you cope with feelings of anger, frustration, and aggression. Practise developing more effective methods for working with your emotions. Howard Zinn, in his book *You Can't Be Neutral on a Moving Train* (1994), titled the epilogue "The Possibility of Hope." There he states that "small acts, when multiplied by millions of people, can transform the world." The small acts of nurses and other health care providers help to nourish the human connections that weave us together. Perhaps we can make a difference in relation to violence—if we are all willing to try.

KEY POINTS

- Violence is a major cause of death and disability in most countries.
- Theories that attempt to explain the nature of violence include the psychiatric/mental illness model, social learning theories, sociological theories, anthropological theories, and feminist theories.
- Characteristics of a dysfunctional family include self-centred members, authority that is inconsistent or lacking, no clearly defined roles, and members who are unable to meet their own or others' needs. Individualism is not encouraged. No common goals are identified. Communications are cold and indifferent. Conflict is perceived as negative, family boundaries are rigid, and family violence occurs.
- *Battering* is a term that describes ongoing physical abuse of someone, usually a woman, child, or older person.
- Trauma is the leading cause of maternal death during pregnancy. Low-birth-weight infants and preterm deliveries are almost doubled in women who have a history of abuse during pregnancy. Inadequate prenatal care is common.
- Since the early 1960s, the number of reported incidents of child abuse or neglect has increased dramatically.
- Abuse of adolescents is often an overlooked type of violence.
- Throughout history, people have chosen certain groups of people to define as being different and therefore deserving of aggressive behaviours.
- The process of recovery from violence is influenced by the severity of the trauma, the resources of the victim, and the help and treatment received by the victim immediately after the traumatic event.
- The essential feature of PTSD is the development of characteristic symptoms after exposure to an extreme traumatic stressor.
- Rape is an act of sexual violence by one person against another that involves the use of power.
- Two major health care goals for victims of violence are to prevent violence from occurring and to provide early recognition and treatment for the violated individuals.
- The first priority of care for every victim of violence is to ensure safety and security. Explain all procedures simply, and ensure cooperation. Allow the patient to maintain as much control as possible.
- Special assessments for a patient who has been involved in violence include documenting the size, shape, colour, and pattern of any wounds, bruises, scars, or other marks, and looking for human bites on the ears, nose, nipples, armpits, back, and genitals.

- By law, health care providers are required to report incidents of suspected or actual abuse or neglect.
- Work to prevent violence in your own life by contacting the sponsors of violent programs on television and

protesting. Support legislative actions designed to reduce violence. Volunteer and educate about the effects of violence on children.

ADDITIONAL LEARNING RESOURCES

Go to your Evolve website (http://evolve.elsevier.com/Canada/Morrison-Valfre/) for additional online resources, including the online Study Guide for additional learning activities to help you master this chapter content.

CRITICAL THINKING QUESTIONS

1. What forms of elder abuse may happen in our society?
2. What are the various forms of bullying that can occur?
3. A 25-year-old single, unemployed mother visits the emergency department (ED) for the third time within the last month with her 6-month-old son. The main complaint is "high temperature." Upon investigation, the 6-month-old boy is found to have a temperature of 38.0°C and no other abnormal findings. The child is somewhat overdressed. His temperature goes down to normal within 30 minutes with no intervention. The last two times he was in the ED, it was a similar presentation. The mother is asking to be seen by a social worker and, as during the previous two times, extensively talks about her own struggles. As with the previous two times, the social worker provides the mother with empathic listening and directions to different community supports. What etiology could be behind that presentation?

REFERENCES

American Academy of Child & Adolescent Psychiatry (AACAP). (2014). TV violence and children. *Facts for Families Guide, 13*(4), 1. https://www.aacap.org/AACAP/Families_and_Youth/Facts_for_Families/FFF-Guide/Children-And-TV-Violence-013.aspx

Center for Biological Diversity. (n.d.). Halting the extinction crisis. https://www.biologicaldiversity.org/programs/biodiversity/elements_of_biodiversity/extinction_crisis/

Cotter, A. (2014). *Homicide in Canada, 2013. Statistics Canada.* https://www150.statcan.gc.ca/n1/pub/85-002-x/2014001/article/14108-eng.htm

Cummings, J., Mintzer, J., Brodaty, H., et al. (2015). Agitation in cognitive disorders: International Psychogeriatric Association provisional consensus clinical and research definition. *International Psychogeriatrics, 27*(1), 7–17. https://doi.org/10.1017/S1041610214001963

Health Link, B. C. (2018). *Date rape drugs.* https://www.healthlinkbc.ca/health-topics/uq2448

Hockenberry, M., & Wilson, D. (2014). *Wong's nursing care of infants and children* (10th ed.). Mosby.

Keltner, N. L., & Steele, D. (2014). *Psychiatric nursing* (7th ed.). Mosby.

Loveisrespect.org. (2017). *Dating abuse statistics. National domestic violence Hotline.* https://www.loveisrespect.org/resources/dating-violence-statistics/

Mental Health Foundation. (2020). *Talking therapies.* https://www.mentalhealth.org.uk/a-to-z/t/talking-therapies

National Initiative for the Care of the Elderly (NICE). (2015). *Into the light: National survey on the mistreatment of older Canadians 2015.* https://cnpea.ca/images/canada-report-june-7-2016-pre-study-lynnmcdonald.pdf

Our World in Data. (2015). *The visual history of decreasing war and violence.* https://slides.ourworldindata.org/war-and-violence/#/title-slide

Paddock, C. (2012). Mental health disorders linked to domestic violence. *Medical News Today, December, 27.* https://www.medicalnewstoday.com/articles/254475.php

Potter, P. A., Perry, A. G., Stockert, P., et al. (2019). *Essentials for nursing practice* (9th ed.). Mosby.

Public Health Agency of Canada. (2018). *Family violence: How big is the problem in Canada?.* https://www.canada.ca/en/public-health/services/health-promotion/stop-family-violence/problem-canada.html

Public Safety Canada. (2018a). *Bullying prevention in schools.* https://www.publicsafety.gc.ca/cnt/rsrcs/pblctns/bllng-prvntn-schls/index-en.aspx

Public Safety Canada. (2018b). *National action plan to combat human trafficking.* https://www.publicsafety.gc.ca/cnt/rsrcs/pblctns/ntnl-ctn-pln-cmbt/index-en.aspx

Public Safety Canada. (2020). *Human trafficking.* https://www.publicsafety.gc.ca/cnt/cntrng-crm/hmn-trffckng/index-en.aspx

Tracy, N. (2019). *Types of child abuse.* https://www.healthyplace.com/abuse/child-abuse-information/types-child-abuse

World Health Organization (WHO). (2002). *World report on violence and health: Summary.* https://www.who.int/violence_injury_prevention/violence/world_report/en/summary_en.pdf

World Health Organization (WHO). (2019). *Violence against health workers.* https://www.who.int/violence_injury_prevention/violence/workplace/en/

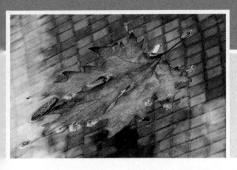

27

Inward-Focused Emotions: Suicide

OBJECTIVES

Upon completion of this chapter, the student will be able to:
1. Explain the range of self-protective behavioural responses.
2. Discuss three myths about suicidal behaviours.
3. Identify two cultural or social factors that relate to suicide.
4. Examine four categories of motivation for attempting suicide.
5. Explain how suicide affects family members and friends.
6. Describe three theories that attempt to explain the causes of suicide.
7. Discuss the occurrence of suicide throughout each life cycle.
8. Outline the process for assessing the suicidal potential of a patient.
9. Choose three therapeutic goals and interventions for patients with suicidal behaviours.
10. Discuss main failures leading to suicide in the hospital setting.

OUTLINE

KEY TERMS

ambivalence (ăm-BĬV-ă-lĕnts) (p. 331)
direct self-destructive behaviours (p. 328)
indirect self-destructive behaviours (p. 328)
medical assistance in dying (MAiD) (p. 334)
parasuicidal (pair-ă-SOO-ĭ-sīd-ăl) **behaviours** (p. 335)
passive suicide (p. 334)
rational suicide (p. 330)
safety plan (p. 337)

self-injuries (p. 328)
suicidal attempts (p. 335)
suicidal gestures (p. 335)
suicidal ideation (Ī-dē-ā-shŭn) (p. 335)
suicidal threats (p. 335)
suicide (p. 327)
suicide precautions (p. 336)
suicidology (SOO-ĭ-sīd-ŌL-ă-jē) (p. 332)

Suicide is the action of intentionally ending one's own life. Historically, suicide has played a part in many societies. In England, suicide was considered an offence against the king. During the 1930s, many people in the United States committed suicide after the stock market crash that began the Great Depression in 1929. During World War II, Japanese kamikaze pilots intentionally sacrificed their lives for political and religious principles. In some societies, suicide is considered acceptable, even honourable. Western societies, however, generally consider suicide to be an inappropriate act committed by desperate or mentally ill individuals.

Suicide has historically served as a solution to life's great obstacles, but it is a long-term solution to a short-term problem. Today we struggle with the dilemmas of rational suicide, freedom of choice, and medical assistance in dying. Discussions about the morality or legality of suicide will grow and fade, but the ending of life by one's own hands continues to occur as people struggle for control over their situations.

CONTINUUM OF BEHAVIOURAL RESPONSES

According to Maslow's hierarchy of needs, safety and security are basic requirements for life. Individuals behave in many ways to secure these needs. Some people respond with behaviours that promote growth, whereas others may live in circumstances or respond in ways that create greater suffering for themselves. Behaviours that are adaptive and help the individual to cope result in a greater understanding and acceptance of oneself. However, maladaptive self-protective responses, if not changed, can eventually lead to self-destruction. Figure 27.1 illustrates the continuum of self-protective responses.

Self-destructive behaviours are classified as direct or indirect. **Direct self-destructive behaviours** are any form of active suicidal behaviour, such as threats, gestures, or attempts to end one's life. In this case, the individual intends to commit suicide. Although they may waver between wanting to live and longing to die, the behaviours communicate an active wish to die.

Many more people, however, engage in indirect self-destructive behaviours, which are more subtle responses to self-protection. **Indirect self-destructive behaviours** are described as any behaviours or actions that may result in harm to the individual's well-being or even death. In this case, people have no actual intention of ending their lives. They may be unaware of the potential for self-harm when engaging in harmful activities and deny the possibility of danger when confronted. Examples of indirect self-destructive behaviours include substance abuse, engaging in inappropriate or dangerous activities, and an inability to change negative thoughts and actions. Because many of these behaviours are legal or socially accepted, people do not realize their potential for harm.

As the continuum of self-protective responses (see Fig. 27.1) moves more toward maladaptive behaviours, indirect self-destructive behaviours progress to active attempts to injure oneself. **Self-injuries** reaffirm to individuals that they are still alive. Pain serves as a reminder of their connection with the body and its physical world. The last and ultimate maladaptive self-protective response is suicide. Suicide is a complex and emotional issue, but it is one with which health care providers must cope. Although overt suicidal attempts receive the most attention, individuals who engage in indirect self-destructive behaviours carry risks as great as those individuals who actually attempt to end their lives.

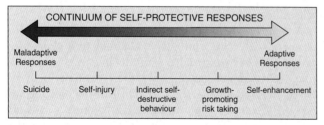

Fig. 27.1 Continuum of self-protective responses. (From Stuart, G. W. [2013]. *Principles and practice of psychiatric nursing* [10th ed.]. Mosby.)

Myths About Suicide

Many half-truths and misconceptions about suicide continue to exist despite educational efforts to promote accurate understanding. Although suicide has always been present in society, little effort was made to understand its nature until the beginning of the twentieth century. Many false ideas about suicide still exist. Table 27.1 explains several of these myths and offers facts to more accurately reflect the nature of suicide.

IMPACT OF SUICIDE ON SOCIETY

Suicide is an international epidemic. The World Health Organization (WHO) reports that "1.5% of worldwide deaths were caused by suicide in 2012, making it the third highest cause of death in the world" (Peebles, 2015). More than 3 000 suicides occur throughout the world every day, making the number of suicide deaths greater than that of people lost through homicide or war.

In 2009, there were 3 890 suicides in Canada, a rate of 11.5 per 100 000 people. The suicide rate for males was three times higher than the rate for females (17.9 vs. 5.3 per 100 000). Married people had a lower suicide rate than that for those who were single, divorced, or widowed. When Canadian suicide deaths are examined across age groups, persons aged 40 to 59 have the highest rates (Navaleenan, 2017).

The true number of persons who end their own lives is unknown because many motor vehicle accidents and other seeming mishaps are actually intentions to carry out a suicide. Because suicide is often preventable, it is important for nurses and other health care providers to be well versed in recognizing and intervening with patients who are distressed.

Cultural Factors

No one knows exactly why a person chooses suicide, but many cultural, social, and individual factors have an influence. The laws, customs, beliefs, values, and norms of a culture usually include a view of suicide. In some cultures, such as ancient Japan, suicide is considered an honourable atonement for transgressions committed during one's life. When a pharaoh (king of Egypt) died, it was an expected custom for the widow(s) to die by suicide and join him on his journey across the heavens.

Religious beliefs and customs affect the incidence of suicide. Certain Christian faiths, for example, forbid suicide under any circumstances, whereas the taking of one's life may be justified in the beliefs of other religious groups. Some cultures believe that, through suicide, they can join loved ones in the afterlife.

Customs and rituals may play a role in suicide. The "evil eye" or voodoo practised by Caribbean islanders is very real for the victim of the curse. In these societies, suicide is not a surprising outcome for an individual who has been hexed or cursed.

Hungary routinely came in first in the WHO's statistics on suicide in past years. However, since 1993, with their cultural upheaval, Russia and the Baltic republics have surpassed

TABLE 27.1 Myths and Facts About Suicide

Myth	Fact
People who talk about it will not commit suicide.	Most people communicate their intent.
One does not need to take a suicide threat seriously.	Every threat of suicide is serious.
A suicide attempt is manipulative behaviour.	Manipulation is usually not a factor.
People who are really serious about suicide give no clues.	Many people communicate warnings of their intent by tidying up their affairs, giving away possessions, or being preoccupied with death.
It is harmful to discuss the subject of suicide with patients.	Most suicidal persons need acceptance and emotional support; discussing the topic demonstrates interest and concern.
Only psychotic or depressed people commit suicide.	Depression is a high-risk factor for suicide, but not all suicidal persons are depressed. Mental illness is a risk factor for suicide.
Suicide occurs only in the lower socioeconomic classes, the poor.	Although poverty is a risk factor, suicide occurs in all socioeconomic classes.
Young children never die by suicide.	Suicidal behaviour is the leading cause of psychiatric hospitalization for young children. Suicide can occur in children as young as 4 years of age.
When people show signs of an improved mood, the threat of suicide is over.	Often energy level and, therefore, a depressed person's capacity to execute a suicidal plan improve faster than a person's mood. This leads to a dangerous situation where a person still has a plan to die due to severe depression and also has the energy to carry out that plan.

Modified from Fortinash, K. M., & Holoday-Worret, P. A. (2011). *Psychiatric mental health nursing* (5th ed.). Mosby.

Hungary in the number of suicides (WHO, 2020). Providers of health care must remember that people hold strongly to their cultural beliefs and practices. An awareness of a cultural group's attitude about suicide may someday help prevent a suicide.

CULTURAL CONSIDERATIONS

In some societies, suicide is an accepted, centuries-old tradition. In Hungary, for example, villages dwindle as their residents choose suicide over the uncertainty of living an isolated, lonely life. When people in Hungary "get fed up, they hang themselves, cut their wrists, or swallow pesticides, just like their fathers and grandfathers did," says Dr. Jorge Ulloa, a psychiatrist who runs a suicide clinic near Budapest.

When they come to Canada, new immigrants bring with them their cultural understanding about appropriate coping strategies for dealing with life's difficulties. For some people, suicide is considered to be a culturally appropriate coping strategy. Care providers must learn about people's cultures and their potentially maladaptive coping strategies and offer alternatives.

Social Factors

Many social influences affect the incidence of suicide. Chief among them is a sense of *social isolation* felt by members of fast-paced, goal-oriented societies. Family and community support systems have dwindled as mobility, politics, and finances have shifted people away from the safety and security of family and friends. The support of kind neighbours and friends has been replaced by the generic, ready-made support of massive and complicated governmental systems. Community mental health services that are government

funded may not always meet the needs of the communities they are located in. This does not mean that they do not exist, but often they are embedded within these community services. If community members are aware of these resources and are directed to access them, early and culturally appropriate intervention outcomes are the expectations (Multicultural Mental Health Resources Centre [MMHRC], 2020).

An inability to meet basic needs has a strong influence on the occurrence of suicide. The social determinants of health are factors that influence social status, and in turn, the inability to afford the basic necessities of life, like shelter, has increased the number of homeless people. It is now estimated that persons with mental illnesses make up more than one third of the homeless population. The risk for suicide, for both healthy and mentally troubled individuals, skyrockets when one is unable to meet food, shelter, and clothing needs. Poverty and homelessness lead to depression and hopelessness. Suicide becomes an acceptable alternative when one is continually hungry, cold, ill, or living in fear.

The availability of weapons, especially firearms, is a significant factor in individuals' ability to carry out suicide. In countries where the ownership of guns is prohibited, suicide rates are lower. To illustrate, in the United Kingdom, owning a handgun is illegal and the suicide rate is less than a third of the rate in the United States, where gun ownership is widespread and defended. The availability of firearms is reflected in a country's statistics on violence and suicide.

Indigenous people in Canada experience disproportionately higher rates of suicide and suicidal ideation compared to their non-Indigenous counterparts. It is estimated that the national rate of suicide among Indigenous people was three times higher than among non-Indigenous Canadians, and that the rate of suicide among Indigenous youth was five to six times higher than among non-Indigenous youth (Kumar & Tjepkema, 2019).

To properly understand the elevated rate of suicide in Indigenous communities, the statistics must be considered alongside its historical context, as noted by the Standing Committee on Indigenous and Northern Affairs (2017, p. 19):

> Hundreds of years of colonization disrupted multiple generations of families, and this has had a lasting and profound effect on Indigenous communities. Legislation such as the *Indian Act* and related federal policies of assimilation established residential schools, created the reserve system, and forcibly relocated different groups of people. The end result was the removal of children from families, the prohibition and resulting erosion of Indigenous languages, cultures, and ceremonies, and the widescale dispossession of Indigenous peoples from their traditional territories. These policies have left a collective trauma on Indigenous communities. These destructive origins place Indigenous peoples at a higher risk of mental distress and suicide than non-Indigenous people.

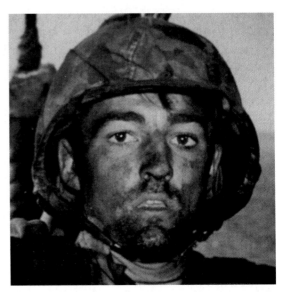

Fig. 27.2 Combat veterans are at risk for suicide. (Copyright © 2007, The History Place. All rights reserved.)

CRITICAL THINKING

A patient who has suffered from a major depressive episode was admitted involuntarily to inpatient psychiatric unit. The patient reported a suicidal plan to use his licensed hunting rifle. The rifle is stored and locked, as per law, in a gun safe in his home.

- Do you think that the rifle can be used to carry out that patient's suicidal plan?
- If so, what steps should be taken to prevent it?

One's state of health can influence suicidal considerations. Losses associated with old age can lead to depression and feelings of futility. Why struggle when tomorrow is a sad repeat of today? Suicide rates climb as age, infirmity, and illness take their toll.

The appearance of human immunodeficiency virus (HIV) and acquired immunodeficiency syndrome (AIDS) has had a profound influence on the suicide rates in many countries. The death-with-dignity philosophy has influenced many AIDS sufferers to choose the time and place of their passing. This form of suicide is called **rational suicide** because the choice to end one's life was made freely and rationally, with a sound mind. Likewise, in the context of a patient's terminal medical diagnosis, the ability to choose how one ends one's life has become an important right. The need to die with dignity has caused an increased awareness of the importance of a patient's rights in this process. However, when mental health concerns are involved, being of sound mind at the time of making that decision has the greatest impact on the legitimacy of this process. Often, the process of rational suicide presents an ethical dilemma.

Other social factors play a role in suicides. Higher suicide rates are seen among survivors of natural disasters or severe acts of aggression, such as ethnic cleansing. Veterans with combat experience (Fig. 27.2) and those with post-traumatic stress disorder (PTSD) suffer higher suicide rates than does the general population. The number, availability, and kind of community-based resources for health promotion and treatment influence a society's mental as well as physical health. Without these resources and the support they offer, the stresses of life can overwhelm a society's citizens.

It is important to be aware of the social changes in this world. Hidden among them are clues to caring for patients who are thinking of ending their lives. Increasing the knowledge base for health care workers is necessary to decrease the attempts of self-harm by veterans, for instance, and for offering early interventions. Research within this population is ongoing to address this issue (Simkus & Van Til, 2018).

DYNAMICS OF SUICIDE

The act of attempting suicide has a profound impact on the lives of families, friends, and communities. When many suicides occur, a whole society becomes affected. Because humans dynamically function in several realms or dimensions at any given time, it is important to consider suicide from a holistic point of view.

Characteristics of Suicide

Suicide is an act of *individual meaning*. The actual reasons for choosing such a final course of action are never known to anyone but the individual. However, it is likely that more than one motive drives a person to suicide.

In the physical dimension, thoughts of suicide produce many of the same biochemical changes in the body as depression. Chronic fatigue and vague complaints are common from both depressed and suicidal individuals. Often suicidal persons will not eat, drink, or rest enough to maintain required energy levels. Recent studies have suggested a link between low serum cholesterol levels and suicide attempts in men. Methods of suicide differ by gender. Men prefer to rely on firearms, hanging, or drowning, whereas women prefer to overdose with pills or inhale carbon monoxide.

The emotional dimension of functioning for the suicidal person often includes feelings of ambivalence, anger, aggression, guilt, helplessness, and hopelessness.

Ambivalence is a state in which an individual experiences conflicting feelings, attitudes, or drives. For the suicidal person, the struggle is between self-preservation (life) and self-destruction (death). Often suicidal individuals threaten or attempt suicide and then behaviourally act out their feelings of ambivalence by seeking treatment.

Anger and aggression are turned inward in suicidal persons. Fears of being abandoned or rejected add to the dynamics. Many persons who feel trapped in frustrating relationships commonly react with rage that becomes self-directed and harmful.

Guilt can also lead to suicide. Suicidal individuals often shoulder the guilt of the world. They may feel sinful and carry around the belief that they must have done something very wrong to deserve their misfortunes. Often personal guilt is exaggerated until the only way to make up for one's transgressions is to offer the final sacrifice—the self.

For the suicidal individual, the emotional dimension is marked by overwhelming feelings of helplessness and hopelessness. Nothing works out the way it was expected. The individual becomes unable to function emotionally. Life is bleak and hopeless as its meaning and purpose slip from one's control. Self-esteem can sink to an all-time low.

In the intellectual dimension, intense emotional suffering leads to distorted thinking and self-defeating thoughts. The self becomes devalued and worth little. Everything is depressing, which leads individuals to a negative and pessimistic view of the future. One's self-talk becomes self-defeating, which soon leads to negative behaviours. Thinking is self-centred rather than oriented toward solving problems. (The focus of cognitive-behavioural therapy is on changing one's perceptions of how one views negative occurrences in life: It is believed that if we alter our negative or distorted beliefs about our experiences, we can experience better outcomes in our situations [Beck Institute for Cognitive Behavior Therapy, 2019].)

The social dimension of functioning includes one's views of others. Many suicidal individuals depend on the frequent feedback of others to reaffirm their self-worth. Self-esteem is low in suicidal people. Their feelings of inferiority, of being less than others, interfere with social relationships and lead to the isolation and loneliness that accompany suicide. For many teens, being bullied can produce such feelings and provide the motivation to end one's own life.

In the spiritual dimension, suicidal individuals grapple with the cultural, religious, and ethical dilemmas associated with one's own demise. Many respond by blaming other people, their society, or their religious practices. Others "make their peace" with the spiritual side of themselves and experience a spiritual calm and serenity before carrying out suicide. Some people believe they will be reunited with loved ones in a new life after leaving this reality.

BOX 27.1 Motivations for Suicide

Cry for help
Refusal to accept a diminished quality, style, or pace of life
Need to affirm the soul
To relieve distress
Preoccupied with suicide
To exercise control

Categories of Motivation

People are motivated to take their own lives for many reasons. Most suicide victims, however, seem to share two major viewpoints. The first is a deep, inner disturbance of hopelessness, despair, poor self-esteem, and feelings of being trapped. The other involves a logic in which the individual considers the act as a way of relieving themselves of the miseries of this life and connecting with a sense of immortality or a life beyond the one they are leaving behind.

There are several categories of motivation for suicide (Box 27.1). The first motive is called "a cry for help." Most commonly suicidal persons bounce between the wish to live and the need to die. They feel trapped in a situation from which they see no other escape. Killing oneself is an effort to break out and take control, to do something about one's life. Suicide may feel like the only form of control for some people. These individuals are communicating their need for the kind of help that will radically change their lives and alter their present existence. The following Case Study illustrates this type of motivation.

CASE STUDY

Azinett was young, alone, pregnant, and scared. She knew she was not welcome at home because her father told her when she left for university, "If you get into trouble, don't come crying to me. You'll have to take care of it by yourself."

Her boyfriend, who swore his love and devotion, denied that he was the father of her baby and then left town. Even her new friends deserted her when they heard she was pregnant. Now the school officials were asking about her plans.

In desperation, Azinett sought to terminate the pregnancy but found that she was "too far along." She decided there was only one course of action that could end her troubles. She really did not want to die, but there seemed to be no other way out. The thought of facing life alone with a new baby was more than she could tolerate.

As she made her final plans, a feeling of calm came over Azinett. She would handle the situation in her own way. At least this way, she rationalized, "I am in control. I am the one who will do something about this."

Later that night, Azinett connected a rubber hose from the exhaust system to the interior of her car, rolled up all the windows, and sat quietly with the motor running. The next morning, when her body was discovered, she held a small note in her hand. It said, "Daddy, I took care of it myself. Love, Azinett."

• What do you think motivated Azinett to die by suicide?
• Why did she feel that this was her only or best course of action?
• If Azinett had come to you for help, what could you have done?

The second motive for considering suicide is the refusal to accept a diminished quality, style, or pace of life. This motive causes persons to carry out rational suicide. They assess their situation in a clear and unemotional manner, consider all the options, and then decide to take steps that will end their lives. Decisions and plans are made logically with little or no emotion. The decision to die by suicide is seen as a logical one. An example would be the 80-year-old man who kills his 78-year-old blind and bedridden wife and then ends his own life after making all the arrangements for their funerals and property settlements.

The third motivation centres around the need to affirm one's soul. These persons believe that there are values more important than life. Suicide is a way of fulfilling one's existence. The 18-year-old who takes his life one summer evening when everything is going well and the future is bright may be searching for that fulfillment.

The fourth motive for suicidal behaviour is to relieve distress related to situations that threaten the intactness of a person. The 70-year-old businessman with prostate cancer who chooses suicide over potentially life-prolonging surgery is an example of this type of motivation.

Last are those individuals who are preoccupied with suicide. They derive comfort knowing that they will control the time and circumstances of their death. These people are usually unwilling to accept life on any terms but their own. They set conditions for living and refuse to continue with life unless it is on their terms. Often suicide is the only form of real control they feel they have.

When working with suicidal patients, it is important to remember that no matter what the motivation, each individual is experiencing deep discomfort and very low self-esteem. Compassion and understanding become valuable therapeutic tools when working with such distressed persons.

THEORIES ABOUT SUICIDE

Suicide is an end result. It is difficult to understand all the factors that lead up to one's decision to end one's life. The study of the nature of suicide is called suicidology. Several theories attempt to explain the causes of suicidal behaviour.

The *psychoanalytical theory* states that all humans have the instinct for life and death within them. Suicidal persons experience much ambivalence between wanting to live and wanting to die. Anger turns inward, and when stressful life events activate their death wish, suicide becomes an option.

Sociological theory considers the relationship between the number of suicides and the social conditions of an area. These theorists believe that suicide rates are affected by group support (or the lack of it), social changes, regulations, religion, legal sanctions or limitations, and philosophical beliefs. In short, the sociological theories consider the effects of social factors on the occurrence of suicide.

Last is the *interpersonal theory*, developed by H.S. Sullivan. Suicide is viewed as the outcome of a failure to work with or resolve interpersonal conflicts.

These three theories form much of the foundation for further studies into the nature of suicide. However, ongoing research into the psychobiological nature of the human being is revealing new information about suicide and its motivations.

New Biological Evidence

Depression, anxiety, and impulsive behaviours are common in suicidal individuals. Because scientists are now able to study the structure and functions of the living human brain, new connections between physical and behavioural activities are being rapidly discovered.

Anxiety and depression are often the forerunners of suicidal thoughts. Researchers have demonstrated that when certain chemicals in the brain (neurotransmitters) are not in balance, people have difficulty regulating their moods. For example, irregularities in a certain neurotransmitter pattern, called the *serotonin system,* have been found in depressed and suicidal persons. According to the US National Institute of Mental Health (NIMH, 2015), "lower levels of serotonin have been found in the brains of people with a history of suicide attempts." These findings have implications for health care providers. As our understanding of the dynamics of suicide grows, so does our ability to recognize the potential for suicide and effectively intervene.

Effects of Suicide on Others

Suicide, like natural death, has a strong effect on those left behind. After the suicide, the lives of the survivors can be filled with questions, anger, sadness, shame, guilt, and health problems. For a spouse, "the death of a spouse by suicide has the potential of severely compromising the psychological well-being of the surviving marital partner" (Constantino, Sekula, Lebish, et al., 2002). The grieving process is further complicated by social attitudes about taking one's own life.

Survivor Guilt

The loss of a loved one through suicide is considered a much more stressful event than the grief reaction to a natural death. Guilt is a main response because survivors often think they could have done something to prevent the suicide. Guilt may also stem from unexpressed anger toward the deceased person for abandoning family and friends. Depression, PTSD with flashbacks, and somatic symptoms are all common among most suicide survivors. Impaired immune system functioning, leading to illness, may accompany the emotional disturbances.

Anger may be expressed as "agonized questioning" that helps the survivors cope with their emotional turmoil and disorganization. Some may hide their resentment, anger, and rage, which can turn into depression. Children often feel responsible for the suicide. Unless they receive much love, support, guidance, and permission to be angry, depression or other behavioural issues may develop.

Socially the stigma of suicide is soon felt. Forced interactions with health care providers, the police, or the media soon after death can bring home the feelings of rejection that are often experienced by the family members of suicide victims. Friends and relatives, unsure of how to help, may withdraw or do nothing. This reaction limits the social contact and support that are so needed after the suicide of a loved one. The survivors of a loved one's suicide may also withdraw from social interactions in order to protect themselves from the gossip and intrusion of inconsiderate others. Thus begins a cycle of guilt, withdrawal, and blame between the survivors and others in their world. With support and understanding, survivors eventually recover and accept the fact that the responsibility for the suicide rests with the individual who died and not with those who are left behind.

Health care providers are not immune to the effects of suicide. When a patient, especially an inpatient, dies by suicide, staff members and other patients may experience guilt, anger, or helplessness. Both patients and staff members need to grieve and express the emotions that follow a suicide. Often other patients on the unit will express anger at the staff, act out, or become self-destructive. Sharing emotions about the suicide gives both staff and patients the opportunity to express themselves and cope with the experience. The survivors of suicide, no matter who they are, must grieve and learn to heal.

SUICIDE THROUGHOUT THE LIFE CYCLE

Attempts to end one's life occur in every age group. Although the motivations for suicide may vary with the person's developmental level, the effort to die remains the same. Understanding how suicide is used at different developmental levels is important. Recognition and treatment of the problems underlying suicidal behaviours are much more effective when begun early.

Suicide and Children

Although depression is usually a component of suicide, with children it may be different. Some experts believe that suicide in children is most often the result of family conflict or disruption. Children learn by exposure. The children of depressed mothers think about and attempt suicide more often than those of emotionally healthy mothers. Children carry out suicide as a cry for help, to change their situation, or to act out a sincere wish to die. Children with existing mental health challenges, such as conduct disorder, attention-deficit/hyperactivity disorder, or psychosis, are at a greater risk for suicide than other children.

Because they are impulsive, suicides in children are usually not planned. Often the loss of a parent triggers suicidal behaviours in children who were not encouraged to grieve. Because very young children cannot understand the concept of death as a permanent state, their wishes to join their lost parent may lead to suicidal behaviours.

The *key* to recognizing the signs of suicidal intent lies in *a change in the child's behaviour.* Any child whose attitudes, behaviours, or habits change dramatically in a short time, especially after a stressful event or situation, is a candidate for suicide.

Suicide and Adolescents

The rate of adolescent suicide has risen dramatically in the past 30 years. The suicide rates for adolescents and young adults have tripled in the past four decades. In 2009, 202 Canadians aged 15 to 19 died by suicide. This represents almost a quarter (23%) of all deaths for this age group (Navaleenan, 2017). Young men are the most affected by violence and suicide in adolescence. Although more adolescent girls attempt suicide, adolescent males are four times more likely to actually die from their attempts. Statistics may not accurately reflect the actual number of adolescent suicides because many suicidal deaths are listed as accidental.

During adolescence, any long-standing family or social problems may continue to worsen as the difficulties of growing up are experienced. If coping skills or resources are insufficient, adolescents, especially those with low self-esteem, may consider suicide an option for solving their problems. Adolescents carry out suicide when they feel there is no other way out of their problems. They see their problems as genuinely unsolvable, now or in the future.

Many factors come into play in adolescent suicide. Depression, poor impulse control, and emotional isolation are related to suicide in adolescents. Dysfunctional or disrupted family interactions, such as divorce or separation of parents, can devastate many teens. Adolescents with anorexia nervosa have higher rates of suicide. Social problems with peers have a strong influence on a teen's emotional state. If one is perceived as different or has unique qualities, the risk of being teased or bullied increases. Sometimes the teen suffers for years, which only adds to the feelings of worthlessness. In fact, so many teens have been bullied to suicide that a new term, "bullicide," has been coined.

The use of drugs or alcohol and a lack of consistent relationships also add to the risk for suicide. When the environment lacks security or presents dangers, many teens feel that their lives will be short and that they will not live until adulthood. The outlook for the future holds little promise with this attitude.

The incidence of suicidal behaviours is also increased in children and adolescents who suffer from chronic disease. Children and adolescents with immune-mediated (type 1) diabetes, for example, have a higher risk for suicide than healthy individuals. Those diabetics who actually try suicide often do so by some method relating to their diabetes, such as overdosing on insulin. Health care providers should routinely assess every patient (including those with medical diagnoses or problems) for the presence of suicidal thoughts. It is crucial to become aware of the risk factors that can play an important role in any individual's choice to die by suicide (Box 27.2).

Some nonsuicidal behaviours are the result of inward-focused emotions. Behaviours such as repeated cutting, scratching, and burning oneself produce the pain that reminds many mentally troubled individuals that they are still alive. However, there is often concern that a completed suicide event may occur in these individuals as a result of impulsive behaviours.

Suicide and Adults

Suicide is a significant problem in adulthood, especially for White men. Women attempt suicide three times more

BOX 27.2   Risk Factors for Suicide

Abuse, neglect, exploitation
Academic pressures, school problems
Accident prone
Chronic or terminal illness, disability, HIV/AIDS
Dysfunctional family relationships
Exposure to suicidal behaviours in others
Family or self-history of anxiety, depression
Family history of suicide
History of alcoholism, substance abuse, or both
Inadequate child-rearing practices
Incarceration, prison, or jail
Living in a rural area
Lack of access to mental health care
Loss of parent or significant other
Low socioeconomic status, poverty, or homelessness
Male gender, unmarried, unemployed
Medications
Member of certain religious cults
Mental health challenges*
Negative outlook for future
Previous suicide attempts*
Profession/occupation: police officer, firefighter, air traffic controller, physician, psychiatrist, college or university student, dentist
Social isolation, lack of social support
Stressful or unhappy personal relationships

AIDS, acquired immunodeficiency syndrome; *HIV*, human immunodeficiency virus.
* Highest risk for suicide.

frequently than men, but men are more successful at completing the act.

In young adults, suicide can occur when individuals are unable to cope with the pressures of adulthood. Some experience problems with interpersonal relationships, whereas others lack personal resources and are poor, hungry, or unemployed. All, however, are dissatisfied with their lives.

The most common method of suicide in Canada is hanging (44%), which includes strangulation and suffocation, followed by poisoning (25%) and firearm use (16%). Males are more likely to die by hanging (46%), while females are more likely to die by poisoning (42%). Males are far more likely to use firearms (20%) than females are (3%) (Navaleenan, 2017).

Loneliness is often a factor in adult suicides. The loss of a family member or significant relationship, whether through divorce or death, can increase the risk for suicide. In addition, certain professions and occupations are associated with higher rates of suicide (see Box 27.2).

Most adult suicides can be prevented if the clues are uncovered early enough. Assess your patients for depression or a recent crisis. Do not hesitate to ask if they ever think about suicide. The answer to that question may offer an opportunity to help save an individual's life.

Suicide and Older Persons

As age increases, so does the rate of suicide. Many studies reveal that the incidence of suicide increases with age. When suicide deaths are examined across age groups, Canadians aged 40 to 59 have the highest rates; 45% of all suicides in 2009 (1 769 out of a total of 3 890) occurred in this age group, compared with 35% for those aged 15 to 39, and 19% for those over age 60. This has been a persistent trend in Canada, yet contrasts with suicide trends in many other countries, where the rate of suicide tends to increase with age (Navaleenan, 2017). The actual number is difficult to determine because only active suicides are counted. Many older persons choose a **passive suicide** by refusing to eat, drink, or cooperate with care.

Most older persons view the timing of death in one of three ways: God controlled, physician and individual controlled, or controlled by the individual alone. Older males have the highest suicide rates within the older population (Stanhope & Lancaster, 2011).

The causes and risk factors of suicide in older people are poorly understood. Although many older individuals who die by suicide have had contact with a health care provider within the month before their deaths, their risk was not identified or treated. Risk factors for suicide in older people are advanced age, male gender, low socioeconomic status, chronic pain or illness, and fear of becoming dependent or helpless. Losses of loved ones and social isolation are common risk factors. A lack of relationships appears to be a driving force behind many suicides. Other researchers believe that intolerable life circumstances are the main motives for suicides in the older population.

Social attitudes about elder suicide differ. Some people think that all suicides among older people are irrational decisions, based on depression or physical illness. They believe aggressive interventions are always required. Others view elder suicide as the last rational decision, the last act of control over one's life.

Older persons tend *not* to communicate their intentions unless directly asked; thus, suicidal attempts in older persons are more successful. One of every two suicide attempts in the older population results in death. These sobering realities must alert every care provider to perform a suicidal risk assessment for all older persons in their care. All health care providers should be alert to behavioural changes, such as appetite, sleep, or activity changes. Social withdrawal and "getting one's affairs in order" strongly suggest the possibility of suicide attempt.

Medical Assistance in Dying

The concept of *rational suicide* in Canada is called **medical assistance in dying (MAiD)**. In June 2016, the Parliament of Canada passed federal legislation that allows eligible Canadian adults to request medical assistance in dying. Clinical personnel can assist in this process without being charged under criminal law. However, physicians, nurse practitioners, and other people who are directly involved must follow the rules set out in the *Criminal Code*, as well as applicable provincial and territorial health-related laws, rules, and policies.

This federal policy may not be consistent with a health care provider's beliefs and values. The federal legislation does not force a person to provide or help to provide medical

TABLE 27.2   Levels of Suicidal Behaviours

Suicidal ideation	Expressed thoughts or fantasies with no definite intent—may express ideas directly or symbolically
Suicidal threats	Verbal or written expressions of intent without actual actions
Suicidal gestures	Actions that result in little or no injury, but communicates the message of suicidal intent
Parasuicidal behaviours	Attempts at suicide with a low likelihood of success
Suicidal attempts	Serious self-directed actions with the intent to end one's life
Death by suicide	The ending of one's life

assistance in dying. In order to be eligible for medical assistance in dying, a person must meet all of the following criteria:
- They must be eligible for health services funded by the federal government or a province or territory.
- They must be at least 18 years old and be mentally competent.
- They must have a grievous and irremediable medical condition.
- They must make a voluntary request for medical assistance in dying that is not the result of outside pressure or influence (Government of Canada, 2020).

In other countries, such as the Netherlands, medical assistance in dying also is an acceptable way to achieve death with dignity. It may seem that the important questions and issues surrounding the control of one's own death are issues for philosophers and medical ethicists. However, health care providers will be addressing many of these questions in daily practice.

THERAPEUTIC INTERVENTIONS

Thoughts about suicide can be described on several levels. Table 27.2 explains each level. Suicide is a serious and preventable public health threat. *Prevention* is the most important health care action for all our patients, especially for those who may be suicidal. Preventing a suicide from occurring means saving a life; therefore, assessment is essential. Prevention requires knowledge of the dynamics of suicide and the ability to recognize the potential for suicidal actions in every patient. The nursing (therapeutic) process is an excellent tool for working with patients who may be considering suicide.

Assessment of Suicidal Potential

Because suicide is becoming more prevalent, it is important to evaluate *every* patient for its potential. To accomplish this, first assess the *risk factors* for the age of the patient. Then *ask* the patient directly if they have any thoughts relating to suicide. Asking patients will not encourage them to take any suicidal actions. On the contrary, it gives them permission to discuss their feelings and attitudes. Box 27.3 offers a list of questions for assessing suicidal intentions. Not every question may be appropriate for every patient, but a series of questions such as these will usually bring out expressions of suicidal thoughts if they are present. Most hospitals in Canada implement at

BOX 27.3   Assessing the Potential for Suicide

"What has been the most difficult moment for you in the recent past?"

"Have things been so bad that you have thought about escaping? If so, how?"

"Are there times when death seems like an attractive option to you?"

"Have you thought of harming or killing yourself?"

"If you were to harm yourself, how would you do it?"

"Do you have access to the items you would need to carry out your plan?" (This includes a gun, medications, a rope, an enclosed garage.)

"Have you thought about or attempted to harm yourself in the past?"

"What has kept you from harming yourself thus far?"

"What might keep you from harming yourself in the future?"

"Do you think you can control your behaviour and refrain from acting on your thoughts or impulses?" This is the **most** important question to ask.

least one of a few evidence-informed standard suicide assessment tools with every patient who is admitted to an inpatient mental health service. These tools are used in addition to a basic mental status examination (MSE). The three most popular assessment tools used today in Canadian practice are the Nurses' Global Assessment of Suicide Risk (NGASR), the Columbia–Suicide Severity Rating Scale (C-SSRS), and the SAD PERSONS screening tool.

Suicide assessment cannot be completed without the assessment of *protective factors,* or characteristics that make it less likely that an individual will consider, attempt, or die by suicide. Typical protection factors include positive social supports, a sense of responsibility for others (such as having dependent children, a partner, or parents [except when the person has postpartum depression or psychosis] or having pets), positive coping skills, a positive relationship with a health care provider, or a religious belief that suicide is wrong.

Because older persons who are taking potent analgesics (pain medications) are at high risk for feelings of depression, it is important to obtain a drug and medication history for every patient. Sometimes something as simple as discontinuing or changing a medication can lift the patient's spirits and decrease suicidal thoughts.

TABLE 27.3   Suicide Assessment

Assessment	Description
Suicide ideation (thoughts)	Patient talks about wanting to be dead, imagines AIDS or other serious illness, seems gloomy, brooding, describes delusion leading to suicide.
History of suicide attempts*	Patient has tried to end own life before; there may be family history of suicide.
Present suicide plan	The more detailed a suicide plan, the more likely it will be carried out.
Availability of items to carry out plan	What weapons (guns, rifles, knives) are available? How difficult is it to obtain such items?
Substance use or abuse	Suicide rates are higher in people who abuse alcohol or other chemical substances.
Level of despair	Ask about the future; when despair is high, hope is low.
Ability to control own behaviour	Inpatient hospitalization is indicated for individuals who are unable to control their suicidal impulses.

AIDS, acquired immunodeficiency syndrome.
*Highest risk.

Hospitalization may be required for the patient's safety and protection if they feel unable to control suicidal behaviours. Suicidal intentions can exist with any medical or psychiatric diagnosis. Patients who are depressed must be carefully monitored for expressions of hopelessness. Table 27.3 lists the basic components of a suicide assessment. Do not hesitate to use this data-gathering tool whenever difficulties in a patient's emotional state are suspected.

When used as part of a health history, the suicide assessment will yield valuable information about the patient's suicidal intentions (if any) along with numerous clues about the individual. Problem statements/nursing diagnoses for suicidal persons are based on each patient's identified challenges and needs (Box 27.4).

! MEDICATION ALERT

Many medications can cause changes in mood. Much publicity has been given to the medication fluoxetine hydrochloride (Prozac), an antidepressant that has been reported to cause violent and suicidal reactions in some individuals.

The adverse effects of certain steroids (e.g., prednisolone) have been known to cause elation and feelings of well-being in some individuals. Administered to others, the same drug can result in severe depression and suicidal thoughts.

While taking antidepressants, some patients regain the energy to plan and carry out a suicide attempt.

Therapeutic Interventions for Suicidal Patients

The first priority for the care of suicidal patients is protection from harm. The patient must be physically prevented from actively attempting suicide. If the risks are so high that a serious attempt may be made, **suicide precautions** are implemented. These precautions are standard interventions to prevent a suicide attempt from occurring and are listed in Box 27.5. Patients with a strong suicidal intent may require constant observation, which requires that a staff member keep the patient in full view at all times.

It is important to note that the increased level of intermediate observation does not actually lead to suicide

BOX 27.4   Problem Statements (Nursing Diagnoses) Related to Suicide

Physical Realm
Risk-taking behaviours
Disturbed body image
Nonadherence
Pain
Risk of self-mutilation
Rape-trauma syndrome
Risk of self-directed violence

Psychosocial Realm
Anxiety
Ineffective coping
Ineffective denial
Complicated grieving
Hopelessness
Powerlessness
Chronic low self-esteem
Impaired social interactions
Spiritual distress

prevention. The use of increased intermediate observation for safety comes from a long-standing (but false) belief that still exists in many mental health facilities. To date, there is no evidence demonstrating that increasing staff levels to conduct different levels of observation (e.g., every hour, every 30 minutes, every 15 minutes, or continuously) leads to more success in preventing a patient's harm to self or others. In fact, increased levels of observation can result in a false sense of security among staff, contribute to the patient's level of distress, increase the patient's feelings of loss of control, and take away nursing time from proper patient care. Fifteen minutes is more than enough time to carry out a suicide, serious mutilation, or assault, or to abscond. For this reason, leading medical health care facilities have concurred that a suicidal patient should not be placed on 15-minute checks. Instead, they suggest that the main things to watch for, that may jeopardize patient safety, are staff failure to adequately assess a patient, lack of timely restraints, lack of repeated and documented assessment,

BOX 27.5   Suicide Precautions

Protect patient from harming themselves.
Determine whether patient has a specific suicide plan.
Determine history of suicide attempts.
Make a safety plan.
Remove dangerous items from the environment.
Place patient in the least restrictive environment that allows for necessary level of engagement and assessment.
Place patient in a room with protective window coverings, as appropriate.
Frequently assess and manage symptoms during suicidal crisis.
Escort patient during off-ward activities, as appropriate.
Demonstrate concern about patient's welfare.
Refrain from criticizing.
Facilitate discussion of factors or events that precipitated the suicidal thoughts.
Facilitate support of patient by family and friends.
Instruct patient and significant others in signs, symptoms, and basic physiology of depression.
Instruct family that suicidal risk increases for severely depressed patients as they begin to feel better.
Instruct family on possible warning signs or pleas for help that patient may use.
Refer patient to psychiatrist, as needed.

failure to provide adequate intervention to alleviate symptoms, failure to remove harmful objects, poor staff training and education, and lack of a cohesive interprofessional team (Jayaram, 2014).

Since 1973, many mental health facilities have practised a "no-suicide contract" with patients, with the hope that such a written or verbal contract may decrease the risk for patient suicides. However, there is no evidence that no-suicide contracts actually work. In fact, there is quite a bit of evidence to suggest that they do not work (Freedenthal, 2018). Instead, collaboration with a patient in developing a **safety plan** is recommended (Centre for Applied Research in Mental Health and Addiction [CARMHA], 2007). Safety plans are different for inpatient and outpatient settings and from person to person. Safety plans can include a description of how the patient will keep their environment safe, how to recognize warning signs, and individual coping strategies; identification of a nonmedical person (family, friend) who can help if coping strategies do not work; if that is not working, which clinicians to call; and if that also is not working, where to go for emergency help (CARMHA, 2007).

One of the most important therapeutic interventions (after ensuring safety) with suicidal persons is to establish a rapport with the patient. Many suicidal people are alone. Most have little self-esteem. Establishing a therapeutic relationship with a health care provider is important for all patients, especially suicidal patients. The focused communications and concerned actions of care providers can help suicidal individuals feel self-worth. With the encouragement and advocacy of their care providers, many suicidal patients are able to develop more effective strategies for living satisfying lives. The Sample Patient Care Plan 27.1 illustrates a patient care plan for an individual who may be suicidal.

Suicide and its associated effects are growing problems in today's society. Many of us will be or have been touched by the suicide of a loved one or friend. It is our duty and responsibility as health care providers to protect our patients, even from themselves, when we must. It is hoped that through our efforts, the tide of senseless loss of life can be turned, and choices will be made to look toward life instead of away from it.

SAMPLE PATIENT CARE PLAN 27.1   Self-Directed Violence

Assessment
History Josef, a 19-year-old man, recently lost his best friend in an automobile accident. For several weeks, he has been saying that he should have been killed instead of his friend. In the past 2 weeks, Josef has refused to work, eat, or engage in any social activities. Yesterday he bought a gun.

Current Findings A depressed-looking young man sitting between two worried parents. Grooming is unkempt; shirt and jeans are ragged and dirty. He volunteers no information but states, "It's not worth it" to the nurse. After obtaining the history from the parents, Josef was admitted to the unit for assessment and observation.

Multidisciplinary Diagnosis

Risk for self-directed violence related to loss of significant other

Planning/Goals

Josef will refrain from making any suicidal gestures or attempts during his inpatient stay.
Josef will discuss his feelings of loss by August 28.

THERAPEUTIC INTERVENTIONS

Interventions	Rationale	Team Member
1. Establish contact and rapport.	Open communication and trust must be established before work can begin	All
2. Establish a personalized safety plan as soon as possible.	Helps identify worsening of symptoms and uses strategies known to be useful in the past to alleviate these symptoms	Psy, Nsg

Continued

SAMPLE PATIENT CARE PLAN 27.1   Self-Directed Violence—cont'd

Multidisciplinary Diagnosis	Planning/Goals	
3. Implement necessary suicide precautions; watch closely.	Protects Josef from self-injury or death, using a safe environment and restraints, as necessary	All
4. Evaluate and document Josef's suicide potential at least twice daily.	Helps assess for changes in seriousness of patient's intent	Psy, Nsg
5. Help Josef identify and discuss sources of distress.	Increases awareness of feelings; helps to plan effective interventions	All
6. Offer emotional support and acceptance.	Encourages Josef to think more highly of himself; helps develop self-worth	All
7. Involve Josef and his family in the treatment plan.	Promotes active decision making; provides emotional support and resources	All
8. Explore coping strategies that worked in the past.	Helps Josef to apply successful coping mechanisms to prevent problems	All

Evaluation During the course of hospitalization, Josef made no attempts at suicide. By August 18, Josef was able to share his sorrow and anger with the unit chaplain.

Critical Thinking Questions
1. What do you think are the benefits or disadvantages of a personalized safety plan?
2. How does the staff offer emotional support and acceptance to Josef when he refuses to verbally communicate?

A complete patient care plan includes several other diagnoses and interventions.
Nsg, nursing staff; *Psy,* psychologist.

KEY POINTS

- Suicide is the action of intentionally taking one's own life.
- Many misconceptions about suicide continue to exist despite efforts to promote an accurate understanding of the problem.
- Many cultural, social, and individual factors influence the occurrence of suicide.
- The act of suicide has a profound impact on the lives of families, friends, and communities.
- Thoughts and actions directed at self-destruction affect every dimension of human functioning.
- There are several categories of motivation for suicide, including a cry for help, a refusal to accept a diminished quality of life, a need to affirm one's soul, an attempt to relieve the distress related to situations that threaten the intactness of a person, a result of psychosis, and an act of those who are preoccupied with suicide.
- Theories that attempt to explain the causes of suicidal behaviour include the psychoanalytical theory, sociological theory, and interpersonal theory.

- New connections between neurotransmitters and behavioural activities are being rapidly discovered.
- After the suicide of a loved one, the lives of the survivors can be plagued with anger, sadness, shame, guilt, health problems, and agonizing questions.
- Some experts believe that suicide in children is most often the result of family conflict or disruption.
- Adolescents carry out suicide when they feel there is no other way out of their problems.
- Adult women attempt suicide more frequently than men, but men are more successful at completing the act.
- Prevention is the most important therapeutic action for patients who may be suicidal.
- Because suicide is becoming so prevalent, it is important for nurses to assess every patient for its potential.
- The first priority for the care of patients who may be suicidal is protection from harm.
- With encouragement and the advocacy of their care providers, many suicidal patients are able to develop effective strategies for living more satisfying lives.

ADDITIONAL LEARNING RESOURCES

Go to your Evolve website (http://evolve.elsevier.com/Canada/Morrison-Valfre/) for additional online resources, including the online Study Guide for additional learning activities to help you master this chapter content.

CRITICAL THINKING QUESTIONS

1. Gregory, 23 years old, is a single, third-year mechanical engineering student who was involuntarily admitted to the inpatient mental health unit in a very agitated state (staring wild-eyed at staff, experiencing fine hand tremors, and appearing fearful). This was following an attempt to kill himself by stabbing himself in the abdomen with a

knife. Fortunately, the wound is superficial and Gregory has been treated with clips and light dressing. Gregory reported that he did it to avoid greater suffering when "the end of the world comes." Gregory reported hearing voices of "Satan" alerting him about that, and about the great suffering that everyone would experience. After some initial treatment with antipsychotic medications, Gregory became more calm and pleasant and denied hearing any voices or any suicidal ideation. Unfortunately, today, the second day of his stay, he is refusing his medical treatment. In a conversation with you, he is visibly agitated, seems scared, and reports that "everybody will die soon, and there will be great suffering." What would be your further assessment at this point and your planned intervention with Gregory?

2. What are the basic suicidal assessment questions you should ask every patient?

3. Stella is a 25-year-old unemployed single female. She lives with her mother, who is divorced. For the past 9 years, Stella has suffered from anorexia, and yesterday she was involuntary admitted to the hospital after attempting to hang herself. In a conversation with you, Stella reports a suicidal ideation to hang herself using the bed linen and the edge of the door to her room. Stella adds that her suffering is so great that she will do whatever it takes to kill herself as soon as she can. What would be your next steps?

REFERENCES

Beck Institute for Cognitive Behavior Therapy. (2019). *Cognitive model: A thought process for developing healthier thinking.* Author. https://beckinstitute.org/cognitive-model/

Centre for Applied Research in Mental Health and Addiction (CARMHA). (2007). *Working with the client who is suicidal: A tool for adult mental health and addiction services.* British Columbia Ministry of Health. https://www.health.gov.bc.ca/library/publications/year/2007/MHA_WorkingWithSuicidalClient.pdf

Constantino, R. E., Sekula, L. K., Lebish, J., et al. (2002). Depression and behavioral manifestations of depression in female survivors of suicide and female survivors of abuse. *Journal of the American Psychiatric Nurses Association, 8*(1), 27–32. https://doi.org/10.1067/mpn.2002.122760.

Freedenthal, S. (2018). *Speaking of suicide. The use of no-suicide contracts.* https://www.speakingofsuicide.com/2013/05/15/no-suicide-contracts/

Government of Canada. (2020). *Medical assistance in dying.* https://www.canada.ca/en/health-canada/services/medical-assistance-dying.html

Jayaram, G. (2014). Inpatient suicide prevention: Promoting a culture and system of safety over 30 years of practice. *Journal of Psychiatric Practice, 20*(5), 392–404.

Kumar, M. B., & Tjepkema, M. (2019). *Suicide among first Nations people, Métis and Inuit (2011–2016): Findings from the 2011 Canadian Census Health and environment Cohort (CanCHEC).* Statistics Canada. https://www150.statcan.gc.ca/n1/pub/99-011-x/99-011-x2019001-eng.htm

Multicultural Mental Health Resources Centre (MMHRC). (2020). *Getting help.* http://www.multiculturalmentalhealth.ca/en/consumers/getting-help/

National Institute of Mental Health (NIMH). (2015). *Suicide in America: Frequently asked questions.* https://www.nimh.nih.gov/health/publications/suicide-faq/tr18-6389-suicideinamericafaq_149986.pdf

Navaleenan, T. (2017). *Suicide rates: An overview.* Statistics Canada. https://www150.statcan.gc.ca/n1/pub/82-624-x/2012001/article/11696-eng.htm

Peebles, G. (2015). *Suicide: A worldwide epidemic. Counterpunch, may 15.* https://www.counterpunch.org/2015/05/15/suicide-a-worldwide-epidemic/

Simkus, K., & Van Til, L. (2018). *2018 veteran suicide mortality study: Identifying risk groups at release.* Veterans Affairs Canada. https://doi.org/10.1097/01.pra.0000453369.71092.69. https://www.veterans.gc.ca/eng/about-vac/research/research-directorate/publications/reports/veteran-suicide-mortality-study2018

Standing Committee on Indigenous and Northern Affairs. (2017). *Breaking point: The suicide crisis in Indigenous communities: Report of the standing committee on Indigenous and Northern affairs.* Parliament of Canada. https://www.ourcommons.ca/Content/Committee/421/INAN/Reports/RP8977643/inanrp09/inanrp09-e.pdf

Stanhope, M., & Lancaster, J. (2011). *Public health nursing: Population-centered health care in the community* (8th ed.). Mosby.

World Health Organization (WHO). (2020). *Mental health: Suicide data: Suicide estimates.* https://www.who.int/mental_health/prevention/suicide/estimates/en/

28

Substance-Related Disorders and Addictive Disorders

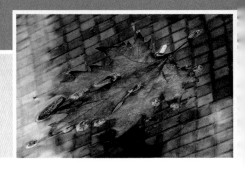

OBJECTIVES

Upon completion of this chapter, the student will be able to:

1. Define three problematic human domains with regard to addiction.
2. Explain how chemical dependency affects persons from different age groups.
3. Describe four serious consequences of substance abuse.
4. Classify seven categories of abused substances and give an example from each group.
5. Identify three reasons why inhalants are abused by adolescents and young adults.
6. Describe signs and symptoms of alcohol withdrawal and intoxication.
7. Describe the three stages or phases of becoming addicted.
8. Compare the three criteria for the diagnosis of a substance-related disorder.
9. Explain what is meant by the term *relapse*.
10. Plan at least four interventions for patients who are diagnosed with substance-related disorders.

OUTLINE

KEY TERMS

The practice of using substances to make oneself feel better is as old as humans themselves. Even animals have been seen eating certain plants that change their behaviours. Alcohol has played a role in many cultures throughout recorded time. Various drugs, potions, solutions, and formulas have been developed as humans attempted to cope with the problems of disease and illness or improve their mood and provide extra energy.

THE ROLE OF CHEMICAL SUBSTANCES IN SOCIETY

Chemical substances are important in modern societies. Without them, we would be unable to produce food, fight disease, or develop products that allow us to live comfortably. The use of different chemical substances has increasingly become a part of everyday life.

Substance Use and Age

The use of chemical substances occurs throughout the life cycle, from the fetus to older adulthood. Even the growing life protected within the mother's uterus is not safe from the effects of chemicals. It is estimated that 10% of pregnant women and 20% of breastfeeding women consume alcohol in Canada, despite huge educational efforts about the effects of alcohol on the fetus and infant (Lange et al., 2016).

There are no safe drugs for pregnant women. Every chemical substance ingested by a pregnant woman poses a potential danger to her unborn child, especially during the first trimester of pregnancy when the developing fetus is highly sensitive. Chemical substances taken during pregnancy can seriously interfere with normal fetal growth and development. They may also alter the placenta itself or interfere with its ability to perform its life-promoting functions.

A common example of the effects of maternal drug use can be seen in infants and children who have **fetal alcohol spectrum disorder (FASD),** which is the result of excessive alcohol use during pregnancy. In Canada, it is estimated that every year about 3 000 babies are born with FASD to mothers who abuse alcohol (Government of Canada, 2017). Children with FASD are smaller at birth, have small heads *(microcephaly),* and fail to develop normally. Figure 28.1 illustrates the physical effects on the child of a chronically alcoholic mother. The less obvious effects include central nervous system (CNS) deficits, various degrees of developmental delays, intellectual impairment, hyperactivity, irritability, and poor feeding habits. These children also have slow rates of growth and certain facial characteristics common to children of alcoholic mothers.

Infants who were exposed to cocaine in utero have sleeping and eating problems, unusual levels of irritability, and high-pitched cries. Other syndromes and developmental problems result from the use of different drugs, but all drugs have one thing in common: *pregnancy and substance use do not mix.*

Children who live with substance-abusing parents are at an increased risk for injuries and developing drug problems themselves. Research has demonstrated that most children of parents who use both legal and illegal chemicals do poorly in school, have difficulty controlling their emotions, and exhibit

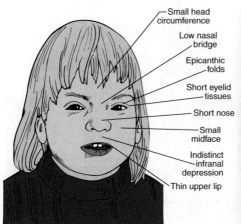
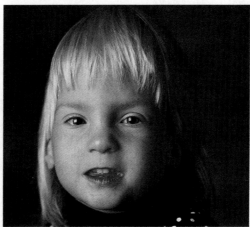

Fig. 28.1 Fetal alcohol spectrum disorder. Milder forms of alcohol-induced effects on the fetus and the infant are known as *fetal alcohol effects.* (Source: From Fortinash, K., & Holoday-Worret, P. [2012]. *Psychiatric mental health nursing* [5th ed.]. Mosby.)

Small head circumference
Low nasal bridge
Epicanthic folds
Short eyelid tissues
Short nose
Small midface
Indistinct infranal depression
Thin upper lip

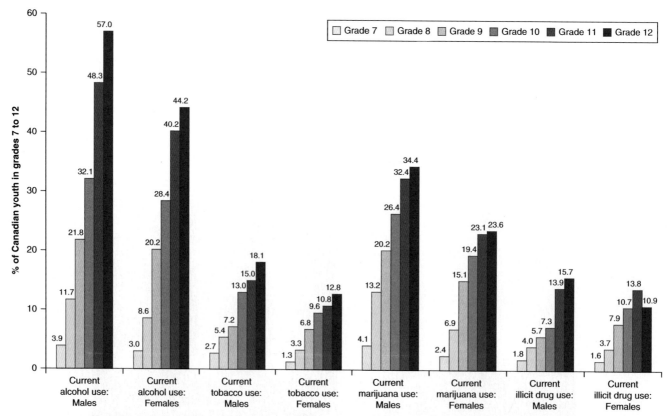

low self-esteem. Many of these children repeat the cycle of substance abuse and of child abuse, which may occur with caregiver abuse, when they reach adulthood. Some choose alcoholic or drug-abusing spouses.

Children can abuse substances as well, but often the substances are legal and easily available. The 9-year-old who demands cola drinks every day demonstrates the same signs of a caffeine addiction as an adult. The 8-year-old boy who has grown up with beer in the house can become an alcoholic just as quickly as his adult counterparts.

Adolescents experiment with a variety of attitudes, behaviours, and lifestyles, and often substance use becomes a part of that experimentation. The younger an individual begins to use substances, the more likely that abuse problems will occur later in life. In Canada, by grade 12, most students are current users of alcohol, tobacco, or drugs. Alcohol is the most prevalent substance used by Canadian youth (usage among male students is 57%, for female students it is 44.2%; see Fig. 28.2) (Leatherdale & Burkhalter, 2012).

Adolescents have various patterns of substance abuse. They may experiment by using drugs on a few occasions. They may use substances (usually alcohol, tobacco, or cannabis) in recreational ways, in social settings for the purpose of relaxation or intoxication. Binge drinking, the consumption of large amounts of alcohol in a short period of time, can lead to alcohol poisoning and death. The US National Institute on

Alcohol Abuse and Alcoholism (2020) defines *binge drinking* as "4 drinks for women and 5 drinks for men, in about 2 hours." If actual addiction occurs, teens are likely to become involved in illegal activities, such as drug trafficking, prostitution, or criminal behaviour.

In adults, substance abuse is common, with about 10% of the adult population regularly abusing alcohol. This statistic is likely an underestimate because episodes of frequent binge drinking are not documented. Other chemicals may be used on a recreational or even daily basis. Substance use and abuse occur most commonly between 18 and 35 years of age, but significant numbers of older persons abuse alcohol and prescription medications.

Older persons are not immune to substance-related problems, but their substance abuse is often misdiagnosed or treated inappropriately. Older drinkers and many older persons not abusing alcohol are inclined to misuse drugs and prescription medications. Polypharmacy (the use of many drugs at the same time) is common among older persons who visit several health care providers. Older substance-abusers are often isolated within their social groups or families. Although the incidence of substance abuse among older persons is unknown, more than 40% of all adverse drug reactions occur in persons older than 65 years of age. This fact should alert health care providers to the possibility of substance abuse in every older patient.

Fig. 28.2 Prevalence of alcohol, tobacco, marijuana, and illicit drug use by grade and sex, Canada, 2008. (Source: From Leatherdale, S. T., & Burkhalter, R. [2012]. The substance use profile of Canadian youth: Exploring the prevalence of alcohol, drug, and tobacco use by gender and grade. *Addictive Behaviors, 37*[3], 320 [Fig. 2].)

Scope of the Problem Today

The abuse of chemical substances presents many problems for people in today's society. Alcohol abuse and drug abuse affect every citizen, in both financial terms and human costs. Infants who have been exposed to cocaine and other drugs are filling health and foster care systems as these children of addicted parents are born. Children of problem drinkers have three times the risk for serious injury as children of non-drinking parents.

Substance abuse and dependence cost society dearly. The use of alcohol and drugs often results in trauma, violence, and mental health challenges. Family and social relationships suffer. Alcohol-related motor vehicle accidents are one of the leading causes of death among people younger than 45 years. Many deaths attributed to falls, drowning, and burns are often related to alcohol and drug use.

People with serious mental illness who also are addicted to or use chemical substances are said to have a **concurrent disorder**.

CATEGORIES OF ABUSED SUBSTANCES

Every chemical, including many substances found in nature, has the potential for abuse. Physicians have long recognized that different types of drugs affect people differently. Nonetheless, drugs may be categorized or classified according to certain shared symptomatology or effects. The categorization process is premised on these long-standing, medically accepted facts. There are 10 categories of **abused substances**: alcohol, caffeine, cannabis, hallucinogens (including phencyclidine [PCP] and its analogues), inhalants, opioids, sedatives (hypnotic) or anxiolytics, CNS stimulants, tobacco, and others. They cause different overdose and withdrawal symptoms and, therefore, require different interventions.

Drugs from each of these categories can affect a person's CNS and impair a person's normal faculties. Each category has disorders related to use, intoxication, and withdrawal. Each category affects the body by working on specific and already existing receptors. Thus, it is important to understand that *all of these substances (or their main components) already exist in the body in some amount naturally, without any consumption.* They play a significant role in daily functions.

1. **Alcohol**: anything that contains ethanol.
2. **Caffeine**: anything that contains caffeine. Caffeine can be found in certain plants, such as cacao, coffee, kola, and tea. Caffeine stimulates the CNS and body metabolism.
3. **Cannabis**: *Cannabis* is the scientific name for marijuana. The active ingredient in cannabis is delta-9 tetrahydrocannabinol, or THC. It influences pleasure, memory, thinking, concentration, movement, coordination, and sensory and time perception. This category includes cannabinoids and synthetics like dronabinol.
4. **Hallucinogens**: Hallucinogens cause the user to perceive things differently than they actually are. Examples include lysergic acid diethylamide (LSD), peyote, psilocybin, MDMA (ecstasy), and PCP.
5. **Inhalants**: Inhalants include a wide variety of breathable substances that produce mind-altering results and effects.

Examples of inhalants include toluene, plastic cement, paint, gasoline, paint thinners, hair sprays, and various anaesthetic gases.

6. **Opioids**: Opioids are a broad group of narcotic pain-relieving drugs. They relieve pain, induce euphoria, and create mood changes in the user. Examples of narcotic analgesics include opium, codeine, heroin, fentanyl, Darvon, morphine, methadone, hydrocodone (Vicodin), and oxycodone (OxyContin).
7. *Sedatives (hypnotic) or anxiolytics*: CNS depressants; similar to alcohol, they slow down the operations of the brain and the body. Examples of CNS depressants include barbiturates, antianxiety tranquilizers (e.g., Valium, Librium, Xanax, Prozac, and Thorazine), gamma hydroxybutyrate (GHB), Rohypnol, and many other antidepressants (e.g., Zoloft, Paxil).
8. *CNS stimulants*: CNS stimulants accelerate the heart rate, elevate blood pressure, and "speed-up" or overstimulate the body. Examples of CNS stimulants include cocaine, "crack," Ritalin, caffeine, amphetamines, and methamphetamine ("crank").
9. *Tobacco*: Nicotine stimulates the adrenal glands, which results in the release of adrenaline. Adrenaline causes the release of glucose and stimulates higher heart rate, ventilation (breathing), and blood pressure. Nicotine also makes the pancreas produce less insulin, keeping the level of glucose high in the bloodstream. Together with the release of dopamine in the reward center, nicotine acts as a simulant. Yet, in high doses it can act as a sedative.
10. *Other (or unknown) substances*: These can be a variety of substances that can cause the same symptoms that meet the diagnostic criteria for substance-use disorder. Usually, these substances are in the following categories: anabolic steroids, nonsteroidal anti-inflammatory drugs (NSAIDs), antihistamines, cathinones (including, Khat, which is popular in the Middle East), and other substances.

Severity of Impact and Legality

All 10 categories of abused substances can create an addiction and cause harm. Yet, the tendency to cause addiction and the severity of the harm to the individual and to society vary among the different substances. Some of them are legal and can be purchased legally, others are considered illegal drugs. As can be seen in Table 28.1, there is no correlation between the severity of substance damage and its legality.

Alcohol

Alcohol has been used since the beginning of recorded time. The effects of beverages containing alcohol are caused by the presence of ethanol (ETOH or CH_3-CH_2-OH), a chemical that results from the fermentation of yeast and grains, malts, or fruits. "Hard liquor," such as whiskey, brandy, gin, and vodka, is derived from distilled spirits, whereas beer and wine are not. The process of distillation increases the alcohol content of the beverage. See Box 28.1 for standard drink sizes in Canada, by type of alcohol.

As with other addictions, individuals must have a genetic predisposition in order to develop an alcohol addiction (**alcoholism**). Unlike other addictions, however, which usually develop very fast (within days to months), alcoholism takes some time to develop, and addiction may take a few years (for younger patients, it may take less time).

Alcoholism is similar to benzodiazepines in terms of its mechanism of addiction and clinical signs. These signs are stronger than those of other narcotic psycho-organic syndromes. Psychological symptoms of alcoholism include *diminished memory* (first short-term and then long-term) and *diminished cognitive function* (until the development of dementia)—both of these are unlikely with other narcotics. In some cases, this may lead to Korsakoff syndrome (Box 28.2). Alcoholism also causes serious damage to internal organs, including paralysis of the CNS, seizures (not only during withdrawal), and damage to the liver, pancreas, duodenum, and stomach. At the beginning, alcohol stimulates insulin production and the patient may present with hypoglycemia (even with hypoglycemic shock). In later stages, pancreatic malfunction will cause diabetes. Alcohol also decreases the potency and affects the genetic integrity of sexual cells, modifying people's heredity.

Dipsomania is constant drinking, from a few days to a few weeks, until the patient reaches a stage of intoxication and cannot drink any more. **Binge drinking** is rapid alcohol consumption in order to achieve quick intoxication. Large doses of alcohol can affect the pumping action of the heart, resulting in cardiac dysrhythmias (irregularities). Surface blood vessels dilate, producing flushing of the skin and rapid loss of body heat. Alcohol also causes numbness of the hands and feet, which creates a false sense of warmth. In large doses, alcohol can actually reduce body temperature. The effects of alcohol on the CNS are directly related to the amount (dose)

TABLE 28.1 Assessing Harm Scores* for Various Substances

Substance	Personal Harm Score	Social Harm Score	Total/ Combined Harm Score
Heroin	2.76	2.72	2.74
Crack cocaine	2.74	2.60	2.69
Crystal meth	2.69	2.54	2.63
Alcohol	2.55	2.70	2.56
Cocaine	2.54	2.33	2.46
Inhaled solvents	2.38	2.18	2.31
Nicotine	2.42	2.23	2.29
Benzodiazepines	2.33	2.17	2.27
Ketamine	2.24	1.97	2.13
Barbiturates	2.25	1.91	2.12
Amphetamine	2.24	1.89	2.11
Methadone	2.19	1.96	2.10
Dihydrocodeine/ Codeine/ Tramadol	2.05	1.89	1.98
Buprenorphine	2.04	1.83	1.96
LSD	2.04	1.87	1.95
Ecstasy/MDTA	2.07	1.74	1.92
Methylphenidate/ Ritalin	1.86	1.62	1.74
Magic mushrooms	1.88	1.60	1.74
Cannabis	1.86	1.61	1.73

*Participants were asked to score each substance for each of the nine parameters, using a 4-point scale, with 0 being no risk, 1 some risk, 2 moderate risk, and 3 extreme risk.
Source: Taylor, M., Mackay, K., Murphy, J., et al. (2012). Quantifying the RR of harm to self and others from substance misuse: Results from a survey of clinical experts across Scotland. *BMJ Open, 2*(4), e000774 (Table 3). https://doi.org/10.1136/bmjopen-2011-000774. https://bmjopen.bmj.com/content/2/4/e000774

BOX 28.1 Standard Drink Sizes in Canada

One standard drink in Canada equals:
341 mL (12 oz) bottle of 5% alcohol beer, cider, or cooler
43 mL (1.5 oz) shot of 40% hard liquor (vodka, rum, whisky, gin, etc.)
142 mL (5 oz) glass of 12% wine

From Rethink Your Drink Canada. (2016). *One standard drink.* http://www.rethinkyourdrinking.ca/

BOX 28.2 Korsakoff Syndrome

Korsakoff syndrome is a chronic memory disorder caused by severe deficiency of thiamine (vitamin B₁), most commonly caused by alcohol misuse. Thiamine helps brain cells produce energy from sugar. When levels fall too low, brain cells cannot generate enough energy to function properly. Given their poor digestion and diet, patients addicted to alcohol commonly have a low level of thiamine. As a result, Korsakoff syndrome may develop.

Korsakoff syndrome is often, but not always, preceded by an episode of Wernicke's encephalopathy, which is an acute brain reaction to a severe lack of thiamine. Wernicke's encephalopathy is a medical emergency that causes life-threatening brain disruption, confusion, staggering and stumbling, lack of coordination, and abnormal involuntary eye movements (see Medication Alert).

Korsakoff syndrome causes problems learning new information, the inability to remember recent events, and long-term memory gaps. Memory problems may be strikingly severe, while other thinking and social skills are relatively unaffected. For example, individuals may seem able to carry on a coherent conversation, but moments later be unable to recall that the conversation took place or to whom they spoke.

Those with Korsakoff syndrome may "confabulate," or make up, information they can't remember. They are not "lying" but may actually believe their invented explanations. Scientists don't yet understand why Korsakoff syndrome may cause confabulation.

Source: Alzheimer's Association. (2019). *Korsakoff syndrome.* https://www.alz.org/media/Documents/alzheimers-dementia-korsakoff-syndrome-ts.pdf

consumed (Table 28.2). Episodes of binge drinking, where large amounts are consumed in a short time, can actually lead to death from acute alcohol intoxication.

> **! MEDICATION ALERT**
>
> An alcoholic patient may often present in the emergency department with low glucose levels. This may require intravenous glucose administration. Entering cells from the bloodstream, glucose will take the rest of already depleted thiamine with it, causing Korsakoff–Wernicke syndrome. Thus, *intramuscular preventative administration of thiamine is recommended.*

Alcohol withdrawal and intoxication both may lead to death. The exact level of alcohol in the blood may not indicate the seriousness of intoxication or withdrawal. For a person who has adapted to very high levels of alcohol in their system, withdrawal symptoms may start at a relatively high level. For a person who is not used to consuming alcohol, a rapid increase in alcohol level from a relatively low level may cause severe intoxication. It is important to assess a patient's history of alcohol use and look for the clinical signs of alcohol intoxication or withdrawal.

Signs of Alcohol Intoxication

There is no official protocol in Canada to assess alcohol intoxication. Medical staff must rely on objective signs: often decreased pulse and blood pressure, different levels of drowsiness to the point of coma, lack of coordination, often nystagmus, often strange behaviour that is uncharacteristic for the person, possible elements of violence, and, at times, fluctuating mood.

Signs of Alcohol Withdrawal

The most popular tool used in Canada for assessing alcohol withdrawal is the Clinical Institute Withdrawal Assessment for Alcohol, Revised (CIWA-AR). The CIWA assesses 10 different parameters from 0 to 7 (except one parameter, which rates from 0 to 4). These 10 parameters are nausea/vomiting, anxiety, paroxysmal sweating (a result of sympathetic nervous system overreaction and not of normal thermoregulation), tactile disturbances, visual disturbances, tremors, agitation, orientation and clouding of sensations, auditory disturbances, and headaches. After determining the final score, a dose of benzodiazepines can be prescribed. Each hospital has its own protocol of frequency and duration for CIWA assessment.

Many of the CIWA parameters are subjective, thus it is very difficult to assess withdrawal correctly. Some sensational parameters can be common to both withdrawal and intoxication. A relatively high alcohol level in the blood can be responsible for both withdrawal and intoxication (depending on the patient's drinking pattern). Thus, the staff's ability to assess objective autonomic signs of withdrawal is also important. These objective signs include elevated pulse, often elevated blood pressure, vomiting, insomnia, diarrhea, very active peristalsis, and visible agitation.

With continued use, tolerance develops, and individuals become dependent on (addicted to) alcohol. Heavy drinkers of longer than 10 years are prone to developing **delirium tremens (DTs)**, a severe form of alcohol withdrawal that involves sudden and severe physical, mental, behavioural, and nervous system changes. Symptoms begin 48 hours to 10 days after the last drink. They worsen quickly and can include changes in mental function, delirium, hallucinations, and seizures. Delirium tremens is a medical emergency. Treatment and close monitoring in the hospital setting are required (close observation of symptoms, vital signs, mental status examination, monitoring of level of consciousness, and initiation of CIWA local protocol).

TABLE 28.2 Effects of Alcohol on the Nervous System

Blood Alcohol Concentration*	Effect on the Body
0.00 g/dL	Sober
0.03 g/dL	May feel a slight buzz, but without having trouble talking, seeing, or keeping one's balance
0.05 g/dL	Feeling buzzed or relaxed
0.08 g/dL	Legally drunk in Canada and the United States One may have trouble balancing, talking, and seeing straight. If the person drinks often, they may not have any symptoms of blood alcohol poisoning at this point, but damage to the brain and liver are still happening.
0.10 g/dL	Impaired judgment, decreased attention, trouble walking, and mood changes
0.15 g/dL	Blackouts and lack of physical control
0.20 g/dL	"Sloppy drunk," vomiting, confusion, staggering around
0.30 g/dL	Unconscious, stupor
0.40 g/dL	Coma or possible death

*Blood alcohol concentrations are given in different ways. Law enforcement agencies use grams per decilitre (g/dL). Health care providers use milligrams per decilitre (mg/dL) or millimoles per litre (mmol/L). For example, the legal limit for ethanol concentration can be stated as 0.08 g/dL, 80 mg/dL, or 17 mmol/L.

Source: University of Rochester Medical Center. (2019). *What do my test results mean?* https://www.urmc.rochester.edu/encyclopedia/content.aspx?contenttypeid=167&contentid=ethanol_blood

If drinking does not stop, death from multiple organ failure (especially the liver) will result, usually after a series of other assorted chronic health challenges.

Caffeine

Caffeine is a CNS stimulant. It is an ingredient in many products found in every supermarket. It is the main active ingredient in coffee, black teas, most cola drinks, other bottled beverages, and energy drinks. However, caffeine is also found in chocolate, diet aids, cold remedies, and over-the-counter pain relievers.

Children are increasingly using caffeine on a regular basis. Energy drinks, which contain large amounts of caffeine, are popular among teens and young adults. Overdose from too many energy drinks has resulted in death due to cardiac problems.

Caffeine stimulates the nervous system, relieving fatigue and increasing alertness and the body's metabolic rate. In large amounts, it can produce tremors, tachycardia, nervousness, and insomnia. The most prominent withdrawal symptom from caffeine is headache.

Caffeine intoxication occurs when high doses are consumed within a short time. Symptoms can last from 4 to 6 hours. They include restlessness, nervousness, rambling speech, high energy levels, agitation, muscle twitching, rapid heart rate, increased blood pressure, and disturbances in heart rhythms.

Cannabis

Cannabis (marijuana) is a term applied to the hemp plant, *Cannabis,* which grows wild in many tropical and temperate climates all over the world. The hemp plant has been used for centuries by many cultures in traditional remedies and other medicines. Historically, it was used to treat pain, decreased appetite, muscle and gastrointestinal tract spasms, asthma, and depression. It has also been used as an antibiotic and a topical anaesthetic. As with many other species of plants, there are male and female cannabis plants. The male plant in the species is used commercially for industrial applications like making rope, clothing, and paper. The female plant produces 50% male and 50% female seeds. It is the female plant that produces the flowers and buds that contain a usable amount of THC. Both male and female plants contain cannabidiol (CBD). CBD and THC molecules are very similar, and both work on cannabinoid receptors located throughout the body. They are part of the endocannabinoid system. Because it is THC that produces the "high" effect, people selectively breed the original hemp plant to get marijuana plants that have high levels of THC.

Cannabis is available in several forms. The dried tops and leaves are called *marijuana.* Hashish (hash) is the dried resin that seeps from the top and leaves, and hash oil is the distilled oil of hashish. All are usually smoked, but they also may be eaten in baked goods and candies.

Marijuana and other cannabis products produce a sense of well-being and relaxation. They alter time perception and affect short-term memory and concentration. Motivation, especially for distasteful tasks, may be decreased. Frequently, an increase in hunger occurs. Large doses can result in feelings of anxiety and paranoia. There are no proven withdrawal signs or symptoms, but anxious mood, irritability, and sleep disturbances have been reported.

Cannabis is legal in Canada following the passage of Bill C-45, the *Cannabis Act,* effective October 17, 2018. Today, only two countries in the world have legalized the use of cannabis for recreational use nationwide: Uruguay and Canada. The following are permitted in Canada under the *Cannabis Act:*

- A person can *purchase* limited amounts of fresh cannabis, dried cannabis, cannabis oil, cannabis seeds, or cannabis plants from retailers authorized by the provinces and territories.
- A person can *possess* up to 30 g of dried legal cannabis or equivalent in nondried form in public.
- A person can *consume* cannabis in locations authorized by local jurisdictions.
- A person can *grow* up to four cannabis plants per household (not per person) for personal use, from licensed seeds or seedlings purchased from licensed suppliers.
- A person can *share* up to 30 g of dried cannabis or equivalent with other adults.
- A person can *make legal cannabis-containing products* at home, such as food and drinks, provided that dangerous organic solvents are not used in making them.

The detailed implementation of the Bill varies across different provinces and territories (Government of Canada, 2018a). In the United States, cannabis products are legal only in some states and the District of Columbia (see Medication Alert). Many other states have authorized its use for medical purposes.

> **! MEDICATION ALERT**
>
> Despite the legalization of cannabis in some jurisdictions of the United States and everywhere in Canada, any Canadian who is known to US Border Security as a user, buyer, seller, or producer of cannabis will be banned from entering the United States. It is important for care providers to be familiar with the laws governing cannabis use in their own province or territory.

A new synthetic cannabis, known as "spice," is being sold as a synthetic marijuana. It is also known as "K2," "Black Mamba," and some other names. A variety of unnamed chemicals are sprayed onto plant material and then smoked. **Spice** is relatively inexpensive, often packaged as incense "not for human consumption" and sold at convenience stores and head shops in colourful packages. It is a much cheaper option than marijuana. Synthetic cannabis has many formulations. As most laboratories are set to detect only original cannabis, they fail to detect these new formulations of synthetic cannabis in urine. This fact makes synthetic cannabis the drug of choice for patients who are mandated to have their urine monitored (e.g., by employers) for cannabis use.

Synthetic cannabis has a much faster onset but shorter duration of action (between 90 and 180 minutes) than that of regular cannabis, and sometimes even has different effects on the human body than those of the natural form. Natural cannabis typically causes orthostatic hypotension and a decrease in blood pressure. Synthetic cannabis, by contrast, can cause a noticeable increase in heart rate and modest increase in blood pressure. Users can also experience serious adverse effects from the unknown chemicals used in these products. Anxiety, paranoia, aggression, and seizures may occur. Spice users, especially new users or those taking high doses, can experience a panic attack or become violently paranoid and attack others or themselves (Zawilska & Wojcieszak, 2014).

Hallucinogens

The hallucinogens are natural and synthetic substances that alter one's perception of reality. The active ingredients of the peyote cactus, mescaline, has been used in the religious ceremonies of certain Indigenous people for many years. The introduction of laboratory-designed hallucinogens in the United States did not occur until the early 1970s. Today they are commonly available. Most doses are taken orally or inhaled, and they are frequently contaminated with toxic chemicals. It is believed that they may temporarily interfere with the actions of neurotransmitters in the brain. These hallucinogens vary in onset, duration of action, and potency, but all produce a sense of altered reality. The three major hallucinogens are LSD, peyote, and psilocybin.

LSD, an ergot fungus, was discovered by accident in the 1930s while researching ergot, a fungus that grows on certain grains. It is sold in tablet, capsule, and liquid forms. The effects of LSD, called a "trip," last about 12 hours.

Peyote buttons are the disc-shaped crowns of the peyote cactus. The active ingredient in peyote is mescaline. The buttons are usually chewed or soaked in water to produce a tea. The effects last about 12 hours. Peyote has been used in some cultural religious ceremonies for centuries.

Psilocybin is found in certain bitter-tasting mushrooms. They are eaten fresh, dried, or steeped in a tea. The hallucinogenic compounds are not inactivated by freezing or cooking. The effects begin within 20 to 30 minutes and last about 6 hours.

Users of hallucinogens experience everything from profound mind-expanding experiences to "bad trips" in which dangerous behavioural reactions occur. The mind-altering effects of hallucinogens include a heightened awareness of reality; distortions in time, space, and body image; feelings of depersonalization; and loss of a sense of reality. Physically, users will have dilated pupils, dizziness, nausea, rapid heart rate, weakness, and an inability to perform tasks such as driving. With severe reactions, convulsions and death have occurred. Flashbacks, which are a return to the psychedelic experience after the drug has worn off, can occur with the use of hallucinogens. The repeated use of hallucinogens can lead to various health problems.

Dissociative Anaesthetics

Phencyclidine (PCP) was originally developed for use as an animal tranquilizer. It is a white crystal powder that is smoked, snorted, or swallowed. When taken by humans, it produces feelings of being separated from one's body and environment (dissociation). It also produces mild depression with low doses and a schizophrenic-like reaction with higher doses. It is highly addictive. Long-term abuse results in memory loss, weight loss, depression, and problems with thinking and speech. PCP is a dangerous drug because it causes people to behave in unpredictable, often violent ways (Table 28.3).

Inhalants

The breathing in of volatile substances or chemical gases (inhalants) is popular among adolescents and young adults for several reasons: They are legal, inexpensive, and easily available, and they have a rapid onset of effect. Unfortunately, the practice is also associated with significant complications, such as sudden death caused by cardiac dysrhythmia or respiratory depression. The use of inhalants can also result in hyperactive motor responses, loss of coordination, and seizures.

The most commonly inhaled substances are alcohol solvents, gasoline, glue, paint thinner, hairspray, and spray paints. Chemicals less frequently used as inhalants include cleaning fluids, typewriter correction liquids, and spray can propellants.

Inhalants are most often used by adolescents in group settings. Several methods are used to inhale the vapours, such as soaking a rag and then holding it to the nose and mouth. The substance may be inhaled directly from the container (huffing) or placed in a bag or other closed container and then inhaled. Soon after inhaling, the individual feels a "high" that is associated with feelings of great well-being (euphoria), excitement, sexual aggressiveness, a lessened sense of right and wrong, and loss of judgement. Signs and symptoms of inhalant intoxication include delusions, hallucinations, anxiety, and confusion.

TABLE 28.3 Signs and Symptoms of PCP Use

Physical Signs and Symptoms	Psychological Signs and Symptoms
Increased blood pressure	Belligerence (wants to fight)
Increased temperature	Bizarre behaviours
Muscle rigidity, ataxia (uncoordinated, staggering)	Delusions, hallucinations, distorted thinking
Repeated jerking	Impaired (poor) judgement
Agitated movements	Impulsive behaviours
Vertical and horizontal nystagmus (eye tremors)	Paranoia, rapid mood swings
Weight loss	Unpredictable behaviours

PCP, phencyclidine.

Although no withdrawal syndrome has been recognized, the repeated use of inhalants can result in profound physical and psychosocial harm.

Opioids (Narcotics)

Opioids have strong pain-relieving actions and are used for medicinal purposes. These substances, called *narcotics* or *opiates,* are obtained by milking a flower called *Papaver somniferum,* the opium poppy. They are commonly prescribed for a variety of painful conditions, coughs, and diarrhea.

The semisynthetic narcotics include heroin, hydromorphone, and thebaine derivatives. The Bayer Company of Germany first marketed heroin in 1898 as a new pain reliever. The *Canada Opium Act* of 1908 made it illegal to sell, produce, and import opium, setting a precedent worldwide. In the United States heroin was legally available to the public until the passage of the *Harrison Narcotic Act* of 1914.

Narcotics are CNS depressants. They occur naturally, semisynthetically, and synthetically. Some natural narcotics have been altered to make new, artificially produced (synthetic) drugs. Natural narcotics are opium, and its principal ingredient, morphine.

The use of opium was documented 4 000 years before Hippocrates, and it continues to be a commonly used substance in many countries today. Opium can be found in several forms. The fluid scraped from the base of the poppy flower and rolled into dark brown chunks is called *raw opium* (Fig. 28.3). Processed opium can appear as a fine white powder. Before the 1900s opium was readily available in Canada and the United States and was a common ingredient in many patent medicines.

Pure **heroin** is a white, bitter-tasting powder that is usually put into solution and injected. Heroin (also known as *dope, dust, junk, smack,* and *horse*) is a depressant. It slows down the activity of the CNS. Today, potent forms of heroin are available. Some are so strong that they need only to be smoked or inhaled to produce the same effect as injecting heroin. Street heroin is found in colours ranging from white to dark brown depending on the additives. An especially potent form is called *black tar heroin* (Fig. 28.4). This crudely processed form of heroin is manufactured in Mexico and may contain as much as 80% impurities. It is

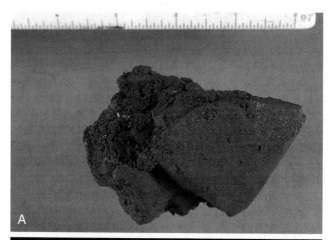
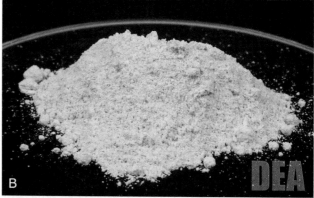
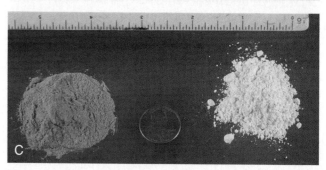

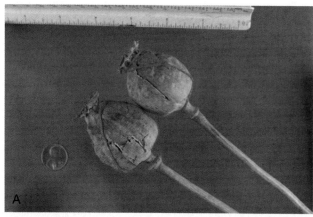
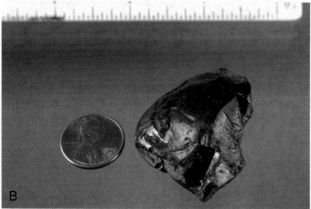

Fig. 28.3 A, Poppy. B, Opium. (Courtesy US Drug Enforcement Agency [DEA].)

Fig. 28.4 A, Black tar heroin. B, Heroin powder. C, Asian heroin. (Courtesy US Drug Enforcement Agency [DEA].)

most commonly diluted and injected. The signs and symptoms of heroin use, overdose, and withdrawal are listed in Table 28.4.

Morphine is one of the most effective painkillers available. It is marketed as a white powder or in solution for injection. It is administered by injection under the direction of a licensed health care practitioner.

Hydromorphone and the thebaine derivatives are semisynthetic narcotics made from opium. A common brand name for hydromorphone is Dilaudid. It is used as an analgesic and is produced in liquid or tablet form. It is shorter acting, more sedating, and up to eight times more powerful than morphine. Although available only by prescription, it is highly sought by addicts. Thebaine derivatives, another opium product, are up to 1 000 times more potent than morphine. Because of the danger of overdose, these drugs are used by veterinarians for the care of large animals only.

Sedatives (Hypnotics or Anxiolytics)

Sedative, hypnotic, or anxiolytic drugs include all benzodiazepines and related drugs, carbamates, barbiturates and barbiturate-like hypnotics, all prescription sleep medications, and most antianxiety medication (Table 28.5).

Benzodiazepines include diazepam, lorazepam, alprazolam, and clonazepam and are known under brand names like Valium, Ativan, and Xanax. Benzodiazepines are used to treat seizures, anxiety, and insomnia.

Carbamates comprise a group of medications developed to help with muscle relaxation. In Canada, for example, methocarbamol can be sold as an over-the-counter oral medicine at a low dose that may be combined with acetaminophen or ibuprofen. A combination product with acetylsalicylic acid and codeine is available in Canada by prescription.

Barbiturates are drugs that help with falling asleep quickly and thus are very useful for surgeries and in other instances where a patient must quickly fall asleep. The two types most popular in Canada are amobarbital (Amytal) and pentobarbital (Nembutal). One that is similar to pentobarbital (but with less breathing adverse effects) is Propofol, which became notorious for causing the death of Michael Jackson. Usually individuals who abuse this group of substances already have other substance-use disorders (e.g., alcohol, stimulants). Of all the categories of substances, this one is particularly lethal in high doses.

Stimulants

Stimulants are another group of commonly abused substances. They include "bath salts," caffeine, cocaine and crack cocaine, ice, methamphetamines, and certain prescription medications, such as amphetamines, appetite suppressants, and methylphenidate (Ritalin).

Amphetamines were originally pharmaceutically manufactured medicines to treat depression, narcolepsy, hyperactivity in children, and obesity. Amphetamines were initially sold without a prescription in inhalers and diet pills. Today they are available only by prescription, but many are illegally manufactured. They are strong stimulants with addictive properties.

Bath salts have nothing to do with bathing. They are a cheap replacement for more expensive stimulants like methamphetamine or cocaine. Just like Spice, they are marketed as "not for human consumption" and are virtually undetectable by a typical drug laboratory. They are made

TABLE 28.4 Signs and Symptoms of Heroin Use, Overdose, and Withdrawal

Heroin Use	Heroin Overdose	Heroin Withdrawal
Constricted pupils	Shallow respirations	Watery eyes
Depression	Clammy skin	Runny nose
Drowsiness	Convulsions	Sweating
Euphoria (feelings of great well-being)	Coma	Muscle cramps
Nausea		Loss of appetite, nausea
Respiratory depression		Chills
		Tremors
		Panic

TABLE 28.5 Prescription Sedatives (Hypnotic or Anxiolytic) Available in Canada

Drug Class	Generic Name	Trade Name	Street Names
Benzodiazepines	alprazolam	Xanax®	Z-bars, bars
	clonazepam	Rivotril®	K-pins
	diazepam	Valium®	Vs, tranks, downers
	flurazepam	Dalmane®	tranks, downers, nerve pills
	lorazepam	Ativan®	nerve pills, tranks, downers
	temazepam	Restoril®	rugby balls, tems, jellies
	triazolam	Halcion®	Up Johns, tranks downers
Nonbenzodiazepine sleep medication	zopiclone	Imovane®	Z-drug
Barbiturates	pentobarbital	Nemutal®	barbs, m&ms, nembies
	amobarbital	Amytal®	angels, blue heavens

From Canadian Centre on Substance Use and Addiction. (2017). *Prescription sedatives* (p. 1). https://ccsa.ca/sites/default/files/2019-04/CCSA-Canadian-Drug-Summary-Prescription-Sedatives-2017-en.pdf

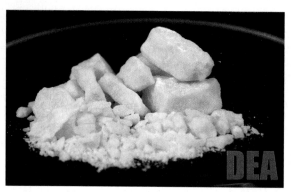

Fig. 28.5 Crack cocaine. (Courtesy US Drug Enforcement Agency [DEA].)

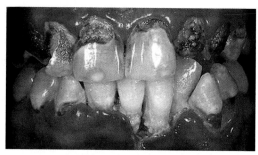

Fig. 28.6 "Meth mouth" in a chronic user. (Courtesy Dr. Stephen Wagner, in Darby, M. L., & Walsh, M. [2015]. *Dental hygiene* [4th ed.]. Saunders.)

from a variety of chemical stimulants and are addictive. The most intense highs come from snorting or injecting. The typical effect includes elevation in mood, decrease in hostility, and increase in empathy. They may cause an increase in body temperature and perspiration. In high doses, however, they can lead to irritation and aggression. Unfortunately, like with other stimulants, this is often followed by depression, psychosis, and suicidal ideation. The typical acute presentation, often in an emergency department, for someone who has ingested bath salts is similar to that for cocaine (with no cocaine detected): acute vasospasm that can lead to death from arrhythmia or renal failure (Gerona & Wu, 2012).

Cocaine is a potent natural stimulant. For centuries, the natives of the South American Andes Mountains chewed the weakly psychoactive leaves of the coca plant to relieve fatigue and hunger. Today coca is grown, processed into cocaine, and shipped to many countries throughout the world.

Cocaine is available "on the street" as a white, crystalline powder that is commonly contaminated with local anaesthetics or sugar. It is either injected or "snorted" by inhaling. Cocaine produces an immediate rush of energy, vigour, and feelings of well-being that last less than 1 hour. The intense pleasurable feelings can lead to a mental dependency that can ultimately destroy one's life as more and higher doses are used. Common signs of cocaine use include changes in eating and sleeping behaviours, a disregard for hygiene, runny nose, and bloodshot eyes. Repeated use can dissolve the nasal septum, resulting in a collapsed nose. Cocaine overstimulates the nervous system. Overdoses can lead to kidney and liver failure, seizures, heart attack, and stroke.

Crack is a type of processed cocaine (Fig. 28.5). Combining cocaine with ammonia or baking soda and heating it removes the hydrochloride molecule and produces chips or chunks of highly addicting cocaine, called *rocks*. These are usually vapourized in a pipe or smoked with tobacco or marijuana. Because of its concentrated form, crack reaches the brain immediately and produces a more intense but shorter-lasting high. Tolerance and addiction develop quickly as users chase the feeling of that first, intense experience. Crack users will ignore family, work, and friends as the drug becomes the priority in life.

Designer drugs (also called *club drugs*) are substances "created by underground chemists who alter the molecular structures of existing drugs" (Hess & DeBoer, 2002). Designer drugs, such as MDMA (ecstasy), STP, and "ice," are easily available in most areas of North America. The designer drug called *ecstasy* is fast becoming the preferred recreational drug of teens and young adults because it allows its users to "party" for long periods of time. Taking this drug, however, can have severe consequences. Because the drug suppresses the need to drink, eat, and sleep, it promotes severe dehydration and physical exhaustion. The leading cause of death among ecstasy users is hyperthermia, a dangerously high body temperature. Kidney or liver failure can result, even after one dose.

Methamphetamine (meth) is one of the most addictive and destructive drugs available today. It is sold in bags of white to pale brown powder that is smoked, snorted, injected, or swallowed. "Crystal meth" is a more potent form of the drug. Users experience a "rush" of euphoria and well-being that lasts for up to 10 to 12 hours. Many users become sexually excited and experience a false sense of energy. They become unusually active, nervous, or anxious. Feelings of power and aggression may be present. Delusions, hallucinations, and paranoia are common.

Because the nervous system is overstimulated, meth users do not eat or sleep for long periods of time (several days). When users do come down or "crash," they may sleep for many hours and be extremely hungry. Weight loss makes users appear thin and gaunt. Once fed and rested, they will begin the cycle again.

Some users will pick at their skin, trying to remove the bugs or hairs they feel moving under their skin. Because meth depresses the immune system, skin sores and injection sites often become infected. Chronic respiratory infections are common. Caustic chemicals in the drug, plus the fact that meth decreases the flow of saliva, causes the rotten, brown, and abscessed teeth known as "meth mouth" (Fig. 28.6). The long-term use of meth causes irreversible harm to the brain, nervous system, heart, blood vessels, lung, liver, and kidneys. Death can also be sudden from a stroke, seizure, or irregular heartbeat.

Tobacco (Nicotine)

Nicotine is present in all forms of tobacco (cigarettes, chewing tobacco, pipe tobacco, cigars, snuff) and certain medications (nicotine patch, nicotine gum). It can produce both relaxation and stimulation: It increases alertness, improves concentration and even memory, increases blood pressure and pulse, and helps to relieve feelings of hunger. Nicotine is frequently used as a method for controlling body weight and is currently a legal inhalant.

Although its popularity is declining, tobacco is still a commonly used substance. Tobacco is either smoked or held between the gum and lip and absorbed through the mucous membranes of the mouth. It is never swallowed because of its toxic effects. Tobacco is addictive, and its continued use is associated with many health complications. In Canada, the United States, and other industrialized countries, the sale of cigarettes and cigars is restricted by age, and smoking is prohibited in the majority of public spaces.

Vaping is the consumption of a vapour. The vapour is a gas condensed into a liquid form (at room temperature) and usually contains nicotine. This liquid is warmed in a portable device (like e-cigarettes) so that it becomes a gas and can be inhaled. The popularity of vaping has grown recently, especially among young adults. The perceived "cleanness" of this method and a huge variety of tastes have made it very attractive not only to former smokers but also to people who otherwise would never try tobacco products. However, vaping has created new, serious medical concerns (e.g., bronchiectasis and emphysema). It is also important to remember that vaping causes the same addiction and damage to health as nicotine from regular smoking (Ghosh, Coakley, Ghio, et al., 2019).

OTHER MEDICATIONS

Many chemicals that were developed to save lives and ease suffering have the potential for being abused. For example, almost all the opium arriving in North America today is broken down into its most useful alkaloids, morphine and codeine. These substances are then refined into powerful pain-relieving medications (narcotic analgesics). They are available only with the prescription of a licensed physician, dentist, or nurse practitioner, but they remain a source of abuse (Box 28.3).

Rohypnol and GHB are CNS depressants, developed by drug companies and abused by teens and young adults. They are odourless, colourless liquids that combine unnoticed with alcoholic and other drinks. Often referred to as "date rape" drugs, they render the victim sedated and helpless during a sexual attack. Often the victim will suffer from "retroactive amnesia, where the person who took the drug can't remember events that occurred while under the influence of the drug" (Helmenstine, 2019). As a result of this unfortunate adverse effect, many sexual assault cases are not reported and go unsolved.

Commonly abused stimulants include the amphetamines, diet pills, and the appetite suppressants. Methylphenidate (Ritalin), a medication used to treat attention-deficit/hyperactivity disorder (ADHD), is another often abused stimulant. The signs and symptoms of stimulant use include changes in personality, anxiety, tension, anger, restlessness, and rapid speech and movement.

Laxatives and diuretics are commonly abused by older persons and by people who are trying to lose weight. Individuals with eating disorders or altered body images often use these drugs to keep themselves excessively thin or to atone for an eating binge. Older persons can develop a dependence on laxatives when they are used too frequently.

CHARACTERISTICS OF SUBSTANCE USE AND ABUSE

It is important to remember the differences between substance use and abuse. Some people can use various chemicals to change the way they feel, but the use does not affect their ability to perform the activities of daily life. This is **substance use**. **Substance (drug) abuse**, however, occurs when use of the chemical interferes with or becomes more important than the activities of daily living.

Stages of Addiction

Many individuals use alcohol, tobacco, or other chemicals and function very well. Those who move from use to dependency (addiction) follow a fairly predictable course. During the *early stage,* individuals are able to use and enjoy their chosen substance. A desire to repeat the first pleasurable experience leads to a frequent pattern of use. One begins to prefer being "high" to other activities.

Soon a habit of excessive use develops as the individual begins to ignore responsibilities and obligations. The person may deny that a problem exists, ignore others' comments, lie to cover up the activity, or conceal the problem by sneaking drinks or doses. During these periods, the individual may also become intoxicated.

Intoxication is defined as a state of maladaptive behavioural or psychological changes resulting from exposure to certain chemicals. With some people who have a genetic predisposition, certain substances or certain types of behaviours create a brain change in the reward (pleasure) centre. This change forces people to repeatedly, uncontrollably, and compulsively seek the intoxication. This behaviour is called **addiction.** (When an addicted individual is not using an addictive substance, it called **abstinence**.) Intoxicated people are frequently belligerent (looking for a fight or an argument) and have wide emotional swings. They often lack sound judgement, and their critical thinking ability is reduced. They will often stagger or show other signs of impaired motor abilities. The actual picture of an intoxicated individual varies greatly. Psychological effects arise from the person's expectations of what the chemical will do and the environment in which the substance is taken.

BOX 28.3 The Opioid Crisis in Canada

In 2016, there were 2 861 apparent opioid-related deaths in Canada, which is equivalent to eight people dying each day, and is greater than the average number of Canadians killed daily in motor vehicle collisions in 2015 (Belzak & Halverson, 2018).

During the *middle (crucial) stage* of addiction, the intoxicating episodes increase as the body attempts to compensate by adapting to the substance. **Tolerance** develops as increased amounts of the chemical are needed to produce the same effects that one dose once produced. *Physical tolerance* occurs when the body has adjusted to living and functioning with the substance in its system. *Psychological tolerance* develops when individuals feel that they cannot function without the use of their chosen chemical substance.

Unfortunately, often when people attempt to stop using some of these substances, they experience negative physical and emotional symptoms. These symptoms are called *withdrawal symptoms*. Therefore, people continue to consume these substances to avoid the negative withdrawal symptoms. This phenomenon is called **dependency**.

By the time one has progressed to the *chronic (late) stage*, tolerance for the chemical is usually quite high. The need for the substance now leads to a loss of control over one's behaviour. Without the chemical, life is miserable. Daily living becomes a nightmare, and all waking effort and energy are focused on obtaining and using the now-required substance.

Substance-Related Disorders and Addictive Disorder

Substance-related disorders consist of two groups: *substance-use disorders* and *substance-induced disorders* (intoxication, withdrawal, and substance-induced mental disorders). Substance-related disorders involve 10 classes of drugs that cause addiction: alcohol, caffeine, cannabis, hallucinogens, inhalants, opioids, sedative, stimulants, tobacco, and other.

In addition to these substances, some types of behaviour may cause a strong addictive effect on individuals who are genetically predisposed to addiction. A few of the disorders involving this excessive behaviour include sex addiction, gambling addiction, shopping addiction, and Internet gaming addiction, but there are also others. Of these, only *gambling addiction* is currently recognized as a disorder in the *Diagnostic and Statistical Manual of Mental Disorders*, 5th edition (*DSM-5*; American Psychiatric Association [APA], 2013). All other types of repetitive excessive behaviour currently do not have enough evidence to support them being recognized as true disorders.

Clinical Presentation

The clinical presentation for a **substance-induced disorder** typically consists of two main presentations: intoxication and withdrawal. These presentations are very different for each category, and even for each substance.

However, the substance-use disorders for each of the 10 previously described categories have very similar clinical presentations. They all have the same 11 diagnostic criteria or recognizable patterns of behaviour. When *at least 2 of the following 11 DSM-5 criteria exist for a 12-month period* and cause significant distress and/or impairment, then a **substance-use disorder** diagnosis can be made (APA, 2013; Mclellan, 2017):

1. The substance is taken for longer than the intended period of time, and in larger amounts.
2. There is an effort to cut down the use of that substance, but without success.
3. A significant amount of time is spent acquiring, using, or recovering from the substance.
4. There are cravings and urges to use the substance.
5. Use of the substance leads to the failure to fulfill basic functions and obligations (school, work, family obligations).
6. The individual continues to use the substance, even when it causes social and/or relationship problems.
7. Important social, family, occupational, or recreational activities are given up or significantly reduced because of substance use.
8. Recurrent use of the substance continues even when it places an individual in physical danger.
9. The use of the substance continues even when it causes or exacerbates physical and/or psychological challenges.
10. More of the substance is needed to achieve the same effect (tolerance).
11. Withdrawal symptoms are manifested when the substance is discontinued, and they can be eliminated when more of the substance is consumed.

Similarity Between Addiction and Other Disorders

To have a better understanding of addiction, we must remember that, in some ways, all diseases are connected to genetic predisposition. All external presentations (the way we look, think, behave, feel, and function, and all our diseases) are influenced by our genetic predisposition, (to the genotype). Without this genetic predisposition, no external factors can cause addiction or mental illness or any other disease (with the exception of different sorts of trauma). In other words, a person must have both of the following components to become ill from an addiction: a genetic predisposition (internal factors or genotype) and an exposure (external factors) to that substance and/or behaviour. If we take one of these components out of the equation, the person will not have that addiction. Currently, there is no way to make gene corrections for these disorders; therefore, we can only treat the symptoms.

Most of the time, psychiatric diseases begin from some kind of trigger (usually stress). All chemical or behavioural addictions also begin from exposure to a chemical or a behaviour.

Both addiction and mental illness are chronic illnesses. This means that the majority of patients will require lifelong treatment and support, as well as good coping skills (recovery model). Thus, in the current stage of modern medicine, we are looking to achieve stable remission and not a cure for mental illness or addiction.

Three Main Malfunctions Leading to Addiction

There are three domains of human activity that may function abnormally, causing addiction. Understanding these malfunctions may help us to understand the phenomena of addiction.

1. *Reward centre and down-regulated mood:* Our mood fluctuates up and down within the norm. At times, our mood correlates with external events, and other times it does not. The majority of patients who suffer from addiction have mood fluctuations that are mainly in the negative spectrum, despite the existence of positive external events. Their mood can be elevated at times but never enough, and never for a very long time. This mood fluctuation can cause problems with relationships and self-esteem. Suddenly, following use of a certain chemical or enacting a certain behaviour, the person may feel happy like never before. This event in an individual's brain creates a strong neuropathway in the reward centre that is already predisposed to it.

2. *Memory:* This unusual happiness stays vivid in the person's memory. Normally, any memory (even a very happy one) will pale and become less vivid over time. However, patients with an addiction have a genetic predisposition through which the memory of this particular happiness that is related to the addiction continues to remain as vivid as if it is just happened.

3. *Frontal lobe:* Patients suffering from addiction are genetically predisposed to lose control over their behaviour and do everything they can to re-experience the same happiness (of which they have a vivid memory), without considering the consequences. Even though withdrawal symptoms are associated with many different drugs' cessation, the main difference with addiction is that the individual is genetically predisposed to experiencing an irresistible urge to seek out that drug or behaviour again.

CASE STUDY

Ernie's father was 15 years old when Ernie was born. His mother, who was 14 years old, gave custody to the father after the first 6 months of Ernie's life. To keep Ernie quiet during his infant and toddler years, his father would blow marijuana smoke into his face. It worked. Ernie would sleep for hours while his father partied.

By the time Ernie was 5 years old, he was drinking beer. At 8 years, he graduated to vodka, gin, and tequila. By 10 years old, Ernie was mixing alcohol with cocaine. School became impossible, so he dropped out at 12 years old. By the time he was 14 years old, Ernie was hustling drugs and trying to sell the sexual favours of three neighbourhood girls.

Where is Ernie today? Fortunately, he overdosed one evening when he was about 17 years old. The nurse in the emergency department, recognizing the potential in this young man, took the time to tell him that he had choices. He was in charge of his own life. Ernie listened. His detoxification was painful. His recovery was slow and difficult, but he persisted, knowing there was something more in life than a fog of consciousness.

Today, despite several setbacks, Ernie has been clean for more than 10 years. He is a university graduate, happily married, and the father of two boys. The strongest thing he drinks now is orange juice.

- How do you think the nurse influenced Ernie's life?

GUIDELINES FOR INTERVENTION

The three most commonly abused types of drugs are alcohol and sedative–alcohol combinations; opiate narcotics, chiefly heroin; and stimulants, chiefly cocaine and amphetamines.

The costs and consequences of substance abuse are high. As individuals progress with drug abuse, their world narrows as they begin to suffer physical deterioration and become isolated from family, occupational, and community relationships.

> **! MEDICATION ALERT**
>
> Remember that older persons are at high risk for becoming drug dependent. When an older person becomes less social and begins to isolate themselves, suspect a problem with drugs. The usual drugs of abuse in the older population are pain medications and drug combinations.
>
> When assessing older patients, have them bring all their medications in a paper bag. These medications should include all over-the-counter and herbal preparations. In this way, an accurate assessment of their medication use can be obtained. Do not forget to ask about alcohol use, especially in combination with their medications.

Absenteeism from work, unpaid bills, and job loss frequently result when substance use is out of control. Involvement with the legal system can occur. Some people deplete their financial resources to obtain their substances. Accidents, trauma, crime, domestic violence, child abuse, prostitution, suicide, disease, and the loss of safe communities are associated with substance abuse. Therefore, it is important for all health care providers to be alert to the possibility of substance-related problems in every patient.

Assessment

The physical examination, patient history, and emotional assessment for any patient suspected of substance abuse should focus on the following aspects:

- *Central nervous system:* Assess for orientation, level of consciousness, balance, gait, and ability to follow instructions.
- *Head and neck:* Examine the eyes, and check pupils and sclera (whites) of the eyes. Note ruddy or pale complexion, distended neck veins, or petechiae (small red dots) on the face. Observe for evidence of injections under the tongue, and inspect the area between the gums and lips.
- *Chest:* Do not forget to take vital signs. Count pulse and respirations for a full minute. Palpate pedal and radial pulses. Observe for any difficulty in breathing. Auscultate the heart for irregular rates or rhythms. Listen to the breath sounds, and note any abnormal sounds.
- *Abdomen:* Inspect the size, shape, and contours of the abdomen. Auscultate all four quadrants, and count the bowel sounds. Check for ascites (water in the abdomen), distention, or enlarged organs. Look for bruising, petechiae,

and other signs of bleeding. Have the patient describe the colour and consistency of their stool.

- *Skin:* Observe and document the size, location, and characteristics of any skin lesions or marks. Check for needle marks on the patient's arms, fingers, legs, and toes. Note the skin turgor and muscle mass of the arms and legs.
- *Nutritional status:* Many chemically dependent persons do not eat regularly and are at risk for malnutrition. Observe the patient's body build and appearance. Ask the patient to list everything they ate yesterday and tell you how meals were prepared. Ask if there have been any recent appetite or weight changes. Inspect the patient's skin colour, hair, and fingernails. If the patient lives alone or is homeless, find out how food is obtained on a daily basis.

The psychosocial assessment includes the following:

- *General appearance:* Is the patient tidy or unkempt? Note the patient's manner and style of dress, jewellery, makeup, hair style, and body marks (e.g., tattoos, symbolic scars).
- *Behaviours:* Note rate of speech, motor activity, and interactions during the interview. Observe for signs of memory loss, difficulty following directions, and problems with communication.
- When exploring alcohol use, remember that individuals tend to minimize the quantity of alcohol used in a day. Have them describe the size of the container that holds the alcohol. Two 4-ounce drinks and two 12-ounce drinks have very different amounts of alcohol.
- *Emotional state:* Watch for signs of depression, emotional instability (mood swings), suspiciousness, anger, agitation, self-pity, or jealousy. Ask patients if they have ever had a hallucination, a blackout (period of time during which the user cannot remember events), any violent impulses, or suicidal ideas.
- *Social support:* Have patients identify the most important people in their lives. Are these people willing to become involved in treatment with the patient? If possible, observe how patients interact with their family and friends. Remember that family members may also need support and treatment.
- *Motivation:* Ask what motivated the patient to seek treatment now. Is the court, their employer, or the family insisting on treatment, or are they seeking relief from the problems associated with substance use? The motivation level of patients plays an important part in their recovery.
- *Diagnostic tests:* Diagnostic testing usually includes standard blood and urine examinations. A complete blood count (CBC), urinalysis, and chemistry panel are done to assess for organ damage. Frequently, tests for hepatitis, human immunodeficiency virus (HIV), tuberculosis (TB), and other infectious diseases are performed. Patients are also assessed for nutritional or bleeding problems. Other diagnostic tests, such as a computed tomography (CT) scan, magnetic resonance imaging (MRI), X-ray films, or an electroencephalogram (EEG), may also be ordered.

Treatments and Therapies

The treatment of substance-related disorders continues to change and grow. Consequently, a broad range of approaches is available today.

Abstinence and Harm Reduction

The aim of both abstinence and harm reduction is to help people reduce the harms they experience because of their substance use. **Harm reduction** is an evidence-informed approach to treating substance use that has the aim of helping people who use legal and illegal psychoactive drugs live safer and healthier lives. Substance use and excessive gambling may affect one's health and legal vulnerability. A reduction in substance use, or abstinence, is not required in order to receive public respect, compassion, or services. A harm-reduction approach assists people who use substances in gaining better control over their health and enables them to take protective and proactive measures for themselves and their families. This approach is the official Canadian "Drug and Substance Strategy" (Government of Canada, 2018b).

In addition, the incidence of psychiatric disorders is very high among substance users. Anxiety and depression are commonly found in patients with substance abuse problems. These disorders must also be treated if the individual is to remain drug-free or reduce their use of drugs.

Nonmedical Treatment

Nonmedical treatment usually comes in the form of therapy. *Individual psychotherapy* is very effective for patients who have certain dependencies (such as cocaine addictions), but it is expensive and therefore unavailable to many people. *Group therapy* can offer peer support from individuals "who have been there," in some cases in the form of one-to-one support with a "sponsor," as in 12-step groups. The person can call their sponsor when their craving is particularly intense. This therapy offers people the opportunity to experiment with and explore their drug-free behaviours with trusted sources. There are also a variety of groups that can help with a specific addiction, such as Alcoholics Anonymous, Cocaine Anonymous, Opium Anonymous, and Gamblers Anonymous.

Medical Treatment

Medical treatment for substance use involves medication that is designed to lessen the craving for a substance and may include opiates like methadone, Subutex, naltrexone, or Suboxone. The goal of opiate use is to normalize the work of the pleasure centre in the brain, prevent withdrawal symptoms, and improve the user's mood and global functioning.

Methadone is a synthetic opioid receptor agonist (it sits on receptors and activates them). Each treatment works for 24 to 36 hours and, unlike narcotics, does not create tolerance (there is no need to increase a dose to reach the same effect). Therapeutic doses do not cause euphoria. Treatment starts at 30 to 40 mg and is increased until opioid withdrawal symptoms (enlarged pupils, tachycardia, increased blood pressure, goosebumps, tears, flulike snot, excessive saliva, increased reflexes, chills, muscle tension, diarrhea, vomiting, abdominal pain, frequent voiding, cold perspiration) disappear. The maximum dose is 120 mg; most patients stabilize at around 80 to 100 mg. At high doses (more than 150 mg), methadone causes an increase of the QT interval. (The QT interval on an electrocardiogram [ECG] represents the work of the heart's ventricular activity. Slow contractions can lead to a drop in blood pressure, syncope, and death. Most psychiatric medications affect the QT interval.) It is very important to perform an ECG before beginning methadone treatment and to continue to monitor symptoms. Methadone can also cause mild sedation.

Buprenorphine, known by the brand name Subutex, is a synthetic opioid partial agonist that is administered sublingually and creates a reaction that prevents withdrawal symptoms. Increasing the dose does not cause euphoria. Subutex is more active in attaching to receptors, much more so than heroin, morphine, methadone, or oxycodone, and thus may push these drugs away from receptors, causing acute withdrawal syndromes. Thus, at the beginning of Subutex treatment, it is important to ensure that withdrawal symptoms have already started and that opioid receptors are no longer occupied by some other opioid drug. Administration of Subutex to a patient on opioids without withdrawal symptoms may cause dangerous withdrawal symptoms.

Treatment starts at a dose of 2 mg and is increased up to 18 to 20 mg, at times to 24 mg, given once per day. Subutex does not increase the QT interval. To achieve a euphoria effect, some patients will take it through the vein. Unlike methadone, there is no danger of overdose with Subutex. Opioid overdose can result if a patient uses heroin after methadone, but overdose will not occur if heroin is taken after Subutex, because Subutex sits very tightly on opioid receptors.

Naltrexone (not to be confused with naloxone, which is used for opioid emergency overdose) is an antagonist opioid receptor, meaning it sits tightly on opioid receptors and prevents them from working. It closes these receptors and does not allow opioid drugs to attach and make receptors work. This effect can cause withdrawal symptoms. In Canada, naltrexone, under the trade name Revia, is used as a treatment for alcohol and opioid dependency. Revia is also used to treat pathological gambling.

Suboxone, a combination of naltrexone and Subutex, is also used to treat addiction. As with Subutex, if a patient takes Suboxone through the vein there will be no euphoria. This makes this medication very safe to use (assuming one can ensure that there is no other opioid in the patient's system). At times it may cause some stimulation of the CNS, so it is not good to administer Suboxone in the evening. There is evidence that Suboxone can help with cocaine dependency as well (Ling, Hillhouse, Saxon, et al., 2016). Suboxone can be given only after withdrawal symptoms are present. Most Canadian clinics and hospitals have an algorithm available on how to administer it. At times, it can be taken once every 2 to 3 days. In Canada, a physician or nurse practitioner must be certified in order to prescribe it.

Naloxone (also known by the brand name Narcan) is the first emergency aid for treating a patient during an opiate overdose (Box 28.4). **Naloxone** is a medication that quickly reverses the effects of overdose from opioids such as heroin, methadone, fentanyl, and morphine.

BOX 28.4 Signs and Symptoms of an Opioid Overdose

Difficulty walking, talking, or staying awake
Blue lips or nails
Very small pupils
Cold and clammy skin
Dizziness and confusion
Extreme drowsiness
Choking, gurgling, or snoring sounds
Slow, weak, or no breathing
Inability to wake up, even when shaken or shouted at

If you suspect an overdose:
1. Know the signs of an overdose.
2. Stay and help. You can help save a life.
3. Call 9-1-1 (or your local emergency help line).
4. Administer naloxone, if you have it.
5. Know that the *Canadian Good Samaritan Drug Overdose Act* protects you from simple drug possession charges.

Naloxone is powerful and starts to work within 2 to 5 minutes. It removes opium from the opiate receptors and occupies them so that opiates cannot work on the brain. The effect is temporary and lasts only for 20 to 90 minutes. However, it can be enough to reverse the effects of opioid overdoses, restore breathing, and save a person's life until professional help arrives.

All across Canada, naloxone can be found in **naloxone kits** for public use in the event of an overdose. These kits are stored in different locations, depending on provincial or territorial guidelines. The kits can be found in pharmacies, community centres, hospitals, and other public places. There are two types of naloxone kits: The first and the most popular is a nasal spray; the second and less popular one contains naloxone that is injectable in any muscle. Each kit has very simple instructions for use.

For alcohol addiction, medical treatments used include Antabuse (disulfiram), antiepileptic mood stabilizers, baclofen, Campral, and Selincro.

Alcohol (CH_3-CH_2-OH) splits into the final products of water (H_2O), carbonic gas (CO_2), and calories. As an intermediate product, it generates acetaldehyde (CH_3-CHO), which is a very toxic product. One of the hypotheses of how alcoholism develops is that alcoholics may drink more because this process of splitting in their system happens faster than in other people's bodies; other people will feel unwell faster with more alcohol intake and stop drinking. **Disulfiram (Antabuse)** prevents acetaldehyde from splitting further to water and carbonic gas, and it causes poisoning. Thus, if a patient takes Antabuse and also drinks, they will feel sick. The idea is that knowing this, the patient will not drink at all. If a person takes Antabuse and drinks, they will be poisoned and, in cases of extended alcohol consumption, may even die. Antabuse is the oldest medication approved in Canada and the United States for alcoholism treatment.

Antiepileptic mood stabilizers, such as carbamazepine (Tegretol), Depalept, or topiramate, help with prevention, especially in cases of alcoholism. Baclofen, a medication whose primary use is to treat muscle spasticity related to neurological damage, is also used for some forms of alcoholism. Campral (acamprosate calcium), a drug that is popular in the United States, is approved for use in Canada. It helps to improve pleasure centre function and to reduce patients' craving for alcohol.

Selincro (nalmefene) is an opioid receptor antagonist. It is the most promising drug for treating alcoholism available in Europe, the United Kingdom, and Israel since 2013 and is on the list of new drugs available in Canada. It has a very mild effect on the liver. Selincro is prescribed starting with one tablet (18 mg) every day for 1 to 3 months, then every other day, and then only as needed (when the patient may be in a situation where alcohol is available).

Regardless of the type of treatment, the first step is for the individual to *recognize the need for help. Denial* is a strong part of most substance-related disorders. For any treatment to be effective, the patient must be truly willing to work toward living without their addiction.

Before treatment of substance-related addiction can actually begin, many people must first go through **detoxification**, the process of withdrawing from a substance, which may require medical supervision. Patients who are addicted to opium, narcotics, alcohol, or sedatives are often hospitalized because of potentially fatal complications associated with withdrawal, such as seizures and respiratory and cardiac problems.

Relapse

Long-term recovery is often marked by periods of relapse. Relapse is the recurrence of substance-abusing behaviours after a significant period of abstinence. In other words, the patient returns to "using" after being "clean" for a period of time. Many treatment therapies and programs concentrate on preventing and treating relapses. It is important to remember that patients who have relapsed feel many distressing emotions. True therapeutic care is given when these patients are accepted and respected, even when they are the least accepting and respecting of themselves. Remember, as a care provider you are a therapeutic agent.

CASE STUDY

Drago is an unemployed 61-year-old with two children and three grandchildren who was widowed 3 years ago. Drago has been admitted to hospital following severe alcohol poisoning. He took his Antabuse but also drank a bottle of vodka the same day. He has suffered from alcohol addiction the last 10 years, since his full-time position at a factory was terminated. He has attempted to stop drinking completely three times; his longest sober period was 3 months. Drago participates in an Alcoholic Anonymous group one to three times per week and takes his Antabuse on and off.

Drago's new physician changes his medication from Antabuse to naltrexone (Revia) and explains to Drago the principles of harm reduction. Drago has also agreed to pass an alcohol test once a month when he comes to see his doctor.

Six months later, Drago has found a part-time job, but he keeps consuming alcohol on a level of about 150 mg of vodka per week at the end of the week. Drago has reported an improved relationship with his immediate family.

BOX 28.5 Problem Statements (Nursing Diagnoses) Related to Substance Abuse

Physical Realm
Nonadherence
Imbalanced nutrition
Risk of injury
Ineffective, risky sexuality patterns
Risk of trauma
Risk of self-directed or other-directed violence

Psychosocial Realm
Anxiety
Intense cravings
Suicidal thoughts
Impaired communication
Ineffective coping
Ineffective denial
Dysfunctional family processes
Hopelessness
Risk of loneliness
Powerlessness
Social isolation
Spiritual distress

BOX 28.6 Key Interventions for Abuse and Dependence Problems

Meet physical needs during detoxification; this intervention is very important.

Address the physiological problems resulting from substance abuse.

Monitor the effects of the therapies prescribed to control the substance use.

Monitor the adverse effects of medications.

Teach patients about the disease and its progression.

Focus on patients' strengths, and help patients build on them.

Help patients learn to problem-solve the dilemmas they fear.

Encourage focus on the present and the future, not on the past.

Behave toward patients in a consistent manner, confronting them in a nonjudgemental, nonpunitive manner if they break the rules of the treatment setting.

Assist patients' families by encouraging them to become involved in group counselling.

Nursing/Therapeutic Process

An important intervention for patients with substance-related problems is to act as a *therapeutic agent*. Practise effective listening skills to gain an understanding of who the patient really is. Use your knowledge of the therapeutic relationship to establish trust and cooperation. Be willing to look beyond the addiction to see the person.

Nursing diagnoses/problem statements that relate to patients with substance abuse problems are based on the individual's identified problems and goals. Box 28.5 lists several such statements. Although the actual care for each patient is individually planned, certain key therapeutic actions are common to all substance-dependent patients (Box 28.6).

Caring for patients with substance-related problems can be challenging. Nurses and other care providers are in valuable positions to influence their patients' well-being. Demonstrations of respect, acceptance, and concern can offer patients the connection that encourages them to work toward freedom from using their particular substance. Personalized approaches allow for discussions about diet, health, problem-solving, and other health concerns. Drug therapists work with patients to develop long-term strategies for coping with their dependency. Patients are offered opportunities for learning and developing new and more effective skills for living. As a care provider, work to become familiar with the subject of substance abuse. Learn as much as you can because you *will* be caring for patients whose problems are related to the use of chemical substances.

SAMPLE PATIENT CARE PLAN 28.1   Ineffective Coping

Assessment
History Mary is a 34-year-old stay-at-home mother with three children and a husband who works long hours. Two years ago, she complained of feeling jittery and tense to her physician. He prescribed a mild sedative, which Mary took religiously every evening before bed. Lately, she has begun to take her "nerve pill" during the day and uses alcohol to help "stabilize" her.

She is being admitted for evaluation and treatment after her husband found her unconscious on the sofa yesterday.
Current Findings A well-groomed woman with flattened speech. Mary answers questions when asked but volunteers no information. She states that she does not belong here because she is not really addicted to anything and resents "being treated like a druggie."

Multidisciplinary Diagnosis

Ineffective coping related to increasing use of sedatives and alcohol

Planning/Goals

Mary will stop or reduce her use of all mood-altering drugs and alcohol for 6 weeks.
Mary will identify and seek help for at least three problems by May 1.

THERAPEUTIC INTERVENTIONS

Interventions	Rationale	Team Member
1. Confront Mary with her substance-abusing actions and their consequences and assist her with identifying the problem.	Denial is common with persons who have a substance-related problem; identifying problems is the first step toward change.	Psy, Nsg
2. Encourage Mary to agree to participate in the treatment program.	Therapeutic interventions are not effective unless the patient wants to cooperate.	All
3. Work with Mary to develop a written contract for behavioural changes.	A personal commitment enhances the likelihood of success.	Psy, Nsg
4. Assist Mary in identifying and adopting more effective coping behaviours.	Encourages problem-solving and the use of more effective behaviours.	Nsg, Psy
5. Assess the social support systems available for Mary.	Supportive significant others are often unavailable for substance abusers.	Nsg, Soc Svc
6. Educate Mary and her family about substance abuse and resources for help.	Knowledge helps Mary and her family cope more successfully with problems.	Nsg, Soc Svc
7. Refer Mary to a treatment centre and provide support until Mary is involved in the program.	Specialized drug treatment programs are likely to be more effective if patients are willing to participate.	Soc Svc

Evaluation During her entire stay, Mary reduced her drug use but expressed many discomforts. Mary was able to identify her drug-using behaviours during her stay but refused to participate in an outpatient treatment program.

Critical Thinking Questions
1. How would the staff confront Mary without making her defensive?
2. What can be done to improve Mary's willingness to participate in treatment?

A complete patient care plan includes several other diagnoses and interventions.
Nsg, nursing staff; *Psy,* psychologist; *Soc Svc,* social services.

KEY POINTS

- Substance use is the ingestion of any chemical that affects the body.
- Addiction is a group of chronic genetic diseases, like most other diseases.
- Abused substances alter the individual's perception by affecting the central nervous system. They are often called *mind-altering drugs* because of their ability to enhance or depress mood and emotions.
- Every mind-altering chemical ingested by a pregnant woman poses a potential danger to her unborn child.
- Children who live with substance-abusing parents are at high risk for injuries and for developing drug problems themselves.
- Adolescent substance use, abuse, and dependence are becoming an ever-increasing problem.
- In adults, substance abuse is common. Substance abuse occurs most commonly between 18 and 35 years of age.
- A significant number of older persons use alcohol and prescription medications.
- Children of problem drinkers have three times the risk for serious injury. Cocaine-exposed and other drug-exposed infants are filling foster care and are often admitted for health care.
- Alcohol-related motor vehicle accidents are one of the leading causes of death among people under 45 years of age. Deaths from falls, drowning, and burns may all be related to substance use.
- Many homeless and mentally ill people use and abuse chemical substances.
- Abused substances include alcohol, diet pills, coffee, tea, cannabis, cocaine, hallucinogens, inhalants, nicotine, opioids, phencyclidine (PCP), and prescription drugs such as sedatives, hypnotics, and antianxiety drugs.
- Many medications have the potential for being abused.
- The use of inhalants has become popular with adolescents and young adults because they are legal, inexpensive, and easily available and have a rapid onset. Significant complications include cardiac dysrhythmia and respiratory depression.
- The movement from use to dependency (addiction) follows a predictable course. In the early stage, use progresses to excessive use. During the middle stage, intoxication progresses to tolerance. In the chronic (late) stage, tolerance progresses to loss of control, dependence, and addiction.
- For a substance-related disorder to be diagnosed, the pattern of substance use must be disabling and lead to significant impaired functioning and distress, and the individual must demonstrate the signs of tolerance, withdrawal, and dependence.
- The assessment of patients with substance-related problems should include a thorough history and physical examination.
- Detoxification is the process of withdrawing a substance under medical supervision. Relapse is the recurrence of the substance-abusing behaviours after a significant period of abstinence.
- The most important intervention for patients with substance-related difficulties is to act as a therapeutic agent. Other interventions are designed to meet physical needs, especially during detoxification; monitor effects of therapies; teach about the disease and its progression; help patients problem-solve; and encourage the patient's family and significant others to become involved.

ADDITIONAL LEARNING RESOURCES

Go to your Evolve website (http://evolve.elsevier.com/Canada/Morrison-Valfre/) for additional online resources, including the online Study Guide for additional learning activities to help you master this chapter content.

CRITICAL THINKING QUESTIONS

1. What are some differences and commonalities between the harm-reduction approach and abstinence?

2. What are the objective symptoms of alcohol withdrawal?

REFERENCES

American Psychiatric Association (APA). (2013). *Diagnostic and statistical manual of mental disorders* (5th ed.). American Psychiatric Publishing.

Belzak, L., & Halverson, J. (2018). Evidence synthesis—the opioid crisis in Canada: A national perspective. *Health Promotion & Chronic Disease Prevention Canada, 38*(6), 224–233. https://doi.org/10.24095/hpcdp.38.6.02

Gerona, R. R., & Wu, A. H. B. (2012). Bath salts. *Clinics in Laboratory Medicine, 32*(3), 415–427.

Ghosh, A., Coakley, R. D., Ghio, A. J., et al. (2019). Chronic e-cigarette use increases neutrophil elastase and matrix metalloprotease levels in the lung. *American Journal of Respiratory and Critical Care Medicine, 200*(11), 1392–1401. https://doi.org/10.1164/rccm.201903-0615OC

Government of Canada. (2017). *Fetal alcohol spectrum disorder.* https://www.canada.ca/en/health-canada/services/healthy-living/your-health/diseases/fetal-alcohol-spectrum-disorder.html

Government of Canada. (2018a). *The cannabis act: The facts.* https://www.canada.ca/en/health-canada/news/2018/06/backgrounder-the-cannabis-act-the-facts.html

Government of Canada. (2018b). *Harm reduction: Canadian drugs and substances strategy.* https://www.canada.ca/en/health-canada/services/substance-use/canadian-drugs-substances-strategy/harm-reduction.html

Helmenstine, A. M. (2019). *Rohypnol (a.k.a. roofies) fast facts.* http://chemistry.about.com/od/drugs/a/rohypnolfacts.htm

Hess, D., & DeBoer, S. (2002). Emergency: Ecstasy. *American Journal of Nursing, 102*(4), 45–47.

Lange, S., Quere, M., Shield, K., et al. (2016). Alcohol use and self–perceived mental health status among pregnant and breastfeeding women in Canada: A secondary data analysis. *BJOG: An International Journal of Obstetrics and Gynaecology, 123*(6), 900–909. https://doi.org/10.1111/1471-0528.13525

Leatherdale, S. T., & Burkhalter, R. (2012). The substance use profile of Canadian youth: Exploring the prevalence of alcohol, drug and tobacco use by gender and grade. *Addictive Behaviors, 37*(3), 318–322. https://doi.org/10.1016/j.addbeh.2011.10.007

Ling, W., Hillhouse, M. P., Saxon, A. J., et al. (2016). Buprenorphine + naloxone plus naltrexone for the treatment of cocaine dependence: The Cocaine Use Reduction with Buprenorphine (CURB) study. *Addiction, 111*(8), 1416–1427. https://doi.org/10.1111/add.13375

McLellan, A. T. (2017). Substance misuse and substance use disorders: Why do they matter in healthcare? *Transactions of the American Clinical & Climatological Association, 128*, 112–130. https://www.ncbi.nlm.nih.gov/pmc/articles/PMC5525418/

National Institute on Alcohol Abuse and Alcoholism. (2020). *Drinking levels defined.* https://www.niaaa.nih.gov/alcohol-health/overview-alcohol-consumption/moderate-binge-drinking

Zawilska, J. B., & Wojcieszak, J. (2014). Spice/K2 drugs—more than innocent substitutes for marijuana. *International Journal of Neuropsychopharmacology, 17*(3), 509–525. https://doi.org/10.1017/S1461145713001247

29

Sexuality and Sexual Disorders

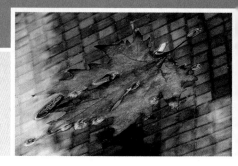

OBJECTIVES

Upon completion of this chapter, the student will be able to:
1. Describe the continuum (range) of sexual responses.
2. Explain how self-awareness affects the care of patients with psychosexual problems.
3. Illustrate how sexuality is expressed through each life stage.
4. Describe sexual orientation.
5. Examine the concept of gender identity.
6. Compare the difference between a sexual dysfunction and a sexual disorder.
7. Define paraphilia, and list three examples of paraphilic behaviours.
8. Apply the nursing process to the care of a patient with a psychosexual issue.
9. Explain the importance of human immune deficiency virus/acquired immunodeficiency syndrome (HIV/AIDS) and sexually transmitted infection (STI) counselling for every patient with a psychosexual issue.

OUTLINE

KEY TERMS

According to Maslow's hierarchy of needs, sex is a basic physiological need. Humans, like most other creatures, have strong sexual drives; but unlike other creatures, human sexual expression is defined by the social customs, norms, and laws of society. A number of terms are used when discussing sex, with several listed in Box 29.1.

People express their sexuality through a variety of thoughts, attitudes, and behaviours. Sexuality is important in every dimension of functioning. The physical dimension of sexuality includes anatomy and physiology—the characteristics that physically define our sex. Sexuality in the emotional and intellectual dimensions encompasses our thoughts,

BOX 29.1 Terms Relating to Sexuality

Human **sexuality** is the combination of physical, chemical, psychological, and functional characteristics that are expressed by one's gender identity and sexual behaviours.
Sexuality comprises the following:

Gender expression: The behavioural portrayal of gender actions and roles

Gender identity: An individual's perception of having a particular gender, which may or may not correspond with their birth sex

Gender role: Cultural and social obligations relating to one's gender

Intersex: Persons who do not meet the medical definition of male or female at birth

Sex: Anatomy and biology that identify one as male, female, or intersex

Sexual orientation: Gender to which one is romantically attracted

Transgender: Individuals whose gender identity and expression are different from their assigned birth gender

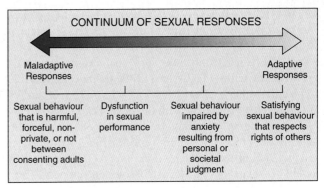

Fig. 29.1 Continuum of sexual responses.

beliefs, and values about sexuality. Socially, interactions with others may range from the intimacy of sexual intercourse, to discussions of sexual attitudes with trusted friends, to passing feelings generated by attractive strangers. Sexuality and its expressions are social in nature.

Cultures have an influence on sexuality. All societies have laws, rules, or customs that regulate sexual behaviour. For example, in North American culture, it is understood that persons involved in sexual activity should be at an age when they can consent to the sexual activity, have a basic understanding of what it means to give consent to sexual activity, and understand the various outcomes that occur from sexual activity (e.g., pregnancy, sexually transmitted infection [STI], shame if sex is nonconsensual). Attitudes, beliefs, and rituals help define what is appropriate sexually. Religious institutions have a strong impact on views of what is right or wrong sexual behaviour. In some cultures, the sexual act is considered a religious ritual, with taboos and regulations governing the experience. Evidence of the practice of *religious prostitution* (the selling of sexual services in exchange for spiritual gain) dates as far back as 5 000 years ago. Cultural attitudes, beliefs, and behaviours toward sexuality and its expressions have changed throughout the years, and they will continue to change in the future.

CULTURAL CONSIDERATIONS

Margaret Mead, in her book *Growing Up in Samoa*, describes children who grow up with few sexual restraints. Although sexual play and experimentation are accepted methods of expression, the pregnancy rate of the islanders is no greater than that among other populations.

In Malaysia, children being born outside of marriage is a common phenomenon. It is the custom for the father to provide for the child's welfare.

THE CONTINUUM OF SEXUAL RESPONSES

Even experts have difficulty agreeing on what is normal sexual behaviour. For years, the norm was defined as a married man and woman who engaged in sexual relations to procreate (have children). Today, a wider range of sexual behaviours is considered to be socially acceptable.

Sexual behaviours can be viewed as occurring along a continuum (Fig. 29.1). At the adaptive end of the spectrum lie satisfying sexual behaviours that respect the rights and wishes of others. As the continuum moves toward maladaptive, sexual behaviours become impaired or dysfunctional. The opposite end of the continuum is marked by sexual actions that are harmful to self or others in some manner.

Perhaps a useful definition of adaptive or healthy sexual responses is sexuality that is:

1. Performed with self, or between two or more consenting adults
2. Satisfying to all
3. Not forced or coerced
4. Conducted in private

Maladaptive or unhealthy sexual responses are those behaviours that do not meet these criteria. They are, in some way or degree, physically or psychologically harmful to the individual or others. Labelling sexual behaviours as healthy or unhealthy must be done with caution because it is easy to pass judgement on those who are perceived to behave differently.

CRITICAL THINKING

- What is the definition of "normal" sexuality?
- How do views compare among a relative, friend, and classmate?
- What is the popular opinion of those who practise what are thought to be different means of sexual expression?
- How do you think your personal beliefs and opinions about sexuality affect your interactions with patients?

Self-Awareness and Sexuality

Nurses and other health care providers, in working with patients, work with the human condition. All care providers must strive to develop an awareness of their own thoughts, attitudes, values, and beliefs regarding sexuality and its modes of expression. *One's self-awareness has a strong influence on discussing sexual issues with patients.* Values that may be unconscious to the care provider are often transmitted loudly and clearly to patients. Nonverbal messages of disapproval decrease the effectiveness of the therapeutic relationship and all other interventions. Individuals who feel judged are not likely to cooperate with the plan of care.

Developing an awareness of your views about sexuality involves the process of defining and clarifying attitudes and values. Each of us carries a sexual point of view, a way of looking at sexuality that was established unconsciously during childhood and adolescence as a part of growing up and interacting with others.

Refer to Chapter 3 for the values clarification process. Apply each of the steps outlined there to the topic of sexuality. Then think about how your values may affect the care of patients with sexual disorders. Know that values are not static; they change as one learns and develops. Remember that when it comes to working with sexually disordered patients, your effectiveness is directly related to personal self-awareness and comfort with different manifestations of a wide range of sexuality. No patient should have to endure the ignorance of their health care provider.

SEXUALITY THROUGHOUT THE LIFE CYCLE

The expression of one's sexuality begins at birth and ends at death. Gender differences define roles in society, attitudes about the dynamics of living, relationships with others, and views of who we are. Gender roles develop as new knowledge, attitudes, and behaviours are added to life experiences. A basic knowledge of sexuality throughout the life cycle is thus important for health care providers.

Sexuality in Childhood

From the moment of birth, children are treated differently on the basis of their biological sex (Hockenberry & Wilson, 2014). Female infants are often dressed in pink, males in blue. Each is assigned a name, which usually indicates a gender. For example, girls are seldom named Bruce or Joseph, and few boys are addressed as Semareh or Sally. Families treat boys differently from girls, even in infancy. Female infants are sometimes considered delicate. They may be handled and spoken to more tenderly, whereas male infants may be stimulated by boisterous voices and play involving motor activity.

Young children are unaware that gender is a permanent attribute. Around the age of 2 years, children learn to label themselves according to their gender. Most respond to being called "good girls" or "brave boys" by the adults in their environment. They soon internalize the label of male or female, boy or girl.

By age 3, most children can accurately label the gender of other persons, but they still believe that their gender can be changed with time if they want. By about age 7, children understand that one's gender is permanent and will not naturally change. Between ages 7 and 9, they learn that one's gender is identified by genital appearance.

Children learn about gender roles in relation to themselves first. Then they apply their learning to members of the same gender. Finally, their knowledge is applied to persons of the opposite gender. Children can identify the simpler aspects of gender roles by age 3. They know, for example, that boys and girls differ in appearance, toy preference, and choice of activities.

By school age, most children identify with the parent of the same gender. However, research has shown that children in same-gender or lone-parent families exhibit no differences in growth and development outcomes, in comparison to those in other or expected household parental relationships (Adams & Light, 2015; Cornell University, 2020). In elementary school, children learn about the expected behaviours associated with each gender role. In the past, this identification involved much stereotyping. Girls could not play certain sports, for example, and boys were discouraged from taking home economics or engaging in other "sissy" activities. Fortunately, this attitude is changing as individual qualities become more important than playing appropriate gender roles.

By the middle elementary school years, children are aware of most aspects of their gender-role stereotypes. Future goals, occupational choices, personality traits, and sexual behaviours are influenced by gender roles that were established early in childhood.

Sexuality in Adolescence

During the early teen years, close relationships with same-gender peers intensify. Through these relationships, children learn about the possibility of intimacy between equals and are exposed to peer standards for appropriate sex-role behaviour (Hockenberry & Wilson, 2014). As time passes, adolescents begin to encounter expectations for mature gender-role behaviour from both peers and adults.

Although 12-year-olds are intensely involved with same-gender friends, opportunities for mixed-group activities and dating increase. Dating activities usually begin in grade 7 or 8 with group social activities, such as dances, picnics, or organized school functions. Group dating moves to double dating, and by the grade 12, most adolescents have been on single-pair dates. Because adolescence is an emotionally stressful time for most individuals, steady dating can offer some relief from insecurity and loneliness and provide a sense of belonging.

Sexual activity among younger adolescents in Canada has become slightly less prevalent in recent years. For teens under 15 years of age, that rate fell from 9.6% in 2003 to 9.0% in 2010. In 2003, among teens aged 15 to 17, 30% reported having had at least one experience of intercourse; for those aged 18 to 19 years, it was 68%, and those aged 20 to 24, 85%. In 2010, the rates were 30%, 68%, and 86%, respectively. During that time, there was a slight increase in condom use, from 62% for sexually active 15- to 24-year-olds in 2003, to 68% in 2010 (Rotermann, 2012). Most teens begin experimenting with sexual activity through kissing and petting. Many teens have experienced multiple sexual relationships by the time they are 19 years old. Unfortunately, some adolescent girls use ineffective or no contraception at all, and some adolescent boys do not use condoms. These practices may lead to STIs, unplanned pregnancy, or both.

Adolescence is a time of intense searching and learning. Much information related to sexuality is gained from peers and other inexperienced or unknowledgeable persons. Nurses should always be alert for the opportunity to assess and correct, if necessary, adolescents' misconceptions about sexuality and its expressions.

Sexuality in Adulthood

Among adults ages 25 to 59, relative *monogamy* (the practice of having only one partner) appears to be most common. The Canadian *Criminal Code* bans polygamy (having more than one marriage partner at a time).

The sexuality patterns of middle-aged adults have changed over the years. More women in their 30s and 40s are bearing children and beginning families. Lone parenthood is also more common today. In 2014, lone-parent families accounted for 20% of families with children under age 16, up from 9% in 1976 (Statistics Canada, 2015).

Sexuality in Older Adulthood

The typical picture of the older person as an asexual and uninterested individual is a myth; nothing could be further from the truth. Older adulthood, for many people, is a time of pursuing one's own interests and desires, including sexuality.

In the past, erectile difficulties and vaginal dryness were obstacles to engaging in sexual intercourse for some people over 50 years of age. Today, thanks to various medications, hormone creams, and vaginal lubrications, these are no longer obstacles to enjoying sexuality in later life.

Sexuality is evident through all the developmental stages throughout life, and although sexual activity may fluctuate in frequency, established sexual patterns can continue. At times, the sexual expression of older persons can be met with cultural and social barriers, attitudes, and expectations. Poor health, medications, disabilities, and the normal aging process all influence one's sexual behaviours and abilities.

Sexuality and Disability

Many persons living with permanent disability are able to enjoy satisfying sexual lives, with some adaptations. In addition, many persons with a disability have no problem with engaging in sexual activities. People who have spinal cord injuries, for example, can still be lovers, partners, and parents. Any condition that affects well-being, mobility, or self-esteem

affects sexuality and its expressions. Health problems such as diabetes, arthritis, cancer, and cardiovascular disease can cause erectile dysfunction (ED).

Men and women who live with disability learn to adapt to their conditions. Most must also cope with negative attitudes and stigma toward disabled people. People with disabilities have the exact same needs as the rest of the population. As a care provider, remember that everyone is an individual first; some of us just happen to have different manifestations of sexuality. Improving the quality of life for people with disabilities involves changing the social attitudes that limit the disabled population.

SEXUAL ORIENTATION

An enduring pattern of emotional, romantic, and sexual attraction to a man, a woman, or both, or the lack of any sexual attraction is one's *sexual orientation*, or sexual preference. In 1948 one of the first researchers into human sexual responses (A.C. Kinsey) developed a scale of human sexual preference, ranging from exclusively heterosexual to exclusively homosexual (Fig. 29.2). He stated that most people were not exclusively one or the other because many had experienced both heterosexual and homosexual expressions of sexuality (Kinsey, Pomeroy, & Martin, 1953).

Sexual orientation is not a person's choice, nor does it result from a person's social environment. For example, with identical twin brothers, one brother may have a heterosexual orientation and the other a homosexual orientation. Thus, sexual orientation is also not a result of genetics. Today we have strong data to suggest that sexual orientation is a result of prenatal epigenetics. In other words, it is the result of changes in gene expressions between fertilization and birth. Fraternal birth order (FBO)—the probability that a boy growing up to be gay increases for each older brother born to the same mother—is a well-documented phenomenon: 15 to 29% of gay men owe their sexual orientation to this effect (Balthazart, 2018).

Currently, there are several recognized modes of sexual orientation (Table 29.1).

In historical terms, same-gender relationships have been around as long as opposite-gender relationships. Cultural and social attitudes toward same-gender relationships have changed as history has evolved.

Most children or teens recognize their sexual orientation with little doubt from a very young age. The process of establishing an integrated or complete identity as a gay man or lesbian is known as *coming out*. Adult support and explanations

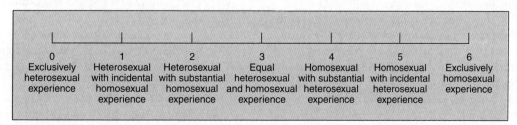

Fig. 29.2 Kinsey's rating scale of sexual preference. (Redrawn from Kinsey, A. C., Pomeroy, W. B., & Martin, E. C. [1953]. *Sexual behavior in the human female.* Saunders.)

TABLE 29.1   Modes of Sexual Orientation

Term	Definition
Heterosexual	People who are attracted to a different gender
Homosexual	People who are attracted to people of the same gender; often referred to as **gay** (applies to both genders) or **lesbian** (applies to female homosexuals)
Bisexual	People who are attracted to both men and women
Pansexual or Queer	People whose attractions span across many different gender identities (male, female, transgender, genderqueer, intersex)
Questioning or Curious	What people who are unsure about their sexual orientation may call themselves
Asexual	People who don't experience any sexual attraction for anyone

CASE STUDY

It is evening in a busy medical-surgical unit. You have just received notice that a 42-year-old man, Jim, is being admitted for injuries suffered in a motor vehicle accident. Because of the severity of his injuries, the physician has ordered that he be visited by immediate family only.

Jim is admitted to the unit and made comfortable. As you glance around for family members who accompanied him from the emergency department, you see only one young-ish-looking man peering anxiously at your patient. "I'm sorry, but immediate family only is allowed in here," you say politely, as you usher him out the door.

Later that evening, Jim begins to respond. He keeps calling out for "my love, J.J." and asking you where J.J. is, so loudly that you are sure everyone on the floor can hear. Finally, Jim quiets down, only after he extracts a promise from you to find J.J. Exhausted, you agree, hoping she would somehow arrive and help to keep this man quiet.

As you open the door to leave the room, the young-ish-looking man from earlier in the evening stands there, almost falling to the floor. With tears in his eyes, he glares intently at you but says nothing. Quietly you ask if his name could possibly be J.J.
• What is the lesson to be learned from this case study?
• How could this experience help you to be more sensitive and therapeutic?

regarding the whole range of human sexuality are extremely important during this time.

Historically, homosexuality was considered a maladaptive mode of sexual expression by many societies. However, studies have revealed that gay men and lesbians commonly function as well in their love relationships as heterosexual persons do. Studies of gay and lesbian couples have found that many couples have long-term relationships with their partners. Many now are legally married.

It appears that both homosexual and heterosexual behaviour styles have much in common. While gay and lesbian

sexuality and bisexuality are now receiving acceptance as modes of sexual expression, many health care providers still carry attitudes and stereotypes that can interfere with the health care provided to gay, lesbian, and bisexual patients. We must all work to develop the self-awareness that enhances our therapeutic effectiveness, especially with persons who have a sexual orientation different from our own.

GENDER IDENTITY

In most societies, official gender identity is based on a person's genitalia: male and female (called the *binary system*). However, in reality, gender is not determined by a person's anatomy. Gender identity is what the person knows they are with regard to their gender. *As with sexual orientation, gender identity is not a person's choice.* There are more than two gender identities (some of the more common genders are male, female, transgender, gender neutral, nonbinary, agender, pangender, genderqueer, two-spirit, third gender, or a combination of these), and different people prefer different terms to refer to themselves. Gender identity is one of the main pillars of who a person is. For any clinician to establish a therapeutic relationship, it is important to get this right. Thus, it is very important *never to assume and always ask the person about their own definition of their gender identity.*

By age 3, most children can identify their gender. It is important for parents to note any discrepancies with a child's assigned-at-birth gender. Children who identify as different from the gender they were assigned at birth may need help and support. Hormone therapy can help prevent the development of unwelcome secondary sex characteristics (certain kinds of fat tissue and muscle growth, hair and voice development, etc.) and ensure development of the true gender secondary characteristics. In cases where more time is required to determine gender identity, hormone therapy can also be used to delay puberty.

Gender Identity Terminology

Gender identity can be described in many ways (as noted above). Some of the more common gender identities a person may encounter include the following:
• **Transgender:** According to the American Psychological Association (2015), "transgender is an umbrella term for persons whose gender identity, gender expression or behaviour does not conform to that typically associated with the sex to which they were assigned at birth." Many of these individuals feel they were born into the wrong sex, and they will go to much time, expense, and discomfort to alter their bodies to more closely match their gender identity. This is most often accomplished with hormone therapy and sexual reassignment surgeries. In Canada, these therapies and surgeries are covered by public health insurance, but different provinces and territories have different approval processes. Wichinski (2015) notes, "Transgender individuals experience a high prevalence of HIV, sexually transmitted infections, victimization, violence, mental health issues, and suicide."

- **Two-spirit:** This term, which originates from Indigenous people in Canada, is commonly used to identify a person who carries the gifts of both males and females, or one who is not specific to any gender.
- **Cisgender:** This term is used to describe someone whose gender matches what they were assigned at birth, based on their visual anatomy.
- **Nonbinary:** A very broad term for identities that fall outside of male/female.
- **Genderqueer:** People who call themselves genderqueer are expressing their identity as being something different from just man or woman; it also can have some elements of both genders.
- **Gender expression:** This is how individuals express themselves to the world (e.g., with clothes, make-up, hair style, shoes, paraverbal communication). Gender expression and gender identity do not always correlate. Thus it is important that care providers not assume what gender identity the person has, but to always ask.
- **Gender fluid:** Some people's gender identity may be fluid or fluctuate from one identity to another or it has become mixed. At times, these changes can be rapid, random, or as a response to the person's environment.
- **Gender neutral:** People who identify as being neither male nor female.

PARAPHILIC DISORDERS

The **paraphilias** are a group of sexual variations that depart from society's traditional and acceptable modes of seeking sexual gratification. When the word *paraphilia* is taken apart, the suffix *philia* means "an attraction to." When used to describe a specific behaviour, the descriptive term replaces the prefix *para*. For example, **pedophilia** refers to a person who is sexually attracted to children (*pedo,* meaning "child").

Paraphilia only becomes a mental health disorder when long-standing, significant distress or impairment is present. People with a paraphilia experience recurrent (over 6 months, at least), intense urges to act on fantasies to achieve sexual arousal. These urges may cause significant distress to these people and make them become a serious physical or psychological threat to others. It is important to note that the majority of people diagnosed with paraphilic disorders are not criminal, as they do not harm other people. The majority do not act on these urges but do suffer from the distress. It is only when a person acts on these urges with a nonconsenting adult or with a child that the person becomes a criminal.

Although few reliable statistics on paraphilias are available, given the inflammatory stigma associated with these disorders, paraphilic disorders may be more common than once thought. A few of the more prevalent paraphilic disorders are as follows:

- Voyeuristic disorder: A person experiencing sexual arousal from observing an unsuspecting person's naked body parts.
- Exhibitionistic disorder: A person experiencing sexual arousal from exposing their own genitals to other unsuspecting persons.

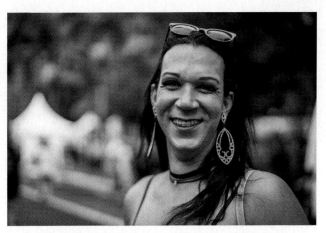

Fig. 29.3 Male transvestite. (iStockphoto/FG Trade.)

- Frotteuristic disorder: A person experiencing sexual arousal from touching or rubbing against a nonconsenting person.
- Sexual masochism disorder: A person experiencing sexual arousal from being humiliated, beaten, bound, or otherwise made to suffer.
- Sexual sadism disorder: A person experiencing sexual arousal from witnessing the physical or psychological suffering of another person.
- Pedophilic disorder: A person experiencing sexual arousal from sexual activities with a prepubescent child (generally aged 13 years or younger).
- Fetishistic disorder: A person experiencing sexual arousal from either the use of nonliving objects or a highly specific focus on nongenital body parts.
- Transvestic disorder: A person experiencing sexual arousal from cross-dressing (Fig. 29.3).

Other Specified Paraphilic Disorders

People who suffer from other specified paraphilic disorders also experience significant distress or impairment but do not meet full criteria for the paraphilic disorders diagnostic class described in the fifth edition of the *Diagnostic and Statistical Manual of Mental Disorders (DSM-5)*. The label "other specific paraphilic disorders" is used when a clinician chooses to communicate a specific reason why the patient's presentation does not meet the criteria for any specific paraphilic disorder. Following are a few presentations of other specific paraphilic disorders:

- Telephone scatologia: Sexual arousal from making obscene phone calls
- Necrophilia: Sexual arousal from a corpse
- Zoophilia: Sexual arousal from having sex with animals
- Coprophilia: Sexual arousal from feces
- Klismaphilia: Sexual arousal from enemas
- Urophilia: Sexual arousal from urine

Unspecified Paraphilic Disorder

People who suffer from unspecific paraphilic disorder also experience significant distress or impairment. However, this label is used when their presentation also does not meet the *DSM-5* criteria for any specific paraphilic disorder, and a clinician chooses not to communicate the reason why the criteria are not met for a specific paraphilic disorder.

Therapeutic Approach

People who have one of the above paraphilic disorders suffer from significant distress and impairment in social, occupational, and many other crucial aspects of life. Given the associated shame and stigma, they tend to avoid seeking help. Without help, their condition may trigger depression, misery, and suicide. It is very important to remember that urges, thoughts, and fantasies are not criminal. If signs of paraphilic disorders are noted, a therapist's responsibility is to explain to the person the lack of criminality in thoughts and fantasies, and the necessity to properly diagnose the disorder.

Different forms of psychotherapy have been developed to specifically target paraphilic disorders, and their effectiveness is growing. A class of medications that has shown good results is antiandrogens, which drastically lower testosterone levels. With professional support and understanding, patients can reduce the intensity of their urges or execute their practice privately. They should also be monitored for their capacity to control their urges to involve nonconsenting individuals. As a care provider it is important to remember that the vast majority of people who suffer from these disorders are law-abiding members of society. A professional and nonjudgemental approach is key to encouraging self-disclosure and requests for help.

If a patient's paraphilic behaviours are out of control and can be harmful to others, inpatient treatment may be required. Individuals who violate the Canadian *Criminal Code* can be incarcerated and may undergo forensic psychiatric assessment and treatment. Penile plethysmography (discussed below) can be part of such an assessment. Upon release from the corrections system, sex offenders who have been convicted of designated sexual offences and ordered by the courts to report annually to police will be registered in the National Sex Offenders Registry. This database is accessible to Canadian police, but not to the public.

Penile Plethysmograph or Phallometry

A man's sexual arousal is physically represented by an erection. That reaction can be measured by calculation of the airflow around the penis when placed in a cylinder. The **penile plethysmograph (PPG)** is a mechanism used to measure the air flow in the cylinder. A phallometric clinic equipped with a PPG machine can aid in determination of sexual orientation and diagnoses of paraphilic disorder. As a stimulus, clinic staff use a set of approved standard images. Some people come to these clinics voluntarily, and some are directed there by court order, after having committed different types of sexual offences.

Even though the majority of such clinics' customers are men, there are some women who require a similar mechanical and objective assessment of their sexual arousal. A vaginal photoplethysmograph is an instrument that can be used to calculate blood flow to the walls of the vagina.

SEXUAL DYSFUNCTIONS

Sexual disorders are those problems that cause long-term distress and impaired functioning in an individual or others who are exposed to the sexual behaviour. These disorders include problems with sexual function, gender dysphoria, and socially inappropriate or illegal methods of sexual expression.

The average person experiences four stages of sexual excitement and pleasure: appetite, excitement, orgasm, and resolution. A **sexual dysfunction** is a disturbance anywhere during these four stages of the sexual response cycle. Its definition also includes any discomfort or pain associated with sexual intercourse. In short, a sexual dysfunction disrupts one's sexual response or experience. Sexual dysfunctions may be lifelong or acquired after a period of normal functioning. They may be limited by certain situations, partners, or types of stimulation, or they may be generalized to every sexual experience. The causes are often related to psychological distress, medication or illicit drug use, and many physical conditions. Arthritis, diabetes, and chronic illness can result in various sexual dysfunctions or alterations in sexual desire. Impaired hormonal functioning and neurological conditions can also lead to difficulties with sexual functioning. Problems in relationships or unrealistic attitudes about sex may also contribute to sexual dysfunction. Table 29.2 describes the most common sexual dysfunctions that occur in men and women.

Very often, a precise etiology of the sexual problem is unknown. It is important to first rule out issues related to a nonsexual mental disorder, a substance's effect, or a medical condition, or whether the dysfunction is resulting from severe relationship distress, partner violence, or other stressors. For diagnosis of all sexual dysfunctions, the dysfunction must be present for more than 6 months and must cause severe distress to the person. Many sexual dysfunctions are treatable, so patients are referred to their physician.

GENDER DYSPHORIA

One of the first things an individual develops is a gender identity, the knowledge that a person has about their gender (which may not correspond with their birth sex). When there is an inconsistency between the child's biological or assigned gender and their gender identity, child **gender dysphoria** can develop.

Children with gender dysphoria are unhappy with their own gender. A persistent desire to become a member of the opposite gender is experienced over time. There is a strong preference for the dress, activities, and roles of the desired gender. Boys will reject rough-and-tumble play and prefer the dress, games, and playmates of girls. Typically, feminine games, toys, and activities are disregarded in favour of more masculine roles in girls with gender dysphoria.

Children of both genders with gender dysphoria have an intense dislike for their sexual anatomy. They want to eliminate their sexual characteristics and trade them for those of the opposite gender. Many truly believe they were born into

TABLE 29.2 Classification of Sexual Dysfunctions

Disorder	Description
Female sexual interest/arousal disorder	Absence of sexual fantasies and desire for sexual activity; inability to attain or maintain sexual excitement during sexual activity; has little sexual arousal
Male hypoactive sexual desire disorder	Absence of sexual fantasies/thoughts and desire for sexual activity
Erectile disorder	Unable to attain or maintain adequate erection during sexual activity
Female orgasmic disorder	Delay in or absence of orgasm following normal excitement
Premature (early) ejaculation	Ejaculation that occurs with minimal stimulation before person wishes it to occur (e.g., within approximately 1 minute of vaginal penetration)
Delayed ejaculation	Marked delay, infrequency, or absence of ejaculation
Genito-pelvic pain/penetration disorder	Pain or anxiety associated with sexual intercourse; may occur in both females and males; may be associated with tightening of pelvic floor muscles
Substance/Medication-induced sexual dysfunction	Significant sexual problems caused by physical effects of medication or substance

the wrong body and reject expectations and behaviours associated with their biological gender. Older children often fail to develop same-gender relationships in school, which can lead to isolation and loneliness.

Adolescents and adults may experience adolescent gender dysphoria and adult gender dysphoria, each of which comes with a strong desire to get rid of one's primary and/or secondary sex characteristics because they are incongruent with one's experienced gender. Mental health challenges are often seen in both adults and children. A gender dysphoria disorder may be diagnosed when the discomforts interfere with activities of daily living.

A number of people with gender dysphoria transition into the desired gender through sexual reassignment therapy. This is accomplished over a long period of psychological counselling, hormonal treatments, and major surgeries. Because decisions made by the individual are irreversible, the process of changing one's sexual identity can take as long as 2 years.

PORNOGRAPHY

Pornography is legal in Canada. However, patients viewing legal pornography may need help with organizing a private environment in which to view it. The exceptions to legal pornography are images showing nonconsenting sexual violence and child pornography.

With regard to child pornography, there is a serious difference between Canadian and other countries' law. Child exploitation to create pornography is prohibited in all countries. But in Japan, for example, anime depicting adolescent girls in sexual acts is legal and also very popular. In contrast, the Canadian *Criminal Code*, Section 163.1, considers *any* visual sexual presentation of a child (including electronic and mechanic) to be child pornography (Government of Canada, 2019). The same law prohibits the production, sale, and possession of sexual toys in the shape of underage people. This is the only instance where paper-based, mechanical, or electronic fantasies and imagination are criminal in Canada. Thus, in Canada, the only legal depiction of naked underage persons is an official picture illustrating the phallometric test, described above.

THERAPEUTIC INTERVENTIONS

Treatment for sexual disorders depends on the cause, the distressing signs and symptoms, and the type of disorder. Group or individual therapy may help patients explore their emotions, behaviours, and coping mechanisms. Cognitive-behavioural therapy (CBT) and recovery groups have been shown to be beneficial. Behavioural therapies, such as positive reinforcement or aversive therapy, focus on changing or managing sexual behaviours in a more acceptable way. Hormonal drug therapy is sometimes used to reduce sexual drives (see Medication Alert box).

! MEDICATION ALERT

Hormones that reduce a person's sexual drive have many adverse effects. As a care provider, it is important to be familiar with each medication and remember to monitor patients routinely for any unusual symptoms.

Many medications prescribed for various medical conditions can cause sexual dysfunction. Examples include the following:

- Antihypertensives
- Antidepressants, anticonvulsants, and other psychotropic medications
- Medications used for conditions of the stomach and small intestine, pain-relieving medications

A complete and accurate history should include an assessment of each patient's medication (including over-the-counter and street drugs) history and current use.

It is important to recognize that thoughts and fantasies are not criminal. Most patients with sexual disorders are not a threat to the public and are treated on an outpatient basis. However, actions that involve nonconsenting adults and underage consenting teens and children *are* criminal.

As a health care provider, if you are uncomfortable with any aspect of a patient's sexuality, your professional judgement and behaviours could be affected. Some psychosexual problems are complex and require the skills of specially educated nurses or sexual therapists. Discuss the situation with your supervisor, because the goal is still to provide the patient with the best possible care. As with other patients, therapeutic interventions remain the same: to accept, assess, intervene, and educate.

Psychosexual Assessment

A thorough understanding of the sexual attitudes and behaviours of patients requires a focused assessment, knowledge, and an understanding that the assessment provides the basis for providing holistic care (Tugut & Golbasi, 2015). Sexuality is a sensitive topic for most people. For this reason, it is important to be aware of the patient's level of comfort when assessing sexual functioning. A basic sexual health history includes the "five P's": **P**artners, **P**ractices. **P**rotection from STIs, **P**ast history of STIs, and **P**revention of pregnancy (Pessagno, 2013). Be sure to obtain the patient's permission before proceeding with the assessment. Be sensitive to the patient's level of comfort.

Barriers to obtaining a sexual history can lie with the nurse or another care provider. They include inadequate training, embarrassment, and a fear of offending the patient. The aim during assessment is that both the patient and care provider will establish enough trust in the therapeutic relationship to honestly share information.

Nursing/Therapeutic Process

Nursing diagnoses/problem statements for psychosexual disorders are based on each patient's identified problems. The primary problem statements for difficulties with sexuality are *sexual dysfunction* and *ineffective sexuality pattern*. Other problem statements are selected to help enhance the patient's physical, emotional, social, and spiritual functioning, and several are listed in Box 29.2.

The quality of care for patients with psychosexual problems depends on each care provider's abilities to remain nonjudgemental and accepting of their patients. The team approach is usually more effective in treating individuals with sexual problems because it helps to maintain objectivity,

---

BOX 29.2   Problem Statements (Nursing Diagnoses) Related to Sexual Disorders

Physical Realm
At risk for injury
Noncompliance
Dysfunctional, ineffective sexuality pattern
At risk for other or self-directed violence

Psychosocial Realm
Anxiety
Ineffective coping
Denial
Dysfunctional family processes
Hopelessness
Loneliness
Powerlessness

---

prevent manipulation, and ensure that therapeutic goals are being met. The Sample Patient Care Plan 29.1 describes treatment for a patient with a sexual dysfunction.

Assessment and treatment are only two important functions of patient care. Advocacy and education are also important in providing effective care for patients with sexual difficulties. Advocacy allows care providers to provide an atmosphere of acceptance in which patients feel safe in discussing sexuality. It also encourages us to discover our prejudices and refine our own values about sexuality.

Perhaps most important is our ability to educate and share information that could spell the difference between life and death for some people. Education about the prevention of HIV/AIDS and other STIs, appropriate methods of preventing unwanted pregnancies, and various means of sexual expression are within the realm of health care. If we are to save a population from the ravages of HIV/AIDS, sexual abuse, and mental illness, we should teach at every opportunity. It is up to us in the helping professions to care for us all.

SAMPLE PATIENT CARE PLAN 29.1 Sexual Dysfunction

Assessment

History Brian, a 31-year-old man, has been treated for chronic depression for the past 2 years. Since his medications were changed 3 months ago, Brian has been complaining of a lack of sexual interest. He has been married for approximately 10 months, and his wife is "worried."

Current Findings An anxious-appearing man. General appearance, speech, motor activity, and interactions are appropriate. Brian describes his problem as a "growing lack of interest" and fears that it will interfere with his marriage.

Multidisciplinary Diagnosis	Planning/Goals
Ineffective role performance related to treatment for depression	Brian and therapist will identify the medications he is taking and list four adverse effects of each medication by April 10. Brian's anxiety will decrease from level 3 to level 2 by April 15 as he works to solve his problems.

THERAPEUTIC INTERVENTIONS

Intervention	Rationale	Team Member
1. Assess degree of sexual frustration and dysfunction; begin with less personal statements.	Builds trust and rapport; helps determine extent of problems and plan effective therapeutic interventions.	Psy, Nsg
2. Reassure Brian that symptoms are troubling but not unique.	Provides reassurance that no physical problems exist.	Nsg
3. Develop a list of every medication (including over-the-counter drugs) that Brian is currently taking.	Certain medications, or combinations of medications, can lead to changes in sexual functioning.	Nsg, Psy
4. Consult with physician for possible dosage regulation of Brian's medications.	Adjustment of dosages may decrease or correct the problem.	Nsg, Psy
5. Educate Brian about each medication's effects on sexual functioning.	Learning to recognize adverse effects early lessens their intensity and offers opportunities for early interventions.	Nsg
6. Refer Brian and his wife for sexual counselling.	Increases knowledge regarding sexuality and its expressions.	Psy

Evaluation Brian listed each medication and demonstrated great interest in learning about their adverse effects. Brian reported a decrease in his level of anxiety as his knowledge of his medications and their effects grew.

Critical Thinking Questions
1. How can a health care provider become more comfortable in obtaining a sexual history?
2. How does learning about the adverse effects of his medications reassure Brian?

A complete patient care plan includes several other diagnoses and interventions.
Nsg, nursing staff; *Psy,* psychologist.

KEY POINTS

- Human sexuality is the combination of physical, chemical, psychological, and functional characteristics that are expressed by one's gender identity and sexual orientation.
- Sexual behaviours occur along a continuum. At the adaptive end of the spectrum are satisfying sexual behaviours that respect the rights of others. As the continuum moves toward fantasies and urges that comprise maladaptive responses, sexual behaviours become impaired or dysfunctional. Individuals may even act on these urges and break the law.
- Healthy sexual responses occur between consenting adults. They are satisfying to all, are not forced or coerced, and are conducted in private.
- The expression of one's sexuality begins at birth and ends at death.
- Many persons living with permanent disabilities are able to enjoy rich and satisfying sexual lives, with adaptation.
- Transgender people are individuals whose gender identity, gender expression, or behaviour does not conform to the sex to which they were assigned at birth.
- Sexual disorders are those problems that cause severe distress and impaired functioning in an individual or others who are exposed to the sexual behaviour.
- A sexual dysfunction is a disturbance anywhere in the sexual response cycle and includes any discomfort or pain associated with sexual intercourse.
- Problems with sexual expression can be caused by medication or illicit drug use and by many physical conditions.
- The paraphilias are a group of sexual behaviours in which there is a persistent sexual arousal to objects, situations, fantasies, behaviours, or interaction with nonconsenting human partners.
- Gender dysphoria is an inconsistency between one's biological gender and their gender identity.
- Treatment of sexual problems depends on the cause, distressing signs or symptoms, and type of disorder.
- If a health care provider is uncomfortable with any aspect of a patient's sexuality, their professional judgement and behaviours may be affected.
- Health care providers need to be sensitive to the patient's level of comfort when assessing sexual functioning.
- The "five P's" of a sexual history focus on **P**artners, **P**ractices, **P**rotection from STIs, **P**ast history of STIs, and **P**revention of pregnancy.
- The quality of care for patients with psychosexual problems depends on care providers' abilities to remain nonjudgemental and accepting of the patient.
- Assessment, treatment, advocacy, and education are important therapeutic activities in relation to caring for patients with sexual difficulties.
- Education about prevention of HIV/AIDS and other STIs and appropriate methods of preventing unwanted pregnancies is an important health care responsibility.

ADDITIONAL LEARNING RESOURCES

Go to your Evolve website (http://evolve.elsevier.com/Canada/Morrison-Valfre/) for additional online resources, including the online Study Guide for additional learning activities to help you master this chapter content.

CRITICAL THINKING QUESTIONS

1. David is a 32-year-old engineer who works at an automobile assembly plant. He is married to Jasmin, a 29-year-old teacher of Asian descent. The couple has two children, aged 1 and 3 years. David was admitted 3 days ago following a serious suicide attempt by hanging. Jasmin found him when she unexpectedly came back home and was able to save him at the last moment. David still has strangulation marks on his neck, and he is under constant observation. There is no known mental illness. After the initial assessment, David remained admitted involuntarily, but with no pharmacological treatment. You have worked with him during your last three shifts and have established a good and trusting therapeutic relationship. David has shared with you that over last 2 years he has suffered gradually intensifying urges to rape "Asian women on the street." What is a potential care plan for David?

2. Jonathan and Myra have brought their 5-year-old daughter, Cheryl, to your outpatient clinic for a consultation. Cheryl persistently refuses to wear dresses and play with dolls and other "girl" toys her parents have bought for her. Instead, she insists on wearing only pants and gravitates to boys in her kindergarten. At the initial conversation, Cheryl tells you that she would prefer to be called "Chuck." What are your findings, and what potential advice could you give to Cheryl's parents?

REFERENCES

Adams, J., & Light, R. (2015). Scientific consensus, the law, and same sex parenting outcomes. *Social Science Research, 53,* 300–310. https://doi.org/10.1016/j.ssresearch.2015.06.008

American Psychological Association (APA). (2015). *What does transgender mean?* https://www.apa.org/topics/lgbt/transgender

Balthazart, J. (2018). Fraternal birth order effect on sexual orientation explained. *Proceedings of the National Academy of Sciences of the United States of America, 115*(2), 234–236. https://doi.org/10.1073/pnas.1719534115, https://www.pnas.org/content/115/2/234

Cornell, U. (2020). *What does the scholarly research say about the well-being of children with gay or lesbian parents?* https://whatweknow.inequality.cornell.edu/topics/lgbt-equality/what-does-the-scholarly-research-say-about-the-wellbeing-of-children-with-gay-or-lesbian-parents/

Government of Canada. (2019). *Definition of child pornography. Justice Laws Website.* https://laws-lois.justice.gc.ca/eng/acts/C-46/section-163.1.html

Hockenberry, M., & Wilson, D. (2014). *Wong's nursing care of infants and children* (10th ed.). Mosby.

Kinsey, A. C., Pomeroy, W. B., & Martin, E. C. (1953). *Sexual behavior in the human female.* Saunders.

Pessagno, R. A. (2013). Don't be embarrassed taking a sexual history. *Nursing, 43*(9), 60–64. https://doi.org/10.1097/01.NURSE.0000431139.82532.b3

Rotermann, M. (2012). *Sexual behaviour and condom use of 15- to 24-year-olds in 2003 and 2009/2010. Health Reports (Catalogue no. 82-003-X).* Statistics Canada. https://www150.statcan.gc.ca/n1/pub/82-003-x/2012001/article/11632-eng.pdf

Statistics Canada. (2015). *Lone-parent families.* https://www150.statcan.gc.ca/n1/pub/75-006-x/2015001/article/14202/parent-eng.htm

Tugut, N., & Golbasi, Z. (2015). Sexuality assessment knowledge, attitude, and skill of nursing students: An experimental study with control group. *International Journal of Nursing Knowledge, 28*(3), 123–130. https://doi.org/10.1111/2047-3095.12127

Wichinski, K. A. (2015). Providing culturally proficient care for transgender patients. *Nursing, 45*(2), 58–63.

30

Personality Disorders

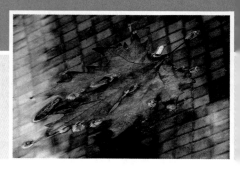

The social realm of functioning is a vital part of being human. People are gregarious, which means they are sociable and in need of the company of others. Although some individuals are able to live in isolation, the vast majority of us need interactions with other people throughout our lives.

Personality is defined as the composite of behavioural traits and attitudes that identify one as an individual.

Personality is a unique pattern of thoughts, attitudes, values, and behaviours. It is established during childhood and developed by adapting to a particular environment and its standards. In part, one's personality is based on one's self-concept (how one feels about oneself). Our personalities define who we are and how we present ourselves to the world.

To find satisfaction in life, people establish relationships with other people. Some relationships assume a special degree of closeness and sharing that become important. These relationships develop intimacy as another person becomes significant in one's life.

Developing intimate relationships requires a willingness to reveal the private side of one's self; the emotions, beliefs, attitudes, dreams, and anxieties that describe one's personal nature. Most people are able to develop and sustain social relationships. Families are established, maintained, and transformed. Relationships outside the family grow and fade as individuals interact and life progresses. For many people, however, the intimacy of important relationships is not achieved because of lifelong patterns of maladaptive thoughts, social responses, and behaviours.

CONTINUUM OF SOCIAL RESPONSES

Interactions with others (social responses) range from autonomy to the disordered behaviours of manipulation, intimidation, aggression, and hysteria. Highly functional people move freely along the continuum, recognizing and balancing their need for intimacy with their need for solitude. Those with ineffective behaviours cope with feelings of dependence and loneliness and the need to withdraw from others. Individuals with personality issues struggle to define and meet their social needs (Fig. 30.1).

PERSONALITY THROUGHOUT THE LIFE CYCLE

Personalities are unique patterns of character that are shaped and influenced throughout life. One's personality is established early in childhood and is moulded through experience. Personality is a set of attitudes, traits, and behavioural patterns that expresses the emotional, intellectual, social, and spiritual realms of an individual. A basic understanding of personality and the factors that influence its development can help health care providers assess and plan for more effective and therapeutic care.

Personality in Childhood

Infants do not see themselves as separate beings until about 18 months of age (Hockenberry & Wilson, 2014). The majority of infants experience their environments as warm, nurturing, and unconditionally accepting. When the infant's needs for food, comfort, safety, and socialization are consistently met, a sense of *trust* and self-worth develops. Infants who are denied love and nurturing have difficulties forming and maintaining significant relationships in adulthood because they have not learned to trust others.

With toddlers, much of their personality is still fluid, changeable, and undefined. As children age, their personality gradually takes shape. Between 18 months and 3 years, toddlers begin to learn to separate from their caregivers and explore the world about them. During this time, they develop a sense of **object constancy**, which is the knowledge that a loved person or object continues to exist even though it is out

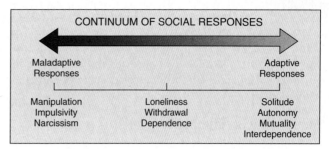

Fig. 30.1 Continuum of social responses.

of sight. For example, a child learns that their toys are still there in the toy chest, even though they cannot see them at this time.

Toddlers often seek out their parents for support, encouragement, and approval. If responses to their independent exploratory behaviours are positive, children build a solid sense of self and develop the capacity for interacting successfully with others. Most researchers believe that, once established, personality traits and temperament are consistent, stable, and generally predictable.

Feelings of morality begin to develop between 6 and 10 years of age. These years are marked by a preoccupation with self, a strong sense of right and wrong, and peer interactions. Trust grows into the capacity for empathy (understanding the feelings and behaviours of others). This is an important ingredient for later relationships. Thinking (intellectual development) moves from the here and now to thoughts of the future. The focus of fantasies changes from imagined objects to real ones, and the use of fantasy becomes a primary way of coping with anxiety.

During the early school years, children learn about cooperation, competition, and compromise. Peer relationships assume more importance, and approval from persons outside the family is sought. Conflicts with parents begin to occur in later childhood as the child's search for independence is tempered by the parents' limits on behaviour. As Stuart (2013) notes, "During this period, a supportive environment that encourages the budding sense of self fosters development of a positive, adaptive self-concept." Without support and encouragement, children's needs for guidance and approval go unmet, which can set the stage for numerous difficulties later in life.

Personality in Adolescence

By the time an individual reaches the teen years, the personality is well established. Relationships with others (especially peers) help adolescents assert their independence from parents. Best-friend relationships offer chances for sharing, clarifying values, and learning about the differences in people. These relationships become interdependent and often include efforts to exclude others. Within their peer group, adolescents support one another in their struggles to assert themselves and cope with the distresses of becoming adults.

As adolescents grow, their relationships expand to include members of the opposite sex. Sexual issues produce anxiety as teens struggle to assume a sexual identity. Sexual activity is experimental and spontaneous. Struggles continue over autonomy within the family. By their early 20s, most individuals have weathered their emotional ups and downs of adolescence and emerge with identities that can carry them into adulthood.

Personality in Adulthood

By young adulthood, most persons are self-sufficient, making decisions, and involved in give-and-take relationships. Occupational choices are made. Families may be started. Self-awareness grows as individuals learn the balance between personal independence and meeting the needs of others. Sensitivity to and an acceptance of the feelings of other persons are critical characteristics of mature relationships in adulthood.

By middle adulthood, most persons are comfortable enough with themselves and their personalities to encourage independence in others. Relationships with friends and significant others grow and evolve. Demands on time and resources change as their children mature, and many middle-aged adults enjoy new freedoms to pursue their own wishes.

Many experts believe that, once established, the personality remains stable and constant. However, adulthood offers opportunities for individuals to look within and decide which aspects of their personality they wish to keep and develop and which aspects they would like to change. People are dynamic, always in physical and psychological motion; and change does occur—even within one's "well-established" personality.

Personality in Older Adulthood

Older persons must cope with loss and change. Old friends are lost, family members move away. Occupational careers end, and friendships from the workplace fade as time passes.

Personality, however, remains intact as an individual ages. Life takes on a deeper meaning as personal accomplishments and contributions to society are reviewed. Older persons who have strong, integrated personalities are able to cope with losses by maintaining what independence they can and accepting their limitations. Strength of personality carries them through life's rougher times.

An important reminder about older persons is that *a sudden change in personality is not a normal sign of aging*. By older adulthood, the personality is deeply entrenched. Patterns of thinking and behaving remain intact until death. As a care provider, do not assume that a personality change in an older person is normal. Changes in emotional control, responses, and levels of interest must be investigated. Many physical and biochemical conditions first appear as subtle changes in personality. The *majority* of sudden-onset personality changes in older persons are caused by physical issues, such as drug reactions or illness. Alert investigations by nurses and all health care providers can often spell the difference between functional living and a diagnosis of dementia or some other psychological condition.

THEORIES RELATING TO PERSONALITY DISORDERS

In medicine, it is difficult to tell the exact point at which a blood pressure reading becomes abnormal. Likewise, it is just as difficult to establish the point at which a normal personality becomes a disordered one. Interest in disordered personalities dates back to the time of the ancient Greeks. During the Middle Ages, individuals who behaved in unusual ways were thought to be possessed by evil spirits. Since then, theories of personality development and disorder have been developed to help understand the complex nature of human beings. Currently, there are four general theories of personality disorders: biological, psychoanalytical, behavioural, and sociocultural.

Biological Theories

As research continues to investigate a connection between behaviour and the body, evidence for this connection has mounted. Studies of families, twins, and relatives of individuals with personality disorders have demonstrated that behaviour and personality are strongly influenced by genetics. Researchers have found that one's **temperament** (the biological bases that underlie moods, energy levels, and attitudes) is genetically linked. Several studies of twins raised in separate environments have shown a remarkable consistency in temperament when tested.

Cardiovascular responses, brain dysfunctions, and biochemical imbalances have been studied as possible physical causes of personality disorders. Other biological evidence is beginning to establish a neurophysical basis for the behaviours seen in individuals with personality disorders. Brain imaging studies suggest a possible physical basis for the failure to appreciate the emotional significance of words and images. Research now suggests that people with some personality disorders show less activity in areas of the brain that help control emotions and aggressive impulses (National Institute of Mental Health, 2017). In other words, the brain mechanism that connects emotions and intellect may be missing or inefficient in persons with personality disorders. As studies into the biobehavioural connections are conducted, new developments will influence the treatment of persons with personality disorders.

Psychoanalytical Theories

According to psychoanalytical theories, infants begin to discover the nature of "good/bad" and "love/hate" as the superego grows. If the mother responds in ways that cause frustration, distress, or pain, the child will have difficulty finding the proper fit between aggression and love. Certain patterns of parental responses, ranging from overinvolvement to neglect, prevent the child from developing a strong sense of self and balance among the three forces of the personality (i.e., ego, id, and superego).

Behavioural Theories

Theorists from the behavioural school of thought see personality disorders as the result of conditioned responses caused by previous events. The separation-individuation theory states that the average 1- to 3-year-old is able to achieve object constancy. Personality disorders occur in persons who are not able to hold a consistent, stable image of the mother when she is absent. This results in fears that range from abandonment and separation to a complete loss of connection with others. Other behaviourists view personality disorders as the result of unmet needs during critical developmental periods.

Sociocultural Theories

Sociocultural theories find the causes of personality disorders embedded in one's culture and society. Research suggests a lack of social cognition, the development of social awareness, may play a role in their etiology (Sharp & Vanwoerden, 2014). A lack of social structure (**normlessness**) and lack of available social roles have been found to be risk factors for the development of personality disorders. Numerous cultural expectations are seen to influence the use of adaptive or maladaptive behaviours.

Sociocultural theorists believe that the foundation for personality disorders is built on society's social and cultural stresses. Many social stressors can lead to difficulties with relationships. Family instability, divorce, and mobility often isolate people from those they love.

PERSONALITY DISORDERS

Narcissus, the son of the river god, was a young and very good-looking man. He was sure that he was the best in the world and that there was nobody who came close to him by any significance. He was the son of a god. Thus, everybody had to accept his superiority in all aspects.

Echo, the beautiful mountain nymph, watched Narcissus walking through the forest near the river bank, down in the valley. She fell in love with him. His body, face, movements—everything was so lovely. She followed him while hiding behind stones of the valley. He noted a small stone falling down and asked, "Who is there?" Echo froze. His voice struck her as the best sound she had ever heard. She hid in a shadow of a rock. She did not know what to say, and only replied back, "Who is there?" When she finally revealed her love to him, he was outraged. He was so angry with her for even thinking that she could be equal to him. What did she think of herself? He was second to none in the world! Echo was devastated by this reaction. Her grief was so great that she ceased to exist. It is only her voice that still lives there in the mountains. If you yell, "Who is there?" you may hear her yelling back to you, "Who is there?"

Narcissus continued with his walks along the river. At one point, he came to the place where the river water was so slow, it was almost not moving. He looked in the water and saw himself. What a beauty! He immediately fell in love with his own image. He stayed in that very place until he turned into a beautiful gold and white flower.

When an individual has an intense and unusual sense of self-importance, this can lead people who love that person to disappear, as happened to Echo in the story above. It also may lead the person to stop being humane, as happened to Narcissus. Clearly, the story ended sadly for both, making it hard for us to judge Narcissus. Other extreme behaviour cannot be judged easily, either. Some people show persistent disregard for the law, order, and their own and other people's lives. Yet, they can be seen by many as noble, or as criminals. Everything depends on culture and circumstances. Just think of the stories of Zorro, Robin Hood, or Aladdin. Thus, it is important for a clinician to discuss people's patterns of behaviour while avoiding judgement and leave punishment to the criminal justice system.

Personality disorders are defined as long-standing, maladaptive patterns of behaving and relating to others. All personality disorders are characterized by continual difficulties with interpersonal relations.

The most important criterion for diagnosing a personality disorder is that behaviours are inflexible, long-standing, and maladaptive, resulting in significant functional impairment (American Psychiatric Association, 2013). The rigid, ineffective behaviour patterns must occur throughout a broad range of occupational, social, and personal situations. The onset of these patterns can usually be traced back to childhood or adolescence, and no medical or other mental health conditions can account for them. Box 30.1 describes the criteria for diagnosing general personality disorder. The definition of **general personality disorder** applies to each of the 10 other specific

---

BOX 30.1 Characteristics of General Personality Disorder

All criteria—A, B, C, D, E, and F—must be present.
A. An enduring pattern of *behaviour that deviates markedly from the person's culture.* This pattern must be manifested at least in two of the following areas:
   1. Cognition: the way in which a person perceives self, others, and events. This way of thinking is persistently different from cultural norms.
   2. **Affect** (emotional response to event): the range of affect, liability, intensity, and appropriateness is consistently outside of cultural norms.
   3. Interpersonal functioning: impaired interpersonal relationships.
   4. Poor impulse control: difficulty in controlling own urges to act.
B. Persistent *lack of flexibility* across all life situations.
C. The person's behaviour leads to a *significant distress or impairment* in social, occupational, or other important areas of functioning.
D. The pattern of behaviour has a *long duration* and goes back at least to the adolescent years.
E. There is *no other mental health illness that can explain* that pattern of behaviour.
F. This persistent pattern of *behaviour cannot be explained by medication effect or other medical condition.*

Adapted from American Psychiatric Association (APA). (2013). *Diagnostic and statistical manual of mental disorders* (5th ed.). American Psychiatric Publishing.

personality disorders. People often can present with a combination of a few personality disorders. Thus, for a clinician, it is good to keep in mind the criteria for general personality disorder as a common denominator.

The fifth edition of the *Diagnostic and Statistical Manual of Mental Disorders (DSM-5*; American Psychiatric Association [APA], 2013) has classified 10 separate personality disorders. For the sake of discussion, personality disorders are grouped into three clusters based on similar behaviours: *eccentric, erratic,* and *fearful.* Table 30.1 lists the main features of each disorder. Remember that individuals can exhibit behaviours from different clusters.

Eccentric Cluster

The eccentric cluster is characterized by *odd* or *strange behaviours.* Persons with disorders in this cluster (group A) find it difficult to relate to others or socialize comfortably. Often they live in isolation and interact only when necessary. Diagnoses in this cluster include paranoid, schizoid, and schizotypal disorders.

Individuals with a **paranoid personality disorder** have developed a pattern of behaviours marked by suspiciousness and mistrust. They often assume that everyone is out to harm, deceive, or exploit them. Family and co-workers are often questioned for hostile intentions. The search for hidden meanings can turn a casual remark into a conflict. Sharing information or becoming close to someone is avoided because it may provide ammunition to be used against them. They are constantly alert for harmful intentions from others.

Often a minor event arouses intense hostility and hostile feelings persist for a long time. Such persons may quickly react with anger to a perceived attack. They can be litigious and may be involved in many legal disputes. They may develop negative stereotypes of others, especially those from different cultural-social groups, and may easily believe in "conspiracies." They can build a tight relationship with other individuals who are like them and believe in similar paranoid ideas.

People with a paranoid personality disorder are unwilling to forgive even the slightest error. Paranoid personality disorders are diagnosed in up to 2.5% of the population. Men are diagnosed with the disorder more often than women, and substance abuse is common. Between 10 and 30% of psychiatric inpatients are diagnosed as having paranoid personality disorders (Fortinash & Holoday-Worret, 2011).

Schizoid and schizotypal personality disorders are marked by an inability to develop and maintain relationships with other people. Individuals with **schizoid personality disorder** lack the desire or willingness to become involved in close relationships. They are society's "loners" who prefer solitary activities and their own company. These people are emotionally restricted and unable to take pleasure in activities, friendships, or social relationships. Often individuals are emotionally detached. There is a coldness and lack of concern for others. Sexual experiences hold little interest. Schizoid personality disorders are slightly more common in men and families with an already diagnosed member.

Persons with **schizotypal personality disorder** have the same interaction pattern of avoiding people as that of schizoid

TABLE 30.1	**Clusters of Personality Disorders**
Cluster/Disorder	**Main Characteristic**
A: Eccentric	
Paranoid	Distrust and suspiciousness; sees others' motives as threatening or malevolent (intend to do harm); may interact in odd or distant ways; untrusting, unforgiving; scheming, secretive; may be emotionally cold and distant
Schizoid	Detachment from social relationships; emotionally cold and distant; absorbed in own thoughts and feelings
Schizotypal	Acute discomfort with close relationships; sensory distortions; very odd behaviours, thinking, dressing, and speech; experiences extreme anxiety in social situations
B: Erratic	
Antisocial	Disregards or violates rights of others; ignores rules of acceptable behaviour; impulsive, irresponsible, aggressive, belligerent; feels no remorse for behaviours
Borderline	Unstable self-image, emotions, moods, and behaviours; stormy interpersonal relationships; unpredictable and self-destructive
Histrionic	Excessive emotional expression and attention-seeking behaviours
Narcissistic	Exaggerated sense of self-importance; grandiose; no empathy or concern for other people or animals; needs constant attention and admiration; exploits interpersonal relationships
C: Fearful	
Avoidant	Social distress, feelings of inadequacy, oversensitive; unwilling to become involved with others
Dependent	Excessive need to be cared for, resulting in clinging, submissive behaviours; wants others to make decisions; requires much reassurance and attention; helpless and uncomfortable when left alone
Obsessive-compulsive	Preoccupation with control, orderliness, and perfection; never satisfied with their achievements; keeps emotions under strict control; dependable, methodical, orderly, and inflexible; has difficulty adapting to change

Data from Mental Health America. (2015). *Personality disorder.* https://www.mhanational.org/

personalities, but behaviours here are characterized by distortions and eccentricities (odd, strange, or peculiar actions). These individuals often have **ideas of reference** (incorrect perceptions of causal events as having great or significant meaning), and they commonly find special, personal messages in everyday events.

Schizotypal people are often superstitious or believe in the paranormal (events outside human understanding). Many think they have special powers to foretell events or read people's minds. Some claim to have magical control over others and to be able to make people do their bidding just by thinking about it. These individuals commonly experience perceptual alterations, such as sensing that there is another person present (when there is not). Speech is often loose and vague, but it can be understood. Often they will use words in odd combinations or in unusual ways.

As with the other disorders in the eccentric cluster, schizotypal personalities are marked by suspiciousness and paranoid ideation—the idea that people are "out to get them," undermine their efforts, or do them harm. Emotional expressions (affect) are usually inappropriate or restricted. Because of unusual mannerisms, style of dress or grooming, and inattention to appropriate social behaviours, these individuals are often considered odd or eccentric. They have problems relating to other people and are very anxious in social situations. They have few, if any, friends because they feel different and just do not "fit in" with others. Schizotypal personality disorders are diagnosed more frequently in men than in women. Signs of major depression also occur in 50% of persons diagnosed with this disorder.

Erratic Cluster

The main characteristic for the group of disorders in the erratic cluster is dramatic behaviour. People with these personality disorders are often overly emotional with unpredictable thinking and behaviours. Each disorder in this cluster (group B) is associated with a dramatic quality in the way in which these individuals conduct their lives. The erratic cluster consists of four separate disorders: antisocial, borderline, histrionic, and narcissistic.

One of our most pressing mental health challenges today is people who have antisocial personality disorders. The central feature of **antisocial personality disorder** is a persistent pattern of disregard for and violation of the rights of others, starting from age 15, as well as three or more of the following features:

1. Failure to follow social norms
2. Repeated lying or conning others for personal profit or pleasure
3. Impulsivity
4. Irritability and aggressiveness; constant fighting and/or assaults
5. Disregard for safety of self or others
6. Consistent failure to sustain any obligations
7. Lack of remorse

CASE STUDY

Ramon was the younger of two boys born to an older, loving couple. As a child, he was always in some type of trouble. When he was about 7 years old, he broke his femur (upper leg) and was required to wear a cast from his chest to his knees for 6 weeks. Although his mother checked on him frequently, he managed mobility. One day Ramon walked out of the house and was seen propelling his encased hips and legs down the street, disinterested in the fact that he could have harmed himself.

By 12 years of age, Ramon was self-centred, demanding, and intolerant of his parents' wishes. He often threatened to burn the house down or kill the dog when he did not get his way. Soon, his father was bailing him out of jail for various minor offences, such as stealing. His parents, unable to control him and afraid for their safety, allowed him to have free run of the house.

At 18 years of age, Ramon joined the Army. By 19 years of age, he had received a general discharge for not following orders. Much to his parents' dismay, Ramon returned home and announced that he would attend the local community college. By this time, however, he was deeply involved with cocaine, alcohol, and a crowd of thrill seekers. His arrest record continued to grow.

One night at a party, Ramon strangled the homeowner's pedigreed Siamese cat. The owner became angry and threatened to have him arrested. Ramon coldly looked into the homeowner's eyes, pulled out a gun, and fired at him.

Later, when asked why he did it, he calmly replied, "What else could I do? That guy was in my face, and his stupid cat was in my way. I didn't hurt him bad."

- What are your reactions to Ramon's behaviours?
- How would your feelings affect the care of this patient?
- Do you think anything could have prevented this event? If so, what?

Antisocial personality disorders are rooted in childhood. Some children have trouble controlling their impulses, so they become disruptive and develop disagreeable ways of coping. Many of these maladaptive behaviours can be seen as early as 4 years of age.

Children with **conduct disorders** usually express their distress by being aggressive toward animals and people. They deceive, lie, steal, destroy property, and break important rules. Many become bullies in school. They are impulsive and quick to anger, and they have no regard for others. If the child is seen by mental health care providers at this time, a conduct disorder is usually diagnosed.

During adolescence, maladaptive behaviours become well established. Truancies from school, open disregard for rules, and thrill-seeking behaviours often get these teens into trouble with authorities and the law. Fighting and physical and verbal abuses are common in teens with antisocial personalities.

Men are more often affected by antisocial personality disorders than women. Commonly they fail to become self-supporting and spend years being impoverished, homeless, or institutionalized. They may abuse chemicals.

A **borderline personality disorder** can be summarized as a pattern of instability in mood, thinking, self-image, behaviour, and personal relationships. Intense fears of being abandoned motivate these individuals to avoid being alone. Relationships are marked by rapid shifts from adoring and idealizing to devaluing and cruel punishment. These extreme shifts are also seen in the area of self-image. Sudden, dramatic changes in career plans, values, types of friends, and even sexual identities are characteristic of these individuals.

The borderline here is that between neurosis and psychosis. **Neurosis** is a pattern of anxiety responses to relationships that are often rooted in childhood responses to conflict with one's parents. The person will worry excessively about how others may perceive them and whether this negative perception will lead to abandonment. During a particularly stressful time, the intensity of this worry and anxiety may cross the border into **psychosis**. In the psychotic stage, the person may have a crystalized paranoid delusion about why people are against them. This thinking may lead to bizarre and even violent behaviour, but typically, the person will cross that border back toward neurosis within 2 hours and without any antipsychotic treatment.

Impulsivity is acting without forethought or regard for the consequences. Persons with borderline personality disorders may gamble, abuse food or drugs, practise unsafe sex with multiple partners, spend money irresponsibly, and engage in self-mutilating or suicidal behaviours. Cutting, burning, pulling out hair, or scratching oneself is common. Of these individuals, 8 to 10% commit suicide.

Although people with borderline personality disorders experience chronic feelings of emptiness, they commonly express intense anger and have frequent displays of aggression or temper. Moods are unstable. Emotions range from great joy to deep depression and change within minutes or hours. They express inappropriate anger and have difficulty controlling their aggression. These individuals become easily bored, so they are always busy.

The most important feature of histrionic and narcissistic personality disorders is attention-seeking behaviours. Individuals with these disorders are often highly emotional and self-centred. They feel inadequate and unappreciated when they are not the centre of attention.

A **histrionic personality disorder** is a pattern of excessive emotional expression accompanied by attention-seeking behaviours. Histrionic persons may be flashy or dramatic in style of dress, mannerisms, and speech in order to draw attention to themselves. They are emotionally shallow and often live in a romantic fantasy world.

A **narcissistic personality disorder** is characterized by a pattern of grandiosity and the need to be admired. These individuals believe they are special, unique, or extra-important. They crave admiration and have unrealistically inflated beliefs about themselves and their accomplishments. They can become extremely angry if criticized or outshone by others. Often, they fantasize about unlimited money, power, or love. They will quickly take advantage of and exploit others without guilt or remorse.

It is interesting to note that more women are diagnosed with histrionic personality disorder, whereas 50 to 75% of persons diagnosed with narcissistic personality disorder are men (Fortinash & Holoday-Worret, 2011).

Psychopaths and Sociopaths

Psychopathy and sociopathy are not medical conditions (in the *DSM-5*) or diagnoses. Yet these terms are very popular in criminology and forensic psychiatry. An individual with psychopathology may carry criteria from some or even all four personality disorders within that cluster. Individuals are often referred to as *psychopaths* or *sociopaths* because they rely on deceit and manipulation to get their way. **Deceit** is lying; it is the act of representing as true something that is known to be false. **Manipulation** is controlling others for one's own purposes by influencing them in unfair or false ways.

The hallmark of psychopaths is a lack of conscience. **Psychopaths** use charm, manipulation, intimidation, and, rarely, violence to control others and satisfy their own selfish needs. They have a stunning lack of conscience and no feelings for others. Because of these traits, it is important that care providers remain alert for these behaviours and investigate sources other than the patient when performing assessments.

Sociopaths have a weak conscience that does not stop them from using others for their own gain. Their capacity to easily rationalize their actions helps them overcome their conscience. However, they can be more impulsive, rage-prone, erratic, and unplanned in their crimes than psychopaths, and this pattern leads more often to apprehension by law enforcement. They have a somewhat lower capacity to manipulate others and generally cannot keep steady work for as long as a psychopath can (Grohol, 2018).

Contrary to popular belief, a psychopath or sociopath is not necessarily violent; for neither is violence required to make a diagnosis of antisocial personality. Most well-educated psychopaths learn to be well adapted externally to social rules. They may go fast and far up the corporate ladder, using manipulation that is natural to them, as well as a disregard for others. Yet, when it comes to physical violence, because of their absolute lack of conscience, psychopaths may demonstrate a significantly higher degree of violence. They can be calculated, cold, serial killers.

By adulthood, psychopaths are usually quite adept at manipulating and deceiving others. They gain money, power, or influence at the expense of others and feel no guilt about their behaviour. They lie, cheat, and con others, and they malinger (pretend to be ill) to achieve their goals.

Psychopaths are often charming. They are glib and clever conversationalists who give compliments and make entertaining statements. An inflated view of their own importance makes them the centre of attention and justifies their living by different rules. Their emotions are shallow, and the relationships they build are superficial. Yet, they may keep these relationships for as long as they can benefit from them.

CASE STUDY

The only reason he was sitting there in the counsellor's office was because she threatened him with divorce. He knew the counsellor would see things his way. After all, she was only a woman, one who could not function without him (although she effectively managed a large business with many employees and he did not work). As the session progressed, the counsellor learned about her many inadequacies. She was expected to return from work to cook, clean, and tend to his needs. No matter how hard she tried, she was unable to live up to "his standards." One of his complaints was about her smoking—not because she was hurting herself, but because of the inconvenience it would cause him if she should become ill and unable to care for him.

In response, his wife assured him that he would never be burdened with caring for her. He reached to slap her, but she avoided his blow and walked out of the room, slamming the door behind her. He looked at the counsellor and said, "Why is she doing this to me?"

- What kind of insight does this person demonstrate?
- Do you think this person believes he has a problem? Why or why not?

Fearful Cluster

The common characteristic of the fearful cluster (group C) is *anxiety*. The three personality disorders in this cluster are avoidant, dependent, and obsessive-compulsive. Each disorder is related to certain expressions of anxiety.

In **avoidant personality disorder**, anxiety is related to fear of rejection and humiliation. To prevent possible rejection, individuals narrow their interests to a small range of activities. They have a minimal support system because they are so afraid of the reactions of others. Their tension does not allow for new friends who may be critical, so they withdraw into a world of isolation and self-pity. These people are hypersensitive to criticism and often feel inadequate and inferior. They are extremely shy in social situations. Often individuals with avoidant personality disorders also suffer from general anxiety, depression, somatic symptom disorder, or illness anxiety disorder.

The anxiety of a person with **dependent personality disorder** is associated with separation and abandonment. People with this disorder carry a deep fear of rejection, which expresses itself as the need to be cared for. To avoid turning people away, they become submissive, over-cooperative, and docile. They do not make demands or disagree with others. When alone, they feel helpless and will go to great lengths to find someone to care for them.

Individuals who have dependent personality disorder refuse to be responsible for their own actions. They are unwilling to begin a task alone, take any independent actions, or assume responsibility for their own daily living activities. Their lack of self-confidence results in the need for excessive reassurance, and they are easily hurt by any criticism or disapproval. Feelings of worthlessness often motivate them to seek out overprotective, dominating, or abusive relationships.

BOX 30.2 Diagnostic Tests to Rule Out Other Medical Conditions Before Personality Disorders Can Be Diagnosed

Complete blood count (CBC), including thyroid function
Screening for HIV and other sexually transmitted infections
Computed tomography (CT) scan
Radiology (X-ray)

Men and women are equally affected, although some studies show a higher incidence among women.

Persons with an **obsessive-compulsive personality disorder (OCPD)** focus their anxiety on uncertainty about the future. They are extremely orderly and preoccupied with details and rules. Some complete many tasks, while others actually accomplish little. Delegating tasks to others is difficult or impossible because no one "can do it as well." There is a "desire to be in control of people, tasks, and situations" (Mayo Clinic, 2020). An excessive commitment to work allows for few friends or social activities. These individuals can be rigid, stubborn, and miserly. They are consumed by the need for perfection, as defined by their own high standards. About two thirds of compulsive personalities are men.

OCPD is not the same as *obsessive compulsive disorder (OCD)*. People with OCD have obsessions (recurrent, anxiety-provoking thoughts) and compulsions (repetitive behaviours to reduce the anxiety related to obsessions). These individuals typically are well aware of their obsessions and compulsions and are looking for help. A patient with OCPD, by contrast, will see their desire to control people and their environment as natural. There are some people who may have both of these conditions (OCPD and OCD) simultaneously.

THERAPEUTIC INTERVENTIONS

Treatment for individuals with personality disorders is complex because these individuals have extremely diverse treatment needs, and no single treatment is appropriate for every patient. Unfortunately, most do not seek treatment or refuse to accept it because of their history of conflict, a basic mistrust of others, and extreme lack of insight.

Treatment and Therapy

Persons with personality disorders may have significant impairments in functioning, but they seldom present for treatment because they are usually unable to recognize their problems. When they do cooperate with treatment, a combination of various *psychotherapies* and *medications* is used. *Hospitalization* may be required when the individual is at risk for harming themselves or others.

First, all physical causes must be ruled out. In-depth histories (including recent injuries), psychological tests, and physical examinations are performed. Diagnostic tests commonly ordered to rule out other medical conditions are listed in Box 30.2. Treatment decisions are guided by the patient's symptoms, complaints, problems, and willingness to cooperate.

At one time, it was thought that personality disorders were untreatable because it was thought that personality was fixed by adulthood. We now know that people continue to evolve and change throughout life. Many individuals respond well to treatment, although the degree of improvement may vary according to the patient's motivation.

A number of psychotherapies have been selected to treat patients with personality disorders. Types of psychotherapy that have been used with success include psychodynamic, cognitive, behavioural, group, and family therapies. Dialectic behaviour therapy (DBT) is a relatively new approach that focuses on reducing harmful behaviours by developing "coping skills to improve affective (emotional) stability and emotional control" (Bienenfeld, 2016).

Schema therapy is a new approach for people with personality disorders. It combines several types of therapies into one integrated system or treatment. Its use is gaining popularity in Europe, where it has been successfully applied to a wide range of different personality disorders. Its focus is to target "enduring and self-defeating patterns that typically begin early in life" (Pearl, 2015). Treatment is designed to help patients recognize and replace long-standing negative thinking, feeling, and behavioural patterns with healthier alternatives.

Care providers work to help patients become more aware of how their perceptions, behaviours, and habits affect their lives. They focus on helping patients modify their behaviours enough to become more successful and appropriate.

Medications are used with great caution in the treatment of people with personality disorders. Antianxiety drugs and antidepressants may be prescribed to help relieve the depression and anger associated with these disorders. Mood stabilizers may help with impulsivity, irritability, and aggression. Antipsychotic medications are only indicated when the patient becomes acutely and dangerously psychotic. Most psychotherapeutic medications are prescribed in limited amounts for short periods because their effectiveness in treating personality disorders is still under investigation.

Nurses must exercise great care when administering medications to individuals with personality disorders. A thorough drug history, including herbal remedies, over-the-counter drugs, and street drugs, is needed. Adherence to medication regimens must be monitored frequently. Safeguards to prevent or reduce the risk for suicide must be in place. If the patient is being treated on an outpatient basis, the amount of any prescribed medication must never be large enough to allow a successful suicide.

It is also important to be alert to the fact that suicidal patients will hoard their medications until they have a lethal dose on hand. Do not hesitate to assess every medicated patient for suicidal thoughts or plans. Be familiar with each class of medications and their adverse effects.

> ### BOX 30.3   Problem Statements (Nursing Diagnoses) Related to Personality Disorders
>
> **Physical Realm**
> Risk-prone behaviours
> Nonadherence
> Ineffective role performance
> Potential for self-mutilation
> Potential for other-directed violence
>
> **Psychosocial Realm**
> Anxiety
> Persistent low self-esteem
> Ineffective individual and family coping
> Ineffective denial
> Disturbed personal identity
> Loneliness
> Impaired social interactions

Nursing (Therapeutic) Process

The goals of care for patients with personality disorders are twofold: (1) to help patients identify and then become responsible for their own behaviours, and (2) to assist patients in developing satisfactory life goals.

While the assessment of every patient should include a mental status examination, for the patient with a personality disorder this is especially important. A nursing history and observation of patient behaviours will reveal how individuals cope with interpersonal relationships and the many aspects of daily life.

The therapeutic relationship is begun at this time, so it is important to remain nonjudgemental. Remember, however, that many patients use manipulation, charm, or other subtle behaviours to achieve their purposes. They often use a technique called **splitting**, which is emotionally dividing the staff by complimenting one group and degrading another. Consistent limit setting and reinforcement can help patients to define their limits, but care providers must keep in mind their own therapeutic boundaries and communicate with one another frequently.

Possible nursing diagnoses/problem statements relating to personality disorders are listed in Box 30.3. Short-term goals are based on each individual's assessed difficulties. They usually focus on the discomforts and ineffective behaviours associated with daily living activities.

Patients with personality disorders often have several difficulties occurring at the same time. The most important ones are identified and linked to the appropriate multidisciplinary and nursing diagnoses. Interventions and evaluations are developed for each diagnosis, based on the individual patient. The Sample Patient Care Plan 30.1 describes the care for an individual with a personality disorder. Caring for these patients can be a challenge, but the process can promote growth in both patient and care provider when they are willing to work together.

SAMPLE PATIENT CARE PLAN 30.1 **Personality Disorders**

Assessment

History Karla was 6 years old when her parents divorced after years of fighting and abuse. Karla, her mother, and her older brother Sam were forced to find shelter in a small hotel room. Shortly after moving in, her mother began to leave Karla alone for long periods. Once, Karla set the room on fire. Another time she strangled the neighbour's canary. On one occasion, she was molested by a drunken visitor.

At 13 years of age, Karla dropped out of school and began living on the streets. Occasionally, she would return home.

Current Findings Today, 19-year-old Karla has been admitted to the medical unit for recovery from repeated attempts to "cut herself apart." She is suicidal and angry, and she has difficulty identifying her actions and their consequences.

Multidisciplinary Diagnosis

Risk for self-directed violence related to feelings of abandonment, depression, and worthlessness

Planning/Goals

Karla will verbally identify the emotions associated with her self-destructive activities by August 15.

Karla will not engage in self-destructive behaviours during her inpatient stay.

THERAPEUTIC INTERVENTIONS

Intervention	Rationale	Team Member
1. Inform Karla that self-harm is not acceptable behaviour while she is here.	Setting limits lets her know which behaviours will not be tolerated	All
2. Have Karla sign a **reverse Q15 minutes observation.** This means she must come to the staff station and sign an observation list every 15 minutes indicating whether she is safe or whether she is in need of protection from herself. According to her wishes, she can be placed in voluntary seclusion or in restraints.	Offers objective data of agreed-on behaviours Offers a means of control of her own form of therapy and limitations	Nsg
3. Establish trust and rapport with Karla.	Allows Karla to identify current behaviours and explore new ones within an atmosphere of safety and trust	All
4. Institute suicide precautions; monitor continuously her environment for safety and her behaviour if acting out.	Provides safety, prevents self-harm, encourages therapeutic relationships	All
5. Assess skin on arms and legs daily for new wounds or signs of trauma.	To monitor for further evidence of self-harm behaviours	Nsg

Evaluation Karla expressed relief at knowing that limits have been set and that she has a sense of self-control over her behaviour 2 days after admission. During the first week, Karla was able to identify her emotions after a dispute with another patient.

Critical Thinking Questions
1. What interventions could help Karla learn about cause and effect relating to her behaviours?
2. What purpose do you think acting out serves for Karla?

A complete patient care plan includes several other diagnoses and interventions.
Nsg, nursing staff.

KEY POINTS

- Personality is the composite of behavioural traits and attitudes that identifies one as an individual.
- The social responses of humans can range from autonomy and interdependence to the ineffective, disordered behaviours of manipulation, intimidation, aggression, and hysteria.
- The human personality is shaped and influenced throughout life.
- Currently, there are four general theories of personality: biological, psychoanalytical, behavioural, and sociocultural.
- Personality disorders are defined as long-standing, maladaptive patterns of behaving and relating to others.
- The eccentric cluster (group A) of personality disorders is characterized by odd or strange behaviours and includes the paranoid, schizoid, and schizotypal personality disorders.
- The erratic cluster (group B) is characterized by dramatic behaviours and consists of antisocial, borderline, histrionic, and narcissistic personality disorders.
- The fearful cluster (group C) of personality disorders is characterized by anxiety and includes the avoidant, dependent, and obsessive-compulsive personality disorders.
- Individuals with personality disorders often also suffer from substance abuse or some other form of mental illness.
- People with personality disorders may have significant impairments, but they seldom present for treatment because they are unable or unwilling to recognize their problems.

- Types of psychotherapy that have been used with success for different personality disorders include psychodynamic, cognitive, behavioural, and group therapies.
- Schema therapy helps patients recognize and replace long-standing negative thinking, feeling, and behavioural patterns with healthier alternatives.

- Medications are used with great caution in the treatment of people with personality disorders to help relieve the distressing symptoms associated with these disorders.
- Goals of care for patients with personality disorders are to help patients identify and then become responsible for their own behaviour and to assist patients in developing satisfactory quality of life.

ADDITIONAL LEARNING RESOURCES

Go to your Evolve website (http://evolve.elsevier.com/ Canada/Morrison-Valfre/) for additional online resources, including the online Study Guide for additional learning activities to help you master this chapter content.

CRITICAL THINKING QUESTIONS

1. What are the main characteristics of personality?
2. The staff notices that an 80-year-old patient's behaviour is rapidly changing. Although he once was outgoing and talkative, he now sits sullenly in his chair. Can this man's personality suddenly change at 80 years of age, or can this change be indicative of something else?
3. A patient automatically assumes that everyone is out to harm, deceive, or exploit her. She often feels deeply injured by others, even when no evidence for this exists. She avoids letting other knows any information about her out of the fear that people will use this information to harm her. Yet, her thoughts do not meet the definition of delusions; rather, they remain a set of beliefs and attitudes. What kind of personality disorder does this scenario describe?
4. The patient is a heavy drinker. He is frequently in bar fights because every time he visits a tavern, someone is "always picking a fight with me." He has a history of being in jail a few times due to theft under $5 000 and destruction of public property. He agrees that these actions are not good but always has a very good explanation for why he had to act that way. What kind of pathology does this scenario describe? What can be done within the team to prevent splitting?

REFERENCES

American Psychiatric Association (APA). (2013). *Diagnostic and statistical manual of mental disorders* (5th ed.). American Psychiatric Publishing.

Bienenfeld, D. (2016). *Personality disorders treatment and management.* http://emedicine.medscape.com/article/294307-treatment

Clinic, M. (2020). *Personality disorders.* https://www.mayoclinic.org/diseases-conditions/personality-disorders/symptoms-causes/syc-20354463

Fortinash, K. M., & Holoday-Worret, P. A. (2011). *Psychiatric mental health nursing* (5th ed.). Mosby.

Grohol, J. M. (2018). *Differences between a psychopath vs sociopath.* PsychCentral. July 8 https://psychcentral.com/blog/differences-between-a-psychopath-vs-sociopath/

Hockenberry, M., & Wilson, D. (2014). *Wong's nursing care of infants and children* (10th ed.). Mosby.

National Institute of Mental Health. (2017). *Borderline personality disorder.* https://www.nimh.nih.gov/health/topics/borderline-personality-disorder/index.shtml

Pearl, M. (2015). *What is schema therapy?.* http://www.schematherapy-nola.com/what-is-schema-therapy

Sharp, C., & Vanwoerden, S. (2014). Social cognition: Empirical contribution. *Journal of Personality Disorders, 28*(1), 78–95.

Stuart, G. W. (2013). *Principles and practice of psychiatric nursing* (10th ed.). Mosby.

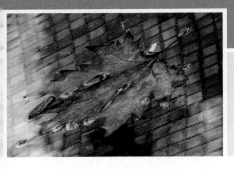

31

Brain Function, Schizophrenia, and Other Psychoses

OBJECTIVES

Upon completion of this chapter, the student will be able to:
1. Describe the basic principles of normal and abnormal brain function.
2. Define psychosis.
3. Describe the signs, symptoms, and behaviours exhibited by a person with schizophrenia and other schizophrenia spectrum disorders.
4. Outline the main pharmacological treatments and mental health therapies for persons with schizophrenia.
5. Describe the therapeutic process applicable to patients suffering from schizophrenia or another psychosis.
6. Plan three nursing responsibilities related to antipsychotic medications.

OUTLINE

KEY TERMS

agnosia (ăg-NŌ-zhă) (p. 392)
akathisia (ĂK-ă-THĒ-zhă) (p. 395)
akinesia (Ă-kĭ-NĒ-zhă) (p. 395)
alexithymia (ă-LĔK-sĭ-THĬ-mē-ă) (p. 390)
alogia (p. 387)
anhedonia (ĂN-hĭ-DŌ-nē-ă) (p. 390)
apathy (p. 390)
bradykinesia (BRĂD-ē-kĭ-NĒ-zhă) (p. 395)
catatonia (p. 387)
cognitive distortions (p. 386)
delusions (p. 387)

derealization (dē-RĔ-l-ĭ-ZĂ-shun) (p. 392)
dyskinesia (DĬS-kĭ-NĒ-zhă) (p. 395)
dystonia (dĭs-TŌ-nē-ă) (p. 395)
extrapyramidal (ĔKS-tr-pĭ-RĂM-ĭ-dăl) **side effects** (EPSEs) (p. 395)
hallucinations (hă-LOO-sĭ-NĂ-shunz) (p. 387)
ideas of reference (p. 391)
illusions (p. 392)
laryngeal-pharyngeal (lă-RĬN-jē-ăl fă-RĬN-jē-ăl) **dystonia** (p. 395)
negative symptoms (p. 387)

neuroleptic malignant (NOOR-ō-LĔP-tĭk mă-LĬG-nănt)
    syndrome (NMS) (p. 396)
oculogyric (ŎK-yoo-lō-JĪ-rĭk) **crisis** (p. 396)
perseveration (pĕr-SĔV-ăr-Ā-shun) (p. 390)
positive symptoms (p. 387)

poverty of thought (p. 390)
psychosis (sī-KŌ-sĭs) (p. 388)
schizophrenia (SKĬT-sō-FRĒ-nē-ă) (p. 388)
tardive (TĂR-dĭv) **dyskinesia** (p. 397)
torticollis (TŎR-tĭ-KŎL-ĭs) (p. 396)

A FEW FACTS ABOUT OUR BRAINS

Here are a few facts about the most interesting organ in our body—the brain—which makes us so special in the animal world.

- The human brain contains 86 billion neurons (cats have about 1 billion) (Voytek, 2013).
- There are anywhere from 1 000 to 10 000 synapses for each neuron (The Human Memory, 2020).
- There are no pain receptors in the brain, so the brain can feel no pain (Greenwald, 2012).
- The weight of the human brain is about 1.4 kg (3 lb).
- While an elephant's brain is physically larger than a human brain, the human brain is 2% of total body weight (compared to 0.15% of an elephant's brain), meaning humans have the largest brain-to-body size (Herculano-Houzel, Avelino-de-Souza, & Manger, 2014).
- At birth, your brain was almost the same size of an adult brain and contained most of the brain cells for your whole life.
- Humans continue to make new neurons throughout life in response to mental activity.
- Your brain uses 20% of the total oxygen in your body (Swaminathan, 2008).
- Sleeping at night may be the best time for your brain to consolidate all your memories from the day (Healthy Sleep, 2007).
- Lack of sleep may actually hurt your ability to create new memories (Healthy Sleep, 2007).
- Just because you do not remember your dreams does not mean that you do not dream. Everyone dreams.
- Scientists who study sleep advise that dreams almost never represent what they actually are. The unconscious mind strives to make connections with concepts you will understand, so dreams are largely symbolic representations (van der Linden, 2011).
- When we blink, our brain has the ability to fill in the brief dark period, which it is essentially unnoticed by our conscious minds, so the whole world does not go dark each time we blink (about 20 000 times a day) (German Primate Center, 2018).

BRAIN FUNCTION

Homo sapiens developed from *Homo erectus* in Africa about 500 000 years ago. It wasn't a very successful animal and at least once was on the verge of total extinction. Like all other mammals unable to live in a community of more than 60 to 80 individuals, with weak muscles, small teeth, and no

other advantages, *Homo sapiens* was losing the environment to other, more capable species.

Suddenly, about 40 000 to 50 000 years ago, something happened that drastically changed *Homo sapiens'* behaviour, allowing communities much larger than 100 individuals to thrive. *Homo sapiens* became so successful that eventually some individuals moved from Africa to populate the entire Earth, despite the obvious lack of any protection against the cold. Not only did groups of *Homo sapiens* expand out of Africa, but they were successful in eliminating all other *Homo*-related species (e.g., Neanderthalensis, Erectus, Cepranensis). We know that there was no meaningful skeletal change in the *Homo sapiens* structure during that time. Despite having advantages of big muscles and strong teeth, *Homo neanderthalensis* was wiped out with the invasion of *Homo sapiens* (Fig. 31.1).

So, what changed? Two main things were definitely new. One was the *Homo sapiens'* capacity to live in groups of more than 100 individuals. Normally, mammals have to know each other personally to understand their position in the group, thereby allowing the group to function. When the number of species in a group grows above their capacity to recognize each other and to collaborate on the basis of that personal

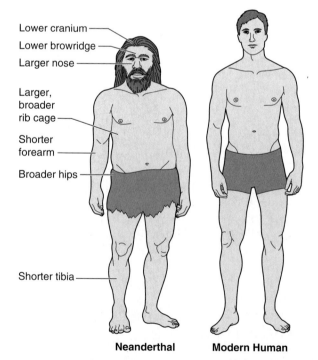

Lower cranium
Lower browridge
Larger nose
Larger, broader rib cage
Shorter forearm
Broader hips
Shorter tibia

Neanderthal   **Modern Human**

Fig. 31.1 Body structure of *Homo neanderthalensis* compared to *Homo sapiens*.

recognition, the group splits. Only *Homo sapiens* can communicate to each other about a third individual (gossip) and in that way maintain the group structure, even in huge numbers. We can develop rules and regulations to assist large populations to function. *Homo sapiens* became able to do this around 50 000 years ago. Around the same time, their population grew, and they spread toward Europe. The large number of individuals in the group allowed for better safety and hunting and, as a result, better survival.

The other thing that changed was *Homo sapiens' unique ability to think about something that does not actually exist in reality.* We can make up stories. For example, things like money, law, morals, the stock market, nationality, and legislative acts are not part of nature. We created them to make our lives better. Not only can we improve the shape of a stone in order to use that stone better, but we can create new tools and mechanisms. A pack of wolves or chimpanzees cannot decide overnight to overcome their leader and institute democracy. But *Homo sapiens* can. The first example of that capacity to make things up was the "Lion Man." The Lion Man sculpture, discovered in Germany, was found to be around 40 000 years old (Fig. 31.2). This makes it the world's earliest figurative sculpture. It depicts something that does not exist: a creature with the body of a man and the head of a lion. Around this same time, *Homo sapiens* began to spread and populate Europe.

What was striking about the Lion Man sculpture is that *Homo sapiens* had a mind capable of imagining, rather than

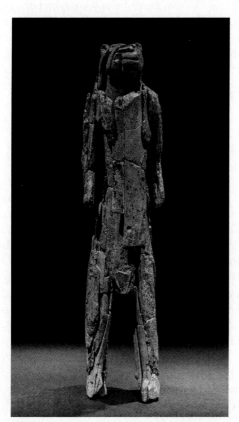

Fig. 31.2 Prehistoric Lion Man sculpture, discovered in Germany 40 000 years ago. (The Lion Man. Stadel Cave, Baden-Württemberg, Germany, 40 000 years old. The oldest known evidence of religious belief in the world. © Ulmer Museum.)

simply representing, real forms. Conservators experimented by making a replica of the Lion Man, calculating that it would take a highly skilled carver at least 400 hours using flint tools (2 months' work in daylight). This means that the carver would have had to be looked after by hunter-gatherers, which presupposes a degree of social organization.

Thus, *Homo sapiens'* ability to think about something that does not exist is a key component of our evolutionary success. This unique ability is the result of our unique brain. At the same time, some of this ability may also be the source for such serious conditions as psychosis. This chapter will explore the basic aspects of this condition and describe diseases related to psychosis.

Normal Brain Function

Our brain information processing and storage are very complicated processes with complex mechanisms. Their full explanation is not a goal of this book. Instead, what follows is a brief description to quickly equip the reader with some basic principles. We hope that the understanding of these principles will help the reader better understand the suffering of a person who has a psychosis and understand how to help to diminish that suffering.

Our brain has many cells. Some are called *neurons*. Each neuron has short branches called *dendrites* and may have one or two long branches called *axons*. The small space between two branches of two or more neurons is called a *synapse*. The information travels inside the branches to the synapse. Within the synapse, the information is transmitted by chemicals called *neurotransmitters*.

Perceptions

From outside our body, information comes to us through our external receptors in different organs: eyes (vision), ears (hearing and balance), nose (smell), mouth (taste), and skin (touch and temperature). This information makes its way to the corresponding brain centre. From the eyes it goes to the vision centre, from the ears it goes to the hearing centre, and so forth.

When a signal reaches the corresponding centre, the centre always tries to compare that signal with already stored codes in our memory and give that new information some meaning. Is that object an apple, a dog, a table, or something else? The information from our internal organs (mostly pain and pressure) is treated in the same way as external information: signals are checked with the memory and sent for quick interpretation by the frontal lobe. In evolutionary terms, the most important thing that these centres can do is to send a message to the frontal lobe (the command centre) as soon as possible. The frontal lobe should alert us of any danger. The speed of that conclusion (to be alert and run away, or to stay peaceful) is more important than the correct meaning.

The frontal lobe needs to be able to identify risk as soon as possible, rather than find out exactly what object caused that risk. For example, some sounds can immediately alarm us without us being able to identify what they are exactly. We can recognize different familiar shapes in objects that have no relationship to these shapes. **Illusion** is our brain's wrong interpretation of the real object. Information comes from external receptors. The interpretation of that information goes to our command centre (frontal lobe); after having been analyzed and compared with memory, this creates our perceptions. Thus, each person's perception from the exact same external information can be different. Indeed, people perceive the same world differently.

A sound may not be heard clearly and an object may not be seen well, but our brain always tries to give meaning and an explanation to the new information, regardless of the quality or source of that information.

Thoughts

Imagine how impulses of information travel back and forth in our brain, and from our memory to our command centre, and within our command centre. These are our thoughts. Our thoughts in the command centre (frontal lobe) are responsible for our behaviour. Luckily for us, we do not need to pay active attention to most of our behaviour. This is because most of our behaviour is automatic and subconscious: We are aware of it, but not really paying attention to it. This allows us to focus attention on other things and to execute subconscious activity at the same time. Neuroplasticity is the capacity of our brain to make new and very stable synapses between different neurons, and then use these new informational highways with high speed and low effort. Among other things, neuroplasticity enables us to form memories and build new automatic behaviours and responses.

In daily life, we perform a lot of automatic—but at the same time very complex—behaviours that do not require the control of consciousness. The majority of these behaviours are the results of learning and constant repetition (e.g., brushing teeth, showering, starting and driving a car). Even stopping at a red light and crossing the intersection on a green light are autonomic, subconscious patterns of behaviour. Most of these actions are so automatic that we do not remember them. We actually master something only when we can do it automatically without thinking about each step of performance. For example, in learning how to ride a bicycle we initially focus our attention on every aspect of this activity, and then once learned, we can do it automatically. These patterns of behaviour quickly and safely help us navigate through life. Automatically, our brain picks up only necessary information from our surroundings to keep up with automatic activity. Our consciousness switches on only when we encounter a nonstandard situation that requires us to find a new and nonautomatic solution (e.g., our normal route to work was blocked, and we had to take a new route). These are examples of automatic thoughts helping us every day.

At the same time, when automatic thoughts are not adaptive anymore, they can cause serious pathology and suffering. These are automatic thoughts that helped before, but now that the environment has changed are no longer helpful. Such thoughts are called **cognitive distortions**. Following are a few typical cognitive distortions (there are many others):

- *Mental filtering* (the person sees only negative things, ignoring the positive)
- *Polarized thinking* (the person automatically decides whether the situation is completely perfect or very bad, based on very limited information)
- *Overgeneralization* (e.g., the person automatically thinks that their first failure or even a small failure will mean failure with all subsequent attempts)
- *Catastrophizing* (when a person automatically exaggerates the importance of a negative event)
- *Personalization* (the person automatically thinks that another person's behaviour somehow is directed at them or that their own behaviour directly affects other people)
- *Fallacy of fairness* (the person automatically applies the judgement of fairness to everything else)
- *Should thinking* (the person automatically thinks about how they should behave and experiences a feeling of guilt if they do not behave that way, or they think about how other people should behave, and then experience anger when they do not behave as expected)
- *Emotional reasoning* (the person automatically thinks that things are the way they feel them)

These thoughts use limited information or clues to quickly alert us about a specific danger. However, when the situation changes and in reality there is no danger, this same limited information with small clues from the environment continues to produce alarming automatic thoughts.

Clinicians use cognitive-behavioural therapy (CBT) to correct automatic and maladaptive thoughts and behaviours like this. This type of therapy switches consciousness back on and destroys the stereotypes and automatic thoughts. From the point of view of neuroplasticity, the result of such therapy would be some deactivation of these super-highways. This process forces thoughts to go slower and occur more consciously, bringing about more accurate and therefore more adaptive information.

To illustrate neuroplasticity and CBT, imagine the pathway that a rabbit makes on the grass. It runs back and forth on the same path day after day. Perhaps this is the shortest distance to food, or there is more food along the way. Over time, the pathway in the grass makes that run easy and automatic. This is an analogy for how cognitive distortion also works. Even if occasionally danger comes close to that pathway, the rabbit will continue to run along that exact pathway again. Now using this pathway will be maladaptive. To avoid encountering danger, the rabbit must practise running through the grass in different directions, consciously choosing a different way each day. If he does this, the old pathway will gradually disappear. This is how neuroplasticity can be changed using CBT. When new danger is encountered the next time, the rabbit will be able to choose the safest way to run away, and the brain will be able to choose a different response.

Abnormal Brain Function

Earlier in this chapter, we saw how the brain applies meaning to external or internal information imperfectly and how maladaptive automatic thoughts can be. There are two other domains in which problems can arise: problems related to conduction of information within the neuron, and problems related to the functioning of synapses. Here, we will focus on the second group of problems: functioning of synapses. We will emphasize a specific neurotransmitter that is used for the conduction of thoughts and perceptions, called *dopamine.* This chemical is released in the junction (synapse) between branches of neurons. Molecules of dopamine are released from the branch of the first neuron. They become attached to the receptors for dopamine on the branch of the second neuron. When enough receptors on the second neuron are occupied, it causes that neuron to fire and conduct an electromagnetic field from that junction to its next junction. At the next junction that second neuron releases molecules of dopamine, causing a third neuron to act, and so on, as the information continues to flow.

Malfunction may occur when the first neuron releases no dopamine, but for some reason there is still dopamine in that junction between the branches. Those unplanned molecules of dopamine attach to the receptors of the second neuron, causing it to initiate electrical activity. When this happens to many neurons, *a massive amount of information is created in the system without coming from the real internal or external world.* Essentially, this can be thought of as meaningless information. If this happens in the frontal lobe, initially, it generates some anxiety because the brain feels something but cannot identify it. There is some information flowing but it does not match anything known and thus has no meaning. Only after some time is that meaningless information crystalizing into a firm thought. The origin of that thought does not come from reality or from a person's memory but from activity created by malfunctions in brain synapses.

Positive Symptoms

For the person experiencing this type of thought, created from initially meaningless information generated as a result of dopamine malfunction, it is as natural as all other thoughts. These types of thoughts are called *delusions.* Delusions are a core concept of psychopathology. While they play a serious role in the diagnosis of a disorder, their definition remains rather ambiguous, as a delusion is a very multifaced phenomenon. **Delusions** are thoughts that do not come from the person's cultural background (religious, political views, culture, and subculture), and it is impossible to convince the person of them being wrong (American Psychiatric Association [APA], 2013, p. 819).

When describing a person's delusion, it is important to avoid generalization (e.g., using terms such as *paranoid, grandiose, bizarre*). The correct way to describe a delusion in clinical documentation is to use the person's own words, (e.g., Mark reported that he is "waiting for the people of South Africa to call him and ask to be their president." He believes that he will be "a great president." He informed me that he is spending his time "preparing himself for that role.").

If dopamine malfunctions in synapses happen on the path of audio information that travels from the ear to the audio centre in the brain, this forces the brain to come up with an audio explanation for the meaningless information. The person is convinced that they hear something. All of our perceptions—visual, audio, smell, taste, and touch—can be compromised in this way. These interpretations of the brain's internal malfunctions as real perceptions, without any external stimulus, are called *perceptual abnormalities* or **hallucinations**.

At times, malfunctioning of the dopamine system and subsequent meaningless information moving throughout the system cause challenges with the flow of original thought. Thoughts become disorganized and may present as disorganized speech. In other cases, the same dopamine system malfunction may not exhibit as delusions, hallucinations, or disorganized speech and may stay undetected. The person may simply not talk, and an observer will not register delusions, hallucination, or disorganized speech. What still can be observed, however, is extremely disorganized behaviour or total lack of movement (**catatonia**).

Delusions, hallucinations, disorganized speech, and disorganized behaviour are called **positive symptoms**; we call them "positive" because they add something to the person's presentation.

The capability that makes us unique in the animal world, creativity (our ability to think about something that does not exist), the one that gave us the enormous advantage discussed at the beginning of this chapter, most probably is the same one that is responsible for delusions: excessive dopamine activity in the synapses. Thus it can be very hard to distinguish clearly between creativity and delusions, especially in art. We can judge some individuals' behaviours as being "delusional" and at the same time see their art or scientific work as genius.

Negative Symptoms

The automatic thoughts discussed above are also compromised during psychosis, creating a serious functional challenge for the person who suffers from it. The informational highways that helped a person react to their environment and do many things are now automatically overloaded with meaningless information. Activities that required no effort in the past are now almost impossible to execute. (For example, try to imagine what it would take for you to brush your teeth without doing it automatically but thinking about each step: stand up, recall where the bathroom is, go there, recall where the toothpaste is, pick it up, recall where the toothbrush is, pick it up, recall that the toothpaste must be opened, open it, recall that it must be squeezed—tired already?)

People with psychosis may have a significant *decline in their activities of daily living (ADLs).* Their emotional response is decreased, and they may experience *avolition* (extreme difficulty with initiating any purposeful activity), **alogia** (diminished speech output), *anhedonia* (decreased ability to experience pleasure), and *asociality* (lack of interest in social interactions). All of these symptoms are called **negative symptoms**. We call them "negative" because they take away from the person's presentation.

Cognitive Symptoms

Some sources identify cognitive symptoms as separate from positive and negative symptoms. These are associated with gibberish information affecting cognition, which can *decrease a person's capacity to concentrate, reason, and form memories.*

Psychosis

The combination of all of the above groups of symptoms (positive, negative, and cognitive) usually leads to an impaired assessment of reality, which is called **psychosis**. This can be a very complex condition that has a variety of clinical presentations. There are many actions or situations that can result in psychosis (i.e., for the brain to produce meaningless information, causing delusions and hallucinations). Some of these include the use of street drugs that affect dopamine production or that act in the same way as dopamine, infections that generate toxins, inflammation and immune reactions, and severe anxiety. In addition, many other medical conditions may have psychosis as a part of their clinical picture.

It is important to remember that anxiety is a very powerful mechanism for boosting the production of unnecessary dopamine. This leads to more meaningless information in the system, increasing the intensity of the psychosis. Thus, *anxiety contributes to the intensity of psychosis.* A calm environment, reassurance of safety, and a trustful relationship with staff are the best nonpharmaceutical tools to support a patient who suffers from psychosis.

THE SCHIZOPHRENIA SPECTRUM

In this chapter, we review schizophrenia and other psychotic disorders. Together with *schizotypal personality disorder* (discussed in Chapter 30), these comprise the schizophrenia spectrum group of disorders. This group is characterized by the presence of positive and negative symptoms. Besides schizophrenia and schizotypal personality, it includes the following: delusional disorder, brief psychotic disorder, schizophreniform disorder, schizoaffective disorder, substance/medication-induced psychotic disorder, psychotic disorder due to another medical condition, catatonia associated with another mental disorder, catatonic disorder due to another medical condition, unspecified catatonia, other specified schizophrenia spectrum and other psychotic disorder, unspecified specified schizophrenia spectrum, and other psychotic disorder. All are discussed in more detail in the next sections.

Delusional Disorder

A *delusional disorder* is characterized by more than 1 month of nonbizarre (reality-based) fixed ideas. The person is able to carry out ADLs, but holds fast to the delusion. Often delusions involve being followed, poisoned, or having their thoughts controlled.

Brief Psychotic Disorder

A *brief psychotic disorder* is a psychotic disturbance that lasts for more than 1 day but less than 1 month. Individuals have delusions, hallucinations, impaired functioning and speech, and disorganized behaviour. They eventually return to their normal state. The episode may have been triggered by negative and positive stressors. For example, it can be triggered by grief or by getting married. It can be triggered by the combination of physical, emotional, and hormonal stress (e.g., having given birth).

Schizophreniform Disorder

A schizophreniform disorder is a schizophrenia-like condition in which a patient suffers from psychosis for more than 1 month but fully recovers for less than 6 months. Thus, from the timeline perspective, it falls between a brief psychotic episode and schizophrenia.

Schizophrenia

Schizophrenia is a condition in which at least two of the criteria listed below are present for the significant portion of a 1-month period of time (unless treated). Among these conditions, criteria 1, 2, or 3 *must* be present:

1. Delusions
2. Hallucinations
3. Disorganized speech
4. Grossly disorganized or catatonic behaviour
5. Negative symptoms

These conditions are responsible for at least 6 months of significant disturbances in major areas of life, such as self-care, work, and relationships (APA, 2013, p. 99).

Nearly 100 year ago, Kurt Schneider, a German psychiatrist, identified a few very specific psychotic symptoms that lead to a quick diagnosis of schizophrenia. Although those symptoms are not official diagnostic criteria, they can be used as red flags for clinicians. Given the importance of these symptoms, these are called "first rank symptoms":

- *Auditory hallucinations*—The person hears their own thoughts. This can be in the form of comments regarding their own behaviour.
- *Thought withdrawal*—The person feels that their thoughts are taken away or controlled by some external authority.
- *Thought broadcasting*—The person feels that their thoughts can go outside of their head and be read by other people.
- *Somatic hallucinations*—The person feels hallucinations regarding body sensations.
- *Delusional perception*—A true perception, to which a person attributes false meaning.
- *Made volitional acts*—The person is certain that their actions or feelings are caused not by themselves but by somebody else or another force.
- *Voices arguing*—The person experiences an audio hallucination, hearing multiple people arguing.

Insight

The schizophrenic person's lack of insight involves unawareness of the symptoms of schizophrenia. Unawareness of symptoms can occur throughout the entire course of illness and is a major predictor of nonadherence to treatment, a high number of involuntary admissions, a high rate of relapses, aggression, and poor outcomes. This lack of insight is not a coping mechanism but rather one of the symptoms of schizophrenia. It is comparable to the lack of awareness of neurological deficits following brain damage, termed *anosognosia*.

Development and Course

Onset of schizophrenia prior to adolescence is rare. The first psychotic episode usually occurs in the early to mid-20s for males and in the late 20s for females. Late onset (after age 40) is rare and mostly occurs in females. Usually, an earlier onset is associated with a worse prognosis. This pattern especially affects males, leading to the prominence of negative symptoms and cognitive impairment even before the development of the first psychotic episode. The cognitive impairment may become stable and remain, even when all other symptoms are in remission. The onset can be abrupt, but the majority of people start to suffer gradually from different clinical signs, mostly depressive symptoms.

In the *prodromal phase,* individuals are usually quiet, passive, and obedient, and they prefer to be alone. They have few or no friends because of their odd, suspicious, or eccentric behaviours. Hallucinations and delusions may be present, but behaviours are not completely disorganized at this point. Family members may report that they can sense the individual "slipping away" in front of their eyes.

Signs, symptoms, and behaviours during the *acute phase* vary widely but include disturbances in thought, perception, behaviour, and emotion. Frequently, individuals lose contact with reality and become unable to function even in the most basic ways.

The *residual phase* follows an acute episode. It is marked by a lack of energy, no interest in goal-directed activities, and a negative outlook. Many of the behaviours seen in the prodromal phase are also present during the residual phase.

After the residual phase, there is a period of relative *remission.* The ability to manage some basic ADLs returns, and the individual experiences some relief from the distresses of psychosis. The course of schizophrenia alternates between acute episodes and periods of decreased symptoms.

Unfortunately, the majority of people with schizophrenia will require some level of support during their lives. They will experience periods of exacerbation and remission. Psychotic symptoms will diminish with time, possibly because of the decline in dopamine activity with advancing age. Negative symptoms tend to persist.

Prevalence

The lifetime prevalence of schizophrenia 0.3–0.7%. Births during late winter and early spring are more prevalent among people with schizophrenia, with males suffering a bit more than females. Females tend to have a later onset, with more positive mood and symptoms, and tend to have a better outcome.

Suicide Risk

Around 5% of people with schizophrenia die by suicide, and about 20 to 40% attempt suicide at least once (APA, 2013;

Fuller-Thomson & Hollister, 2016). Many more have suicidal ideations.

Aggression

Aggression and some sort of hostility can be associated with schizophrenia, but spontaneous or random assaults are uncommon. Aggression is mostly associated with young males, lack of adherence to treatment, history of violence, and substance abuse. The majority of people with schizophrenia are not aggressive and are victims of aggression and abuse more often than those in the general population.

Interview Tips and Strategies for Patients With Schizophrenia

There are two general interview approaches to use with people who suffer from schizophrenia:

1. Purposefully explore the entire psychosis region in one interview section.
2. Explore the psychosis in little bits, as the patient spontaneously raises it.

Following are some examples of specific questions that could be asked for gracefully raising the topic of psychosis:

- "When you are feeling really bad, do your thoughts ever get so painful that they sound like a voice to you?"
- "Have you ever had experiences or thoughts that seems odd to you or perhaps even frightening?"
- "Do you sometimes have thoughts or feelings that seem almost like you are having nightmares while you are awake?"
- "Do you sometimes feel like you have special talents that others do not have, like the ability to read minds or send your thoughts into other people's minds?"

Uncovering Dangerous Psychotic Process

Some symptoms of psychosis may lead a person to act violently. Clinicians may uncover the potential for the dangerous behaviour and act to ensure the safety and security for all (which may include providing a person with antipsychotic medication before their psychosis discharges in a dangerous way).

There are three main scenarios that are associated with an increased risk of aggression or violence in patients who have a psychosis (Scott & Resnick, 2013):

1. *Command auditory hallucinations* (negative voices, talking in the third person). It is important to determine the following about the patient's hallucinations:
   - Whether they are dangerous or not dangerous (i.e., do they pose a danger to the patient or to others?)
   - The intensity of the hallucinations
   - The degree of control of the hallucinations and their closeness to the patient
2. *Alien control* (usually via some kind of technology) (see the Case Study that follows): This is the type of delusion where a person believes that some external force controls their behaviour. The risk is high when such "control" is accompanied by a threat. This is also called "threat/control-override symptoms" (Nederlof, Muris, & Hovens, 2011).

3. *Hyperreligious ideation:* These are particularly dangerous during the postpartum period of psychotic depression because they may lead to filicide (child killing by a parent) (Knabb, Welsh, & Graham Howardat, 2012).

These three psychotic processes most often include an intent to act violently against the self or others. People are typically open about these delusions and their plans "to protect" themselves, "religion," or the "whole world." They should be taken very seriously. Uncovering and monitoring the intensity of these delusions on an ongoing basis allow proactive intervention, diminish suffering, and ensure safety for both staff and patients.

Following are some examples of questions the clinician can ask a patient to uncover dangerous psychotic processes:
- "Do you feel a need to protect yourself?"
- "Have you needed to take actions against somebody who tried to harm you?"

If any danger to staff or patients is identified, proactive intervention should occur in two domains: environmental and medical. The staff must ensure immediate safety. Depending on the situation, this can include a range of activities, starting with simply establishing an increased distance between the staff and the patient until mechanical restraints can be applied (as a last resort). That action must be followed by pharmacological antipsychotic intervention to decrease the intensity of delusions and diminish the suffering of the person experiencing the psychosis. These actions must be carried out proactively and before a patient acts on their delusions. (The difference between emergency pharmacological intervention and chemical restraint is described further below.) Thus, uncovering these delusions along with constant active monitoring of their intensity, especially during the active phase of the disease, is a high priority for staff.

CASE STUDY

Rob was a model child, cooperative, pleasant, and enjoyable—until he turned 17 years old. It all seemed to start when he began a campaign to see every science fiction movie ever made. Soon he was speaking an "interplanetary space language" that no one other than himself could understand.

About 6 months into his outer space-oriented lifestyle, Rob quit school and began to spend his days "attending intergalactic conferences of great minds." His family became worried when Rob refused to bathe or change his clothes for weeks at a time. Often, they would enter the room to find Rob arguing animatedly with the lamp or listening with interest to the wall. When an outburst of unprovoked anger resulted in injuries to his younger sister, the family sought counselling.

- What do you think is the family's first priority with Rob?
- What do you think would be the mental health care team's first priority?
- What signs do you think would indicate a need for an inpatient psychiatric setting?

CULTURAL CONSIDERATIONS

In India, a man with schizophrenia is often considered a "wise man" because of his ability to speak with spirits. He is usually honored and sought out for his advice.

In Haiti, many people believe that humans can communicate with spirits and deities (gods) and have religious ceremonies to induce spirit possession. The group considers being possessed not as a shameful experience but as a privilege. Psychotic persons are believed to be victims of the "evil eye," called maldyok, or to be possessed by supernatural beings. Their behaviour is tolerated by members of the community, but they are expected to consult native healers "who treat with amulets, packets of herbs and spices, liquids, baths, powders, rubbing, and massage" (Giger & Davidhizar, 2020).

Speech Disturbances

Language difficulties involve incorrect usage. Speech includes a number of unusual characteristics: clang associations, concrete thinking, echolalia, flight of ideas, loose associations, ideas of reference, mutism, pressured speech, neologisms, verbigeration, and word salad. Table 31.1 explains each term and provides an example of each communication difficulty.

Other Characteristics of Schizophrenia: Clinical Picture

Thought processes in people with schizophrenia vary widely, from contact with reality to fantasy thinking. Negative experiences are remembered more than positive ones. Individuals may demonstrate **perseveration**, the repeating of the same idea in response to different questions, or **poverty of thought**, a lack of ability to produce new thoughts or follow a train of thought. People with chronic schizophrenia have little insight into their problems. Often their judgment is impaired. Usually there is a general decline in intellectual abilities as the disorder progresses.

In the emotional realm, persons with schizophrenia experience a range of inappropriate emotions. *Affect,* the outward expression of one's emotions, is described as blunted, flat, inappropriate, or labile. Other emotional responses include **alexithymia**, a difficulty in identifying and describing emotions; **apathy**, a lack of concern, interest, or feelings; and **anhedonia**, the inability (or decreased ability) to experience pleasure in life.

Behaviourally, individuals with schizophrenia display little impulse control and an inability to manage anger. They may injure themselves and others or act in response to hallucinations commanding them to do something. A lack of energy or motivation (avolition) often leads to poor performance at work or school, unemployment, and homelessness. The inability to cope with depression, added to a lack of social supports, leads to a high risk for suicide. Many patients refuse to adhere to treatment by not taking their medications. Others abuse alcohol and street drugs. Such individuals with concurrent disorders can present many challenging health care situations.

TABLE 31.1 Speech Disturbances in Schizophrenia

Speech Problem	Description
Clang associations	Repeating words or phrases that sound alike or substituting a word that sounds like the appropriate word *Example:* "Honey, money, sunny" or "I need some honey to buy the paper."
Concrete thinking	Inability to consider the abstract meaning of a phrase; frequently tested by having patients interpret proverbs *Example:* "A stitch in time saves nine" may mean "sew the holes in your clothes" to a person with schizophrenia.
Echolalia	Repeating words of another after one has stopped talking *Example:* Nurse: "How is your day going?" Patient: "Day going, day going, day going."
Flight of ideas	Rapid change in topics with a rapid flow of speech *Example:* "The sky is blue. The dog is dead, and I have two eyes."
Ideas of reference	The belief that some events have special personal meaning *Example:* "The United States is sending satellites into space so that they can spy on me."
Loose associations	Thinking characterized by speech that moves from one unrelated idea to another *Example:* "I'm hungry, but the desert has no rain so it's cold outside."
Mutism	Refusal to speak
Neologisms	Words or expression invented by the individual *Example:* "The ispy is not happy when the fulgari is green."
Verbigeration	Purposeless repetition of phrases *Example:* Patient repeats for days: "Prepare to launch the orbiter."
Pressured speech	Rapid, forced speech *Example:* "I must prepare. There's no time to waste. Can't talk now."
Word salad	A random, jumbled set of words that have no connection or relationship to one another *Example:* "Hot happies are spying on me but no men love short feet."

Socially, persons with schizophrenia are usually unable to establish or maintain relationships with others. Self-esteem is low, and gender identity confusion may exist. They tend to have few friends and little interest in hobbies or other activities. Social behaviours are often inappropriate. Many prefer to be alone because of hallucinations or feelings of paranoia. The few family and social relationships that do exist usually follow a rocky course. Refer to Table 31.2 and review the description of symptoms of schizophrenia.

CRITICAL THINKING

The prodromal negative signs and symptoms of schizophrenia often begin in adolescence. As the teen's behaviour becomes more bizarre and positive signs appear at the beginning of their 20s, friends and family become uncomfortable with and afraid of the individual, so they respond by limiting their interactions with the person.
- What are the perceptions about people who are unable to share reality?
- How do people react to a close friend who was diagnosed with schizophrenia?
- How should one cope with being afraid of someone whose behaviours are out of contact with reality?

Schizoaffective Disorder

Schizoaffective disorder is diagnosed when depression or mania is also present. Patients show signs of a mood disorder as well as schizophrenia. Usually the moods of people with schizophrenia are flat and unreactive. Persons with schizoaffective disorder, however, experience changes in mood. The disorganized behaviours of schizophrenia are still present, and emotions may move from depression to elation. A person must also have at least one episode of delusions or hallucinations for 2 or more weeks in the absence of a major mood change. The prognosis for schizoaffective disorder is better than for schizophrenia (APA, 2013, p. 105).

Substance/Medication-Induced Psychotic Disorder

Persons with substance/medication-induced psychotic disorder experience delusions, hallucinations, or both and have evidence of substance intoxication or withdrawal.

Psychotic Disorder Due to a Medical Condition

Persons with psychotic disorder due to a medical condition experience delusions, hallucinations, or both and have evidence that these are the consequences of another medical condition.

Catatonia Associated With a Mental Disorder

The essence of any catatonia is a psychomotor disturbance that significantly changes motor activity and engagement. The change usually involves a decrease in activity and engagement, but it can also involve an increase. Therefore, catatonia can be challenging to recognize and diagnose. During the particularly active phase, a person may be in need of supervision to avoid self-harm or harm to others and to ensure proper nutrition.

TABLE 31.2 Clinical Symptoms of Schizophrenia

Perceptual	Intellectual	Emotional	Behavioural	Social
Hallucinations: May be commanding; content can match delusions 1. Auditory 2. Visual 3. Tactile: For example, may feel surrounded by spider webs 4. Olfactory and gustatory: May refuse to eat because food smells or tastes bad 5. Tactile **Illusions**: False perceptions because of misinterpretations of real objects **Altered internal sensations:** 1. Formication: Sensation of worms crawling around inside 2. Chill: Feeling of chills in the marrow of one's bones **Agnosia:** Failure to recognize familiar environmental stimuli such as sounds or objects seen or felt; sometimes called "negative hallucinations" **Distortion of body image:** Relating to size, facial expression, activity, detail, exaggeration, or diminution of body parts **Negative self-perception:** Relating to ability and competence	**Delusions:** Unusual ideas, not reality based: 1. Omnipotence 2. Persecution 3. Control **Derealization:** Loss of ego boundaries; cannot tell where own body ends and environment begins; feeling that the world around one is not real **Ideas of reference:** Notion that other people or the media are talking to or about one **Errors in recall of memory:** Caused by incorrect categorization **Difficulty sustaining attention:** 1. Unable to complete tasks 2. Errors of omission **Incorrect use of language:** 1. Neologisms (invented words) 2. Incoherence, verbigeration 3. Echolalia, word salad 4. Concrete, restricted vocabulary 5. Poor comprehension 6. Loose associations **Flight of ideas:** Abrupt change of topic in a rapid flow of speech	**Labile affect:** Range of emotions: 1. Apathy, dulled response 2. Flattened affect 3. Reduced responsiveness 4. Exaggerated euphoria 5. Rage **Inappropriate affect:** Laughing at sad events, crying over joyous ones **Disruption in limbic functioning:** Inability to screen out disruptive stimuli and loss of voluntary control of response	**Little impulse control:** 1. Sudden scream as a protest of frustration 2. Injury to a body part believed to be offensive 3. Responds to command hallucinations **Inability to manage anger:** Anger and lack of impulse control lead to violence: verbal aggression, destruction of property, injury, homicide **Substance abuse:** Dulls painful psychological symptoms **Nonadherence to medication:** Lack of insight	**Poor peer relationships:** 1. Few friends as a child or teen 2. Preference for solitude **Low interest in hobbies and activities:** 1. Daydreamer 2. Not functioning well in social or occupational areas 3. Preoccupied and detached 4. Behavioural autism **Loss of interest in appearance:** 1. Careless grooming 2. Introversion **Not competitive in sports or academics:** 1. Poor adjustment to school 2. Withdrawal from activities **May suffer from:** 1. Attention deficit–hyperactivity disorder 2. Somatic symptoms

Modified from Fortinash, K. M., & Holoday-Worret, P. A. (2011). *Psychiatric mental health nursing* (5th ed.). Mosby.

Catatonia can be associated with a mental disorder or with other medical conditions, including neurodevelopmental, autoimmune, and others. Each time catatonia is diagnosed, it must be indicated with which mental or medical condition it is associated.

To diagnose this disturbance, at least 3 of the following 12 psychomotor features must be present (APA, 2013, p. 119):

1. *Stupor*—no psychomotor activity at all
2. *Catalepsy*—fixated prolonged passive body position or posture
3. *Waxy flexibility*—tendency to remain in immobile position; attempt to change that position by an examiner will face a resistance
4. *Mutism*—no or very little verbal response
5. *Negativism*—oppositional or no response to simple instructions
6. *Posturing*—spontaneous and active maintenance of the body against gravity
7. *Mannerism*—a very bizarre, almost caricatural and repeated movement or action
8. *Stereotypy*—repetitive, frequent, and non–goal-directed movements
9. *Agitation*—serious agitation with no external stimuli
10. *Grimacing*—making a face that looks like one is in pain or shows other facial expressions without stimuli
11. *Echolalia*—mimicking another person's speech
12. *Echopraxia*—mimicking another person's movements

TABLE 31.3 Criteria for Involuntary Admission and Community Options

Jurisdiction	Definition of Mental Disorder	Harm Criterion	Deterioration as Alternative to Harm	Need for Treatment	Incapable of Treatment Decision	CTO/ Leave
British Columbia	Specific	Broad	Yes	Yes	No	Leave
Alberta	Specific	Broad	Yes	No	No	CTO
Saskatchewan	Specific	Broad	Yes	Yes	Yes	CTO
Manitoba	Specific	Broad	Yes	Yes	No	Leave
Ontario	Broad	Bodily	Yes (partial)	No for bodily harm Yes for deterioration	No for bodily harm Yes for deterioration	CTO & Leave
Quebec	Broad	Bodily	No	No	No	CTO
Nova Scotia	Specific	Broad	Yes	Yes	Yes	CTO
New Brunswick	Specific	Broad	No	No	No	No
Prince Edward Island	Specific	Broad	No	No	No	Leave
Newfoundland	Specific	Broad	Yes	Yes	Yes	CTO
Yukon	Specific	Bodily	No	No	No	Leave
Northwest Territories/ Nunavut	Specific	Bodily	No	No	No	No

CTO, community treatment order. CTO jurisdictions also provide for leave.
Data from Gray, J. E., Hastings, T. J., Love, S., & O'Reilly, R. L. (2016). Clinically significant differences among Canadian mental health acts, 2016. *Canadian Journal of Psychiatry, 61*(4), 222–226. https://www.ncbi.nlm.nih.gov/pmc/articles/PMC4794956/

Catatonic Disorder Due to a Medical Condition

This disorder is diagnosed in the same manner as catatonia, but there is evidence that the catatonia is associated with a particular medical condition.

Unspecified Catatonia

With unspecified catatonia, the person has clinically severe distress but presents some, but not all, of the criteria for catatonia. There is also no known underlying mental or medical condition, or there is not sufficient information.

Other Specified Schizophrenia Spectrum and Other Psychotic Disorder

The patient has significant distress in the main aspects of their life due to schizophrenia spectrum symptoms, but these do not meet the full criteria of any of the above-listed conditions. This diagnosis is used when a clinician chooses to specify why this condition does not meet any of schizophrenia spectrum disorders.

Unspecified Schizophrenia Spectrum and Other Psychotic Disorder

This diagnosis is the same as above, but the clinician chooses not to communicate the reason why this condition does not meet any of the criteria for schizophrenia spectrum disorders.

THERAPEUTIC INTERVENTIONS

Because of impaired judgement and the lack of insight, many individuals with schizophrenia do not voluntarily try to receive treatment. Thus, often an admission is involuntary. (The criteria for involuntary admission are different in different Canadian jurisdictions, as outlined in Table 31.3). The treatment is most often provided by a multidisciplinary mental health care team. The core team consists of psychiatrists, nurses, psychologists, and psychiatric social workers. Dietitians, occupational therapists, recreational therapists, medical general practitioners, pharmacists, and spiritual advisors may join the team, when needed.

Individuals are admitted to an inpatient unit during acute psychotic episodes, when they are a danger to themselves or others, or for stabilization of disorganized or inappropriate behaviours or to diminish their suffering from psychotic symptoms. The goals of inpatient care are to *stabilize the patient, prevent further decline* in functioning, and *assist the patient in coping* with the disorder. Long-term goals include psychosocial and vocational rehabilitation. When available, family members are included in the care and education of the patient.

Treatments and Therapies

Patients with acute psychoses are treated with a combination of therapies and medications. The multidisciplinary treatment team may recommend social skills training, supported housing and employment, and vocational rehabilitation, in addition to personal, family, or behavioural therapy. Stress reduction and early interventions are also important in the treatment of schizophrenia. Commonly used psychotherapies include the following:

- *Cognitive-behavioural therapy (CBT)* to identify and change ineffective patterns of thinking and behaviour

- *Cognitive enhancement therapy (CET)* to "a combination of computer based brain training and group sessions" (National Alliance on Mental Illness [NAMI], 2016) to organize thoughts and increase intellectual (cognitive) functions
- *Supportive therapy* to teach patients how to live with psychosis in more healthy ways
- *Family psychoeducation* and support to help teach individuals and their families how to bond, problem-solve, collaborate, and learn from each other

Psychotherapies may focus on different areas of treatment, but each relies on the patient's willingness to work and the therapeutic interactions with care providers.

Pharmacological Therapy

Medications used to treat psychosis are called *antipsychotic* or *neuroleptic medications* (listed in Table 31.4). The main function of the medication is to penetrate the blood–brain barrier (BBB) and to attach itself to the receptors of the postsynaptic neurons. Unlike dopamine, this attachment generates no further activity for that neuron; the "gibberish information" from the presynaptic (first) neuron will be not able to go toward that second neuron. This is because molecules of dopamine released by the first neuron will not find a place to attach to the second neuron. Thus, molecules of the medication and those of dopamine compete for the attachment to receptors. Having a stronger *affinity* (the likelihood to attach to a receptor and stay), molecules of medication win this competition. The result is a diminishing intensity of psychosis, but also various adverse effects when medication blocks other receptors that should keep working. One of the goals of any new antipsychotic medication is to be as selective and specific as possible and target only those receptors that need to be blocked.

Antipsychotic medications slow the central nervous system (CNS). These effects include an emotional quieting, slowed motor responses, and sedation. Antipsychotics exert their influence on the body by interrupting the dopamine (neurotransmitter) pathways in the brain, thus producing a calming effect throughout the entire nervous system. After an antipsychotic medication is taken, hallucinations and delusions decrease, thought processes change, and hyperactivity subsides. Mental clouding clears, and previously withdrawn people begin to socialize.

Antipsychotic medications interact with many other chemicals. When used in combination with other medications, an enhanced effect is produced that increases CNS depression. The adverse effects and reactions of these medications are numerous and can be troublesome for the patient. Refer to "Antipsychotic (Neuroleptic) Medications" in Chapter 7 for a discussion of adverse effects and adverse reactions.

Nursing (Therapeutic) Process

Caring for patients with psychoses requires a team effort. First, a thorough physical and mental assessment is obtained. Histories include a description of the patient's most distressing problems and a complete review of systems if the patient is able to communicate appropriately. Interpersonal relationships and support systems are also explored when possible.

The mental status examination is performed (see Chapter 9). Risks for violence and suicide are assessed, and a past medication history is taken (see "Uncovering Dangerous Psychotic Processes" earlier in the chapter). Box 31.1 provides several important general principles for working with patients with schizophrenia and other forms of psychoses.

The basic goals of care are to assist patients in controlling their symptoms and achieving the highest possible level of functioning. For this to happen, patients and their families

TABLE 31.4 Medications Used to Treat Psychosis (Antipsychotics)

Class	Examples
Typical antipsychotics	chlorpromazine (once marketed as Largactil) flupenthixol (Fluanxol) afluphenazine (Modecate) haloperidol (Haldol) loxapine (Loxapac) perphenazine (Trilafon) pimozide (Orap) trifluoperazine (Stelazine) thiothixene (Navane) zuclopenthixol (Clopixol)
Atypical antipsychotics	risperidone (Risperdal) quetiapine (Seroquel) olanzapine (Zyprexa) ziprasidone (Zeldox) paliperidone (Invega) aripiprazole (Abilify) clozapine (Clozaril)

BOX 31.1 Interventions for Patients With Psychotic Disorders

Ensure and maintain safety.
Establish a trusting interpersonal relationship.
Confirm the patient's identity.
Apply empathic listening.
Assist the patient in communication to help the patient understand and be understood.
Decrease psychosocial stressors and demanding situations.
Help the patient manage anxiety.
Encourage responsibility for self.
Promote adherence to prescribed therapeutic regimen.
Assist with activities of daily living.
Promote social interaction, if the patient is interested.
Regulate activity levels.
Encourage and praise socially acceptable behaviours.
Encourage family involvement and understanding.
Teach the patient to identify stressors and how to recognize, manage, and prevent symptoms.
Educate patient and family about adverse effects and toxic effects of antipsychotic medications.

Modified from Fortinash, K. M., & Holoday-Worret, P. A. (2011). *Psychiatric nursing care plans* (5th ed.). Mosby.

must be actively involved in the treatment. The expected outcome is for the patient to live, learn, and work at the maximum possible level of success. Short-term goals relate to keeping the patient safe, restoring adequate nutritional and rest habits, establishing and maintaining contact with reality, and fostering open communication. The Sample Patient Care Plan 31.1 describes the care for a patient with schizophrenia.

Special Considerations

Because antipsychotic medications affect the body's nervous system, they are potentially harmful chemicals. Several special assessments, interventions, and evaluations are required for patients who are receiving these powerful chemicals. Some adverse effects are harmless, and some are uncomfortable. Others are life-threatening. The most common adverse

SAMPLE PATIENT CARE PLAN 31.1 SCHIZOPHRENIA

Assessment

History Terry, a 22-year-old man, was found wandering naked in the streets talking to himself. He seems preoccupied and appears to be listening to voices. Further history is unobtainable because Terry is unable to communicate in a way that can be understood at this time.

Immediate Presentation A wild-eyed, unkempt young man who is preoccupied. Clothes are ragged and dirty. Speech is unintelligible; he carries on animated conversations with himself. Since admission, 24 hours ago, Terry has refused to eat, drink, or bathe because "someone is trying to poison" him. He is polite but responds only when addressed. No family or friends can be located.

Multidisciplinary Diagnosis

Disturbed sensory perception related to social isolation and lack of adequate support systems

Planning/Goals

Terry will communicate in a logical manner within 7 days after admission.

Terry will carry out his activities of daily living independently within 15 days after admission.

THERAPEUTIC INTERVENTIONS

Interventions	Rationale	Team Member
1. Establish therapeutic relationship; be available, listen actively; do not pass judgement.	Trust must be established if therapy is to be effective	All
2. Establish and reinforce a daily routine.	Increases security by knowing what to expect; helps refocus on the activities of daily living	Nsg, All
3. Use clear, direct statements when talking; make sure body language is in keeping with the message being sent.	Unclear or confusing communications can increase Terry's distorted perceptions	All
4. Intervene with active hallucinations; move Terry to a quiet area, focus on reality, assure patient that he will be safe, identify needs filled by the hallucination.	Decreases sensory input; helps divert attention to reality, provides reassurance; helps decrease anxiety	Nsg, All
5. Accept and support Terry's feelings and appropriate expressions of emotion.	Communicating empathy and understanding decreases anxiety.	All
6. Encourage Terry to take his medications routinely.	Medications must be taken regularly to control psychotic symptoms.	Nsg, MD
7. Utilize prn (as-needed) medication to control acute symptoms, diminish Terry's suffering, and ensure safety.	Usually, antipsychotic medication is started at a low dose and gradually increased. It can take up to 7 days to see a good effect of these scheduled medications. Thus, the use of prn medication to control acute symptoms is especially important during the beginning of the treatment.	Nsg, MD
8. Carefully monitor Terry's response to his medications.	Early recognition prevents serious adverse effects and complications from occurring.	Nsg
9. For discharge planning, explore the possibility of placement in an assisted living home.	A stable and predictable environment decreases acute psychotic episodes.	Soc Svc

Evaluation Seven days after admission, Terry stated that his hallucinations had diminished significantly in their intensity, and he is not sure if they are real anymore. Fifteen days after admission, Terry was independently eating, drinking, and performing his own activities of daily living, but he still required routine encouragement to bathe.

Critical Thinking Questions
1. How does a lack of support system influence Terry's mental illness?
2. How important is a group home for Terry after he is discharged from the inpatient environment?

A complete patient care plan includes several other diagnoses and interventions.
MD, physician; *Nsg,* nursing staff; *Soc Svc,* social services.

effects of antipsychotic medications are alterations in the CNS and peripheral nervous system functions.

CNS alterations include **extrapyramidal side effects (EPSEs)**, best described as "abnormal involuntary movement disorders [that] develop because of a medication-induced imbalance between two major neurotransmitters, dopamine and acetylcholine, in portions of the brain" (Keltner & Steele, 2018). When taking these medications, as many as 75% of patients experience EPSEs. Low-potency antipsychotics, such as chlorpromazine (Thorazine), are more likely to cause sedation and anticholinergic adverse effects (dry mouth, blurred vision, urinary retention). High-potency antipsychotics, such as haloperidol (Haldol), are less sedating and anticholinergic, but they have an increased risk for EPSEs.

EPSEs include akathisia, akinesia, dyskinesia, dystonia, and medication-induced parkinsonism. The most serious adverse effects are neuroleptic malignant syndrome and tardive dyskinesia. All these symptoms arise from a lack of the neurotransmitter dopamine in the brain and the subsequent blocking of nerve transmissions.

Akathisia is an inability to sit still. Patients experiencing akathisia report that they feel nervous and jittery or have lots of nervous energy. Assaultive behaviours can result if they are forced to remain in one position for even a short time. Many patients stop taking their medications because of these adverse effects. The best treatment for akathisia is to reduce the dose of antipsychotic medication. Nurses must be careful not to evaluate the signs and symptoms of akathisia as a worsening of the patient's psychosis. If a prn (as-needed) antipsychotic drug is administered at this time, it will cause an increase in the patient's symptoms.

Akinesia means the absence of movement, both physically and mentally. Actually, patients who are experiencing this unwanted effect demonstrate **bradykinesia** (slowing of body movements and a diminished mental state). Patients lack spontaneity and do not try to move or speak. They may assume bizarre postures and maintain them for long periods of time. These patients require careful assessment because many of the behaviours associated with EPSEs are similar to the behaviours for which the patients sought treatment. Astute care providers who routinely observe their patients' behaviours stand a better chance of distinguishing between medication-induced and psychosis-induced behaviours.

Dyskinesia is characterized by involuntary abnormal skeletal muscle movements. They are usually seen as jerking motions and sometimes seriously interfere with the patient's ability to walk and perform other voluntary movements.

Dystonia is impaired muscle tone. Dystonic reactions produce rigidity in the muscles that control gait, posture, and eye movements. When dystonia involves the muscles that control eye movements, the eyes involuntarily roll to the back of the head. This adverse effect is called **oculogyric crisis**; it is a frightening experience for the patient. Another unsettling dystonic reaction is **torticollis**, in which contracted cervical muscles force the neck into a twisted position.

The most serious and potentially life-threatening adverse effect is **laryngeal-pharyngeal dystonia**. When the muscles of the throat become rigid, the patient begins to gag, choke, and become cyanotic. Respiratory distress and asphyxia result if immediate intervention does not occur. Anticholinergic drugs are used to treat all of these reactions.

Medication-induced parkinsonism is a term used to describe a group of symptoms that mimic those of Parkinson's disease. Tremors, muscle rigidity, and difficulty with voluntary movements are seen in patients with Parkinson's disease and some individuals undergoing antipsychotic medication therapy. Other unwanted CNS effects include seizures, which can occur at any time during therapy. The medication clozapine (Clozaril) appears to be associated with a higher incidence of seizures, so patients taking this medication must be carefully monitored for signs of seizure activity.

Neuroleptic Malignant Syndrome

Neuroleptic malignant syndrome (NMS) is a potentially fatal EPSE of antipsychotic medications. The condition is poorly understood and frequently goes undiagnosed. Death can occur from respiratory failure, kidney failure, aspiration pneumonia, or pulmonary emboli. Although NMS is usually associated with high-potency antipsychotics, it can occur with many other dopamine-altering medications.

NMS occurs more often when two or more psychotherapeutic medications are combined. When lithium is used with a psychotherapeutic medication or depot (oil-based, long-acting) injections are given, patients are assessed frequently for signs of NMS. The development of NMS may occur suddenly after a single dose or after years of medication treatment. It is often associated with other extrapyramidal reactions, such as dystonia and akathisia.

Symptoms of NMS begin with a sudden change in the patient's level of consciousness and a rapid onset of rigid muscles. Often there is associated respiratory difficulty, tremors, and an inability to speak. The cardinal sign of NMS is a high body temperature. Temperatures can reach as high as 42°C, but usually range between 38° and 40°C. The temperatures of all patients receiving psychotherapeutic medications must be frequently and routinely monitored. Without intervention, the patient's physical condition declines rapidly (see Medication Alert).

! MEDICATION ALERT

Frequently monitor patients taking antipsychotics for:
- Sudden change in level of consciousness
- Rapid onset of rigid muscles
- Respiratory difficulty
- Tremors
- Inability to speak
    Cardinal sign of neuroleptic malignant syndrome (NMS):
- High body temperature (38–42°C)
    Autonomic nervous system signs and symptoms:
- Rapid, laboured respirations
- Tachycardia
- Rapid changes in blood pressure
- Increased perspiration (diaphoresis)
- Incontinence
    Central nervous system signs and symptoms:
- Sudden agitation
- Confusion
- Delirium
- Combativeness
- Rigid posturing
    Without intervention, the patient's *physical condition declines rapidly.*

BOX 31.2 Signs and Symptoms of Tardive Dyskinesia

Protrusion of the tongue (flycatcher sign)
Puffing of cheeks or tongue in cheek (bonbon sign)
Grinding of teeth, chewing, lateral jaw movements
Lip smacking, puckering
Grimacing, making faces, tics
Blinking, squinting
Impaired gag reflex (choking, aspiration)*
Shrugging of shoulders
Thrusting of pelvis
Twitching of trunk, legs, and arms
Toe movements, foot tapping
Impaired diaphragmatic movements (breathing difficulties)*

* Life-threatening symptoms.

Signs of autonomic nervous system dysfunction are evident in NMS: tachycardia, rapid changes in blood pressure, increased perspiration (diaphoresis), incontinence, and rapid, laboured respirations. CNS alterations include sudden agitation, confusion, delirium, combativeness, and rigid posturing. Severe muscle rigidity leads to tissue breakdown, an increased white blood cell count, and possible kidney failure.

No specific treatment exists for NMS. Supportive measures, including intensive respiratory care, are instituted and all medications that may have caused the development of NMS are stopped.

Subclinical (mild) cases of NMS have been reported. Care providers should suspect NMS in any patient with signs or symptoms of pneumonia or urinary tract infection. Patients who have diaphoresis, tachycardia, an elevated white blood cell count, or any muscle rigidity may be experiencing NMS. Sudden changes in consciousness should always be investigated and reported.

Those who care for patients taking psychotherapeutic medication must be aware of the potential for the development of NMS. An action as simple and routine as obtaining vital signs may save a patient's life. Do not hesitate to notify your supervisor or physician if a patient develops a sudden fever, changes in blood pressure, sudden changes in alertness, confusion, or altered levels of consciousness.

Tardive Dyskinesia

Tardive dyskinesia is a serious, irreversible adverse effect of long-term treatment. The word *tardive* means "appearing later." *Dys* means "difficult," and *kinesis* means "movement" in Greek. Therefore, the literal translation of "late difficult movement" explains the condition.

Tardive dyskinesia is a drug-induced condition that produces involuntary, repeated movements of the muscles of the face, trunk, arms, and legs. Many patients exhibit the signs of tardive dyskinesia after several months or years of medication treatment. Others develop signs and symptoms after discontinuing their medications.

After a period of antipsychotic medication use, the body attempts to compensate for the lack of dopamine by developing extra-sensitive receptors in the brain. When the brain is stimulated by dopamine, it overreacts and produces abnormal muscle movements. Older people, especially women, and those who have had a stroke are at the greatest risk for developing tardive dyskinesia, but symptoms are most severe in young men.

The signs and symptoms of tardive dyskinesia usually involve the facial muscles first. Box 31.2 lists the major signs and symptoms. Appendix B (at the end of the book) lists an assessment tool. People who experience the effects of tardive dyskinesia are frightened at their lack of control. In addition, the sight of a person engaged in these unusual movements and behaviours can be unnerving for care providers. Sensitive, caring staff can help to ease the patient's distress.

This condition is difficult to treat, and the effects are persistent. At this time, tardive dyskinesia is considered irreversible except in the very early stages. Nursing measures for tardive dyskinesia include routine assessments and measures to prevent injuries. Patients with impaired gag reflexes may require soft foods. Be sure suction devices are readily available. Teach every patient and family member how to recognize the signs and symptoms of tardive dyskinesia.

Anticholinergic Effects

Most medications are not effective for the treatment of tardive dyskinesia, but some success has been reported with the drugs bromocriptine, reserpine (Serpasil), and clonazepam. Vitamin E has been found to be effective in reducing symptoms.

Undesired effects of antipsychotic drugs also influence the peripheral nervous system. The anticholinergic effects of dry mouth, blurred vision, urinary retention, and photophobia (sensitivity to bright light) are common, especially during the first few days of therapy. Tachycardia is a more serious adverse effect and can cause sudden death.

Hypotension is another potentially serious adverse effect. Nurses must protect patients from falls during the first few weeks of therapy because the hypotensive response is greatest when patients stand or change positions suddenly. These episodes of low blood pressure cause a rapid heart rate (tachycardia) as the body attempts to adapt to a lower blood pressure. Antipsychotic medications are contraindicated in patients who have a history of low blood pressure, cardiac irregularities, or heart failure. Table 31.5 lists the major adverse effects of antipsychotic medications.

TABLE 31.5	Adverse Effects of Antipsychotic Medications, and Nursing Care
Adverse Effects	**Interventions**
Peripheral Nervous System Effects	
Constipation	Encourage high-fibre diet; increase water intake; give laxatives as ordered.
Dry mouth	Give sip of water frequently; provide sugarless hard candies, sugarless gum, and mouth rinses.
Nasal congestion	Give over-the-counter nasal decongestant if approved by physician.
Blurred vision	Advise patient to avoid potentially dangerous tasks. Reassure patient that normal vision typically returns in a few weeks when tolerance develops. Pilocarpine eyedrops can be used on a short-term basis.
Mydriasis	Advise patient to report eye pain immediately.
Photophobia	Advise patient to wear sunglasses outdoors.
Hypotension or orthostatic hypotension	Ask patient to get out of bed or chair slowly. Patient should sit on the side of the bed for 1 full minute while dangling feet, and then slowly rise. If hypotension is a problem, measure blood pressure before each dose is given.
Tachycardia	Tachycardia is usually a reflex response to hypotension. When intervention for hypotension (previously described) is effective, reflex tachycardia usually decreases. With clozapine, hold the dose if pulse rate is greater than 140 pulsations per minute.
Urinary retention	Encourage voiding whenever the urge is present. Catheterize for residual fluids. Ask patient to monitor urine output and report output to nurse. Older men with benign prostatic hypertrophy are particularly susceptible to urinary retention.
Urinary hesitation	Provide privacy, run water in the sink, or run warm water over the perineum.
Sedation	Help patient get up early and get the day started.
Weight gain	Help patient order an appropriate diet; diet pills should not be taken.
Agranulocytosis	A high incidence of agranulocytosis (1–2%) is associated with clozapine. White blood cell count (WBC) should be taken weekly.
Central Nervous System Effects	
Akathisia	Be patient and reassure patient who is "jittery" that you understand the need to move. Because akathisia is the chief cause of nonadherence to antipsychotic regimens, switching to a different class of antipsychotic drug may be necessary.
Dystonias	If a severe reaction, such as oculogyric crisis or torticollis occurs, give antiparkinson medication (e.g., benztropine mesylate [Cogentin]) or antihistamine (e.g., diphenhydramine [Benadryl]) immediately, as needed, and offer reassurance. Call physician at once to obtain an order for intramuscular administration. For less severe dystonias, notify physician when an order for an antiparkinson medication is warranted.
Drug-induced parkinsonism	Assess for the three major parkinsonism symptoms—tremors, rigidity, and bradykinesia—and report to physician. Antiparkinson medications may be indicated.
Tardive dyskinesia	Assess for signs by using the Abnormal Inventory Movement Scale. Medication holidays may help prevent tardive dyskinesia. Anticholinergic agents will worsen tardive dyskinesia. Young men taking large doses of high-potency antipsychotic medications (e.g., haloperidol) may be prescribed prophylactic antiparkinson medications.
Neuroleptic malignant syndrome (NMS)	Be alert for this *potentially fatal* adverse effect. Routinely take temperature and encourage adequate water intake in all patients on a regimen of antipsychotic medications; routinely assess for rigidity, tremor, and similar symptoms.
Seizures	Seizures occur in approximately 1% of patients receiving antipsychotic medication treatment. Clozapine causes an even higher rate, up to 5% of patients taking 600–900 mg/day. Use seizure precautions. Document and report any seizure activity.

Nursing Responsibilities

Nurses have three major responsibilities when caring for patients who are receiving antipsychotic medication therapy. The first relates to medication administration. Nurses should review the desired actions, adverse effects, and incompatibilities for each medication prescribed. If the medications are to be administered intramuscularly, a large muscle mass is chosen and the patient warned of a burning sensation on injection. It is important to rotate injection sites. If liquid preparations are ordered, be sure to follow the instructions for dilution. Some neuroleptic drugs cannot be mixed with water, so read the manufacturer's instructions before diluting any liquid medication. *Read all labels carefully.*

Some injectable medications are water based, and others are oil based. Oil-based medications are *never* given intravenously. They are intended for intramuscular use only. The drug class called the *phenothiazines* can cause contact dermatitis, so avoid getting these drugs on the skin. Wash your hands after every contact and wear gloves if you frequently handle phenothiazines.

The second major nursing responsibility is to monitor patient responses to each medication. During the first 1 to 2 weeks of therapy, assess the patient's vital signs as ordered, record fluid intake and output, and routinely assess skin condition. Assess frequently for signs or symptoms of adverse effects.

All care providers must constantly remain vigilant to the occurrence of adverse effects with each medication prescribed. In addition, nurses must thoroughly assess patients before administering any prn (as-needed) medication because a medication will actually worsen symptoms if the nurse is not able to discern an adverse effect from a behaviour. Patients who are receiving antipsychotic medications are at risk for developing NMS and tardive dyskinesia. Accurate identification of their signs and symptoms early can help prevent permanent conditions from occurring.

The third nursing responsibility, patient and family education, has a direct effect on the patient's level of functioning. One of the primary tasks of nurses is to assist patients in coping with their ADLs. When the patient and family are willing to learn about the patient's medications, treatment can be more successful. Box 31.3 lists the most important points of patient and family education.

Keep these general guidelines in mind. Get to know the patients for whom you are caring. The more you know about each person, the better you will be able to tell the difference between behaviours that are from the effects of medication and those that belong to the patient. The proper nursing assignment based on the primary nursing team care model (discussed in the next chapter) can help in attaining that knowledge. Antipsychotic medications are powerful. They demand to be treated with respect and require knowledge from those who receive them and those who work with them.

Caring for persons with psychoses is one of the most challenging areas of mental health care. Hospitalization and education are only the beginning steps in a long road toward optimal functioning. Relapse is common. Continued treatment and support are needed for family members and patients alike if we are to cope with the devastating effects of schizophrenia and other serious psychotic mental illnesses.

BOX 31.3   Patient and Caregiver Education: Antipsychotic Medications

Review the expected benefits and possible adverse effects of medication therapy with patient and caregivers. Review extrapyramidal side effects. Because there is no effective treatment for tardive dyskinesia, signs or symptoms should be reported immediately. Fine vermicular (wormlike) movements of the tongue may be the first sign of this adverse effect.

Instruct patient and family to *report any new signs or symptoms.*

Help patients understand that several weeks of medication use may be necessary before a benefit is received.

Instruct patients to swallow extended-release forms whole; do not crush or chew.

Warn patients to avoid driving or operating hazardous equipment and notify the physician if vision changes or sedation occurs.

Instruct patient to report signs of agranulocytosis, including sore throat, fever, and malaise. Tell patients to report signs of liver dysfunction, including jaundice, malaise, fever, and right upper quadrant abdominal pain.

These medications may interfere with the body's ability to regulate temperature. Warn patients to avoid prolonged exposure to extreme temperatures, allow for frequent cooling-off periods when exercising or in hot environments, and dress warmly for exposure to the cold.

Review possible endocrine adverse effects with patient and family. Assess carefully and tactfully for these adverse effects. Provide emotional support as appropriate. If adverse effects are intolerable, consult the physician for possible medication or dosage change.

Instruct patients to monitor weight (if possible). If weight gain is a problem, counsel about low-calorie diets. Refer to a dietitian as needed.

Stress the importance of informing all health care providers of all medications being taken.

Warn patients to avoid over-the-counter medications unless first approved by the physician.

Caution patients to avoid drinking alcoholic beverages while taking antipsychotics.

Warn diabetic patients that antipsychotics may alter blood glucose levels. Monitor blood glucose levels carefully. Consult the physician about changes in dietary or medication treatment for diabetes.

Tell patients not to discontinue therapy abruptly or without discussion with the physician.

Instruct patients to keep these and all medications out of the reach of children.

The medications may produce false-positive pregnancy results. Women who suspect they are pregnant should consult the physician. Women may desire to use contraceptive measures while taking these medications; counsel as appropriate. As always, pregnant or lactating women should avoid use of all drugs, if possible.

If additional medications are prescribed to treat adverse effects of antipsychotic agents, review their use and adverse effects with the patient and family.

KEY POINTS

- A psychosis is a disorder in which there is an inability to recognize reality, relate to others, or cope with life's demands.
- Neurobiological responses can range from adaptive contact with reality to disorganized thoughts, emotions, and behaviours.
- The onset of acute symptoms most often occurs in men during their mid-20s and women in their late 20s.
- Schizophrenia can have its first onset in people in their 40s and 50s. Older persons with psychosis have long-standing difficulties. Many suffer from irreversible adverse effects of long-term antipsychotic medications use, as well as other chronic medical problems.
- Scientific evidence currently points to biological (physical) causes for psychotic behaviours.
- Schizophrenia is a group of related mental health disorders characterized by disordered perceptions, thinking, and behaviour.
- Most of our actions follow automatic subconscious thoughts. This automatic mechanism is often compromised during psychosis, making it very difficult to execute otherwise simple activities (ADLs).
- Other psychotic disorders include brief psychotic disorder, delusional disorder, and psychoses related to medical conditions or medication use.
- The treatment goals for inpatient, short-term care are to stabilize the patient, prevent further decline in functioning, and assist the patient in coping with their disorder.
- Long-term goals include psychosocial and vocational rehabilitation when possible.
- Patients with acute psychoses are treated with a combination of therapies and medications.
- Antipsychotic medications, which may take weeks to become effective, help to stabilize behaviours.
- Psychosocial therapies include personal therapy, social skills training, vocational rehabilitation, behavioural therapy, stress reduction, and family education.
- Several special nursing assessments, interventions, and evaluations are required for patients who are receiving powerful antipsychotic medications.
- Nursing responsibilities with antipsychotic medications relate to medication administration, monitoring patient responses, and patient and family education.

ADDITIONAL LEARNING RESOURCES

Go to your Evolve website (http://evolve.elsevier.com/Canada/Morrison-Valfre/) for additional online resources, including the online Study Guide for additional learning activities to help you master this chapter content.

CRITICAL THINKING QUESTIONS

1. How can psychosis disrupt automatic thinking and behaviour?
2. The patient has been taking Haldol (haloperidol) 4 mg every evening. Yesterday, the patient received a dose of IM Clopixol Acuphase (zuclopenthixol) 75 mg. (This medication is active for 72 hours following the injection.) During today's assessment, just before the patient's next evening dose of Haldol, the nurse notes a temperature of 39°C, muscle rigidity, and confusion. As the nurse, what would you suspect, and what should you do?
3. A patient with schizophrenia tells the nurse that he is the Prime Minister of Canada. How would you support that patient?
4. How might different perceptual abnormalities affect a person's understanding of reality and affect behaviour?

REFERENCES

American Psychiatric Association. (2013). *Diagnostic and statistical manual of mental disorders* (5th ed.). American Psychiatric Publishing.

Fuller-Thomson, E., & Hollister, B. (2016). Schizophrenia and suicide attempts: Findings from a representative community-based Canadian sample. *Schizophrenia Research and Treatment*, 1–17. 3165243 https://www.ncbi.nlm.nih.gov/pmc/articles/PMC4764754/

German Primate Center. (2018). Why it doesn't get dark when you blink: Understanding how perception and memory interact. Science News. September 24 https://www.sciencedaily.com/releases/2018/09/180924110425.htm

Giger, J. N., & Davidhizar, R. E. (2020). *Transcultural nursing: Assessment and intervention* (8th ed.). Mosby.

Greenwald, B. (2012). Can the brain itself feel pain? *Brainline*. https://www.brainline.org/author/brian-greenwald/qa/can-brain-itself-feel-pain

Herculano-Houzel, S., Avelino-de-Souza, K., & Manger, P. R. (2014). The elephant brain in numbers. *Frontiers in Neuroanatomy*, 8, 46. https://doi.org/10.3389/fnana.2014.00046. https://www.ncbi.nlm.nih.gov/pmc/articles/PMC4053853/#__ffn_sectitle

Keltner, N. L., & Steele, D. (2018). *Psychiatric nursing* (8th ed.). Mosby.

Knabb, J. J., Welsh, R. K., & Graham-Howard, M. L. (2012). Religious delusions and filicide: A psychodynamic model. *Mental health. Religion & Culture*, 15(5), 529–549. https://doi.org/10.1080/13674676.2011.594998

van der Linden, S. (2011). *The science behind dreaming*. Scientific American. July 26 https://www.scientificamerican.com/article/the-science-behind-dreaming/

National Alliance on Mental Illness (NAMI). (2016). Schizophrenia. https://www.naminycmetro.org/diagnoses-mental-health/schizophrenia/

Nederlof, A. F., Muris, P., & Hovens, J. E. (2011). Threat/control-override symptoms and emotional reactions to positive symptoms as correlates of aggressive behavior in psychotic patients. *The Journal of Nervous and Mental Disease*, 199(5), 342–347. https://doi.org/10.1097/NMD.0b013e3182175167

Scott, C. L., & Resnick, P. J. (2013). Evaluating psychotic patients' risk of violence: A practical guide. *Current Psychiatry*, 12(5), 29–50. https://www.mdedge.com/psychiatry/article/65126/schizophrenia-other-psychotic-disorders/evaluating-psychotic-patients-risk

Sleep, H. (2007). *Sleep, learning, and memory*. Harvard Medical School. http://healthysleep.med.harvard.edu/healthy/matters/benefits-of-sleep/learning-memory

Swaminathan, N. (2008). Why does the brain need so much power? *Scientific American*. April 29 https://www.scientificamerican.com/article/why-does-the-brain-need-s/

The Human Memory. (2020). Brain neurons and synapses. https://human-memory.net/brain-neurons-synapses/

Voytek, B. (2013). Are there really as many neurons in the human brain as stars in the Milky way? *Scitable*. May 20 https://www.nature.com/scitable/blog/brain-metrics/are_there_really_as_many

32

Chronic Mental Health Disorders

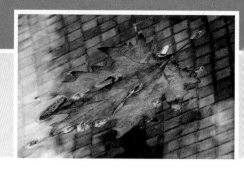

OBJECTIVES

Upon completion of this chapter, the student will be able to:
1. Explain how deinstitutionalization has affected the delivery of mental health care in Canada.
2. Describe the experience of mental illness from a patient's viewpoint.
3. Outline three psychological and three behavioural characteristics of chronic mental illness.
4. Explain how children and adolescents can be affected by chronic mental health challenges.
5. Examine the connection between human immunodeficiency virus (HIV)/acquired immunodeficiency syndrome (AIDS) and mental illness.
6. Describe the structure of an inpatient mental health care unit (staffing, equipment, assignment, electronic health record).
7. Summarize the care for patients with multiple mental health challenges.
8. Discuss three principles of psychiatric rehabilitation.
9. Apply the nursing (therapeutic) process to patients with chronic mental health disorders.
10. Plan seven basic interventions for patients who are chronically mentally disordered.

OUTLINE

KEY TERMS

Some mental illness follows an individual throughout life. *Chronic* means long-lasting, persistent, or continual. Most chronic mental health challenges follow a wavy course, marked by periods of relapses and remissions. **Relapses** are periods of dysfunction accompanied by an increase in the signs, symptoms, and seriousness of a mental health symptom.

Remissions are times of partial or complete disappearance of symptoms. The course for chronic mental health challenges follows this up-and-down pattern.

Many mental health conditions are acute. They begin abruptly, increase in intensity, and then subside after a short time. Persons with phobias, anxiety disorders, or depression often respond well to therapeutic interventions and have no further problems. However, for a certain group of individuals, mental illness becomes a way of life.

Chronic mental illness is the presence of one or more recurring psychiatric disorders that result in significantly impaired functional abilities. Individuals with chronic mental health challenges are often referred to as chronically mentally ill (CMI) or seriously mentally ill (SMI). Many people with chronic mental illness are contributing members of society, struggling to hold on to some degree of mental health. They are our relatives, our friends, and members of our community.

SCOPE OF MENTAL ILLNESS

Chronic mental disorders are disabling for people in every society and culture. Each year, millions of individuals seek help for mental health issues. In 2012, 17% of Canadians aged 15 and older—approximately 4.9 million individuals—perceived themselves as having needed mental health care in the past 12 months (Statistics Canada, 2013). When the social costs of lost productivity, shortened lives, disrupted families, and implementation of criminal justice are factored in, the total costs are enormous.

The costs in terms of suffering cannot be estimated. Society encourages people to recover from acute mental disorders and resume normal daily activities, but it tends to ignore the needs of those persons who are (and will be) unable to cope independently with life. Chronic mental illness carries with it social stigma, and being labelled "crazy" keeps many people from seeking help.

Individuals with chronic mental health challenges have much higher rates of suicide. Many individuals handle their distressing symptoms by using alcohol, street drugs, or other chemicals. They must then deal with an addiction in addition to their illness. Remember, however, that every individual who is CMI is a real person who is coping with personal problems, plus suffering from the stigmas of being labelled mentally ill.

PUBLIC POLICY AND MENTAL HEALTH

Individuals with chronic mental illness are cared for in the community. They are expected to provide for their basic needs, protect themselves, and seek help for their problems—all rather complex behaviours. The reality is that most people with chronic mental illness are unable to meet these expectations without some assistance.

Effects of Deinstitutionalization

Historically, people with psychotic behaviours were treated by having their movements physically restrained or moving them to a secluded area. When antipsychotic medications became available, in the 1960s, people no longer had to be physically controlled. Psychiatric hospitals began to discharge long-term patients into the community through a practice called "deinstitutionalization." The thought was that most people released from the psychiatric hospitals could live in the community with the proper support and aftercare. Unfortunately, the aftercare, which was a critical part of the

overall plan for providing community psychiatric services, often failed to be implemented. Changing political parties, political manoeuvring, and varying government policies have ignored the population suffering from chronic mental illness. Today, the consequences of our government mental health policies can be seen in the ever-increasing numbers of homeless persons and prison inmates.

EXPERIENCE OF CHRONIC MENTAL ILLNESS

What is it like to have a chronic mental illness? To face each day knowing the struggle ahead, or wonder if this day will bring acceptance and hope or another slide into "madness"?

Persons who face mental illness must cope with problems that are unknown to the rest of us. Individuals are often lumped into a group labelled CMI and are stripped of their identity, dignity, convictions, and feelings. They lack choice, respect, and control, and they are expected to cooperate with therapies that make them feel sick. Box 32.1 provides a glimpse into the world of one individual who suffers from chronic mental illness. It is hoped that this true account will serve as a reminder that every patient is truly a unique individual and should always be viewed as such.

Meeting Basic Needs

The issues facing the mentally troubled population are the same as those with which the rest of us must cope: adequate food, shelter, and clothing; gainful employment; meaningful relationships; and access to health care. Many people with chronic mental illness, however, must strive to meet their needs on a daily basis. Because their disorders prevent them from planning or logically carrying out an activity, many individuals with chronic mental illness are homeless, hungry, and unable to care for themselves. They are found everywhere, some chatting amiably with or responding to voices in their heads.

The individuals with chronic mental illness who do manage to provide for their own basic needs must struggle with the labels and expectations of others. Often it is difficult for them to remain employed for long periods because of occasional relapses. As one CMI patient put it, "I am an effective, loyal worker for over 90% of the time, but the 10% of the time I have troubles is all that's remembered."

Poverty and mental illness often go hand in hand. Most mentally troubled persons are unable to plan or use their money wisely. Because about half of CMI persons abuse alcohol or drugs, few dollars are spent on life's necessities.

Access to Health Care

Historically, people with severe or chronic mental health challenges were most often treated (or at least provided with custodial care) through psychiatric hospitals all across Canada. With ongoing innovative therapy and new medications, many could return to their communities and function effectively. However, community support was often not available after hospitalization, and many individuals once again fell victim to their psychoses. Only this time the tightened admission policies of most institutions did not allow most of

---

BOX 32.1   A Patient's Reflection on Being Chronically Mentally Ill

The following reflection was excerpted from the words of Betty Blaska (1991, pp. 173–175):

You spend the whole first evening and night crying. You don't want to be here. There must be a mistake. . . . You're only 18, very young, very naive. You're not yet a CMI. Next day the "staffing" (as they call it) is very intimidating. All the head brass of the hospital are there. They laugh at you. You tell them you don't want to stay. They patronize you: "Oh, we think we will just keep you here for a while." You don't know it yet, but you're on the way to becoming a CMI.

The first time you experience dystonia from the neuroleptics they've given you, you are extremely frightened. Your tongue is rigid, and you're unable to control its movements. You rush to the nurses' station, where they are huddled inside this little cage's protective walls. They won't leave for fear of contamination. They are puzzled by your presence and seem greatly inconvenienced by it. You can't speak because of your tongue's movements. They wait impatiently for you to tell them what's wrong. And you wonder what's wrong with them. Can't they see your predicament? But no. It's not that they don't see. They don't feel. Because you don't count. You're on the way to becoming a CMI.

Your first discharge from the psych ward finds you loaded up on major tranquilizers, neuroleptics, and other psychoactive substances. Your follow-up therapist sees you for a while and then announces that he won't continue with you unless you come in with your family for family therapy sessions—all eight of you. But they're scattered all over the state. And they don't want to come

in because they hate shrinks almost as much as you do. They've been belittled, browbeaten, and laughed at by the MHPs. And so your therapist refuses to see you at all, saying, "If it's important enough for you to see me, you'll get your family to come in." . . . And he also refuses to refill the [prescriptions]. So you go through withdrawal. And you end up back on the same psych ward. And then they say to you, accusingly, "Why did you go off your medications?" It's then you realize: You're a CMI.

You've been in and out of the hospital, on and off a cadre of psychoactive drugs. In doses you complain are too high. In combinations you complain are too much. . . . And the myriad of drug side effects—nausea, diarrhea, and dizziness. Vision so bad you can't cross the street because you can't judge the cars' distance from you. Drug-induced psychoses so bad you can't leave your bed or look out the window for the terror you feel. Blood pressure so low you can't stand for very long, and your voice so weak you can't be heard across a telephone wire.

So, you're without a job. And they send you to a place called DVR—Division of Vocational Rehabilitation. They "help" you get a clerical job. Never mind that you don't want to do that kind of work. Never mind that you have a degree—or two. Or that you have dreams. They "help" you get a clerical job because, yes, you've guessed it, you're a CMI. A woman CMI. But the men CMIs are just as lucky. They get to become janitors!

- With what labels (stigmas and stereotypes) is this person coping?
- How has reading this reflection changed your impressions of the experience of persons who are mentally ill?

CMI, chronically mentally ill [person]; *MHP*, mental health professional.
Excerpted from Blaska, B. (1991). First person account: What it is like to be treated like a CMI. *Schizophrenia Bulletin, 17*(1), 173–176. https://doi.org/10.1093/schbul/17.1.173

---

the CMI population to return, so they were forced to cope with their disorders as best they could. Other mentally ill persons became involved in the *revolving door syndrome,* a cycle of repeated short hospital admissions and discharges. This in-and-out-of-the-institution pattern is also called *recidivism.*

Many individuals self-medicate to relieve distressing symptoms. Many young mentally ill individuals are *polysubstance* abusers; that is, they use a variety of chemical substances, sometimes in combination. For example, meth is often used in combination with alcohol or heroin.

Individuals with chronic mental illness are often unable to plan for or manage their health care because of their illness. Many refuse shelter or treatment because of their paranoia, believing people will harm them. It is estimated that at least half of the mentally ill population suffer from untreated medical disorders. People with mental illness live an average of 10 to 15 fewer years than the general population.

People who want to receive treatment often find that services are inadequate or unavailable. Even when admitted to an institution, their stay may not be long enough to improve their condition. Outpatient services are the basis for supporting mentally ill persons in the community. However, they may not be available, or the individual may refuse treatment. Access to comprehensive mental health care remains a

problem today. Thus health care providers must be prepared to recognize and assist those individuals whose only crimes are being too disordered to effectively care for themselves.

CHARACTERISTICS OF CHRONIC MENTAL ILLNESS

Each person's experiences with mental illness are unique. Diagnoses serve only to group and label certain behaviours. The real meaning of being "depressed" or "schizophrenic" is found only within the individual who suffers from the distresses associated with the particular label.

Many mentally troubled persons are given more than one psychiatric diagnosis. Individuals who have schizophrenia frequently suffer from severe depression after an acute psychotic episode. Suicidal gestures increase as depressed persons begin to stabilize from their medications and see the hopelessness of their situations. Persons with personality disorders may have disturbing phobias or anxiety. However, the experience and suffering of living with these disorders are unique to each individual. Certain features are common to all persons who must live with mental illness. For the sake of discussion, these characteristics are divided here into three categories: behavioural, physical, and psychological characteristics.

Behavioural Characteristics

The nature of one's mental disorder determines the level of disability. Persons who suffer from chronic mental illness often have difficulty with behaviours and activities required for successful living. Impaired judgement, lack of motivation, altered realities, or disruption of automatic thinking often leads to an inability to perform even the most basic activities. Individuals may lack personal grooming habits, table manners, or expected social behaviours. They may have difficulty relating to others. Often, they are unable to function socially or occupationally. Assaultive behaviours or criminal activities may be present. The majority of individuals with chronic mental illness depend on others for their care. Many times, this involves living with family members or in group homes. For those who try to live independently, it all too often means a life of homeless shelters and mean, nameless streets. If the shelters take in too many people to allow for physical distancing, these individuals can be more vulnerable to contracting a community-spreading illness such as COVID-19.

The sexual behaviours of chronically mentally disordered persons place them at increased risk for contracting and sharing sexually transmitted infections, such as HIV/AIDS. Plus, behavioural changes can result from HIV infection if the virus invades the nervous system.

Violence is an unfortunate aspect of many chronically mentally troubled people's lives. Most individuals with serious mental illness are nonviolent. However, the inability to solve problems, make sound judgements, or control emotional behaviours can make some individuals a threat to the safety and well-being of others. Family members, especially children, frequently become the targets for anger and aggression. Many potentially dangerous individuals are released back into the community under the banner of self-determination and individual rights.

Physical Characteristics

The appearance of a person with chronic mental difficulties may vary from being tidy and appropriate to weather conditions and social situations, to being unkempt, and being over- or underdressed for the weather (e.g., individuals may be layered in various articles of clothing in high heat or strip to their underclothes in freezing weather). Personal hygiene is often lacking, as evidenced by strong body odours and soiled clothing. Malnutrition is common. Some may be obese due to metabolic changes that are caused by their medications. Chronic medical challenges are also common.

Psychological Characteristics

Individuals who suffer from chronic mental illness have several intellectual, emotional, social, and spiritual features in common. Intellectually, *altered thought processes* disrupt the ability to think clearly, solve problems, or make plans. Hallucinations, delusions, and obsessive thoughts are unwelcome intrusions that routinely disrupt the flow of reality-based thinking. Fear,

mistrust, and paranoia can complicate the picture by presenting problems with daily living activities.

Chronic *low self-esteem* follows the label of mental illness everywhere. The ability to make logical sense out of life is hampered by the many distresses of being mentally ill. Even when one is adapting effectively, the stigma of being odd, crazy, or eccentric is wrapped around each action. Other people feel uncomfortable around CMI individuals and avoid interacting with them, thus reinforcing the differences between "sick" and "well."

Mentally troubled people often see themselves as helpless, ineffective, and incapable of change. The experience of a small success will often prevent them from making any further attempts because they "just know" that they will eventually fail. When self-concept is low, it is difficult to convince someone that a brighter future can exist.

Depression is a partner of many mental health disorders. Depressive episodes can occur when an individual is coping with stress or in association with a psychotic episode. Even when mentally troubled persons are functioning effectively, depression can be a companion for many of them. Thus, in the health care system, nurses need to assess each patient for the presence of depressive symptoms.

Loneliness is the suffering that results when one is isolated from others. Many people need connections with other people, and they suffer when removed from the company of others. Individuals with chronic mental health challenges are usually very lonely. Their basic needs for love and belonging go unmet, and they respond by becoming more emotionally paralyzed.

Starved for social interaction, some persons with chronic mental illness go to great lengths, such as criminal or violent activity, to gain attention. Others withdraw from society, fearing further rejection, and live a life of mistrust and solitude. Those who do have social interactions often are unable to express themselves, make decisions, or adapt to certain social roles. As the distress of attempting to cope socially increases, many find that retreating into their illness is easier than struggling with the complexities of interacting with other people. That said, some CMI individuals prefer to be lonely and feel very uncomfortable with anyone's attempt to socialize with them.

Another characteristic of chronic mental illness is *hopelessness,* the catalyst for suicide. The struggle for mental health consumes much energy. Feelings of worthlessness plague self-esteem and lead to depression. Hopelessness brings with it the feeling that there are no solutions to one's problems, that life is destined to remain distressful, and that the only way to relieve the pain is to destroy the sufferer.

SPECIAL POPULATIONS

Chronic mental health problems can begin at any stage in life, but they are usually not noted until early or middle adulthood. Children, adolescents, adults, and older people all suffer from the difficulties of chronic mental illness, but each group poses some unique and special problems that affect their abilities to respond to mental health interventions.

Children and Adolescents Living With Chronic Mental Illness

The seeds of many adult mental health challenges are planted in childhood. Some children must learn to cope with psychological impairments early in life. Children with intellectual disability (an IQ below 70 with impairment in functioning) have problems with the intellectual and emotional aspects of life. Also, people who are mildly or moderately intellectually disabled "are believed to be more susceptible to mental illness" (Fortinash & Holoday-Worret, 2011). Emotional problems, such as anxiety or depression, often accompany the challenges faced by these individuals. Conflicts between expectations and actual abilities may result in the development of a personality disorder or psychosis.

Children with *autism spectrum disorder (ASD)* live in a world of their own. They do not develop the ability to respond to and communicate their needs, and they remain dependent on others, sometimes throughout their lives. Without the help and care of others, these children could not survive reality.

Health care providers play important roles in the care of autistic individuals and their families. Occupational therapy teams and nurses focus on the skills needed for daily activities. Psychologists and special education teachers measure functional abilities and encourage skill development, and psychiatrists monitor patients' overall progress. The most important specialist is a behaviour therapist (BT). The BT applies principles of behaviour analysis to shape and channel an autistic individual's behaviour into more socially appropriate forms. Early intervention is a key component for success. All care providers provide emotional support and information.

Children who are at risk for developing chronic mental health problems include those who have been neglected, who have been repeatedly abused or mistreated, or who have witnessed or experienced violence. Children with conduct disorders, attention-deficit/hyperactivity disorder (ADHD), and depression also have a greater risk of developing a chronic mental health disorder.

During adolescence, many maladaptive behaviours become ingrained, and new ones are developed. All parts of an individual are related. Adolescents who have chronic physical health problems, such as arthritis, diabetes, or cystic fibrosis, commonly experience psychological problems as well. Teens with diabetes have high rates of depression and suicidal behaviours.

Several chronic mental health challenges often develop during adolescence. Eating disorders, personality disorders, and schizophrenia can begin during the teenage years. Depression can become a long-standing challenge for adolescents who have not learned to cope successfully. The road to chemical dependency most frequently begins during adolescence. The effects of post-traumatic stress can lead some teens to stress-reducing but maladaptive behaviours that, over time, become daily patterns of ineffective functioning.

Older Persons Living With Chronic Mental Illness

Older persons with chronic mental illness fall into two groups: those who have had mental health challenges for decades, and those diagnosed with a mental disorder after age 50 years. The most common acquired mental health challenges in older adulthood are Alzheimer's disease and other neurocognitive disorders. As many as 20% of persons over the age of 80 suffer from some form of dementia (Fortinash & Holoday-Worret, 2011). Depression is another frequent chronic mental health challenge of older persons, especially if accompanied by sensory losses and communication impairments.

Increased drug abuse, violence, and chronic behavioural problems leave many adults incapable of raising their children, forcing older family members (often grandparents) to assume the primary responsibility and care for their grandchildren.

At a time when individuals should be looking forward to personal freedom and decreased responsibilities, the prospect of spending another 15 to 20 years raising more children can be overwhelming. Health care providers can work to address the issues of grandparents experiencing the strain of caring for the children of parents with addictions. The mental health of at least two generations depends on timely and supportive health care interventions.

Persons With Multiple Disorders

The word **comorbidity** (co-occurring) refers to the presence of two or more mental health disorders. Individuals with a **concurrent disorder** are suffering from two mental health disorders, one of which is usually substance related. The depressed person who uses cocaine is an example. Substance abuse and mental illness result in an interactive process that is seen in physical, psychological, and behavioural patterns that differ from those patterns in persons with an addiction or a serious mental illness that does not co-occur with each other.

Research shows that more than 50% of those seeking help for an addiction also have a mental illness, and 15 to 20% of those seeking help from mental health services are also living with an addiction (Canadian Centre on Substance Abuse, 2009). These people present a significant challenge for treatment because of the complexity of their disorders. The multidisciplinary treatment team appears to be the most promising approach for helping patients with co-occurring disorders cope with their problems in each area of functioning.

PROVIDING CARE FOR PEOPLE WHO ARE CHRONICALLY MENTALLY ILL

People with chronic mental health challenges are found everywhere in society. Currently the majority of mental health care is provided within the community, outside the world of the institution. For this reason, most interactions between health care providers and their patients address some issues or problems relating to mental health. Inpatient treatment settings are used only when required.

Inpatient Settings

Persons with chronic mental health challenges are hospitalized only when their behaviours pose a threat to themselves or others. Even then, it is often for only a short time. The immediate goal of care for patients is to help them control their behaviours. The average length of stay for mental illness is about 10 days. Inpatient treatment settings for the CMI population include the acute care hospital or psychiatric unit of an acute care facility.

The pattern of admission, a short institutional stay, discharge, a short community stay, and readmission (recidivism) remains a problem for both health care providers and their patients.

Outpatient Settings

Once an acute psychiatric episode has subsided, many CMI patients are discharged to halfway houses or other group-living environments. Aftercare programs range from partial hospitalization to sheltered living arrangements or home care, depending on the size, economics, and support of the community and its resources.

CULTURAL CONSIDERATIONS

When chronic mental health patients are cared for in community group housing situations, make sure to perform a complete cultural assessment. People from different cultures have different points of view about mental illness. Living with people from other cultures requires open communication and a willingness to accept other points of view. These qualities are often difficult to achieve, especially when one is mentally troubled.

Many people with chronic mental illness live with their families, who require much support to cope effectively. In some communities, CMI individuals live with therapeutic families in foster care programs. Unfortunately, more mental health care is needed in settings such as homeless shelters, health clinics for the poor, and prisons.

Psychiatric Rehabilitation

The concept of **psychiatric rehabilitation** focuses on assisting individuals with serious mental illness to effectively cope with their life situations. A multidisciplinary approach includes the special talents of physicians, psychologists, nurses, occupational therapists and physiotherapists, dietitians, and other specialists.

Each realm of human functioning is addressed during treatment. Physically, patients are assessed for and taught the skills needed to perform activities of daily living, including proper nutrition, activity, and rest habits. Emotional problems are explored, and patients are taught how to identify their feelings, control their anger, and reach their goals. Intellectually, patients are encouraged to problem-solve and set goals. Occupational or vocational training allows individuals the opportunity for employment.

Involvement with psychiatric rehabilitation programs also offers opportunities for people with severe mental illness to meet their often-neglected social needs. Many programs provide group therapies and opportunities to learn more socially appropriate behaviours.

THERAPEUTIC INTERVENTIONS

Persons with chronic mental disorders should be treated in the "least restrictive environment." This is defined as a setting that encourages the greatest degree of freedom, self-determination, autonomy, dignity, and integrity. However, the concept is not easily implemented when patients are unable or unwilling to seek out or consent to treatment and the funding for mental health care remains unstable.

Treatments and Therapies

The two basic goals for patients who live with chronic mental illness are to achieve stabilization and maintain the highest possible level of daily functioning. Achieving these two goals would indicate the achievement of recovery. The concept of **recovery** in mental health refers to living a satisfying, hopeful, and contributing life, even when a person may still be experiencing ongoing symptoms of a mental health challenge or illness (Mental Health Commission of Canada, 2019). According to the World Health Organization (WHO, 2017), there are 10 key components of recovery:

1. *Inclusion:* This is important for recovery because people need to be able to access the same opportunities as any other person and be included in the community.
2. *Relationships:* These include friends, partners, family members, mental health and other practitioners, and peers, including peer supporters and groups in the community. All of these relationships have an important role in supporting people in recovery.
3. *Hope:* This is universally seen as key to recovery, and without it people can give up their recovery journey.
4. *Belief:* Believing that a change in one's situation is possible is central to the recovery approach and can be fostered by hope-inspiring relationships.
5. *Identity:* Redefining or rebuilding identity is a central component of recovery because people often lose their sense of self when they are given a diagnosis.
6. *Meaning and purpose:* This can vary for everyone, but it is important that recovery supports people to rebuild and find meaning in their lives.
7. *Dreams and aspirations:* The recovery approach helps empower and support people to develop and achieve their dreams and aspirations in life.
8. *Control and choice:* Recovery focuses on respecting a person's right to exercise their legal capacity to make their own choices and on providing support to do so whenever this is seen as helpful by the person.
9. *Managing ups and downs:* Recovery enables people to develop skills that are required to manage negative moments in life and any associated triggers.
10. *Positive risk-taking:* This is essential for recovery, as it allows individuals to learn and grow from their experiences; it is important that people are supported while embarking on positive risk-taking.

These components are used to guide the planning of patients' recovery plans.

Therapies and recovery plans are designed for the individual based on identified problems, available resources, and the patient's willingness to cooperate. Various individual and group therapies, along with certain medications, are usually recommended by the treatment team after a complete health assessment and consultation with the patient.

With support and assistance, many individuals who live with chronic mental illness are able to function outside the institution. However, a number of problems or situations can disrupt their stability and trigger a relapse.

Pharmacological Therapy

Persons with chronic mental disorders are treated with a variety of medications depending on symptoms and distress levels. Antianxiety agents and antidepressants are often prescribed to improve emotional comfort. Antipsychotic (neuroleptic) medications are prescribed to help control hallucinations and other symptoms of psychosis.

Medication therapy is an important part of treatment. However, the adverse effects of many of these medications are uncomfortable, and patients often stop taking them as soon as the acute symptoms subside. Several antipsychotic medications are available in long-acting injectable forms, sometimes indicated as *decanoate*. One of the most powerful predictors of medication refusal is one's insight into the illness, and most individuals with severe mental illness have little insight.

All care providers, especially nurses, must carefully monitor patients routinely for adherence to medications.

Nursing (Therapeutic) Process

The first step in working with severely mentally disordered patients is to obtain the most complete database possible. Mental health challenges affect every area of functioning, and nurses must perform thorough histories and assess patients' physical status, perceptions, and behaviours.

After each member of the treatment team completes their assessment, patient issues are identified, and therapeutic interventions are designed. Nurses focus on helping patients cope with each activity of daily living. Multidisciplinary and nursing diagnoses are chosen, and basic interventions are agreed on by the treatment team and (when possible) the patient. Nursing diagnoses for CMI patients are selected according to the patient's identified challenges.

Therapeutic interventions are then designed to help the patient solve the identified problems. Although each patient requires a unique combination of interventions, several fundamental therapeutic actions apply to all patients. Table 32.1 lists each intervention and its rationale. A care plan for a CMI patient is presented in Sample Patient Care Plan 32.1 on p. 411.

TABLE 32.1 Basic Interventions: Chronic Mental Illness

Nursing Interventions	Rationale
Relating to Risk of Danger	
Assess risk for harm to self or others. Uncover dangerous psychotic processes.	Proactively ensures safety and prevents violence. Provides prn pharmacological intervention and/or psychological support and/or environmental protection, preventing any potential damage to patient and to staff
Encourage patient to notify staff when feeling angry or when destructive thoughts begin.	Helps prevent violence before it actually occurs
Gently and in a nonthreatening way, orient patient to their immediate environment and to the rules.	Reduces risk of violence, decreases patient anxiety
Sensory/Perceptual Alterations	
Assess for intensity of delusions and hallucinations.	Helps to determine level of psychosis
Ask patient to share the meaning of their hallucinations or delusions.	To determine patient's point of view and intent
Teach patient distraction techniques, such as whistling, clapping hands, mindfulness.	Offers patient strategies for controlling hallucinations
Activities of Daily Living	
Establish a schedule for grooming, eating, sleeping.	Increases self-esteem, encourages responsibility, and helps patient appear more socially acceptable
Stay in the patient's environment (see discussion of mobile nursing stations on p. 410); monitor intake, output, personal hygiene activities.	Allows for earlier intervention and proper documentation of symptoms and assessment of executed interventions
Communication	
Use active listening; establish trust; encourage conversation; praise attempts to speak clearly and effectively.	Helps to assess patient's communication style and patterns; increases understanding of and respect for patient
Social Skills	
Encourage good social skills, such as table manners, personal grooming, and appropriate communications and behaviours.	Promotes patient's acceptability by other persons; increases self-esteem; helps to teach effective social behaviours

prn, As needed.
Modified from Fortinash, K. M., & Holoday-Worret, P. A. (2011). *Psychiatric-mental health nursing* (5th ed.). Mosby.

Documentation and Transfer of Accountability

After all data about a patient are obtained and organized, the data should be recorded, monitored, and passed on to the next care provider through a formal **transfer of accountability (TOA)**, to include the following information:

- *Main mental status abnormalities*: appearance, affect, mood (including numeric assessment from –10 to +10), thoughts (including delusions, homicidal and suicidal ideation) and the correlation between them; perceptions, thought form and speech, insight, any PTSD symptoms (flashbacks, depersonalization, avoidance, nightmares, etc.).
- *Sleep*: register sleep pattern during every shift (day, evening, and night)
- *Appetite*: can be registered as a monitoring of consumed portions (not eating, quarter, half, three quarter, full, double, food from home, etc.)
- *Formal suicide assessment* (if applicable) by an evidence-informed tool. The two most popular in Canadian hospitals are the Nurses' Global Assessment of Suicide Risk (NGASR) and the Columbia–Suicide Severity Rating Scale (C-SSRS). The NGASR is simple and easy to administer, but is not valid for child and adolescent assessment. The C-SSRS is more comprehensive, includes protective factors, and is good for assessing children and adolescents, but requires more skill and time to administer and to interpret.
- *Formal assessment of violence* (if applicable) by an evidence-informed tool. The Dynamic Appraisal of Situational Aggression: Inpatient Version (DASA IV) is popular for simplicity, but there are others.
- *Formal assessment of group participation* (if applicable): refused, passive, active
- *Formal assessment of cooperation* with prescribed medications: for example, whether the patient was cooperative, required encouragement, or refused.
- *Formal assessment of pro re nata (prn) or "as needed" medication use and their effect*: what health symptom was it used for, when, and what was the result?
- *Vital signs (VS) assessment* (if applicable, or per unit protocol)
- *Weight and change from the previous data* (if applicable, or per unit protocol)
- *Bowel movements (BM)* every shift: no BM, normal BM, diarrhea × N times, etc.
- *Use of passes off the unit* (if applicable): used N times and came back on time, not used, used and was late N minutes, etc.
- *Activities of daily living (ADLs) assessment* every shift: performed well, required assistance, refused, etc.

All of the above areas must be well registered, but there is no need to spend a lot of time reading all information upon TOA. It is enough to pass on only abnormal information. Thus, the TOA can be very comprehensive and quick to use at the same time.

Electronic Health Record

Many medical facilities are replacing their paper-based documentation with an electronic health record (EHR). It is imperative for any EHR be able to support the above *structured input of information and quick dynamic presentation of abnormalities*.

Structured input is based on prewritten standard answers to all or most of the described-above formal assessments. Thus, without the need for narrative input, nurses can document standard and massive amounts of information quickly. This improves not only the speed of their documentation but also the quality. Everything not captured by that structured documentation can be captured separately as a narrative. In having most of the information stored in a standard structural format, the EHR can then be used to pull out only abnormal results and attach them to the time. This creates a one-page summary or table of all abnormalities and their dynamics. The real benefit of such a document is that these *data can be compared with the same patient's historical data and available treatment algorithms and can suggest an evidence-informed treatment*. This approach allows quick TOA and supports informed decisions about a patient's care.

Organization of Nursing in Mental Health Care

Staffing. Mental health units should be staffed with a very diverse nursing staff who have some extra mental health education. Patient–nurse therapeutic relationships are one of a few key components of treatment. Nursing staff diversity (in terms of cultural background, age, gender, sexual orientation, etc.) is very helpful for ensuring success in building therapeutic relationships with patients of varying backgrounds. Basic mental health education and skills are required in order to make a correct assessment and provide earlier intervention, especially with acute and dangerous symptoms.

It is advisable that the manager of a mental health nursing team be a nurse with a lot of knowledge of and skills in mental health, including front-line experience. This experience enables the manager to lead staff by establishing trust (because the person is very familiar with front-line nurses' experiences), role-modelling, solving complex cases, and educating on the basis of their own experience and knowledge.

Assignment: The Primary Nursing Model. Since low levels of anxiety and good therapeutic relationships are so valuable for a patient's recovery, it is important to establish a system where the patient usually receives care from the same group of nurses. Therefore, it is advisable that each patient have a few nurses (5 to 7) in a sequenced group that are assigned to work with the patient in an ordered manner. The first nurse in that lineup would work with the patient when that nurse is present. The second nurse in the lineup would work with that patient only when the first nurse is not present. The third nurse in the sequence would work with the patient only when the first two nurses are off, and so on. This type of system ensures that a patient has the opportunity to establish a good relationship with that group of nurses, particularly with those few in the first two or three positions in the nursing sequence. Nurses who are first for that patient can then be positioned further down the line for other patients. This model of nursing assignment is called the *primary nursing care model*.

The assignment should not be forced; nurses should be allowed to sign their name to a new patient voluntarily or to take their name off a patient assignment at any time. It is advisable that a positive countertransference process be used to determine the nurse–patient assignment (when a nurse feels that their connection with a patient can be positive).

The Nurse in Charge of the Shift. A typical mental health unit can be acute 24/7. Most nursing interventions are collective, that is, they are performed as a group. Therefore, use of the *collective leadership model is preferable*. This model ensures that any nurse can act as a nurse in charge of the shift, 24/7, which not only allows schedule flexibility but also supports a sense of group accountability and is instrumental to having a team approach. This can be achieved by rotating all main nursing staff through the nurse-in-charge position at each shift (day, evening, and night). By contrast, the pattern of having one particular nurse in charge for, say, all morning shifts can be detrimental to the sense of collective nursing leadership and may lead to poor competency of other nurses when they are required to perform that role.

Therapeutic Environment and Nursing Work Station. *Mobile nursing stations (MNSs)* on wheels equipped with a computer and locked cubbies for medications have revolutionized the inpatient environment. Durable, with a low centre of gravity and a powerful, long-lasting battery, MNSs can safely stay in the inpatient environment and can even take some casual physical abuse. MNSs enable nurses to observe patients, make documentation (in the EHR), and dispense medication in a patient's environment. This means there is no need for nurses to stay in a centralized nursing station (sometime called *interprofessional station*) at all times. Equipped with MNSs and mobile phones, nurses are now a part of the therapeutic inpatient environment. They may return to the nursing station for meetings, change of shift, changing or adding medications to MNS storage, or for other activities, but nurses can and should spend the bulk of their time in patients' environments.

Following are a few immediately noticeable benefits of having nurses spend more time in the patient environment:

- Nurses' capacity to identify symptoms worsening improves dramatically. The consequent early intervention prevents suffering and more acute presentation of mental health symptoms such as violence and suicidality.
- Nurses' capacity to build a therapeutic relationship with patients is increased. Nurses are much more physically approachable; it is much easier for the disturbed individual to initiate contact with a nurse who is sitting in the same room than to ask for attention through the nursing station door or window.
- Patients tend to act differently in a nurse's presence. They tend to behave in more socially acceptable ways and tend to put more effort into executing ADLs.
- A more constant nursing presence in patients' environments helps them to maintain hope and self-esteem.

The Myth of Intermediate Observation. Unfortunately, many medical care facilities still engage in old practices without any evidence or cost-efficiency analysis regarding their effectiveness. Such practices continue simply because this is how things have been done historically. In 2007, the Agency for Healthcare Research and Quality of the US Department of Health and Human Services released a very detailed and extensive report, *Making Health Care Safer II: An Updated Critical Analysis of the Evidence for Patient Safety Practices*, on large numbers of older health care practices. Among these was the practice of different types of "nursing observation" (which can range from constant observation to intermediate observation at varying time intervals). The conclusion of this report was that there is no evidence for their efficacy or efficiency (RAND Corporation, 2007).

In many places, nursing staff are required to perform *close observation* (also called *intermediate observation*). Typically, in Canada, this means that a nurse physically observes a patient every 15 minutes and documents the observation. However, there is no evidence that this action helps to prevent violence or suicidality in patients, and there is no evidence that this intervention can diminish the intensity of the patient's symptoms or patient suffering. Thus, especially in places with limited nursing resources, this practice takes nursing time away from providing evidence-informed care, resulting in less symptom control and a greater risk of patient violence and suicidality. Nonetheless, when staff believe such close observation can be a reasonable practice, it is important to ensure that there are opportunities for medical or environmental interventions and to increase therapeutic engagement to control patients' symptoms and diminish suffering.

In some cases, patients may require reassurance or frequent contact with a staff member in order to feel safer. This should be incorporated in the patient care plan and done as often as needed. This is a therapeutic intervention and not an "observation" limited to a particular time (e.g., when the patient is awake or when the patient comes to the nurse at certain time intervals to report symptoms and seek reassurance).

The Myth of Chemical Restraint. All across Canada, the use of restraints to ensure personal and public safety is typically regulated by some sort of provincial act and by local hospital policies. These acts and policies recommend use of any type of restraint only *"as a last resort."* They also specify the use of pharmacological measures to control a person's behaviour as a "chemical restraint" that also should be used only as a last resort. These acts typically relate to use and limitation of patient restraints.

At the same time, the use of pharmacological intervention to treat a patient's symptoms, including in emergency situations when neither the patient nor the patient's substitute decision maker can make an informed decision, is regulated by a different set of provincial acts, called the *Consent and Capacity Act*. In a typical mental health care setting, a patient's behaviour that poses a danger to themselves or others is a result of that patient's mental health symptoms. Therefore, the acute pharmacological intervention provided, sometimes against the patient's will, is intended to control these symptoms. This intervention must be provided as soon as possible to diminish the patient's suffering and ensure safety.

Unfortunately, the stigma of mental illness is still very powerful and is responsible for the general population (and even some hospital staff) believing that mentally ill patients can control their symptoms and behaviour. Thus, when patients are not able to do so, staff who have this incorrect belief provide pharmacological intervention and emergency treatment to a mentally ill patient only as a last resort, when suffering is already so unbearable that the patient becomes a danger to themselves or others. This attitude denies the patient acute and emergency treatment in a timely manner.

The point here is that, outside of very rare circumstances, pharmacological intervention in mental health care must be used as soon as possible to avoid patient suffering and ensure safety. *The use of the pharmacological intervention in mental health emergencies to treat symptoms of mental illness is not considered application of a chemical restraint.*

Mental Health Care in the Community

Care plans for long-term psychiatric patients are adapted to the particular care setting—be it the home, community day care centre, clinic, or institution. If the mental health care services are well coordinated, care plans move with the patient when care providers or settings change. This method encourages continuity of care that is so important for coping with severe mental challenges.

Once patients return to the community, mental health centres provide them with the ongoing care needed to help them function effectively. Community mental health centres with strong financial bases are able to provide their patients with services such as medical care, medication supervision, individual and family therapy, crisis intervention services, family support services, skills training, and vocational counselling or training, in addition to continued emotional support and encouragement. With long-term therapeutic and community support, many individuals with severe mental illness and their families are able to cope with the numerous challenges associated with their disorders.

SAMPLE PATIENT CARE PLAN 32.1   **Chronic Mental Illness**

Assessment

History Markus is a 34-year-old man with a history of at least 11 admissions to psychiatric units of various general hospitals. Today, he is being readmitted after he was found wandering the streets arguing with himself and threatening to kill someone else if they didn't "stop calling me names." He was medicated with 1 mg of haloperidol (Haldol) intramuscularly in the emergency department.

Current Findings An unkempt man with a strong body odour and soiled clothing; speech is slow and disjointed; responds verbally without external stimuli. Emotional state (affect) is flat except for verbal responses to hallucinations. Markus states that he is and has been hallucinating for the past 3 days. The hallucinations are auditory; the voices want Markus to kill himself. He thinks they may be right because during the time he is in the community, he feels forced to spy on other people for CSIS, and the voices tell him that he is better off dead than being a spy. When asked what made him take to the streets, Markus replied that he thought he could "out walk the out talk." He has not taken his prescribed medications since he last saw his therapist about 4 weeks ago.

Multidisciplinary Diagnosis	Planning/Goals
Disturbed sensory perception related to impaired perceptions	Markus will seek out a staff member when he feels like he is losing control over his auditory hallucinations.
	Markus will not harm himself or others.
	Markus will report the decrease in intensity of auditory hallucinations within 4 days after admission.

THERAPEUTIC INTERVENTIONS

Interventions	Rationale	Team Member
1. Orient Markus gently but frequently to place, time, and current activity.	Provides reassurance about safety; decreases anxiety level	All
2. Speak slowly; use clear, simple messages.	Helps to increase Markus's understanding, thus decreasing his anxiety	All
3. Reassure Markus often that he is safe here and will not be harmed by the voices or other people.	Helps Markus trust the safety of his environment, presents reality as safe	All
4. Listen to and accept descriptions of his feelings, hallucinations.	Conveys respect for and acceptance of the person and encourages communication	All
5. Set limits on aggressive behaviours; utilize prn medication as early as possible.	Promotes a safe environment for all patients and staff, helps Markus to be responsible for his own behaviours. Administering medication early helps to avoid suffering and prevents Markus from acting on his delusions and hallucinations.	Nsg, All

SAMPLE PATIENT CARE PLAN 32.1   Chronic Mental Illness—cont'd

Multidisciplinary Diagnosis	Planning/Goals	
6. Encourage Markus to take his medications; make a copy of the daily medication schedule and encourage Markus to follow it.	Medications help control psychotic symptoms, reduce anxiety, improve functioning. Developing a daily medication routine in the hospital helps increase medication adherence after discharge	Nsg, MD
7. Develop discharge planning for Markus to return to his foster home.	A stable and predictable environment helps decrease acute psychotic episodes	Soc Svc

Evaluation After the fourth day of hospitalization, Markus sought out staff members when his hallucinations became very intense. With the exception of one acting-out episode, Markus was able to follow all the unit's rules. Reports of hallucinations have decreased from "continually" on admission to once or twice per week the second week of his stay.

Critical Thinking Questions
1. What strategies would help increase Markus's adherence to taking his medications?
2. What discharge planning does Markus require?

A complete patient care plan includes several other diagnoses and interventions.
CSIS, Canadian Security Intelligence Service, *MD,* physician; *Nsg,* nursing staff; *Soc Svc,* social services.

KEY POINTS

- Each person's experiences with mental illness are unique, but most chronic mental health challenges are characterized by periods of relapses and remissions.
- Chronic mental disorders are disabling for people in every society and culture.
- As a result of deinstitutionalization, many individuals who are chronically mentally ill are homeless, hungry, and unable to care for themselves.
- Access to comprehensive mental health care remains a problem in Canada today.
- Psychological characteristics of persons who are chronically mentally ill include altered thought processes, chronic low self-esteem, depression, hopelessness, loneliness, and suicidal behaviours.
- Behavioural characteristics of individuals who are chronically mentally ill include the inability to perform activities of daily living; being dependent on or living with family; employment difficulties; ineffective independent living; and sexually active, violent, or criminal behaviours.
- Physical characteristics may vary from average to bizarre. Dress may be unusual; personal hygiene is often lacking. Malnutrition is common.
- Chronic mental health disorders can begin at any stage in life, but they are usually not noted until early or middle adulthood.
- The social epidemic of violence, crack cocaine, and other drug use has resulted in a new group of primary care providers: grandparents who are raising their grandchildren.
- Substance abuse and mental illness result in an interactive process that is seen in physical, psychological, and behavioural patterns uniquely different from those of persons with an addiction or serious mental illness that does not co-occur each other.

- Individuals who are chronically mentally ill are at a high risk for contracting HIV infection owing to current behaviours and past histories.
- Because all areas of human functioning are deeply interwoven, mental health nursing is a critical component of every nursing practice.
- Nurses focus on helping the patient who is chronically mentally ill cope with each activity of daily living.
- The basic goals for chronically disordered mental health patients are to achieve stabilization and be maintained at their highest level of daily functioning.
- Psychiatric rehabilitation is a multidisciplinary treatment approach that focuses on assisting patients with serious mental illness in coping effectively with their life situations.
- The primary nursing care model is a basic mental health care model that supports the building of therapeutic relationships, quality of assessment, and early intervention.
- The proper observation and documentation of patient symptoms, delivery of care, and transfer of accountability for patients are key staff responsibilities.
- Persons with chronic mental disorders are treated with a variety of medications depending on symptoms and distress levels.
- Emergency pharmacological intervention to treat symptoms of mental illness, with or without a patient's consent, should be provided as soon as possible to avoid damage or serious suffering for the patient. Pharmacological intervention in this type of scenario is not considered a chemical restraint.
- Once returned into the community, chronically mentally ill people require aftercare or rehabilitation services.
- The mental health of a society depends on the mental health of each of its individual citizens.

ADDITIONAL LEARNING RESOURCES

Go to your Evolve website (http://evolve.elsevier.com/Canada/Morrison-Valfre/) for additional online resources, including the online Study Guide for additional learning activities to help you master this chapter content.

CRITICAL THINKING QUESTIONS

1. What are the main lifelong struggles that an individual who is chronically mentally ill may have?
2. What should the modern inpatient mental health environment look like? What components should it have to promote recovery and safety?
3. As a staff member working in the inpatient unit, what must you observe, document, and pass on to the next care provider?

4. A patient was apprehended by the police after demonstrating a high level of violence. He is hostile, angry, and suspicious and has refused any prescribed medication. He thinks that the staff is a group of imposters who will disassemble his body. He has told the staff that he will do everything possible to fight "right now." However, he has not acted in a physically violent manner on the floor since his admission a few hours ago. As a nurse on the unit, what will you do?

REFERENCES

Blaska, B. (1991). First person account: What it is like to be treated like a CMI. *Schizophrenia Bulletin, 17*(1), 173–176. https://doi.org/10.1093/schbul/17.1.173

Canadian Centre on Substance Abuse. (2009). Concurrent disorders: Substance abuse in Canada. https://ccsa.ca/sites/default/files/2019-04/ccsa-011811-2010.pdf

Fortinash, K. M., & Holoday-Worret, P. A. (2011). *Psychiatric mental health nursing* (5th ed.). Mosby.

Mental Health Commission of Canada (MHCC). (2019). What is recovery? https://www.mentalhealthcommission.ca/English/what-we-do/recovery

RAND Corporation, University of CaliforniaSan Francisco/StanfordJohns Hopkins University & ECRI Institute. (2007). *Making health care safer II: An updated critical analysis of the evidence for patient safety practices.* Agency for Healthcare Research and Quality U.S. Department of Health and Human Services (AHRQ Publication No. 13-E001-EF March 2013).

Statistics Canada. (2013). Canadian Community Health Survey: Mental health, 2012. https://www150.statcan.gc.ca/n1/daily-quotidien/130918/dq130918a-eng.htm

World Health Organization (WHO). (2017). Promoting recovery in mental health and related services. jsessionid=D2D54019D-C0429E9CD9938C8907406C6?sequence=1 https://apps.who.int/iris/bitstream/handle/10665/254810/WHO-MSD-MHP-17.10-eng.pdf

33

Challenges for the Future

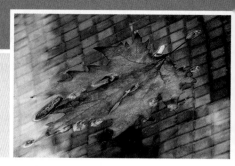

OBJECTIVES

Upon completion of this chapter, the student will be able to:

1. List three challenges that health care providers face in delivering mental health care in Canada.
2. Describe the roles, functions, and interactions of the mental health care team.
3. Examine three obligations of the therapeutic partnership for the patient and the care provider.
4. Describe three expanded roles for nurses who care for people who are mentally ill.
5. Examine two challenges involved with the change process.

OUTLINE

KEY TERMS

change process (p. 421)
competent (KŎM-pĕ-tĕnt) (p. 418)
culture-bound disorders (p. 417)
deinstitutionalization (p. 415)
homelessness (p. 416)
mental health care team (p. 418)

nurse case managers (p. 420)
planned change (p. 421)
psychosocial (sī-kō-SŌ-shŭl) (psychiatric) rehabilitation (p. 415)
unplanned change (p. 421)

The need for mental health applies to us all. Every person experiences periods of emotional turmoil and crises, and, at some point, we all need a little assistance to help us cope. When one is experiencing physical illness, it produces emotional stresses ranging from indifference to crisis behaviours. Nurses and other health care providers help provide the nurturing that all patients (not only those with mental illnesses) need. In addition, they are now challenged to provide that care within ever-changing health care delivery environments.

CHANGES IN MENTAL HEALTH CARE

Mental disorders rank first among illnesses that cause disability worldwide (Whiteford, Degenhardt, Rehm, et al., 2013). One in three Canadians will be affected by a mental illness during their lifetime (Pearson, Janz, & Ali, 2015). The loss of productivity and constantly increasing costs for treatment generate challenges for any economy.

Health care is currently undergoing many changes. Escalating costs in several countries, including Canada, are forcing health care officials and policy makers to take a close look at where and how health care funds are spent. Social changes, such as an aging population, and overburdened federal and provincial budgets are exerting their influence on today's health care system. Refugees who are arriving from different conflict zones are showing signs and symptoms of post-traumatic stress disorder (PTSD). Men and women are returning from armed conflicts with physical and mental wounds that change lives. Mental health care so urgently needed by many is often unavailable.

The influences of many cultures and new technologies are changing the way we look at health and illness. Patients may not speak the same language as their health care providers, creating a greater need for translators as well as care providers who speak the languages of their patients. Technological advances are opening new areas of exploration, and discoveries about the biochemical nature of humans are challenging the foundations of our thinking about illness and health.

The treatment and prevention of mental illness (and other health issues) are caught up in the web of change. As a result, all health care providers will be challenged to deliver effective, cost-accountable care. This challenge will call for creativity and innovation. Change is a certainty, and adaptability is a necessity.

Change in Settings

Historically, most psychiatric care was limited to the inpatient setting, either a unit at the local community hospital or at a long-term care facility. It was recognized that institutionalized care was not only wrong but inhumane and fiscally irresponsible, and that community-based care is the preferable model. In the 1950s, chlorpromazine started to be used in the United States as the first medication for positive symptoms of schizophrenia and for mania episodes of bipolar I disorder. A greater orientation toward community care and the availability of medication that was able to cope with the main acute symptoms of mental illnesses (psychosis and mania) marked the beginning of a movement that we now call *deinstitutionalization*. **Deinstitutionalization** is the gradual closing of long-term mental health facilities and the transfer of their patients' care to communities, which took place from the 1960s to the late 1990s. This process continues today in some places.

Most psychiatric long-term care institutions are now closed. In most places, however, communities underestimated the financial investment that such care would require. In Ontario, for example, a recent Ombudsman report indicated a serious gap in mental health care services that was created by the closing of long-term care facilities and by multiple community agencies struggling to respond to the needs of mentally ill patients and their families (Dubé, 2016). Mental health departments at hospitals are full, and local emergency departments are becoming havens for persons who are experiencing crisis. Some individuals with acute problems are denied care and told to return when "something happens" or "during working hours."

Changes in the system that once supported mentally ill patients have now moved these individuals into community health care systems, but the specialized "aftercare" that was promised is commonly not adequately provided, even today.

As a result of this unsupported release of patients, many mentally troubled persons became sick again and eventually homeless. Seriously mentally ill individuals now comprise 24–50% of the homeless population (Munn-Rivard, 2014). Jails and prisons have evolved into holding facilities for people with mental disorders. More than 20% of inmates have had past problems with mental illness. Many mentally ill individuals are jailed just to get them off the streets. Others are found living at the fringes of society, sleeping in abandoned buildings, and depending on the generosity of others for food and clothing. Thus the treatment settings for people with mental illness have changed, following patients from the institution to the street, jail, neighbourhood clinic, or local physician's office.

Mental health care is an important component of overall health. Its provision must be addressed if we are to become capable, adaptable, and functional people. Health care providers must become skilled in assessing and working with patients suffering from mental or emotional disorders, no matter where the setting or what the situation.

Challenges Created by the Canadian Health Care System

Among other developed countries, Canada has a very unique health care system. It is publicly funded to provide hospital care, physician care, and prescribed diagnostic tests inside and outside hospitals. Medications are covered only during hospitalization. However, for any nonphysician out-of-hospital care (nurses, psychologists, occupational therapists, behavioural therapists, physiotherapists, and others) and any medications prescribed on an outpatient basis, Canadians must pay out of pocket or have private insurance that can cover these expenses. Different provinces have different drug plans for the no-income population.

Another important aspect of our system (with some rare exemptions) is that all Canadian physicians are private companies (usually incorporated) paid by the provincial Health Insurance Plan on a fee-for-service (FFS) basis. For example, the more operations a surgeon completes, the higher will be their income. The more times a family physician sees a client, the higher will be that physician's income. The more times a psychiatrist sees a client, the higher will be their income. If a physician does more tasks for which compensation is high, performs fewer tasks for which the compensation is low, and performs none of the tasks that are not financially compensated, then their income will be high. The client does not pay at all; these services are paid for by 100% public money. In each province, there is a different FFS payment scheme (information about these is public and available online; for example, the following URL presents the example for Ontario: http://www.health.gov.on.ca/en/pro/programs/ohip/sob/physserv/sob_master20181115.pdf).

Typically, in psychiatry, the highest fees are paid for initial assessments, reassessments, and one-on-one therapy. Lower fees are paid for group therapy and competency hearings.

Data from Manchandra, R., Chue, P., Malla, A., et al. (2013). Long-acting injectable antipsychotics: Evidence of effectiveness and use. *Canadian Journal of Psychiatry, 58*(5, Suppl 1), 5S–13S. https://doi.org/10.1177/088740341305805s02

Team meetings, communication with other staff members, family education, and calls to a patient are usually not covered in the fees. Essentially, in using the specific FFS system described above, physicians are directed to focus more on acute care, less on supportive treatment, and are paid nothing for focusing on prevention. No other developed country does this.

The Royal College of Physicians and Surgeons of Canada as well as provincial colleges set medical ethical codes, and all physicians must abide by the Hippocratic Oath. However, the main goal of any private company is the constant increase and stability of its net revenue, and since all Canadian physicians are private companies, that is also their goal. Practising preventive medicine directly contradicts that goal. This situation creates a conflict of interest for physicians between the goal of increasing revenue and following the Hippocratic Oath.

In the majority of developed countries, physician remuneration works in the opposite way: most of the physicians (with some rare exemptions) are on a global base salary (GBS), therefore they are free from the above conflict of interest. It must be noted that the US health care system is not a good example, because it has extremely poor health outcomes for its extremely high expenses.

Long-Acting Injectables

There are two main routes by which to administer antipsychotic medication: oral (tablets or pills) and injectable. Depending on the formulation of an oral medication, usually it should be taken once to a few times per day. Injectable medications that exist in a long-acting form can be taken once every 2 to 4 weeks.

A worldwide study of almost 30 000 patients with schizophrenia showed a 20 to 30% reduction in relapse when long-active injectable (LAI) antipsychotic medications were used in patients (Tiihonen, Mittendorfer-Rutz, Torniainen, et al., 2016). Even if relapse does happen for the patient on LAI, the intensity of the symptoms will be less and the need for hospitalization decreased. A large hospital study clearly indicated that use of LAIs resulted in a 19% lower likelihood of rehospitalization following a relapse in schizophrenia and significantly fewer visits to the emergency department. In addition to clinical benefits, LAI provides significant cost savings because of reduced hospitalizations (Lafeuille, Gravel, Lefebvre, et al., 2013; Lafeuille, Laliberte-Auger, Lefebvre, et al., 2013). See Box 33.1 for information regarding rates of LAI use in different countries.

In an open letter, published in the *Canadian Journal of Psychiatry,* about the Canadian practice of not prescribing LAI antipsychotics, despite their proven benefits to prevent relapses and readmissions, psychiatrist Dr. J. Peter Weiden said, "Come on, Canadian colleagues, you can do better than this!" (Weiden, 2013).

CRITICAL THINKING

- Do you think the low rate of LAI use in Canada has anything to do with how the Canadian health care system is structured?
- Based on the uniqueness of the Canadian health care system, what other statistical differences would you anticipate that Canada has in relation to other developed countries' health care systems?

Homelessness

One of society's greatest challenges today is homelessness. Many families live just one paycheque away from poverty. They can financially cope for the present, but if one stressor is added, their whole living situation becomes threatened.

Homelessness means to be without a permanent residence or without a place to live. Historically, homeless people were unmarried, intermittently employed, and White male adults with an average age of 50 years. However, they seldom actually slept in the streets because of the availability of community shelters. Today, the homeless population is much more diverse, and for various reasons, including lack of shelter availability, many homeless people live on the street.

Loss of control over the daily events of their own lives can lead homeless people toward a loss of self-worth, learned helplessness, and depression. The health status of the homeless population, both mental and physical, is poor. Many were relatively adjusted when they were discharged from an institution or housed in a stable environment, but when their medications ran out and the aftercare was not available or provided, the psychiatric challenges returned. Without adequate support, resources, and encouragement, many chronically mentally ill individuals find it almost impossible to take steps to improve their lives.

Homelessness has become a national tragedy that in some way affects us all. The trauma of losing one's home, adjusting to life in a shelter or on the street, and struggling for a way out produces both psychological and emotional distress. Stress disorders are common among the homeless population, even among persons with previously high levels of functioning.

Adults with serious and chronic mental illness have an impaired ability to function in daily life. Self-care activities, interpersonal relationships, and abilities to work or attend school are commonly compromised. Financial resources are usually very limited.

Homeless mentally ill persons are in poorer health. They struggle with more barriers to employment and tend to have less contact with family or friends than homeless individuals without mental difficulties.

However, health care challenges for the homeless population can be addressed. As the providers of health care, we must find new ways of working with this population if we are to protect and encourage the health of all people.

The *Canadian Charter of Rights and Freedoms*

The *Canadian Charter of Rights and Freedoms* is a part of the Canadian Constitution. Section 15 of the *Charter* declares that every person in Canada—regardless of race, religion, national or ethnic origin, colour, sex, age, or physical or mental disability—is to be considered equal. The *Charter* also allows for the existence of certain laws or programs aimed at improving the situation of disadvantaged individuals or groups. For example, programs or acts to improve employment opportunities for people with mental or physical disabilities may be protected under subsection 15(2) (Government of Canada, 2018).

To improve employment opportunities for people with a variety of disabilities, Canada passed the *Employment Equity Act*. The purpose of this Act is to achieve equality in the workplace so that "no person shall be denied employment opportunities or benefits for reasons unrelated to ability and, in the fulfilment of that goal, to correct the conditions of disadvantage in employment experienced by women, Aboriginal peoples, persons with disabilities and members of visible minorities by giving effect to the principle that employment equity means more than treating persons in the same way but also requires special measures and the accommodation of differences" (Government of Canada, 2019).

Under the *Employment Equity Act,* an employer must not only provide equal opportunity to people with disabilities but also must provide necessary accommodations for such employees. For employees with mental health challenges, these accommodations can include things like a flexible schedule, certain flexible working hours, a unique breaks regimen, working from home, or other reasonable accommodations.

CRITICAL THINKING

You are working in a community hospital. Today, you find out that one of your co-workers, who told you that he has a history of mental illness has been assigned to your care team. You have never worked with this person before today.
- What is your initial reaction?
- How do you think this will affect the activities of the workplace?

Cultural Influences

The world is shrinking in terms of its interconnectedness. In the past, a person would grow, live, procreate, and die within one community or geographic region. Today, world travellers work in one part of the globe and commute to another area to raise their families. Waves of immigrants and refugees move from their homelands to other countries in search of better lives. Rapid forms of transportation move thousands of people around the world in a matter of hours instead of days. As more individuals become computer literate and users of global computer networks, our world will become even more interconnected. Because of these changes, health care providers are encountering persons from various cultural backgrounds with greater frequency. Learning to interact effectively and respectfully is a challenge that faces all the world's citizens, but for health care workers, this is especially important.

The mental health challenges of a culture can have a universal quality. There are some behaviours, such as those associated with depression, which all cultures define as mental health disorders. Other disorders may be specifically limited to members of a certain group. These types of problems are called **culture-bound disorders** because they appear to be related to specific cultures. For example, the Latin-American disorder *susto* is an emotional anxiety that results from "soul loss."

Health, illness, and mental illness are defined differently throughout various cultures. The person who talks to himself may be considered "a nut" in one society and may be revered as a holy man in another. Their behaviours might be exactly the same, but the social setting in which they take place differs. The point here is that mental illness, to a large extent, is culturally defined. To work effectively with patients from other cultures, one must discover how these patients define mental illness.

As displaced individuals adapt to their new cultures, they combine elements of both the home and host culture into their daily lives. The result is a unique blend of both worlds, a "third culture." Bicultural patients require a thorough cultural assessment to discover their individual frames of reference (how they view the world). Only then can therapeutic interventions be planned with an expectation of success. An effective therapy in one culture is not always successful when applied in another culture.

As more people emigrate throughout the world, care providers will encounter many patients whose first language is not English or the provider's native language. This can present many challenges, especially when a psychiatric component is involved. Even when the patient speaks or understands some English, the stresses of illness (and the complexities of a modern health care system) can increase anxiety, and patients often attempt to communicate by reverting back to their native language. Often these communications can be misunderstood and result in poor treatment outcomes. If mental health care providers are to deliver effective care, they must be aware of the cultural backgrounds of their patients and develop plans of care with each patient's unique cultural heritage in mind. Caring for culturally diverse patients is another challenge in that services are only as effective as patients perceive them to be.

THE MENTAL HEALTH CARE TEAM

Mental illness has a multifaceted nature that includes physical disorders, social factors, psychological issues, and spiritual concerns. In an attempt to meet the many patient needs and to provide care in both inpatient and community settings, interdisciplinary mental health care teams were introduced. A **mental health care team** is a group of professionally trained specialists who develop and implement comprehensive treatment plans for patients with mental and emotional challenges.

Team Members

The ideal composition of an interdisciplinary (also called *multidisciplinary*) mental health care team is the patient, a physician, a psychologist, a nurse, a dietitian, a social worker, a representative of the patient's spiritual beliefs (e.g., minister or priest), an occupational therapist, and other specialists, as needed. The main function of the team is to coordinate care as the patient moves from inpatient to community settings and through the health care system. Refer to Table 2.3 in Chapter 2 for a description of each team member's role in the health care team.

Interdisciplinary Interactions

Members of the mental health care team communicate frequently because scarce services must be allocated and patients need effective care. Some care teams meet often to monitor patient progress, review the patient's use of services, and establish treatment goals. Others may interact by phone or e-mail. All work with patients and with one another is to meet defined goals. To illustrate: Nurses who care for hospitalized patients begin discharge planning on admission and communicate with the care team throughout the patient's hospitalization. Discharge planners and social workers communicate with community members who provide services. When patients are ready for discharge, the care team is able to help with a smooth transition for the patient back into the community because the interactions of each team member focus on the treatment goals.

Mental Health Care Delivery Settings

In the past, mental health care was obtained in the psychiatrist's office or the inpatient setting. Mental health care is currently delivered in three general settings: the institution, the community, or the home. Mental health units in general hospitals and inpatient mental facilities are examples of institutional settings. Mental health specialists are found in many community settings. Many of these specialists work in neighbourhood clinics or with social service agencies. There is a huge variety of outpatient care delivery models across Canada. Their financial support can be very different (e.g., support from a provincial health care insurance plan, city budget, local ethnic and/or religious organization).

CHANGE AND MENTAL HEALTH PATIENTS

Throughout history, mental illnesses have been labelled as being somehow "different" from physical maladies. At one time, people with mental illnesses were considered possessed. Consequently, they were neglected, abused, and confined without hope of improvement.

As new psychiatric theories arose, attitudes toward mentally ill persons changed, but they were still viewed as victims who somehow caused their own problems. During this time, the role of the patient was to be a passive recipient of care. Therapies were designed and delivered without regard to appropriateness, and patients were expected to cooperate. Relationships between patients and care providers ranged from patronizing to adversarial.

Today, both the providers and consumers of mental health care are striving to change these attitudes and practices. Involving patients in treatment means that every party involved must assume an active role. This interaction involves the building of trust, mutual respect, and acceptance.

Competency

Are people with mental illness capable of making decisions about proper care and treatment of their disorders? The larger answer is that society struggles to balance individual rights with the need to protect its citizens. Meanwhile, the legal system and those who work with mentally ill individuals are often challenged to provide the answer to this complex question.

To be considered **competent**, an individual must be able to (1) make a choice, (2) understand important information, (3) appreciate their own situation, and (4) apply reasoning. Studies reveal that while mental illness can coexist with competent decision making, as many as 50% of individuals with mental illness show seriously impaired judgement. Many hospitalized patients with severe symptoms, such as paranoia or disorganized thought, are incompetent. In this context, it may be useful to apply the four measures of competence when assessing a patient's decision-making abilities. It may help solve the dilemma of discerning which patients are able to make reasonable treatment decisions.

The challenge of meeting patient needs without violating their rights is especially true for patients with mental health challenges. Previously, when people were discharged from institutions into their "least restrictive environments," their rights to freedom, autonomy, and self-determination were protected. However, the concept of the least restrictive setting begins to break down when patients are unable to provide the essentials of daily living for themselves and are in need of treatment.

Individuals are not exercising their rights to freedom when they wander the streets aimlessly, out of touch with reality. They are able to determine little for themselves and have virtually no ability to direct their own lives. In these cases, an institutional setting may prove to be a more beneficial environment.

Empowerment of Patients

The traditional role of a patient was to be passive; patients were expected to accept the physician's diagnosis, therapies, and comments without question. They were also expected to be motivated, cooperative, and follow treatment regimens to get well. As a result, people became increasingly detached from their own responsibility for their health care and discontented with the system that delivered that care.

By contrast, today's patients have become more responsible and active consumers of health care, but many health care services remain tied to old models relying on the passive patient. Individuals entering the current health care system are beginning to exercise their right of self-determination. They seek out information about their conditions, weigh the pros and cons of each treatment option, and select those that best suit them. Because the consumer's role has moved from a passive to an active one, the term *client* becomes more appropriate than the passively connoted term *patient*. Hopefully, the relationship between care providers and clients develops into a dynamic interchange, with therapeutic goals that are mutually acceptable. Many health care facilities across Canada are now using the terminology of *client* instead of *patient*, reflecting the more active role that their service consumers now play. Thus, in Canada, as a care provider you will see both terms used.

Obligations of Patients

To receive the most effective care, patients must fulfill certain obligations. These responsibilities are few, but they are important for the success of treatment. First, patients must be truthful. Often people are uncomfortable about sharing personal information. They may expect that health care providers will pass judgement on their actions or refuse care. Nevertheless, honest, complete data are essential for planning care. Second, patients have an obligation to be responsible for their own behaviours. Even people who periodically lose contact with reality are capable of assuming some responsibility for their behaviour. Third, patients have an obligation to cooperate with treatment—that is, assuming patients want to "get well." Consumers of mental health care services who are willing to assume the obligations of truthfulness, responsibility, and cooperation can play an active role in successful diagnosis and treatment of their symptoms. Within the therapeutic relationship, care providers also have certain obligations.

Obligations of Care Providers

As patients assume certain obligations, so do the care providers who work with them. From the psychiatrist to the allied team members and administrative personnel, each person assumes specific responsibilities when working with patients. However, all health care providers share the following obligations.

First and most important, it is essential to *accept* the patient "as is." As care providers, we do not have to like or approve of any behaviour, but the *person* must be accepted as a worthy human being, capable of change. Do not pass judgement on them. We are here to help, not to conjure up emotionally based opinions.

Second, it is important to demonstrate *respect* for patients. Refer to patients by name. Ask permission before entering their living space, if necessary. Show approval for gains made in therapy. Express concern for their well-being, and remember to be polite. All of these behaviours demonstrate respect

TABLE 33.1 Obligations of the Therapeutic Partnership	
Patients	**Care Providers**
To be truthful	To accept the patient as a person capable of change
To be responsible for one's own behaviours	To demonstrate respect for and acceptance of the person
To cooperate with treatment	To empower patients To educate patients

for patients much more clearly than words. Even the most disturbed person responds to respectful care.

Third, *empower* patients. Much mental illness is associated with patients' feelings of lack of control over their lives. Care providers who recognize this can provide small but frequent opportunities for decision making and success. As patients choose among various options, they are exercising some control over their environment. Hopefully, decisions gradually move from making choices to solving problems. During the process, each success provides encouragement for the next step and a sense of control.

Fourth, mental health care providers, especially nurses and therapists who work closely with patients, have the added obligation to provide educational opportunities. Unless patients are comatose, they are capable of learning. New knowledge enables people to change. Education is an intervention that helps mentally troubled patients attain increased control of their lives, and empowered patients are more willing to explore and change their behaviours.

Table 33.1 summarizes the obligations of the therapeutic partnership.

Health care providers in Canada are also expected to comply with federal privacy rules. The *Personal Information Protection and Electronic Documents Act* (PIPEDA) provides national standards for protecting the privacy of an individual's health information and regulates how personal health information is disclosed and used by the private sector. The basic obligation of health care providers is to protect the patient's privacy. Each province has its own act that regulates the use and protection of personal health information by health care providers. In Ontario, for example, the *Personal Health Information Protection Act* (PHIPA) ensures that a patient's health information remains protected.

Studies have demonstrated that patients who feel they have some control over their situation report fewer symptoms and less discomfort. They have speedier recoveries and are able to participate in activities of daily living sooner than patients who perceive they have little or no control. In short, patients need to be active participants in their own care.

Providers of Care

Membership in the health care profession is also changing. In the past, only physicians, nurses, and family members provided mental health care. Today, several allied health team members (e.g., occupational therapists, behavioural therapists, recreational therapists) and personal support workers (PSWs) provide many services that were once exclusively within the realm of psychiatry. Because each provider works within a narrow specialty, it becomes the nurse's responsibility to ensure that safe, coordinated health care is being delivered to patients. Nurses need to understand and exercise their roles in coordinating health care.

The services of PSWs are just as important in the inpatient mental health care setting as they are in acute care. Certified PSWs help nurses with patient care and treatments. PSWs may have some advanced training.

Many inpatient mental health programs depend on the PSW's abilities. Those who demonstrate an acceptance of others, compassion, cultural awareness, patience, and a gentle sense of humour are selected to be part of the mental health care team. The main function of supportive PSWs is to act as helping individuals. PSWs on the floor help patients with activities of daily living and communication, provide reassurance, assist with therapeutic recreation, alert nurses about changes in patients' symptoms and, overall, contribute to the unit's therapeutic environment.

Expanded Role for Nurses

The profession of nursing has undergone many changes in the past 40 years. The "handmaiden to the physician" model has been replaced by the role of a professional, with all its accompanying rights and obligations. Contemporary nurses are considered experts in the area of assisting people in coping with the effects of health challenges in everyday living. They are guided by each province's or territory's college and professional standards of care.

Nurses participate fully as members of the treatment team. They also provide education for patients and their significant others and coordinate the activities of various therapeutic interventions and support agencies. Nurses' roles are continuing to evolve; the challenge that every nurse faces is to grow with change.

As mental health care moves into the community, new roles are opening up for nurses. Hospitals no longer employ the majority of nurses because attempts to control costs have decreased the numbers of nurses per institution. Patients are being discharged from acute care facilities earlier. They require nursing services in their homes and communities. Because nurses help people to adjust to and cope with the changes in daily living that result from their illness or condition, nurses practise in a number of challenging new settings.

Preventive health care is another main responsibility. Routine screening for weight, hypertension, and response to medications provides nurses many opportunities to instruct patients in more healthful living activities. Weekly lectures and discussions about proper nutrition, sexually transmitted infections, and current health issues are planned and conducted by nurses. Realistic goals are set to encourage patients to commit to meeting their needs, and much support by all members of the staff helps patients regain their self-esteem.

Nurses also collaborate with physicians to plan and implement programs for people with serious mental illness. **Nurse case managers** collaborate with psychiatrists to develop treatment plans tailored to each patient's special needs. Patients are encouraged to share their concerns with their nurse case manager, who evaluates the need for psychiatric consultation. Nurses and psychiatrists meet weekly for discussions and decisions about each patient's medications, therapies, and referrals.

Nurses in this setting provide intake assessments and referral services, initial and ongoing medication services, supportive counselling, and individual and group education. They act as advocates for patients interacting with family, the legal system, or other parts of the health care system. Because of the nurse case manager's support and guidance, patients with severe mental illness are able to function more adequately within their community, and costly and unnecessary psychiatric consultations are reduced. The nurse–physician collaborative practice model may prove to be one solution to the challenge of delivering mental health care to patients within their home environments.

Psychosocial (psychiatric) rehabilitation is another area in which nurses are expanding their roles. Evolving as a social model of treatment rather than a medical model, psychosocial rehabilitation is a way of assisting people with mental health challenges in readjusting and adapting to life in the community. In these settings, nurses are able to use their full range of skills without the focus being placed on illness or disability. Wellness, wholeness, and the abilities of the individual are emphasized. Vocational, educational, residential, social, and personal adjustment services are offered. Patients are encouraged to exercise freedom of choice and become self-directed. Individual care plans, called *personal service plans,* are developed but controlled by patients who identify the goals that are important to them. Patients choose resources and support people with guidance from the treatment team (referred to as a "service delivery team").

Self-help is a fundamental concept of psychosocial rehabilitation. Care team members offer social and vocational coaching, but patients must act for themselves. The belief that all people have the inherent capacity for change and the focus on what the patient can do have resulted in some remarkable successes. Nurses who practise within these settings truly work with persons in their environment to maximize wellness.

As health care moves into the community, the need for mental health clinical nurse specialists will continue to grow. Mental health (psychiatric) home care nurses focus on prevention and wellness care. They collaborate with other professionals and serve as the patient's advocate within the mental health delivery system. Patients who are facing the crises of illness are assisted with both their physical and emotional difficulties. Because nurses are able to intervene during the early stages of dysfunction, the services of mental health home care nurses are proving to be successful as well as cost-effective.

MANAGING CHANGE IN THE HEALTH CARE SYSTEM

Life is a dynamic process, so all living things undergo change. Seasons, plants, people, and processes all change. All providers must keep pace with continual changes in health care,

BOX 33.2 Reasons Why People Resist Change

1. Problems are known and comfortable.
2. Change brings about discomfort.
3. Change disrupts the status quo.
4. Individuals feel their self-interests are threatened.
5. Individuals have inaccurate perceptions about the nature or implications of the change.
6. Individuals may believe the changes will not be beneficial.

TABLE 33.2 Coping With Unplanned Change

Nursing Action	Comments
Do not panic.	Remain calm no matter what happens. Keep your own reactions under control by staying in the "thinking" mode. Remember that decisions made during high stress are more likely to be ineffective. Stay calm.
Analyze the situation.	Define the problems that are occurring as a result of the change. Assess why the change is happening now, and consider its possible effects. Assess resources and limitations.
Reset priorities.	Determine what needs to be done. List needs in order of importance, and then communicate and act.
Match resources with priorities.	Match what needs to be done with the best available resource. Resources are always limited. Do the best you can with what you have.
Continuously evaluate.	This step is even more important when the change is unplanned. Monitor individuals and groups as they progress through the change process. Monitor the situation's dynamics. Be prepared for the possibility of other changes.

new therapies, theories, medications, and more. Therefore, it is important to understand the characteristics of change and how to successfully cope and adapt.

The **change process** is defined as the series of steps that result in a difference. Change itself is inherently neither good nor bad. It is the reactions of the people involved in the change process that label or judge a change.

People often resist change because it implies uncertainty, which brings about a disturbance in the status quo. We all resist change to some extent to maintain our equilibrium and keep things "the way they are." People resist change for several reasons. Although major problems may be present in the current situation, they are known and comfortable. Change can bring about discomfort when the status quo is disrupted. Individuals may feel that their self-interests are threatened. They may have inaccurate perceptions about the nature or implications of the changes or become so threatened that they begin to use psychological defence mechanisms to defend their viewpoints. Some people resist change because they truly believe the changes will not be beneficial (Box 33.2). Dealing effectively with change requires a period of transition and psychological adaptation. Understanding the change process can help both care providers and patients adapt to the continuing process of change.

The Change Process

There are two basic types of change: *planned change* and *unplanned change* (Morrison, 1993). **Planned change** is the deliberate effort to make things different within a system. Changes are carefully planned and implemented slowly and deliberately. When done appropriately, planned change meets with minimal hostility and resistance. Planned change is always the ideal, but seldom the reality. **Unplanned change** is unexpected, not anticipated, and usually not desired. Change happens whether it is planned or unexpected. In health care settings, unplanned changes are daily occurrences. "Expect the unexpected" is a statement often made by managers and supervisors in the workplace to describe unplanned change.

Whether change is unanticipated or expected, intense reactions may be provoked in some people. Although reactions to change are highly individual and can range from simple acceptance to outright hostility, most reactions can be generalized into three categories: anxiety, mistrust, and loss. All of these reactions affect mental health patients.

When the comfort of a daily routine is lost, people (especially those with mental health challenges) become anxious. Planned changes for these patients must be implemented slowly, in small steps, giving time for adjustment. Unexpected change, however, does not allow for this luxury, and anxiety levels may increase.

Mistrust develops when people are unclear about what is happening. Once individuals feel threatened, resistance develops and an "us versus them" attitude evolves. To keep mistrust at a minimum, it is important to maintain open communications with all those involved in the change. Listen to everyone's concerns, and provide what information you can.

Change also involves loss when one gives up old, comfortable attitudes or behaviours. Phrases such as "in the old days" or "the way we used to do it" are expressions associated with loss. Replacing loss with hope by focusing on possible benefits can help people to cope with change, especially if it is unexpected. Nursing actions for coping with unplanned changes are offered in Table 33.2.

Mental health care providers must be especially adept at coping with unexpected changes. Change affects us all, but adaptability, healthy emotional responses, and a willingness to support ourselves and others go a long way toward meeting the challenge of coping successfully with changes in today's busy world.

OTHER CHALLENGES

Life today is filled with myriad personal, professional, and social challenges. Personally, we are constantly challenged to move calmly through the struggles of everyday living. Professionally, we are charged with all the obligations and responsibilities of a helping professional, not to mention our duty to the people who become our patients. Socially, we are confronted with many complex relationships and interrelated social problems.

The Challenge to Care

Patients remember the health care workers who cared for them, who listened, who held their hand, and who supported them when times were rough. Caring is the essence of nursing and the power of the health care professions. Do not become so involved in the physical aspects of providing care that you forget to nurture the art of caring for people. Scientific evidence is lending new support for the actions that make up the art of caring.

Connections between the mind and body are an intricate network that responds as a whole. Emotions are responses of a whole person, complete with physical and psychological reactions. Certain therapeutic actions, such as touch, have been found to reduce anxiety levels and may play a role in actually boosting the immune system by decreasing the immunosuppressive effects of stress. Therapeutic touch can decrease pain and promote wound healing. We have known all along that caring is a powerful weapon in the search for health and wholeness.

A Look to the Future

All areas of human functioning are deeply interwoven. Physical illnesses are always accompanied by some level of emotional, intellectual, social, and spiritual distress. The opposite is also true. Therefore "psychiatric" or "mental health" care is a critical component of every therapeutic situation. Caring for the physical body is not enough. For high levels of wellness and adaptation, the whole individual—every aspect of the dynamic being we call "the patient"—must be considered with every therapeutic action.

Health is defined by the patient's criteria for wellness. Health care providers emphasize patients' strengths and their abilities to adapt and to change. By working with patients' personal definitions of health, the focus is on their goals, and an understanding of the interactions between them and their complex and changing environments is gained.

Nurses help patients adjust to the activities of daily living. Because of this, nurses are in a position to shift the focus of health care from one that concentrates on deficits and deficiencies to one that considers the possibilities and positive achievements that are within the grasp of each patient. This health-oriented point of view allows for successful interventions by concentrating on solutions that draw on patients' strengths and supportive resources.

The health care professions are undergoing change. Because mental distress or illness affects every aspect of a person's life, the care needs of individuals with acute and chronic mental health challenges are many. Issues affecting mental health policies are currently being explored, but too few resources are available for treating the numerous individuals who require care. As a result, nurses and other health care providers must consider every interaction with their patients as an opportunity to encourage high levels of mental health. If we are to make progress with the social problems of crime, violence, abuse, homelessness, and poverty, we must treat each mentally troubled person as our most important patient because the mental health of a society depends on the mental health of each of its individual citizens.

It is an exciting time to be a health care provider. To gain the most benefit in this role, maintain a positive attitude. Do your best and strive to learn. Numerous challenges await us. The knowledge you have gained in this text will help you to meet future challenges brought on by things like pandemics. Perhaps one of the greatest will be to bring the caring into the community that ensures health care services will be available to every individual.

KEY POINTS

- Challenges facing health care providers are escalating costs, sociocultural changes, and advances in technology.
- Treatment settings for people with mental illness have evolved from the residential institution to the street, jail, neighbourhood clinic, community hospital, and local physician's office.
- Homelessness can lead to significant physical and emotional distress, and homeless people often suffer from poor mental and physical health as a result.
- The *Canadian Charter of Rights and Freedoms* states that people with mental health challenges have the same rights and opportunity for employment as other people.
- Learning to interact respectfully and effectively with people from cultures different from their own is an important challenge for health care workers.

- The interdisciplinary (multidisciplinary) mental health care team consists of the patient, physician, psychologist, nurse, dietitian, social worker, chaplain, occupational therapist, and other specialists, as needed. The main function is to coordinate care as the patient moves from inpatient to community settings and through the health care system.
- The role of the patient has changed from being a passive participant to an active consumer of health care services.
- To be considered competent, an individual must be able to make a choice, understand important information, appreciate their own situation, and apply reasoning.
- Patients are obligated to be truthful, responsible, and cooperative with care.
- Care providers are obligated to accept the patient "as is," demonstrate respect, empower patients, and educate.

- Expanded roles for nurses include positions in centres for homeless people, collaborating with physicians as case managers, working with psychosocial rehabilitation teams, and meeting the needs of special populations.
- Change, the process of making something different or becoming different, is inherently neither good nor bad.

- Care providers are in a position to shift the focus of health care from one that concentrates on deficits and deficiencies to one that considers the possibilities and positive achievements that are within the grasp of each patient.

ADDITIONAL LEARNING RESOURCES

Go to your Evolve website (http://evolve.elsevier.com/Canada/Morrison-Valfre/) for additional online resources, including the online Study Guide for additional learning activities to help you master this chapter content.

CRITICAL THINKING QUESTIONS

1. How do population changes (e.g., immigration, refugees, and aging) affect the needs and delivery of mental health care?
2. What are some unique qualities of the Canadian health care system, and how might these affect service delivery?
3. What are the basic obligations of a patient and of a health care provider?
4. How does empowering patients improve their responses to care?

REFERENCES

Dubé, P. (Ombudsman of Ontario). (2016). *Nowhere to turn: Investigation into the Ministry of Community and Social Services' response to situations of crisis involving adults with developmental disabilities.* Toronto: Ombudsman Ontario. https://www.ombudsman.on.ca/Media/ombudsman/ombudsman/resources/Reports-on-Investigations/NTT-Final-EN-w-cover.pdf

Government of Canada. (2018). Rights of people with disabilities. https://www.canada.ca/en/canadian-heritage/services/rights-people-disabilities.html#a1c2

Government of Canada. (2019). *Employment Equity Act* (S.C. 1995, c. 44). Justice laws website. https://laws-lois.justice.gc.ca/eng/acts/E-5.401/page-1.html#h-215135

Lafeuille, M. H., Gravel, J., Lefebvre, P., et al. (2013). Patterns of relapse and associated cost burden in schizophrenia patients receiving atypical antipsychotics. *Journal of Medical Economics, 16*(11), 1290–1299. https://doi.org/10.3111/13696998.2013.841705

Lafeuille, M. H., Laliberte-Auger, F., Lefebvre, P., et al. (2013). Impact of atypical long-acting injectable versus oral antipsychotics on rehospitalization rates and emergency room visits among relapsed schizophrenia patients: A retrospective database analysis. *BMC Psychiatry, 13.* article number 221. https://bmcpsychiatry.biomedcentral.com/articles/10.1186/1471-244X-13-221

Morrison, M. W. (1993). *Professional skills for leadership: Foundations of a successful career.* Mosby [Seminal Reference].

Munn-Rivard, L. (2014). *Current issues in mental health in Canada: Homelessness and access to housing (Publication No. 214-11-E).* Canada: Library of Parliament. https://lop.parl.ca/staticfiles/PublicWebsite/Home/ResearchPublications/InBriefs/PDF/2014-11-e.pdf

Pearson, C., Janz, T., & Ali, J. (2015). Mental and substance use disorders in Canada. https://www150.statcan.gc.ca/n1/pub/82-624-x/2013001/article/11855-eng.htm

Tiihonen, J., Mittendorfer-Rutz, E., Torniainen, M., et al. (2016). Mortality and cumulative exposure to antipsychotics, antidepressants, and benzodiazepines in patients with schizophrenia: An observational follow-up. *American Journal of Psychiatry, 173,* 600–606. https://doi.org/10.1176/appi.ajp.2015.15050618

Weiden, J. P. (2013). Why are Canadians complacent about long-acting injectable antipsychotic therapies? Come on, Canada, you can do better!. *Canadian Journal of Psychiatry, 58*(5, Suppl. 1), 3S–4S. https://doi.org/10.1177/088740341305805s01

Whiteford, H. A., Degenhardt, L., Rehm, J., et al. (2013). Global burden of disease attributable to mental and substance use disorders: Findings from the Global Burden of Disease Study 2010. *Lancet, 382*(9904), 1578–1586. https://doi.org/10.1016/S0140-6736(13)61611-6

A APPENDIX

Mental Status Assessment at a Glance

1. Appearance
   Manner of dress

   _____

   Personal grooming

   _____

   Facial expressions

   _____

   Posture and gait

   _____

2. Speech
   Manner of response (frank, evading, cooperative, etc.)

   _____

   Choice of words (to assess general intelligence, education, levels of function, thought processes)

   _____

   Speech disorder

   _____

3. Level of consciousness
   Level of alertness

   _____

   Orientation (time, place, person)

   _____

4. Attention span
   Ability to keep thoughts focused on one topic

   _____

   Repeat a series of numbers

   _____

   Serial sevens (ask patient to subtract 7 from 100, 7 from 93, and so on)

   _____

5. Memory
   Immediate memory (ask patient to repeat words after 15 minutes)

   _____

   Recent memory (ask patient about yesterday's activities)

   _____

Remote memory (ask patient about dates of birth, marriage, schooling)

_____

6. Understanding abstract relationships
   Understanding of proverbs (concrete or abstract)

   _____

   Ability to understand similarities (e.g., "How are a bicycle and an automobile alike?")

   _____

7. Arithmetic and reading ability
   Simple addition, subtraction, multiplication, and division (ask patient to make change)

   _____

   Ability to read newspaper, magazine

   _____

8. General information knowledge
   Discuss newspaper or magazine article

   _____

   General information questions (e.g., "How many days in a year? Where does the sun set?")

   _____

9. Judgement
   Responses to family, work, financial problems

   _____

   Responses to "What would you do if . . ." questions

   _____

10. Emotional status
    Ask, "How do you feel today?" or "How do you feel about . . ." questions

    _____

    Affect (mood)

    _____

    Current situation and coping behaviours

    _____

A Simple Assessment of Tardive Dyskinesia Symptoms

Patient Identification _____

Date _____

_____ 1. Observe the patient unobtrusively at rest (e.g., in the waiting room). (Have patient sit in a hard, firm chair without arms.)

_____ 2. Ask if there is anything in his or her mouth (i.e., gum, candy). If yes, please remove it.

_____ 3. After observing the patient, rate according to the severity of symptoms:
   0 = Absent
   1 = Questionable
   2 = Present and easily controlled
   3 = Present and barely controlled
   4 = Present and not controllable

_____ 4. Ask if any movements in mouth, face, hands, or feet are noticed. If yes, ask how much they interfere with daily activities.

_____ 5. Examine patient with hands and feet exposed to observe movements in the extremities.

_____ 6. Ask patient to sit with feet flat on floor and hands hanging unsupported. (Assess body movements.)

_____ 7. Ask patient to open mouth. (Observe tongue at rest within mouth.) Do this twice.

_____ 8. Ask patient to protrude tongue. (Observe abnormalities of tongue movement.) Do this twice.

_____ 9. Ask patient to repeatedly touch the thumb to each finger sequentially in both hands. (Observe tongue and face.)

_____ 10. Flex and extend patient's left and right arms (one at a time).

_____ 11. Ask patient to stand up. (Observe in profile. Observe all body areas again, hips included.)

_____ 12. Ask patient to walk with arms resting comfortably at his or her sides. (Observe hands, legs, and face.)

_____ 13. Have patient walk a few paces, turn, and walk back to chair. (Observe hands, gait, and body movements.) Do this twice.*

_____

*Activated movements.

Data from Sandoz Pharmaceuticals, East Hanover, NJ; Fleischhacker, W. W., Bergmann, K. J., Perovich, R., et al. (1989). The Hillside Akathisia Scale: A new rating instrument for neuroleptic-induced akathisia. *Psychopharmacology Bulletin, 25*(2), 222–226; and Brasic, J. R. (2012). *Tardive dyskinesia.* http://emedicine.medscape.com

Canadian Standards for Psychiatric-Mental Health Nursing

Standard I: Provides Competent Professional Care Through the Development of a Therapeutic Relationship

A primary goal of psychiatric-mental health (PMH) nursing is the promotion of mental health and the prevention or diminution of mental disorder. The development of a therapeutic relationship is the foundation from which the PMH nurse can "enter into partnerships with clients, and through the use of the human sciences, and the art of caring, develop helping relationships" (Registered Nurses' Association of Ontario [RNAO], 2002).

The nurse:

1. assesses and clarifies the influences of personal beliefs, values, and life experience on the therapeutic relationships and distinguishes between social and therapeutic relationships;
2. works in partnership with diverse and heterogeneous populations, families, and relevant others to determine goal-directed needs and to establish an environment that is conducive to goal achievement;
3. uses a range of therapeutic verbal and nonverbal communication skills that include empathy, active listening, observing, genuineness, and curiosity;
4. recognizes the influence of age, culture, class, ethnicity, language, stigma, and social exclusion on the therapeutic process and negotiates care that is sensitive to these influences;
5. mobilizes and advocates for resources that improve community integration and increase the ability of diverse and heterogeneous populations and their families, including those isolated geographically, to access mental health services;
6. understands and responds to human reactions to distress and loss of control that may be expressed as anger, anxiety, fear, grief, helplessness, hopelessness, and humour;
7. recognizes and respects the client's expert and unique knowledge, and facilitates the client's behavioural, developmental, emotional, or spiritual change, while acknowledging and supporting the client's participation, responsibility, and choices in their care;
8. respects the client's and family's lived expertise and unique knowledge in promoting recovery;
9. fosters mutuality of the relationship by reflectively critiquing therapeutic effectiveness through client and family responses and feedback, clinical supervision, and self-evaluation;
10. understands the nature of chronic illness and applies the principles of health promotion and disease prevention when working with clients and families in the promotion of recovery.

Standard II: Performs/Refines Client Assessments Through the Diagnostic and Monitoring Function

Effective assessment, diagnosis, and monitoring is central to the nurse's role and depends on theory as well as on understanding the meaning of the health or illness experience from the perspective of the client. The nurse explains the assessment process to the client and provides feedback. Knowledge is integrated with the nurse's conceptual model of nursing practice, which provides a framework for processing client data and for developing client-focused plans of care. The nurse makes professional judgements based on evidence and recognizes and includes the client as a valued partner.

The nurse:

1. collaborates with clients and with other members of the health care team to gather holistic, client-centred assessments through observation, engagement, examination, interview (using respectful, recovery focussed language), and consultation while attending to confidentiality and pertinent legal statutes;
2. assesses, documents, and analyzes data to identify health status, potential for wellness, health care deficits, potential for risk to self and others; alterations in thought content and/or process, affect behaviour, communication and decision-making abilities; substance use and dependency; and history of trauma and/or abuse (emotional, physical, neglect, sexual, or verbal);
3. formulates and documents a plan of care in collaboration with the client, family, and mental health team that supports recovery and reintegration/social inclusion in the community through discharge planning and provision for ongoing support, all while recognizing variability in the client's ability to participate in the process;
4. refines and expands client assessment information by assessing and documenting significant change(s) in the client's status and by comparing new data with the baseline assessment and client goals;
5. assesses and anticipates potential needs and risks, collaborating with the client to examine their environment for risk factors such as self-care, housing, nutrition, economic support, psychological state, and social interactions;

6. determines the most appropriate and available therapeutic modality that meets the client's needs, and assists the client to access necessary resources.

Standard III: Administers and Monitors Therapeutic Interventions

The nature of mental health problems and mental disorders raises specific practice issues for the PMH nurse in the assessment and administration of therapeutic interventions. Many clients are at risk for harm to self or others, either directly or through neglect (including self-neglect). Every effort will be made to include the client in all aspects of decision-making. The PMH nurse will be alert and respond to adverse reactions.

The nurse:

1. utilizes and evaluates evidence-based interventions to provide ethical, culturally competent, safe, effective, and efficient nursing care consistent with the mental, physical, spiritual, emotional, social, and cultural needs of the individual;
2. provides information to clients and families/significant others in accordance with relevant legislation;
3. assists, educates, and empowers clients to select choices which support informed decision-making and provides information about the possible consequence(s) of the choice;
4. supports clients to draw on their own assets and resources for self-care, daily living activities, resource mobilization, and mental health promotion;
5. determines clinical intervention, using knowledge of clients' responses;
6. uses technology appropriately to perform safe, effective, and efficient nursing intervention;
7. uses knowledge of age-specific implications of psychotropic medications and administers medications accurately and safely, monitoring therapeutic responses, reactions, untoward effects, toxicity, and potential incompatibilities with other medications or substances and provides medication education with appropriate content;
8. utilizes therapeutic elements of group process;
9. incorporates knowledge of family dynamics, cultural values, and beliefs in the provision of care;
10. collaborates with the client, health care providers, and community members to access and coordinate resources such as employment, education, and volunteering, and seeks feedback from the client and others regarding interventions;
11. encourages and assists clients to seek out mutual support groups and to strengthen social support networks as needed;
12. seeks out the client's response to, and perception of, nursing and other therapeutic interventions and incorporates it into practice;
13. ensures care for individuals of different populations (e.g., incarcerated individuals, individuals with intellectual disabilities) from therapeutic and rehabilitative perspectives.

Standard IV: Effectively Manages Rapidly Changing Situations

The effective management of rapidly changing situations is essential in critical circumstances that may be termed psychiatric emergencies. These situations include risk factors for self-harm, aggressive behaviours, and rapidly changing mental and physical health states (Canadian Standards for Psychiatric-Mental Health Nursing [SERPN], 1996).

The nurse:

1. utilizes the therapeutic relationship throughout the management of rapidly changing situations;
2. assesses the client using a comprehensive holistic approach for actual or potential health issues, problems, risk factors, and/or crisis/emergency/catastrophic situations;
3. knows about resources required to manage actual and potential crisis/emergency/catastrophic situations and plans access to these resources;
4. monitors client safety and utilizes continual assessment to detect early changes in client status, and intervenes accordingly;
5. implements timely, age-appropriate, and client-specific crisis/emergency/catastrophic interventions as necessary;
6. uses trauma-informed care when managing crisis situations with clients to minimize further trauma and interference with recovery objectives;
7. commences critical procedures when necessary which, in an institutional setting, includes suicide precautions, emergency restraint, elopement precautions, and infectious disease management and, in a community setting, includes community support systems such as police, ambulance, and crisis response resources;
8. utilizes a least restraint approach to care;
9. develops and documents the management plan of care and intervention;
10. coordinates care to prevent errors and duplication of efforts where rapid intervention is imperative;
11. evaluates the effectiveness of the rapid responses with the client and modifies critical plans as necessary;
12. involves, with client collaboration, the family and significant others to identify the precipitates of the event and to plan ways to minimize risk of recurrence;
13. participates in process review with the client, family, health care team, and other service providers as needed;
14. utilizes safety measures to protect client, self, and colleagues from potentially abusive situations in the work environment;
15. participates in and implements activities that improve client safety in the practice setting.

Standard V: Intervenes Through the Teaching-Coaching Function

All interactions are potentially teaching/learning situations. The PMH nurse attempts to understand the life experience of the client and uses this understanding to support and promote learning related to health and personal development. The nurse provides health promotion information to individuals, families, communities, and different populations.

The nurse:

1. collaborates with the client to determine learning needs, emphasizing and supporting the client's potential for recovery;
2. plans and implements health promotion education with the client while considering the context of the client's life experiences, readiness, culture, literacy, language, preferred learning style, and available resources;
3. explores options and resources with the client to build knowledge for making informed choices related to health needs and for accessing the system as needed;
4. incorporates knowledge of diverse learning models and principles, including the principles of recovery, when creating learning opportunities for clients;
5. provides guidance, support, and relevant information (with appropriate critiques) to clients, families, and significant others;
6. documents the teaching/learning process (assessment, implementation, client involvement, and evaluation);
7. determines with the client the effectiveness of the educational process and collaboratively develops or adapts it to meet learning needs;
8. engages in teaching/learning opportunities as a partner with clients, families, and community agencies.

Standard VI: Monitors and Ensures the Quality of Health Care Practices

The nurse has a responsibility to advocate for clients' rights to receive the lease restrictive form of care and to respect and affirm clients' rights to self-determination in a safe and equitable manner. The PMH nurse must be informed about relevant legislation, its interpretation, and its implications for nursing practice.

The nurse:

1. identifies philosophies, attitudes, values, and beliefs of the workplace culture that affect the nurse's performance, safety, and compassion, and responds appropriately;
2. understands how the determinates of health affect community well-being and PMH nursing practice;
3. understands relevant legislation and its implications for nursing practice, and utilizes it appropriately;
4. expands and incorporates knowledge of innovations and changes in mental health psychiatric nursing practice to ensure safe, confidential, and effective care;
5. ensures and documents ongoing review and evaluation of PMH nursing care activities;
6. participates in dialogue and critical reflection about the interdependent functions of the team within the overall plan of care;
7. advocates for the client within the context of the health care environment;

8. advocates for continuous improvement to the organizational/systemic structures consistent with the principles of safe, ethical, and competent care;
9. recognizes the dynamic changes in health care locally and globally and, with stakeholders, supports strategies to manage these changes.

Standard VII: Practices Effectively Within Organizational and Work-Role Structure

Psychiatric-mental health nursing care occurs in both community and hospital settings. For the PMH nurse, care requires a therapeutic relationship involving reflective, ethical, and evidence-based practice within complex and dynamic situations. The PMH nurse must be able to plan and implement collaborative care, apply recovery principles, promote mental health, consult with community members, and advocate for the mental health of their clients and others.

The nurse:

1. collaborates with clients/families/significant others and other stakeholders to facilitate safe, supportive, and respectful environments for all persons;
2. actively participates to sustain and promote a climate which supports ethical practice and a moral community;
3. understands and utilizes quality outcome indicators and strives for continuous quality improvement;
4. seeks to utilize constructive and collaborative approaches to resolve differences among members of the health care team which may impact care;
5. participates in developing, implementing, and critiquing mental health policy which fosters recovery and continuity of care;
6. advocates and supports a nursing leadership role;
7. supports and helps to mentor and coach newly graduated nurses;
8. utilizes knowledge of collaborative strategies for social action in working with consumer and advocacy groups;
9. pursues opportunities to reduce stigma and to promote social inclusion and community integration for clients.

Source: Extracted from Canadian Federation of Mental Health Nurses. (2014). *Canadian Standards for Psychiatric-Mental Health Nursing* (4th ed., pp. 7–12). Author. https://live-cfmhn.pantheonsite.io/wp-content/uploads/2019/05/2014-Standards-of-Practice-Final-1.pdf Gloria McInnis-Perry (PhD), Ann Greene (MEd), Elaine Santa Mina (PhD), et al. © 2014 Canadian Federation of Mental Health Nurses. Reprinted with permission.

REFERENCES

Registered Nurses' Association of Ontario (RNAO). (2002). *Best practice guidelines: Crisis intervention.* Author. http://rnao.ca/sites/rnao-ca/files/Crisis_Intervention.pdf.

Society for Education and Research in Psychiatric-Mental Health Nursing (SERPN). (1996). *Educational preparation for psychiatric-mental health nursing practice.* Author.

A

abstinence   Not engaging in an addictive behaviour or use of an addictive substance.

abuse   The improper usage or treatment of a thing (e.g., abuse of a substance, harm to an individual).

abused substances   Chemicals that affect the central nervous system and thus alter an individual's perceptions; also referred to as mind-altering substances.

acceptance   Act of receiving or undertaking what is being offered.

acquired immunodeficiency syndrome (AIDS)   A chronic, potentially life-threatening infection caused by the human immunodeficiency virus (HIV), AIDS damages the immune system and prevents the body from warding off infection and disease.

acting out   Use of inappropriate, detrimental, or destructive behaviours to express suppressed or denied emotions.

active listening   A communication concept that embodies an intentional empathetic form of listening aimed at understanding collaboratively constructed meanings. A care provider commits to giving their full attention to the patient as well as the topic being discussed, thereby temporarily suspending their own reactions as they listen to understand.

acupuncture   Insertion of fine needles into the skin at specific points on the body, known as meridians, in order to treat illness.

addiction   Physical dependence on a drug or a behaviour despite the physical and psychosocial issues associated with it.

adolescence   The period of life between 11 and 21 years of age.

adulthood   The period of life lasting from about 18 to approximately 65 years of age.

advocacy: The process of providing a patient with information, support, and feedback so that they can make an informed decision.

affect   The outward manifestation of a person's feelings or emotions.

affective   Pertaining to emotion, mood, or feeling.

affective disorders   Psychiatric disorders that have mild to severe impact on emotional states, from deep depression to elation.

affective loss   In dementia, the loss of mood, emotion, and personality.

ageism   The practice of stereotyping older persons as feeble, dependent, and unproductive.

aggression   A forceful attitude or action that is expressed physically, verbally, or symbolically.

aging   The process of growing older.

agitation   Behaviour that is verbally or physically offensive.

agnosia   The inability to recognize familiar environmental objects or people (stimuli).

agoraphobia   The avoidance of people, places, or events from which escape would be difficult (especially open or public places) and in which a panic attack may therefore occur.

akathisia   The inability to sit still, commonly caused by antipsychotic medications.

akinesia   The loss or impairment of voluntary movement.

alcohol   Ethanol (ETOH); the result of the fermentation or distillation of yeast and grains, malts, or fruits.

alcoholism   Chronic disease caused by prolonged or excessive alcohol use.

alexithymia   Difficulty in identifying and describing emotions.

allopathic   Using Western medical and surgical methods to treat disease and injury; follows the disease model.

alogia   Diminished speech output.

alternative medicine   Practices and treatments that are used instead of conventional (allopathic) medicine. Also known as complementary medicine.

Alzheimer's disease (AD)   A progressive, degenerative disorder that impedes the functioning of brain cells and synapses, resulting in impaired memory, thinking, and behaviour.

ambivalence   A state in which an individual experiences conflicting feelings, attitudes, or drives.

amnesia   Loss of memory that cannot be explained by normal forgetfulness.

amphetamines   Class of drugs that act as central nervous system stimulants.

anger   Normal emotional response to a perceived threat, frustration, or distressing event; occurs in response to an individual's frustration level or feelings of being threatened or losing control.

anhedonia   Loss of interest or pleasure from previously enjoyed activities.

animal therapy   A relatively new therapy that involves providing specially trained service animals to assist veterans with combat-related post-traumatic stress disorder (PTSD).

anorexia nervosa   A severe disturbance in eating behaviour that results in a person weighing much less than a healthy weight.

anticipatory grief   The process of grieving before an actual event occurs.

antipsychotics   Medications used to treat the symptoms of major mental disorders.

antisocial personality disorder   A personality disorder that is characterized by persistent antisocial, irresponsible, or criminal behaviour, often impulsive or aggressive, with disregard for any harm or distress caused to other people, and an inability to maintain long-term social and personal relationships.

anxiety   A vague, uneasy feeling experienced by individuals in response to a stressor.

anxiety disorder   Psychic tension that interferes with a person's ability to perform activities of daily living.

anxiety state   State that occurs when one's coping abilities are overwhelmed and emotional control is lost.

anxiety trait   Learned component of the personality in which an individual reacts to relatively nonstressful situations with anxiety.

apathy   Lack of feelings, emotions, concern, or interests.

aphasia   A disorder in which the language function is defective or absent; inability to speak or understand verbal messages.

apnea   absence of airflow into the lungs.

aromatherapy   The use of certain essential oils to promote health and well-being.

asexual   Persons who experience no sexual attraction for anyone.

assault   Any behaviour that presents an immediate threat to another person.

assertiveness   The ability to directly express one's feelings or needs in a way that respects the rights of other people and retains the individual's dignity.

assessment   The first step of the nursing process, which includes the gathering, clustering, and analysis of data relating to a patient.

attention-deficit/hyperactivity disorder (ADHD)   A cluster of behaviours associated with inattention and impulsive actions.

attitudes   Ideas that help make up one's points of view or outlook.

autism   A pervasive developmental disorder of the brain. Symptoms appear during the first 3 years of life and include disturbances in physical, social, and language skills; abnormal responses to sensations; and abnormal ways of relating to people, objects, and events.

autonomic nervous system (ANS)   The system responsible for regulating the internal vital functions of the body, such as the cardiac and smooth muscles.

autonomy   The ability to direct and control one's own activities and one's destiny.

avoidance behaviours   Refusal to cope with anxiety-producing situations by ignoring them.

avoidant personality disorder   Extreme anxiety related to a fear of rejection and humiliation; to prevent possible rejection, individuals narrow their interests to a small range of activities and have a small support system, if any.

Ayurveda   A healing system developed in India that focuses on the innate harmony of the body, mind, and spirit.

B

bath salts   A cheap replacement for more expensive stimulants like methamphetamine or cocaine; marketed as "not for human consumption" and are virtually undetectable by a typical drug laboratory. They are made from a variety of chemical stimulants and are addictive—the most intense highs come from snorting or injecting; the typical effect includes elevation in mood, decrease in hostility, and increase in empathy. They may cause an increase in body temperature and perspiration. In high doses they can lead to irritation and aggression, often followed by depression, psychosis, and suicidal ideation.

battering   Repeated abuse of someone, usually a woman, child, or older person.

battery   Unlawful use of force on a person.

behaviour   Manner of conducting oneself; one's actions.

belief   A conviction that is mentally accepted as true regardless of whether or not it is based in fact.

beneficence   Actively doing good.

bereavement   Emotional and behavioural state of thoughts, feelings, and activities following a loss.

binge drinking   The consumption of large amounts of alcohol in a short period of time; can lead to alcohol poisoning or death. Often defined as 4 drinks for women and 5 drinks for men in a period of about 2 hours.

binge eating disorder   Uncontrolled ingestion (over a certain period of time) of an amount of food that is larger than most individuals would eat in similar circumstances.

biofeedback   A process that provides visual or auditory information about autonomic body functions.

bipolar disorder   Behavioural issues associated with sudden, dramatic shifts in emotional extremes.

bisexual   A person who is attracted to and engages in sexual activities with more than one sex or gender.

body image   A person's subjective concept of their physical appearance.

borderline personality disorder   Instability in mood, thinking, behaviour, personal relationships, and self-image.

bradykinesia   The slowing down of body movements and mental state.

bulimia nervosa   Uncontrolled ingestion of large amounts of food (*binge eating*), followed by inappropriate methods to prevent weight gain (*purging*).

bullying   Repeated use of aggressive behaviours to intentionally intimidate another person. Includes actions within a relationship between a dominant and a less dominant person or group where an imbalance of power is manifested through aggressive actions that are physical or psychological; negative interactions occur that are direct (face-to-face) or indirect (gossip, exclusion); and negative actions are taken with an intention to harm physically (e.g., punching, kicking, biting), verbally (e.g., threats, name-calling, insults), and by social exclusion (e.g., spreading rumours, ignoring, gossiping).

C

caffeine   The active ingredient in coffee, tea, and other beverages that stimulates the central nervous system.

calculation   The ability to solve mathematical problems.

cannabis   Leaves and flowers of the plant Cannabis, also called *marijuana*.

caring   Concern for the well-being of a person, demonstrated through attentive listening, comforting, honesty, acceptance, and sensitivity.

case management   Assignment of a health care provider to assist a patient in assessing health and social service systems and to ensure that all required services are obtained.

cataplexy   A sudden episode of bilateral muscle weakness and loss of muscle tone that lasts for seconds to minutes.

catastrophic reactions   Minor anxieties or frustrations that cascade into severe behavioural reactions in which the person becomes increasingly confused, agitated, and fearful and may wander, become noisy, act compulsively, or behave violently.

catatonia   Total lack of movement.

catchment area   A delineated geographic region used for the planning of health care services.

central nervous system (CNS)   The brain and spinal cord, which together control all the motor and sensory functions of the body.

cephalocaudal   A pattern of growth and development in which the head of an organism develops first, followed by the extremities, and then the feet.

change process   A series of steps that result in a difference.

chelation   A treatment using the chemical EDTA, which binds to heavy metals and removes them from the body.

chemical dependency   Psychophysiological state of being addicted to drugs or alcohol; also called *addiction*.

chiropractic   A treatment that uses hands-on manipulations to improve the relationship between body structure (the spine) and function.

chronicity   Long-term, persistent difficulties; in chronic mental disorders, periods of relative comfort and ease of functioning, alternate with relapses into acute psychiatric states.

chronic mental illness   The presence of one or more recurring psychiatric disorders that results in significantly impaired functional abilities.

cisgender   Someone whose gender matches what they were assigned at birth, based on their visual anatomy.

civil law   Private law that addresses relationships between individuals.

closed system   Set of interacting, related units with rigid, impermeable boundaries that close out information and energy and eventually shorten survival.

cocaine   Processed extract of the coca plant that causes central nervous system stimulation and intense feelings of well-being.

codes of ethics   Statements encompassing the set of rules to which practitioners of a profession are expected to conform.

cognition   Activities of the mind characterized by knowing, learning, judging, reasoning, and memory.

cognitive   Pertaining to the mental processes of comprehension, judgement, memory, and reasoning.

cognitive-behavioural therapy (CBT)   A type of psychotherapy in which negative patterns of thought about the self and the world are challenged in order to alter unwanted patterns of behaviour or to treat mood disorders such as depression.

cognitive distortions   The ways in which the mind convinces a person of something that is not true. These inaccurate thoughts typically work by reinforcing negative thinking or emotions (e.g., telling ourselves things that sound rational and accurate, but that merely serve to make us feel bad about ourselves). Examples include overgeneralization, catastrophizing, personalization, polarized thinking, and emotional reasoning.

commitment   A personal bond to some course of action.

communication   Reciprocal exchange of information, ideas, beliefs, feelings, and attitudes between two persons or among a group of persons.

communication disorders   Difficulties with expressing and receiving messages, pronouncing words, and stuttering that interfere with a child's development.

communication style   Rituals connected with greeting and departure, the lines of conversation, and the directness of communication.

community mental health centres   Outpatient settings in which a comprehensive variety of mental health services are made readily available to all members of a community.

community support systems (CSS) model   An organized network of caring and trained people committed to assisting chronically mentally ill people with meeting their needs within the community.

comorbidity (co-occurring)   Two medical or psychiatric disorders present at the same time.

compassion fatigue   A syndrome that caregivers may develop when they internalize pain or anguish related to other people in their work environment.

competent   A state of being able to make a choice, understand important information, appreciate one's own situation, and apply reasoning.

complementary medicine   Practices and treatments that agree, or "work with," allopathic therapies.

complicated grief   A persistent yearning for a deceased person and other related symptoms that often occur without the signs of depression but are associated with impaired psychological functioning and disturbances of mood, sleep, and self-esteem.

compulsion   A distressing recurring behaviour that must be performed to reduce anxiety.

compulsive overeating   A pattern of eating to lessen emotional discomfort, anxiety, or distress.

conative loss   Loss of the ability to make and carry out plans.

concurrent disorder   People with serious mental illness who are also addicted to or use substances; a situation in which an individual is suffering from two mental health disorders at the same time.

conduct disorders Persistent patterns of unacceptable behaviours that include defiance of authority, engaging in aggressive actions toward others, refusal to follow society's rules and norms, and violation of the rights of others.

confidentiality The sharing of patient information only with those persons who are directly involved in the care of the patient.

confusion A disruption in higher brain functions resulting in the inaccurate interpretation of stimuli.

congruence In interpersonal communication, the agreement between verbal and nonverbal messages.

consistency Behaviours that imply being steady and regular; dependable.

consultation A process in which the assistance of a specialist is sought to help identify ways in which to cope effectively with patient management issues.

contract law A division of private law that focuses on agreements between individuals or institutions.

controlled substances Certain drug classes manufactured, distributed, and dispensed according to the federal regulations of the 1996 *Controlled Drugs and Substances Act.* These drugs currently include narcotics, stimulants, depressants, hallucinogens, and some tranquilizers.

conversion disorder A somatic symptom disorder in which an individual presents with issues related to the sensory or motor functions.

coping mechanisms Any thought or action that is aimed at reducing stress.

countertransference A barrier in the therapeutic relationship based on a nurse's or therapist's emotional responses to the patient.

crack A type of processed cocaine made by combining cocaine with ammonia or baking soda and heating the mixture to remove the hydrochloride molecule, resulting in chips or chunks of highly addicting cocaine, called *rocks.*

criminal law A division of public law designed to protect the members of a society.

crisis A period of severe emotional disorganization resulting from a lack of appropriate coping mechanisms or supports.

crisis intervention Short-term, active therapy that provides emotional first aid for victims of trauma, with the goal of assisting individuals and families in managing the immediate crisis situation and returning to precrisis levels of functioning.

cultural assessments Tools that allow us to learn how patients perceive and cope within their worlds.

cultural competence The process of continually learning about the cultures of patients/clients that health care providers encounter and developing cross-cultural therapeutic health care skills.

culture A set of learned values, beliefs, customs, and behaviours that is shared by a group of interacting individuals.

culture-bound disorders A combination of psychiatric and somatic symptoms that are considered to be a recognizable disease only within a specific society or culture.

cyber-bullying Intimidation and bullying behaviour that occurs via Internet communications.

cyclothymic disorder A pattern of behaviours involving repeated mood swings, alternating between hypomania and depressive symptoms.

D

data collection Activities that elicit, retrieve, or discover information about a certain subject.

deceit Lying; the act of representing as true something that is known to be false.

defamation Any false communication that results in harm.

defence mechanism Unconscious, intrapsychic reaction that offers protection to the self from a stressful situation.

deinstitutionalization The gradual closing of long-term psychiatric hospitals and the transfer of their patients to community mental health centres, which took place from the 1960s to late 1990s and continues today in some places.

delirium A change of consciousness that occurs over a short period of time.

delirium tremens (DTs) A severe form of alcohol withdrawal that involves sudden and severe physical, mental, behavioural, and nervous system changes.

delusions False beliefs that are resistant to reasoning or change.

dementia Loss of multiple abilities, including short- and long-term memory, language, and the ability to understand (conceptualize).

demonic exorcisms Religious ceremonies in which patients were physically punished to drive away the possessing spirit.

denial A psychological defence mechanism in which one refuses to acknowledge painful facts.

dependency Addiction; when people continue to consume substances to avoid negative withdrawal symptoms.

dependent personality disorder Anxiety associated with separation and abandonment with a deep fear of rejection that expresses itself as the need to be cared for.

depersonalization A feeling of unreality and alienation from the self, with ego and self-concept disorganization. Also called *derealization.*

depression An emotional state characterized by feelings of sadness, disappointment, and despair.

derealization The loss of ego boundaries; an inability to tell where one's body ends and the environment begins. It is a sense of being outside oneself, a detachment from the body, as if one were watching a movie. The body takes on an unreal quality. A person may feel absent or like they are an external observer. Also called *depersonalization.*

designer drugs Substances created by underground chemists who alter the molecular structures of existing drugs.

detoxification The process of withdrawing a substance under medical supervision.

development Increasing ability in skills or functions.

dietary supplement: A "dietary ingredient" supplement to the diet.

dipsomania Constant drinking, from a few days to a few weeks, until the patient reaches an intoxication stage and cannot drink any more.

direct self-destructive behaviours Any form of active suicidal behaviour, such as threats, gestures, or attempts to intentionally end one's life.

discharge planning The process by which a nurse helps a patient cope with the hurdles of illness or surgery through early identification of and intervention for potential issues after the patient's discharge from a health care facility.

disease Condition in which a physical dysfunction exists.

disinhibited social engagement disorder A pattern of culturally inappropriate, overly familiar behaviour with strangers.

dissociation Disconnection from full awareness of self, time, or external circumstances.

dissociative disorder A disturbance in the normally interacting functions of consciousness: identity, memory, and perception.

dissociative identity disorder (DID) The presence of two or more identities or personalities that repeatedly take control of an individual's behaviour.

dissociative trance disorder A disorder in which trances cause clinically significant distress or impairment. Dissociative trance disorders are listed in the *DSM-5* under the category of "other dissociative disorders."

disturbed communications Interference in communication related to the sending or receiving of messages, inadequate mastery of the language, insufficient information, or no opportunity for feedback.

disulfiram (Antabuse) A chemical that produces uncomfortable and possibly serious physical reactions when taken with alcohol; used in the treatment of alcoholism.

domestic violence Aggressive behaviours directed toward significant others.

drug-induced parkinsonism Group of symptoms that mimic Parkinson's disease, including tremors, muscle rigidity, and difficulty with voluntary movements.

duty to warn The duty to protect potential victims from possible harm by a psychiatric patient.

dying process The experience of progressing through several psychological stages before the actual moment of death; allows a person to cope with the overwhelming emotional reactions associated with losing a loved one.

dynamics Interactions among the various forces operating in any system.

dyskinesia The inability to execute voluntary movements.

dyslexia   An impaired ability to read, sometimes accompanied by a mixing of letters or syllables in a word when speaking.

dysthymia   Daily moderate depression that lasts longer than 2 years.

dystonia   Impaired muscle tone.

E

eating and feeding disorder   Ongoing disturbance in behaviours associated with the ingestion of food.

eating disorders   Severe disturbances in eating behaviours that can result in a person's body being far below or above a healthy weight.

ego   In psychoanalysis, the part of the psyche that experiences and maintains conscious contact with reality; the rational part of the personality; the seat of mental processes such as perception and memory; develops defence mechanisms to cope with anxiety.

elder abuse   Any action on the part of a caregiver to take advantage of an older person, their emotional well-being, or their finances/property.

electroconvulsive therapy (ECT)   Artificial induction of a grand mal seizure by passing a controlled electrical current through electrodes applied to one or both temples.

electromagnetic fields (EMF)   Energy used in modalities such as magnetic resonance imaging (MRI) and radiation therapy to treat illness.

elopement   Unannounced leaving or running away from an inpatient health care institution.

emotion   An instinctive or intuitive reaction to various stimuli, based on an individual's perceptions.

emotional abuse   The rejection, criticism, terrorizing, and isolation of a significant other.

empathy   The ability to recognize and share the emotions and states of mind of another and to understand the meaning and significance of that person's behaviour.

encopresis   Fecal incontinence in a child older than 4 years of age who has no physical abnormalities; includes the repeated, usually voluntary, passage of feces in inappropriate places.

enuresis   Involuntary urinary incontinence of a child 5 years of age or older.

environmental control   The ability of an individual to perceive and control their environment.

equilibrium   Attempt of a system or organism to maintain a steady state or balance within itself and among other systems.

ethical dilemmas   Uncertainties or disagreements about the moral principles that endorse different courses of action.

ethics   A set of rules or values that govern right behaviour.

ethnicity   A broad term that refers to the socialization patterns, customs, and cultural habits of a particular group.

excoriation disorder   Repeated picking of the skin with fingers, needles, or other objects despite efforts to stop.

exploitation   Use of another individual for selfish purposes, profit, or gain.

expressive therapy   The use of creative activities to explore and transform difficult emotional and medical conditions.

extended family   A household group consisting of parents, children, grandparents, and other family members.

external losses   Those losses outside the individual that relate to objects, possessions, the environment, loved ones, and support.

extrapyramidal side effects (EPSEs)   Abnormal involuntary movement disorders caused by a medication-induced imbalance between two major neurotransmitters, dopamine and acetylcholine, in portions of the brain.

eye movement desensitization and reprocessing (EMDR)   A treatment that uses controlled eye movements to help reprocess traumatic memories.

F

factitious disorder   Signs and symptoms that are intentionally produced so that one can assume the sick role. Also called Munchausen's syndrome.

factitious disorder imposed on another   The deliberate production of signs and symptoms in another person. Situations most often involve a caregiver (mother, babysitter) who induces signs of illness in a child and then presents the child for medical care. Also called *factitious disorder by proxy*.

failure   Lack of success; neglect or omission.

false imprisonment   Detention of a competent person against their will.

feedback   Responses and intrapersonal communications of each person when messages are being sent and received.

felonies   Crimes that are punishable by imprisonment.

fetal alcohol spectrum disorder (FASD)   A disorder seen in infants and children as the result of maternal excessive alcohol use during pregnancy.

fidelity   The obligation to keep one's word.

flashbacks   Vivid recollections of an event in which the individual relives a frightening, traumatic experience.

flooding   A method for treating phobias that rapidly exposes patients to the feared object or situation and keeps up the exposure until anxiety levels diminish.

forensic evidence   Objective information that is obtained from a victim and used in a court of law to determine the guilt or innocence of an alleged perpetrator of violence.

fraud   The act of giving false information with the knowledge that it will be acted on.

fugue   Escape from reality; dissociative fugue: sudden, unexpected travel, with an inability to recall the past.

functional assessment   Analysis of each patient's abilities to perform the activities of daily living.

G

gangs   Groups of people, generally adolescents, who act, look, and dress alike; share the same values; and follow similar codes of conduct.

gay   A homosexual person (male or female).

gender dysphoria   An inconsistency between an individual's biological sex assigned at birth and their gender identity.

gender expression   The behavioural portrayal of gender actions and roles.

gender fluid   A situation in which a person's gender identity is fluid or fluctuates from one identity to another, or becomes mixed. At times, these changes can be rapid, random, or as a response to a person's environment.

gender identity   An individual's internal sense of being male, female, both, or neither male nor female.

gender neutral   Individuals who identify as being neither male nor female.

genderqueer   Individuals who use this label identify with a gender other than male and female; they can also express elements of both genders.

gender roles   Cultural and social obligations and patterns of behaviour relating to one's gender.

general adaptation syndrome   The generalized defence of the body in response to stress that consists of three stages: alarm, resistance, and exhaustion.

generalized anxiety disorder (GAD)   A disorder that is diagnosed when an individual's anxiety is broad, long-lasting, and excessive. It is primarily a disturbance in the emotional area of functioning. Eventually it affects every other aspect of one's world. People with generalized anxiety disorder are worried and anxious more often than not.

general personality disorder   A personality disorder that includes the following criteria: an enduring pattern of behaviour that deviates markedly from the person's culture and goes back to at least the adolescent years; a persistent lack of flexibility across all life situations; behaviour that leads to significant distress or impairment in social, occupational, or other important areas of functioning; no other mental health illness explains this pattern of behaviour, and this persistent pattern of behaviour cannot be explained by the effects of medication or another medical condition. This category encompasses specific personality disorders such as borderline, obsessive-compulsive, avoidant, schizotipal, antisocial, and narcissistic.

gentle persuasive approach   An approach to dealing with dementia in individuals that reframes the challenging behaviour associated with dementia and reinterprets it as a self-protective/defensive or responsive behaviour that occurs as a result of unmet needs; staff are encouraged to assess the meaning of the behaviour and work alongside the resident or patient.

genuineness   The quality of being open, honest, sincere; actively involved.

gerontophobia   The fear of aging and refusal to accept older individuals into the mainstream of society.

gregarious   Sociable, in need of the company of others.

grief The set of emotional reactions that accompany a loss.

grieving process The experience of coping with a significant loss.

growth The increase in physical size that follows organized and orderly patterns.

H

hallucinations False sensory inputs with no external stimuli in the form of smells, sounds, tastes, sight, or touch.

hallucinogen Chemical substance that alters one's reality.

harm reduction An evidence-informed approach to substance use that aims to help people who use legal and illegal psychoactive drugs to live safer and healthier lives; an important but controversial approach to health promotion that is based on user input and demand, compassionate pragmatism, and a commitment to offering alternatives in order to reduce risky health behaviours, accept alternatives to abstinence, and reduce barriers to treatment by providing user-friendly access to addictive substances.

health A state of physical, emotional, sociocultural, and spiritual well-being in which the psychological realms are in balance with the physical self in a state of homeostasis.

health–illness continuum A broad spectrum or scale by which a person's level of health can be described, ranging from total wellness to severe illness.

heroin A semisynthetic narcotic of opium.

heterosexual A person who expresses sexual desire or preference for members of the opposite sex.

histrionic personality disorder A pattern of excessive emotional expression accompanied by attention-seeking behaviours.

hoarding disorder The persistent difficulty in parting with or discarding possessions, regardless of their value, because of the intense anxiety this act generates. Persons may hoard certain items, but to the person with hoarding disorder, accumulating possessions becomes a way of life.

holistic health care A philosophical concept that considers all aspects of human functioning and help patients achieve harmony within themselves and with others, nature, and the world.

homelessness The situation of an individual, family, or community without stable, permanent, and appropriate housing, or the immediate prospect, means, and ability of acquiring it; encompasses a range of living situations: (1) unsheltered: those who are absolutely homeless and living on the streets; (2) emergency sheltered: those who are staying in overnight shelters for people who are homeless; (3) provisionally accommodated: those who are staying in temporary accommodations; and (4) at risk of homelessness: those who are not homeless but whose current economic and/or housing situation is precarious or does not meet public health and safety standards.

homeopathy A therapeutic method that uses natural substances in microdoses to relieve symptoms.

homeostasis Tendency of the body to achieve and maintain a steady internal state.

homicides The taking of others' lives; murders.

homosexual A person who expresses sexual desire or a preference for members of their own sex.

hope Multidimensional dynamic life force characterized by an anticipated and confident yet uncertain expectation of achieving a future good.

hospice Care for people with terminal illnesses or conditions and for their loved ones ones; hospice care prioritizes comfort and quality of life by reducing pain and suffering.

hospitalization The placing of an ill or injured person into an inpatient health care facility that provides continuous nursing care and an organized medical staff.

humoral theory of disease Hippocrates' view that illness was the result of an imbalance of the body's humors of blood, phlegm, black bile, and yellow bile.

hypersomnia A condition characterized by prolonged sleep episodes or frequent daytime sleeping that occurs daily for at least 3 months. Excessive sleepiness is severe enough to cause significant impairment of activities of daily living and is not caused by any other physical or mental health disorder. Also called *hypersomnolence disorder*.

hypersomnolence disorder A condition characterized by prolonged sleep episodes or frequent daytime sleeping that occurs daily for at least 3 months. Excessive sleepiness is severe enough to cause significant impairment of daily living activities and that is not caused by any other physical or mental health disorder. Also called *hypersomnia*.

hypertensive crisis Condition in which the blood pressure rises to extreme levels; commonly caused by an interaction between monoamine oxidase inhibitors and other substances.

hypnosis The induction of a relaxed, trancelike state in which an individual is receptive to appropriate suggestions.

hypomanic episode A period during which an individual experiences an elevated level of mood or irritability, increased energy or activity, and at least three of the following symptoms: inflated self-esteem or grandiosity; decreased need for sleep; more talkativeness than usual; objective flight of ideas or subjective experience of racing thoughts; distraction by unimportant or irrelevant stimuli; significant increase in goal-directed activity and psychomotor agitation; uncharacteristic involvement in high-risk activities.

hypopnea Reduction in airflow, which occurs during breathing-related sleep disorder.

I

id In psychoanalysis, the part of the psyche functioning in the unconscious and the source of instinctive energy, impulses, and drives; based on the pleasure principle; has strong tendencies toward self-preservation.

ideas of reference Incorrect perceptions of causal events as having great or significant meaning; finding special, personal messages in everyday events.

identity diffusion Failure to bring various childhood identifications into an effective adult personality.

illness A state of social, emotional, intellectual, and physical dysfunction.

illness anxiety disorder A disorder in which individuals have been preoccupied with worry or anxiety for at least 6 months about getting a serious illness. They may excessively seek medical attention and extra tests, or they may do the opposite and try to avoid medical checkups because of the intense worry that a serious illness will be discovered.

illusions False perceptions of actual stimuli.

impulse control Ability to express one's emotions in appropriate or effective ways.

impulsivity A pattern of behaviour in which actions are taken without forethought or regard for the consequences.

incest Inappropriate sexual activities with one or more members of one's family.

incongruent communications Interactions in which the verbal messages being sent do not match one's nonverbal communications.

indirect self-destructive behaviours Any behaviours that may result in harm to an individual's well-being or death, in which people have no actual intention to end their lives.

inferiority A feeling of being inadequate or less than others.

informed consent The process of presenting information to patients about the benefits, risks, and adverse effects of specific treatments, thus enabling patients to make voluntary and competent decisions about their own care.

inhalants Chemical substances that are introduced into the body by breathing in through the nose and mouth.

inpatient psychiatric care A health care facility that provides 24-hour/day care within a structured and protective setting.

insight The power or act of seeing into a situation; understanding the inner nature of things.

insomnia The inability to fall asleep.

insomnia disorder A disorder of a severe impairment due to the inability to fall asleep, maintain a sound sleep, and/or return to sleep after awakening early.

integrative medicine Uses the most effective practices and treatments from both conventional and alternative medical systems with an emphasis on the interrelationship among body, mind, and spirit.

integrity A state of wholeness, of being complete.

intellectual development disorder A diagnosis by the American Psychiatric Association that identifies children who function significantly below the average intellectual level for their age group and are limited in their abilities to function; also called *intellectually delayed*.

intermittent explosive disorder (IED)   A failure to resist aggressive impulses that result in the destruction of property or assault of another living being.

internal losses   Physical or emotional losses that involve some part of oneself.

interpersonal communications   Interactions that occur between two or more persons consisting of the verbal and nonverbal messages that are sent and received during every interaction.

intersex   Persons who do not meet the medical definition of male or female at birth.

interview   Purposeful, organized conversation with a patient.

intoxication   The state of being under the influence of a chemical substance or drug.

intrapersonal communications   Messages that are sent and received within oneself.

invasion of privacy   Violation of a person's space, body, belongings, or personal information.

involuntary admission   A request for mental health services that is initiated by someone other than the patient.

involvement   The process of actively interacting with the environment and the persons within it.

J

judgement   The ability to evaluate choices and make appropriate decisions.

justice   Implies that all patients are treated equally, fairly, and respectfully.

K

kleptomania   A recurrent urge to steal, typically without regard for need or profit.

Korsakoff syndrome   A chronic memory disorder caused by severe deficiency of thiamine (vitamin B_1), most commonly caused by alcohol misuse. Thiamine (vitamin B_1) helps brain cells produce energy from sugar—when levels fall too low, brain cells cannot generate enough energy to function properly.

L

la belle indifférence   Lack of concern or indifference about the nature or the implications of the signs and symptoms of a somatoform disorder.

laryngeal-pharyngeal dystonia   A life-threatening adverse effect of antipsychotic medications that occurs when the muscles of the throat become rigid and the patient begins to gag, choke, and become cyanotic. Respiratory distress and asphyxia result if immediate intervention does not occur.

laws   Controls by which a society governs itself.

learning disorder   Problems with learning to read, write, or calculate.

lesbian   A woman who expresses sexual desire or preference for other women.

liability   The concept that care providers are legally responsible for their professional obligations and behaviour. It includes the obligation to remain competent, maintain a current knowledge base, practise at a level appropriate to one's education, and practise unimpaired by drugs, disability, or illness.

libel   Written communication that results in harm.

libidinal energy   Also called *libido*; psychic energy or instinctual drive associated with sexual desire, pleasure, or creativity.

life space   The psychological field or space in which one moves, including oneself, other people, and objects.

limit setting   The process of consistently reinforcing the established structure (rules, routine) of the therapeutic setting.

lithium   A naturally occurring salt used to treat mania.

lobotomy   A surgical procedure that disconnects the frontal lobes from the thalamus in the brain, resulting in a decrease in violent behaviours and mood swings.

loss   Actual or potential state in which a valued object, person, or body part that was formerly present is lost or changed and can no longer be seen, felt, heard, known, or experienced.

lunacy   Medieval term meaning a mental disorder caused by or relating to the moon.

M

machismo   Compulsive masculinity evidenced by a preoccupation with physical strength and athletic prowess; the person attempts to demonstrate daring or violent and aggressive behaviours.

magical thinking   A disorder of thought content; the false belief that one's thoughts, actions, or words will cause or prevent a specific consequence in some way that defies commonly understood laws of causality.

major depressive episode (MDE)   Diagnosed when there is a combination of the following symptoms (for which one of the first two symptoms must be present) for at least 2 weeks and cause significant distress and impairment to an individual: observed/reported feelings of sadness, emptiness, or hopelessness; loss of interest or pleasure; significant weight loss or gain or frequent change in appetite; frequent insomnia or hypersomnia; frequent fatigue or loss of energy; frequent psychomotor agitation or retardation; frequent feelings of worthlessness and guilt; decreased ability to think or concentrate, or decisiveness; recurrent thoughts of death or suicidal ideation.

malingering   Somatoform disorder in which one produces symptoms to meet a recognizable, external goal.

malpractice   Failure to exercise an accepted degree of professional skill or learning, resulting in injury, loss, or damage.

mania   Extreme emotional state characterized by excitement, great elation, overtalkativeness, increased motor activity, fleeting grandiose ideas, and agitated behaviours.

manic episode   An emotional state in which a person has an elevated, expansive, and sometimes irritable mood accompanied by a loss of identity, increased activity, and grandiose thoughts and actions unsupported by reality.

manipulation   Controlling others for one's own purposes by influencing them in unfair or false ways.

marriage   A legal state that bonds two people as a single-family unit.

masochism   Sexual arousal achieved by being the recipient of pain, humiliation, or suffering.

massage   The manipulation of muscles and connective tissue to relax the body and enhance well-being.

maturation   The process of attaining complete physical and psychosocial development.

maturity   The ability to accept responsibility for one's actions, delay gratification, and make priorities; the period in life from the end of adolescence until death.

medical assistance in dying (MAiD)   Legislation that provides individuals who may be experiencing intolerable suffering due to a grievous and irremediable (incurable) medical condition with the option to end their life with the assistance of a doctor or nurse practitioner. Medical assistance in dying is provided only to legally eligible patients.

meditation   A term describing various techniques that share four common elements: concentration, retraining the attention to one item while excluding all other thoughts, mindfulness, and an altered state of consciousness.

memory   The faculty of the brain responsible for recalling past events, experiences, and perceptions.

memory loss   A natural part of the aging process related to the inability to recall certain details or events.

mental health   A relative state of mind in which a person who is healthy is able to cope with and adjust to the recurrent stresses of everyday living in an acceptable way.

mental health care team   A group of professionally trained specialists who develop and implement comprehensive treatment plans for patents with mental or emotional issues.

mental illness   Any disturbance of psychic equilibrium that results in maladaptive behaviours and impaired functioning.

mentally healthy adult   A person who can cope with and adjust to the recurrent stresses of daily living in an acceptable way.

methadone   Narcotic used to treat long-term heroin addiction.

methamphetamine (meth)   One of the most addictive and destructive drugs available today, it is sold in bags of white to pale brown powder that is smoked, snorted, injected, or swallowed.

misdemeanors   Crimes that are punishable by fines or imprisonment of less than 1 year.

model   Example or pattern that provides a matrix or framework for a theory.

monoamine oxidase inhibitors (MAOIs) Antidepressant medication that has serious adverse reactions and dietary and medication interactions.

mood The subjective state of an individual's overall feelings.

mood disorder A prolonged emotional state that influences one's whole personality and life functioning.

morals Attitudes, beliefs, and values that define one's basis for right or wrong behaviour.

mortality The condition of being subject to death.

mourning The process of working through or resolving one's grief.

multidisciplinary mental health care teams Teams composed of psychiatrists, social workers, psychologists, nurses, and other health care providers who share their expertise and develop comprehensive therapeutic patient care plans.

Munchausen's syndrome See *factitious disorder.*

mutuality The process through which the patient assumes an appropriate level of autonomy without blocking the provision of necessary health care services.

N

naloxone A medication that quickly reverses the effects of an overdose from opioids such as heroin, methadone, fentanyl, and morphine. It is a powerful medication that starts to work within 2 to 5 minutes of administration by removing opium from the opiate receptors and reoccupying them so that opiates cannot work on the brain.

naloxone kits Kits containing naloxone that are stored in different public locations (depending on provincial or territorial guidelines)—often pharmacies, community centres, hospitals, and other public places—that can be applied in the event of an emergency opiate (e.g., fentanyl) overdose. There are two types: (1) a nasal spray (this type is the most popular one) and (2) naloxone that is injectable into any muscle. Each kit has very simple instructions for use.

narcissistic personality disorder A pattern of behaviour characterized by ideas of grandiosity and the need to be admired; the belief that one is special, unique, or extra important.

narcolepsy An uncommon sleep disorder in which an individual has repeated attacks of sleep.

narcotics Natural, semisynthetic, or synthetic chemical substances that act as central nervous system depressants.

naturopathy A whole medical system that views disease as an alteration in the process by which the body heals itself.

negative symptoms In schizophrenia, behaviours that indicate a lack of adaptive mechanisms, including flat affect, poor grooming, withdrawal, and poverty of speech.

neglect The lack of meeting a dependent person's (usually a child's) basic needs for food, clothing, shelter, love, and belonging.

negligence Omission or commission of an act that a reasonable and prudent person would or would not do.

neurocognitive disorder (NCD) Conditions related to loss of multiple cognitive abilities (dementia) or a few or even a single cognitive ability (complex attention, executive function, recognition of emotions, learning, and memory).

neuroleptic malignant syndrome (NMS) A serious and potentially fatal extrapyramidal side effect of antipsychotic or neuroleptic medications.

neuron The basic unit of the nervous system whose function is to transmit electrical information to other nerve cells.

neuropeptides Neurotransmitters composed of strings of amino acids that interact with the endocrine, immune, and nervous systems.

neuroplasticity The principle that brain circuits are constantly changing in response to what we actually do in the world. As we think, perceive, form memories, or learn new skills, the connections between neurons also change and strengthen.

neurosis A pattern of anxiety responses to relationships often rooted in childhood responses to the conflict with one's parents. There is an excessive amount of worry about how others may perceive the person and whether this negative perception may lead to abandonment.

neurotic behaviours Behaviours that are recognized by the person as unacceptable, recurrent, and persistent. The behaviours may be odd or unusual, but they are within socially acceptable limits. The individual is in contact with reality and able to carry out activities of daily living.

neurotransmitters Chemicals found in the nervous system that facilitate the transmission of energy and act as the body's chemical messenger system.

nicotine The addictive, active ingredient in tobacco.

nocturnal sleep-related eating disorder (NSRED) Binge eating during sleep; the person has impaired consciousness while preparing food and eating it, with little or no memory of these actions the next morning. During the sleep eating episode, the individual quickly consumes a bizarre selection of high-calorie foods and nonfood items, such as cleaning products, animal food, or cigarettes.

nonadherence An informed decision made by a patient not to follow a prescribed treatment program.

nonmaleficence The ethical principle of do no harm.

nontherapeutic communications Messages that hinder effective communications.

nonverbal communication Messages that are sent and received without the use of words, including one's intrapersonal communications; the messages created through the body's motions and the use of touch, space, and sight; unspoken interpersonal communications; and behaviours such as eye movement, gestures, movement of the body, expressions, posture, and eye contact.

normlessness A lack of social structure; a situation in which the social norms regulating individual conduct have broken down or are no longer effective as rules for behaviour.

norms Established rules of conduct that arise from a culture's behavioural standards.

nuclear family Household unit consisting of two parents and their offspring.

nurse case manager Professional nurse who works with psychiatrists to develop treatment plans tailored to each patient's unique needs.

nursing (therapeutic) process An organizational framework for the practice of nursing that uses the steps of assessment, nursing diagnosis, planning, implementation, and evaluation for the delivery of patient care.

nurture An act or process that promotes the development of persons or things.

O

obesity Abnormal increase in body fat; body weight that is more than 20% above one's ideal weight.

object constancy Awareness that a person or item still exists even though it cannot be perceived (seen, touched) at the time.

obsession Persistent, recurring, inappropriate, and distressing thoughts.

obsessive-compulsive personality disorder Extreme anxiety about the uncertainty of the future; extremely orderly and overly preoccupied with details; devoted to work, with few leisure activities, and is consumed by the need for perfection.

oculogyric crisis Dystonic reaction, usually an adverse effect of psychotropic medication, in which the eyes involuntarily roll to the back of the head.

open system A set of interacting, related units with permeable boundaries through which matter, energy, and information pass.

opioids A broad group of narcotic pain-relieving drugs that can also induce euphoria and create mood changes in the user; examples of narcotic analgesics include opium, codeine, heroin, fentanyl, Darvon, morphine, methadone, hydrocodone (Vicodin), and oxycodone (OxyContin).

oppositional defiant disorder (ODD) a childhood disorder that is characterized by negative, defiant, disobedient, and often hostile behaviour primarily toward adults and authority figures.

outpatient mental health care A health care setting that provides comprehensive services for mentally ill patients within their home environments.

P

pain management A series of nursing interventions designed to assist patients in identifying, defining, and controlling pain.

panic attack A brief period of intense fear or discomfort accompanied by various physical and emotional reactions.

paranoid personality disorder A suspicious system of thinking with delusions of persecution and grandeur; a pattern of behaviours marked by suspiciousness and mistrust.

paraphilias A group of sexual variations that depart from society's traditional and acceptable modes of seeking sexual gratification.

parasomnias Sleep disorders characterized by abnormal behavioural or physical events during sleep.

parasuicidal behaviours Unsuccessful attempts and gestures of suicide that are associated with a low likelihood of success.

parasympathetic nervous system A branch of the autonomic nervous system designed to conserve energy and calm the sympathetic nervous system's excitability. Its main functions are to monitor and control the regulatory processes of the body, which it accomplishes by governing smooth muscle tone and glandular secretions; also responsible for the body's "freeze" response.

passive aggression Indirect expressions of anger through subtle, evasive, or manipulative behaviours.

passive suicide The act of taking one's own life by refusing to eat, drink, or cooperate with care.

pedophilia Fondling of and/or other types of sexual activities with a prepubescent child (usually under age 13 years and having not yet developed secondary sex characteristics).

peer groups A group of people of similar age, interests, and developmental levels.

penile plethysmograph (PPG) A mechanism used to measure air flow in a cylinder at a phallometric clinic to help determine sexual orientation and diagnoses of paraphilic disorder. As a stimulus, clinic staff use a set of approved standard images. Some people come to these clinics voluntarily, and some are directed there by court order because of sexual offences.

perception The use of the senses to gain information.

peripheral nervous system (PNS) The 31 spinal nerves that originate in the spinal cord in addition to the 12 pairs of cranial nerves; this system is further divided into a motor system and an autonomic system.

perseveration Repeating of the same idea in response to different questions or interactions.

personal identity The composite of behavioural traits and characteristics by which one is recognized as an individual.

personality The unique pattern of attitudes and behaviours that each individual develops to adapt to a particular environment and its standards.

personality disorder An enduring pattern of inner experience and behaviour that deviates markedly from the expectations of an individual's culture, is pervasive and inflexible, has an onset in adolescence or early adulthood, is stable over time, and leads to distress or impairment.

personality fusing A type of identity fusion in which individuals are so desperate to define themselves that they attempt to bind their self-concepts to another person.

personality map A full description of all alters (their full identity, triggers for appearance, views, and attitudes), used in treatment for a person who suffers from dissociative identity disorder.

personifications According to Harry Stack Sullivan, the distorted images of certain relationships that spill over or transfer into other relationships.

pervasive developmental disorders Issues severe enough to affect several areas of a child's functioning (including difficulty with social interaction skills, communication skills, and learning) that their behaviour differs from that of other children of the same age and developmental level.

phencyclidine (PCP) Drug developed for use as an animal tranquilizer; in humans, produces mild depression with low doses and a schizophrenic-like reaction with higher amounts.

phobia An extreme fear of people, animals, objects, situations, or occurrences.

phototherapy Exposure of patients to full-spectrum light for certain periods during the day for the relief of depressive symptoms that occur during the winter months.

physical abuse Injury inflicted on a child, ranging from minor bruises and lacerations to severe trauma and death.

physiological stress response Mechanism that protects mammals during times of threat or illness; responsible for fight-or-flight response; a biochemical survival system designed to provide the body with the energy for fighting or fleeing.

pica Eating disorder characterized by ingestion of nonfood items, such as hair, string, or dirt, for more than 1 month.

planned change The deliberate effort to make things different within a system. Changes are carefully planned and implemented slowly and deliberately.

polypharmacy The simultaneous use of multiple medications by a single patient, to treat one or more conditions.

polysomnogram Device that monitors a patient's electrophysical responses during sleep and includes such measurements of brain wave activity (electroencephalogram [EEG]), muscle movement (electromyogram [EMG]), and extraocular eye movements (electrooculogram [EOG]).

pornography Videos, photographs, writings, and other media containing the explicit description or display of sexual organs or sexual activity with the intention of causing sexual arousal.

positive symptoms In schizophrenia, the signs related to maladaptive thoughts and behaviours, including hallucinations, speech issues, and bizarre behaviours.

postpartum depression A condition characterized by symptoms of tearfulness, irritability, hypochondria, sleeplessness, impairment of concentration, and headache in the days and weeks after childbirth.

post-traumatic stress disorder (PTSD) Problems that develop after a person experiences a psychologically distressing event; characterized by an oversensitivity to or overinvolvement with the stimuli that recall the traumatic event.

poverty Inability to secure the basic necessities of life, such as food, shelter, and clothing.

poverty of thought Lack of ability to produce new thoughts or follow a train of thought.

prayer An active process of appealing to a higher spiritual power.

prejudice Displacement of unacceptable impulses and behaviours onto a culturally different group.

primary gain Physical signs and symptoms of an illness used to relieve an individual's anxieties by masking inner emotional turmoil.

principle Standard or code that guides actions.

professional (nurse) practice acts A series of regulations that identify the limits and scope of practice and act as the legal framework for practice in that province or territory.

prostitution The practice of engaging in sexual activity in exchange for payment.

proximal-distal The pattern of growth and development in which growth occurs from near to far, midline to distal.

psyche The vital or spiritual aspect of an individual as opposed to the body or soma; total components of the id, ego, and superego, including all conscious and unconscious aspects.

psychiatric rehabilitation Multidisciplinary services that assist people with mental health issues to readjust and adapt to life in the community as actively and independently as possible; includes personal adjustment and social, residential, educational, and vocational services. Also called *psychosocial rehabilitation*.

psychoanalysis Founded by Sigmund Freud, a branch of psychiatry devoted to the study of the psychology of human behaviour; also a therapy for certain emotional disorders that investigates the workings of the mind.

psychobiology The study of the biochemical foundations of thought, mood, emotion, affect, and behaviour.

psychogenic disorders Physical illnesses that are believed to arise from emotional or mental stressors, or from psychological or psychiatric disorders.

psychoneuroimmunology (PNI) The study of interactions among the body's central nervous system, the immune system, and aspects of the personality.

psychopath A person with an antisocial personality disorder and a pervasive pattern of disregard for and violation of the rights of others, often using deceit and manipulation.

psychophysical disorders Disorders in which stress-related issues result in physical signs and symptoms.

psychosis   An inability to recognize reality, relate to others, or cope with life's demands. Also called *psychotic disorder*.

psychosocial (psychiatric) rehabilitation   Multidisciplinary services that assist people with mental health issues to readjust and adapt to life in the community as actively and independently as possible; includes personal adjustment and social, residential, educational, and vocational services. Also called *psychiatric rehabilitation*.

psychosomatic illnesses   Popular term that describes emotionally (*psycho*) related physical (*somatic*) disorders.

psychotherapeutic medications   Chemicals that affect the mind and treat the symptoms of mental-emotional illness.

psychotherapy   Any of a large number of related methods of treating mental-emotional disorders by psychological techniques rather than by physical means.

psychotic behaviours   Behaviours that are characterized by personality disintegration, reduced awareness, and an inability to function within socially acceptable limits. The individual is not in contact with reality and is unable to carry out their activities of daily living.

puberty   Period in life at which the ability to reproduce is developed, beginning with a 24- to 36-month growth spurt and ending when the reproductive system is mature.

public law   Focuses on the relationship between the government and its citizens.

purging   Recurring inappropriate behaviours used to prevent weight gain; usually associated with bulimia.

pyromania   An obsessive desire to set fire to things.

Q

Qi Gong   A system of movement, regulation of breathing, and meditation designed to enhance the flow of *qi* (energy) throughout the body.

R

rape   Unlawful sexual activity involving the penetration of the mouth, vagina, or anus, carried out through the use of force without a person's consent.

rape-trauma syndrome   A nursing diagnosis related to PTSD that encompasses the essentials of care for the victims of this violent experience; the psychological trauma experienced by a rape victim that includes disruptions to normal physical, emotional, cognitive, and interpersonal behaviour.

rapport   A dynamic process involving an energy exchange between a nurse and a patient, serving as the background for all other nursing actions.

rational suicide   An act of purposefully ending one's own life after conscious and rational deliberation.

reactive attachment disorder   A disorder of early childhood or infancy characterized by inappropriate attachment behaviour, in which a child almost never seeks out comfort, protection, or support from an attachment figure. The main feature is underdeveloped attachment between the child and caregiver.

reasonable and prudent care provider   Principle by which the law judges a caregiver's actions by comparing what other caregivers would do in similar situations.

recidivism   Relapse of a symptom, disease, or pattern of behaviour.

recovery   Living a satisfying, hopeful, and contributing life, even when the person may still be experiencing ongoing symptoms of a mental health challenge or illness.

refeeding syndrome   When the body uses its own fat tissue and amino acids to survive during prolonged starvation and lack of carbohydrate sources for energy; complications include heart failure, abnormal heart rhythms (dysrhythmias), respiratory failure, muscle breakdown, and death.

reflection   The process of looking into one's own mind. An analysis of self: one's feelings, reactions, attitudes, opinions, values, and behaviours. It is also a process for observing and analyzing one's behaviour in various situations. Reflection allows us to "step out" of the interaction and watch our own behaviours.

refugee   A person who, because of war or persecution, flees from their home or country and seeks refuge elsewhere.

Reiki   A life force energy that flows through one's body.

relapse   The recurrence of substance-abusing behaviours after a significant period of abstinence; periods of dysfunction accompanied by an increase in the signs, symptoms, and seriousness of a mental health challenge.

religion   A defined, organized, and practised system of beliefs and practices usually involving a moral code.

religiosity   Delusions of great spirituality; belief that one has powers to communicate with God or be a spirit.

remissions   In chronic mental illness, times of partial or complete disappearance of symptoms.

resistance   Patient attempts to avoid recognizing or exploring anxiety-provoking material.

resource linkage   The process of matching a patient's needs with the most appropriate community services.

responding strategies   Therapeutic techniques that relate to a nurse's actions or interventions while communicating.

responsibility   The state of being answerable for acts or decisions and the ability to fulfill obligations.

restless legs syndrome   A sensorimotor, neurological sleep disorder that is characterized by an urge to move the legs in response to intolerable sensations (e.g., creeping, crawling, tingling, burning, itching). Individuals with the disorder suffer from significant distress and impairment due to this urge to move their legs. The urge increases during times of rest, is intensified in evenings or at night, and moving the legs actually relieves the urge. Also called *Willis-Ekbom disease*.

restraint   A limitation on a patient's movement. There are three general classifications of restraint used in Canadian health care settings: environmental, chemical, and physical.

reverse Q15 minutes observation   A safety mechanism used for mental health patients whereby patients who are at risk of harming themselves must report to the nursing station and sign an observation list every 15 minutes to indicate whether they are safe or in the need of protection from themselves.

right   Power, privilege, or existence to which one has a just claim.

risk factor assessment   Interview tool to identify risk factors that potentially present an immediate threat to the patient.

role   Expected pattern of behaviours associated with a certain position.

role performances   Socially expected behavioural patterns.

rumination disorder   An uncommon problem of childhood that involves the regurgitation and rechewing of food.

S

safety plan   A plan used in mental health care that can include a description of how the patient will keep their environment safe, how to recognize warning signs, individual coping strategies, who is a nonmedical person (family, friend) to help if coping strategies do not work; if that is not working, who are the clinicians to call; and, if that also is not working, where to go for emergency help.

schizoid personality disorder   A condition that leads an individual to feel a lack of desire or willingness to become involved in a close relationship, instead preferring solitary activities; such a person is emotionally restricted, and communicates emotional detachment, coldness, and a lack of concern for others.

schizophrenia   A condition associated with disturbing thought patterns, behaviours, and loss of contact with reality to the extent it impairs functioning.

schizotypal personality disorder   Interaction pattern of avoiding people, with behaviours characterized by distortions and eccentricities (odd, strange, or peculiar actions).

seasonal affective disorder (SAD)   Levels of mild to moderate depression experienced during long winter days; symptoms begin to lift with the coming of spring and longer days.

secondary gain   A situation in which the payoff for remaining ill outweighs the advantages of recovery, with patients profiting or avoiding unpleasant situations by remaining ill.

secondary resistance   Occurs when a patient is motivated by drives other than the need to regain health. Many times, the payoff for remaining ill outweighs the advantages of recovery.

selective mutism   The hallmark of selective mutism is a repeated, consistent failure to speak when one is expected to do so as well as when one is able to speak in other situations.

self-awareness   Consciousness of one's own individuality and personality.

self-concept   The attitudes, notions, beliefs, and convictions that make up an individual's self-knowledge, including perceptions of personal characteristics and abilities, interactions with other people and the environment, values associated with experiences and objects, and goals and ideals.

self-esteem   Individual's judgement of their own worth.

self-ideal   Personal standards of how one should behave.

self-injuries   Attempts to harm or hurt oneself.

sensitive periods   Certain times during which children are more affected by influences (positive or negative) within their environment.

sensorium   Part of the consciousness that perceives, sorts, and integrates information.

sex   Anatomy and biology that identify one as male, female, or intersex.

sexual abuse   Any sexual activity that occurs without consent, with children being especially vulnerable.

sexual disorder   Disturbances in sexual desire or functioning that cause marked distress and interpersonal difficulties.

sexual dysfunction   A disturbance anywhere in the four stages (appetite, excitement, orgasm, resolution) of the sexual response cycle.

sexuality   The combination of physical, chemical, psychological, and functional characteristics that are expressed by one's gender identity and sexual behaviours.

sexual orientation   An individual's sexual and romantic attraction to others. Also called *sexual preference*.

shaken baby syndrome   Vigorous manual shaking of an infant who is being held by the extremities or shoulders, leading to whiplash-induced intracranial and intraocular bleeding and no external signs of head trauma.

sick role   The actions and behaviours of a person who is ill and excused from everyday responsibilities.

signal anxiety   A learned anxiety response to an anticipated event.

situational crisis   An event or situation for which one is unprepared, resulting from environmental factors outside the individual.

situational depression   Depressive responses tied to a specific event or situation that can be traced to a recognizable cause.

slander   Verbal communications that result in harm.

sleep-related hypoventilation   Periods of decreased respirations during sleep resulting in elevated carbon dioxide levels in the blood.

sleep terror   Terror/panic arousals from sleep without the ability to respond to others or to be comforted by others.

sleep–wake disorder   A condition or issue that repeatedly disrupts an individual's pattern of sleep.

sleepwalking   Rising from the bed while asleep and walking around with no ability to respond to others.

social isolation   Removal of or withdrawal from the company and companionship of other people.

sociopath   A person with an antisocial personality disorder and a pervasive pattern of disregard for and violation of the rights of others, often using deceit and manipulation. (See *psychopath*.)

soma   The body, as distinguished from the mind or psyche.

somatic symptom and related disorders   Disorders for which the common denominator in all patients who suffer from them is intense suffering and impairment resulting from somatic symptoms (formerly called *hypochondriasis*).

somatic symptom disorders   Conditions in which a person's persistent symptoms suggest the presence of a medical illness for which no physical causes can be found.

somatic therapies   Physical interventions that affect behavioural changes (e.g., electroconvulsive therapy).

somatization   The act of focusing anxieties and emotional conflicts into physical symptoms.

somatoform disorder   Disorder in which a child or adult has the signs and symptoms of illness or disease without a traceable physical cause.

speech cluttering   Disorder of speech and language processing that results in unorganized, unrhythmic, and frequently unintelligible speech.

spice   Unnamed chemical combinations sprayed onto plant material and then sold and smoked as a synthetic marijuana. It is also known as K2.

spiritual dimension   A broad term that includes an individual's belief in a higher power and a sense of meaning and purpose in life.

spirituality   The belief in a power greater than any human being.

splitting   The act of emotionally dividing staff members or other people by complimenting one group and degrading another; performed by patients.

standards of practice   A set of guidelines that provide measurable criteria for care providers, patients, and others to evaluate the quality and effectiveness of health care; also called *standards of care*.

stereotype   Oversimplified mental picture of a cultural group.

stigma   A sign or mark of shame, disapproval, or disgrace, of being shunned or rejected.

stimulants   A group of commonly abused substances that includes bath salts, caffeine, cocaine and crack cocaine, ice, methamphetamines, and certain prescription medications such as amphetamines, appetite suppressants, and methylphenidate (Ritalin).

stressor   A nonspecific response of the body to any demand placed on it.

substance (drug) abuse   Inappropriate use of psychoactive substances (e.g., drugs, medications, or toxins), leading to dependence, addiction, or withdrawal.

substance-induced disorder   A disorder diagnosed when an addictive substance is taken for a longer than intended period of time and in larger amounts; there is an effort to cut down the use of that substance without success; a significant amount of time is spent acquiring, using, or recovering from the substance; there are cravings and urges to use the substance; use of the substance leads to a failure to fulfill basic functions and obligations (e.g., school, work, or family obligations); the individual continues to use the substance even when it causes social or relationship difficulties; important social, family, occupational, or recreational activities are given up or significantly reduced because of substance use; recurrent use of the substance continues even when it places an individual in physical danger; the use of the substance continues even when it causes or exacerbates physical and/or psychological issues; more of the substance is needed to achieve the same effect (tolerance); and withdrawal symptoms are manifested when the substance is discontinued, and they can be eliminated when more of the substance is consumed.

substance use   The act of taking a chemical substance.

substance-use disorder   Occurs when a person's use of alcohol or another substance (drug) leads to health issues or challenges at work, school, or home.

suicidal attempts   Self-directed actions that are intended to do serious harm to oneself or end one's own life.

suicidal gestures   Suicidal actions that result in little or no injury to oneself but communicate a message.

suicidal ideation   Thoughts or fantasies of suicide that are expressed but have no definite intent.

suicidal threats   Expressions of the intent to take one's life but without any action.

suicide   The act of intentionally taking one's own life.

suicide precautions   Standard interventions to prevent a suicide attempt from occurring.

suicidology   The study of the nature of suicide.

sundown syndrome   A group of behaviours characterized by confusion, agitation, and disruptive actions that occur in the late afternoon or evening. The cause is unknown, but sundowning is associated with dementia, loss of cognitive functions, and physical or social stressors.

superego   In psychoanalysis, the part of the psyche, functioning mostly in the unconscious, that develops when the standards of the parents and society are incorporated into the ego.

surveillance   The process of watching over adolescents to determine whether they are safe, are behaving within acceptable limits, are making good decisions, or are in need of adult intervention.

sympathetic nervous system   The division of the autonomic nervous system that prepares the body for immediate adaptation through the fight-or-flight mechanism.

systematic desensitization (SD)
A psychiatric therapy that helps patients learn to cope with one anxiety-provoking stimulus through gradual exposure until the stressor is no longer associated with anxiety. This step-by-step method progressively removes the anxiety from the distress-causing event and allows patients to develop more effective ways of perceiving their anxiety.

T

tardive dyskinesia Drug-induced condition that produces involuntary, repeated movements of the muscles of the face, trunk, arms, and legs; usually occurs after a long period of antipsychotic medication use.

temperament Genetically linked biological bases that underlie moods, energy levels, and attitudes.

terminal illness Illness or condition likely to result in death.

territoriality The need to gain control over an area of space and claim it for oneself.

theory A statement that predicts, explains, or describes a relationship among events, concepts, or ideas.

therapeutic communications Interactions that focus on the patient, foster the therapeutic relationship, and are specifically designed to achieve patient outcomes.

therapeutic environment (milieu) Inpatient psychiatric setting that provides safe, stable surroundings that are structured to enhance the patient's response to treatment.

therapeutic relationship A series of interactions initiated by the nurse with the purpose of providing corrective interpersonal experiences.

therapeutic touch A healing technique based on the practice of the laying on of hands, where the healing energies of the therapist encourage the patient's body energies to return to a balanced state.

thought content What an individual is thinking.

thought processes How a person thinks, analyzes the world, and connects and organizes information.

tolerance Relating to drug use, a state in which increased amounts of a chemical are needed to produce the same effects that were once produced by a single dose.

tort law Division of private law that relates to compensation for a legal wrong committed against the person or property of another.

torticollis A condition involving the contraction of the cervical muscles of the neck that causes the head to tilt down.

traditional Chinese medicine (TCM) A whole medical system based on the view that the body is a delicate balance of opposing forces, termed *yin* and *yang*.

trance A state resembling sleep in which consciousness remains but voluntary movement is lost, as in hypnosis.

transference A patient's emotional response to the nurse based on earlier relationships with significant others.

transfer of accountability (TOA) Exchange of information about a patient (e.g., via a change-of-shift report), to nurses working on next shift.

transgender Individuals whose gender identity and expression are different from their assigned sex at birth.

trauma-informed care Practices that promote a culture of safety, empowerment, and healing. Refers to care focused on the patient's past experiences of violence or trauma and the role it currently plays in their lives. When a history of trauma is present, health care staff must be aware of this and avoid approaches and situations that may retraumatize or aggravate trauma symptoms in patients.

traumatic stress reaction A series of behavioural and emotional responses following an overwhelmingly stressful event.

trephining The act of cutting holes in the skull to encourage evil spirits to leave.

trichotillomania A disorder that involves repeated, persistent pulling of hair from the body despite efforts to stop.

trust A risk-taking process in which an individual's situation depends on the future behaviour of another person.

two-spirit A term that originated with Indigenous peoples in Canada and is commonly used to describe a person who identifies as having both a masculine and a feminine spirit or one who does not identify with any gender.

U

unplanned change Change that is unexpected, not anticipated, and usually not desired. Change happens whether it is planned or unexpected. In health care settings, unplanned changes are daily occurrences.

unresolved grief Unhealthy or ineffective grief reactions. People who experience unresolved grief are unable to shift their attention from their loss to the realities of everyday life. They become so preoccupied with the loss that they are unable to function effectively. Long-standing, unresolved grief can result in depression and complicated grief. Also called *dysfunctional grief* or *complicated bereavement*.

V

value A dearly held belief about the worth of an idea, behaviour, or item.

values clarification A method of discovering one's own values by assessing, exploring, and determining what those personal values are and how they affect personal decision making.

vaping The consumption of a vapour. The vapour is a gas condensed into a liquid form (at room temperature) and usually contains nicotine. This liquid is warmed in a portable device (like e-cigarettes) so that it becomes a gas and can be inhaled.

vascular dementia (VaD) A condition that occurs as a complication of cardiovascular disease causing extensive or very small cerebral vascular accidents (CVAs) when not enough blood is nourishing the brain to keep it functioning properly. The course of VaD may be characterized by a steep decline of function and long periods with no changes.

veracity The duty to tell the truth.

verbal communication A mode of communication involving sounds and words, including the spoken and written word, use of language and symbols, and arrangement of words or phrases.

victimization Process of causing harm; children suffer more victimizations than do adults, including more conventional crime, more family violence, and some forms unique to children, such as family abduction, neglect, and abuse.

violence Any behaviour that threatens or harms another person or their property.

voluntary admission When the patient originates the request for mental health services.

W

whole medical systems Medical systems that are built on complete systems of theory and practice, including Western medicine, osteopathy, homeopathy, naturopathy, Ayurveda, and traditional Chinese medicine.

Page numbers followed by *f* indicate figures; *t*, tables; *b*, boxes.